CPEN

Certified Pediatric Emergency Nurse Review

Fourth Edition - (updated 2021)

Scott L. DeBoer RN, MSN, CEN, CPEN, CCRN, CFRN, EMT-P

Founder

Pedi-Ed-Trics Emergency Medical Solutions, LLC

Emergency / Critical Care Transport Nurse Educator

Editors

Julie Bacon MSN-HCSM, RN-BC, NE-BC, CPN, CPEN, C-NPT (Editions II-IV)

Emily C. Dawson MD, FAAP (Editions III-IV)

Lou Romig MD, FAAP, FACEP (Editions I, II, & IV)

Michael Seaver RN, BA (Editions I-IV)

"You make 'em, I amuse 'em"
Dr. Seuss

© Copyright 2021 - Pedi-Ed-Trics Emergency Medical Solutions, LLC

www.PediEd.com

ACKNOWLEDGEMENTS

Lisa DeBoer... President of Pedi-Ed-Trics Emergency Medical Solutions, LLC and my wife. Thank you for continuing to be an inspiration and blessing to me, our children, and so many others.

Joshua DeBoer, age 23, and Nina DeBoer, age 21... Thank you for all of your help with computer and culinary services. I couldn't have completed this book and the accompanying live and online CPEN review courses without you. I'm so proud of the young adults you are becoming!

This review book is designed to provide accurate information in regard to the subject matter. The handbook and its recommendations are based upon the author's review of current nursing and medical research as noted in the bibliography. In publishing this book, neither the author, nor the editors/publisher are engaged in rendering nursing, medical, or other professional services. If nursing, medical, or other expert assistance is required, the services of a competent professional should be sought.

© Copyright 2021 – Pedi-Ed-Trics Emergency Medical Solutions, LLC

All rights reserved. Reproduction in whole or part by any means whatsoever without written permission of Pedi-Ed-Trics Emergency Medical Solutions, LLC, is prohibited by law.

ISBN 978-0-578-79429-7

Certified Pediatric Emergency Nurse (CPEN) Review IV

Table of Contents - Certified Pediatric Emergency Nurse (CPEN) Review IV

CPEN Examination Content List	10-13
CPEN Recertification Information	14-19
Chapter 1: **Emergency Assessment of Crashing Kids**	21-73
Chapter 2: **Emergency Care of Crashing Kids**	75-125
Chapter 3: **Respiratory Emergencies - Working & Wheezing**	127-176
Chapter 4: **Cardiovascular Emergencies - Congenital Hearts to CPR**	177-215
Chapter 5: **Neurological / Psychiatric Emergencies - Neuro Nightmares & Dysfunctional Dilemmas**	217-278
Chapter 6: **Environmental Emergencies - Drowning, Drugs, Bugs Bites & Radical Rashes**	279-338
Chapter 7: **Abdominal & OB / Neonatal Emergencies - Bellies, Births & Babies**	339-379
Chapter 8: **Endocrine Emergencies - Hormones & Haagen-Dazs**	381-399
Chapter 9: **Orthopedics & Pain Management - Bumps, Breaks, Morphine, & Monitoring**	401-443
Chapter 10: **Miscellaneous Medical Emergencies - Remaining Reminders**	445-490
Chapter 11: **Medical Maladies & Trauma Trivia**	491-595
Chapter 12: **So New... Who Knew? Even More Pediatric Potpourri**	597-783
Test Taking Tips	786-787
Requests From the Mother of a Catastrophically Injured Child	788
The Miracle Toddler Diet	789
How To Raise Mom & Dad	790
God Created Children	791

Editors - 4th Edition
Certified Pediatric Emergency Nurse (CPEN) Review IV

Julie Bacon MSN-HCSM, RN-BC, NE-BC, CPN, CPEN, C-NPT

Program Manager & Chief Flight Nurse

Johns Hopkins All Children's LifeLine and Transfer Center

Clinical Advisory Chair: Florida EMS for Children

St. Petersburg, Florida

(Editions II - IV)

Emily C. Dawson MD, FAAP

Pediatric Emergency Medicine & Critical Care Attending Physician

Chicago, Illinois

(Editions III - IV)

Lou Romig MD, FAAP, FACEP

Pediatric Emergency Medicine Attending Physician

Tampa, Florida

(Editions I, II & IV)

Michael Seaver RN, BA

Senior Healthcare Informatics Consultant

Grayslake, Illinois

(Editions I - IV)

Certified Pediatric Emergency Nurse (CPEN) Review IV

Reviewers / Contributors - 4th Edition

Justin R. Allen DNP, RN, CEN, NRP, CCEMTP
Observable Media
Emergency Department Consultant
Boone, North Carolina

Michael Austin FP-C, EMT-P
Critical Care Flight Paramedic
UF Health Jacksonville: TraumaOne Flight Services
Critical Care Educator: The Rescue Company 1
Jacksonville, Florida

Pamela D. Bartley BSN, RN, CEN, TCRN, CCRN, CFRN, CTRN, CPEN
CEO of PDB Nurse Education, LLC
Prosperity, South Carolina

Ashley Bauer MSN, MBA, APRN, FNP-C, CFRN, C-NPT
Chief Creative Officer: FlightBridgeED, LLC
Partner: FOAMfrat, LLC
Partner: EMSPOCUS, LLC
Scottsville, Kentucky

Eric Bauer MBA, FP-C, CCP-C, C-NPT
Chief Executive Officer: FlightBridgeED, LLC
Partner: FOAMfrat, LLC
Partner: EMSPOCUS, LLC
Scottsville, Kentucky

Maria Broadstreet RN, MSN, CPNP-AC/PC
Pediatric Critical Care Nurse Practitioner
Ann & Robert H. Lurie Children's Hospital of Chicago
Chicago, Illinois

Maricar Cabral RN, CCRN
Pediatric ER Nurse Educator
Joe DiMaggio Children's Hospital
Hollywood, Florida

Daniel Carlascio NRP
EMS Educator
Linenhurst, Illinois

Nicholas P. Comeau MSN, RN, CCRN, TCRN, CPN
Nursing Professional Development Specialist II
Cone Health: Greensboro, North Carolina
Clinical Nurse II: Pediatric Intensive Care Unit
North Carolina Children's Hospital
UNC Health: Chapel Hill, North Carolina

Rosanne Conliffe MSN, RN, RNC-NIC
Pediatric Nurse Educator
Gainesville, Florida

Dawn Coval BSN, RN
Clinical Nurse Educator: Emergency Department
Metro Health: University of Michigan Health
Wyoming, Michigan

Trinity Czarnik
Graphic Artist
St. John, Indiana

Certified Pediatric Emergency Nurse (CPEN) Review IV

Lisa DeBoer NREMT-P/PI, CET
President
Pedi-Ed-Trics Emergency Medical Solutions, LLC
Dyer, Indiana

Brett A. Dodd RN, MSN, CEN, CCRN, CFRN, CPEN, TCRN, CNML, CHSE
Trauma Education, Injury Prevention, and Outreach Coordinator
Cedars Sinai Medical Center
Los Angeles, California

Steven Donahue MS, BSN, RN, CEN
Clinical Nurse IV: Emergency Department
Paoli Hospital: Main Line Health
Paoli, Pennsylvania

James C. DuCanto, MD
Staff Anesthesiologist
Advocate Aurora St. Luke's Medical Center
Milwaukee, Wisconsin

Kelly Carlson Eberbach DNP, MBA, RN, CPN, CPEN
Clinical Nurse Educator: Emergency Department
Nursing Professional Excellence
Nemours Children's Hospital
Orlando, Florida

Amanda Grindle MSN, RN, CNL, CCRN, CPN
Clinical Program Manager for Hospital Readiness
Children's Healthcare of Atlanta
Atlanta, Georgia

Robert P. Harris RN, CFRN, CTRN, TCRN, CEN, CPEN, C-NPT, CCRN
Author: The Flight Nurse Bible
San Diego, California

Bruce Hoffman MSN, CFRN, FP-C, CCP-C, NR-P, C-NPT
Chief Operating Officer
FlightBridgeED, LLC & The FlightBridgeED Podcast
Ellington, Connecticut

Judie Holleman, MSN, APRN, CCRN, PCPNP-BC, CPNP-AC
Pediatric Nurse Practitioner: Section of Neurosurgery
The University of Chicago Medicine & Biological Sciences
Chicago, Illinois

Samuel Ireland AAS, CC-P, FP-C
FOAMfrat
Milwaukee, Wisconsin

Kristin Ireland AAS, RRT, EMT
FOAMfrat
Milwaukee, Wisconsin

Lindsay Jackson MS, CPNP-AC, APRN
Lead Advanced Practice Provider: Cardiac Intensive Care Unit
Ann & Robert H. Lurie Children's Hospital of Chicago
Chicago, Illinois

Steven J Jewell BSN, RN, CEN, CPEN, USN, (ret.)
Critical Care Registered Nurse
Brooke Army Medical Center: Department of Emergency Medicine
Fort Sam Houston, Texas

Certified Pediatric Emergency Nurse (CPEN) Review IV

Bill Justice NRP, TEMS-I
Associate Director
University of Oklahoma Center for Pre-Hospital and Disaster Medicine
Tulsa, Oklahoma

Brenna Kouzoukas MSN, RN, FNP-BC, CCRN, CFRN
Flight Nurse: University of Chicago Medicine UCAN
Chicago, Illinois

Michael R. Lovelace RN, CCRN, CEN, CFRN, CPEN, CTRN, NHDP-BC, NREMT-P, TCRN
Trauma Lead / Educator
University of Alabama Hospital Emergency Department
Birmingham, Alabama

Stuart McVicar RRT, C-NPT, EMT-P
Transport Respiratory Therapist
American Family Children's Hospital
Madison, Wisconsin

Justin Milici MSN, RN, CEN, CPEN, TCRN, CCRN, FAEN
Clinical Editor
Elsevier Clinical Solutions
Dallas, Texas

Bradford Nash EMT-P
Paramedic/Firefighter
Abington, Pennsylvania

Christine O'Neill BSN, RN-BC
Director of Clinical Education
410 Medical, Inc.
Denver, Colorado

Mark Piehl MD, MPH, FAAP
Pediatric Intensivist: WakeMed Children's
Medical Advisor: WakeMed Mobile Critical Care
Associate Professor of Pediatrics
University of North Carolina School of Medicine
Chief Medical Officer: 410 Medical
Raleigh, North Carolina

Velvet Reed-Shoults MBA, MHA, RN, CEN, TCRN, CBIS, CLNC
Director of Clinical Outreach
Northwest Health System
Bentonville, Arkansas

Michael Rushing BSN, RN, NRP, CEN, CPEN, CFRN, TCRN, CCRN-CMC
AHA Coordinator
Baptist Health Care
Pensacola, Florida

Michael J. Schwien BS, BSN, RN, CEN
Staff Nurse: Emergency Department
Main Line Health: Lankenau Medical Center
Wynnewood, Pennsylvania

Sherri Sommer-Candelario RN, BSN, RN-BC, CCRN, CPEN
Supervisor: Transport/ECMO
Kapi`olani Medical Center for Women & Children
Honolulu, Hawaii

Certified Pediatric Emergency Nurse (CPEN) Review IV

Christopher R. Speaker APN, FNP-BC, CPN
Nurse Practitioner: Division of Pediatric Surgery
Ann & Robert H. Lurie Children's Hospital of Chicago
Chicago, Illinois

Carlos Tavarez BSN, CFRN, CEN, TCRN, CTRN, EMT-P, FP-C, CCT-P, WEMT
Flight Nurse/Paramedic
Orlando Health Air Care
CEO: The Rescue Company 1
Orlando, Florida

Lynn Sayre Visser MSN, RN, PHN, CEN, CPEN
Author: Fast Facts for the Triage Nurse and Rapid Access Guide for Triage and Emergency Nurses
Editor: Journal of Emergency Nursing blog
Loomis, California

Michelle R Webb MSN, CRNA, TNS, CEN, PHRN, CFRN
Senior Nurse Anesthetist
UnityPoint Health Methodist
Peoria, Illinois

Sara Webb MSN, C-FNP, C-PNP, EMT-P, C-NPT
Neonatal-Pediatric Transport Nurse: LifeLine
Pediatric Surgery Advanced Nurse Practitioner
Johns Hopkins All Children's Hospital
St. Petersburg, Florida

Lori Wertz MN, RN, CPEN
Clinical Education Specialist
Pediatric Intensive Care Unit
Phoenix Children's Hospital
Phoenix, Arizona

Clark Wilkerson MBA, BSC, EMT-P, NAEMS-E
Division Chief / Training Officer
Bentonville Fire Department
Bentonville, Arkansas

Mary Willner BS, BSN, CEN, TCRN, CPEN
Senior Staff Nurse: Emergency Department
Hennepin County Medical Center
Minneapolis, Minnesota

Allen C. Wolfe Jr., MSN, APRN, CNS, CCRN, CFRN, CTRN, CMTE
Senior Director of Clinical Education
Life Link III
Minneapolis, Minnesota

Reviewers / Contributors - Prior Editions

Kathleen Adams RCP, RRT-NPS

Amy Baxter MD, FAAP, FACEP

Kelly Begley AAS, CCEMT-P

Marlene L. Bokholdt MS, RN, CPEN

Teri Campbell RN, BSN, CEN, CFRN

G. Patricia Cantwell, MD

John R. Clark JD, MBA, NREMT-P, FP-C, CCP-C

Craig Felty RN, BSN, CEN, EMT-P

Christopher George, EMT-P

Bradley Goettl RN, BSN, CEN, CPEN, EMT-P

Kelley Holdren RN, BSN, CFRN

Judie Holleman MSN, RN, CPNP

Kelly Houde RN, MSN, CEN, CPEN

Stacie Hunsaker RN, MSN, CEN, CPEN

Lisa Koser MSN, ACNP-BC, CPNP-AC, CCRN, CEN, CFRN, C-NPT, EMT-P

Thelma Kuska BSN, RN, CEN, FAEN

Cynthia Lafond RN, DNP

Bonnie Lundblom RN, BSN, CCRN, CPEN

Patricia Manning

Stuart McVicar RRT, C-NPT, EMT-P

Loreen Meyer RN, BSN, CCRN

Tracy Meyer RN, BSN, CFRN, NREMT-P

Justin Milici, RN, MSN, CEN, CPEN, CFRN, CCRN, TNS

Suzanne Mindlin, JD

Lynn Mohr MS, RN, PCNS-BC, CPN

Eddie Norton, EMT-P

Annemarie O'Connor MSN, FNP-BC, APN/CNP

Curtis Olson BSN, BA, RN, EMT-P, CEN

Cheryl Perry RN, BSN

Cheryl Querry RN, SANE-A

Steven Rogge RN, BSN, CEN, CFRN, CCRN, FAWM

Sean G. Smith, BSN, RN, Paramedic, FP-C, C-NPT, CCRN-CMC, CFRN, CEN, CPEN

Christopher Speaker RN, MSN, APN, FNP-BC, CPN

Michelle Webb RN, MS, CRNA

Lori Wertz RN, MN, CPEN

Tim Wolfe, MD

Certified Pediatric Emergency Nurse
Detailed Content Outline

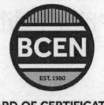

A CPEN® is a registered nurse who possesses advanced critical thinking and highly developed skills in providing emergency care to pediatric patients and their families. The CPEN® is able to apply these skills autonomously, demonstrating the ability to assess, analyze, intervene, and evaluate ill or injured pediatric patients in the emergency setting.

The following concepts are integrated throughout the examination, appropriate to the stated task:

- Collaboration with other health care providers
- Communication
- Conflict management
- Critical incident stress management (debriefing)
- Discharge planning
- Diversity
- Ethical Considerations
- Evidence-based practice
- Family-centered care
- Growth and development
- Health promotion and injury prevention
- Medication administration
- Pain management
- Patient safety
- Pharmacology

© 2018. BCEN. All rights reserved.

Certified Pediatric Emergency Nurse Detailed Content Outline

1. Triage Process and Assessment — 31

A. Emergency Intake
  1. Visual assessment (sick vs. not sick)
  2. Pediatric Assessment Triangle (PAT)
  3. Triage priority based on acuity and resources
  4. Isolation
B. Emergency preparedness
  1. Decontamination (e.g., chemical or biological agents)
  2. Mass casualty
C. History and Physical
  1. Primary survey
  2. Secondary survey
  3. Behavioral status and risk for harm (e.g., risk-taking behaviors, self-harm, violence)
  4. Developmental milestones
  5. Children with special needs
  6. Sexual orientation and gender identity
  7. Caregivers' perception of child's baseline and current status
D. Pain
  1. Developmentally appropriate assessment and reassessment of pain
  2. Non-pharmacological and pharmacological interventions
  3. Procedural sedation
E. Family
  1. Family functioning and dynamics (e.g., coping strategies, support systems, parenting skills, learning style)
F. Legal Issues
  1. Consent for treatment
  2. Preservation of forensic evidence
  3. Chain of custody
  4. Government regulations
     a. EMTALA
     b. HIPAA
     c. Mandatory reportable situations (e.g., child abuse/neglect, infectious diseases)

2. Medical Emergencies: Respiratory, Cardiovascular, and Neurological — 32

A. Respiratory
  1. Upper Airway
     a. Foreign body
     b. Infections (e.g., croup, epiglottitis)
     c. Inhalation injuries
     d. Congenital conditions (e.g., stenosis, malacia)
     e. Artificial airway (e.g., tracheostomy)

2. Lower Airway
   a. Foreign body
   b. Infections (e.g., bronchiolitis, pneumonia)
   c. Reactive airway disease/asthma
   d. Congenital conditions (e.g., cystic fibrosis, chronic lung disease)
B. Cardiovascular
   1. Shock (i.e., hypovolemic, cardiogenic, distributive, obstructive)
   2. Rhythm disturbances
   3. Infections (e.g., myocarditis)
C. Neurological
   1. Infections (e.g., meningitis)
   2. Seizure
   3. Shunt dysfunction
   4. Headache, migraine, and tumor
   5. Stroke
   6. Congenital conditions (e.g., hydrocephalus, arteriovenous malformation)
D. Post-resuscitative care

3. Additional Medical Emergencies

A. Gastrointestinal
   1. Foreign body
   2. Obstructions (e.g., pyloric stenosis, intussusception, volvulus, constipation)
   3. Infections (e.g., gastroenteritis, appendicitis, pancreatitis)
   4. Inflammatory bowel disease (e.g., Crohn's disease, ulcerative colitis)
   5. Gastrointestinal bleeding
   6. Nutrition (e.g., failure to thrive, formula intolerance, obesity, fluid-electrolyte imbalance, GERD)
   7. Congenital conditions (e.g., tracheoesophageal fistula)
B. Genitourinary
   1. Infections (e.g., UTI, STI, PID, epididymitis, pyelonephritis)
   2. Male genitourinary emergencies (e.g., testicular torsion, priapism, phimosis)
   3. OB/GYN emergencies (e.g., ectopic pregnancy, vaginal bleeding, emergent delivery, ovarian cysts, ovarian torsion)
C. Maxillofacial
   1. Foreign body
   2. Infections (e.g., peritonsillar, abscess, strep throat, mastoiditis)
   3. Hemorrhage (e.g., epistaxis, post-T&A bleed)
D. Ocular
   1. Foreign body
   2. Infections (e.g., periorbital cellulitis, conjunctivitis)
E. Musculoskeletal
   1. Foreign body (e.g., impalements)
   2. Infections (e.g., osteomyelitis, septic arthritis)
   3. Congenital conditions (e.g., osteogenesis imperfecta)
F. Integumentary
   1. Foreign body
   2. Infections (e.g., cellulitis)
   3. Rash (e.g., hives, petechiae, infestations)
G. Hematology/Oncology
   1. Hematology (e.g., sickle cell, bleeding or clotting disorders, ITP)
   2. Oncology (e.g., fever and neutropenia, tumor lysis syndrome)
H. Endocrine/metabolic (e.g., congenital adrenal disorders, glucose disturbance)
I. Sepsis
J. Allergic reactions and anaphylaxis

Certified Pediatric Emergency Nurse (CPEN) Review IV

4. Special Considerations	27

A. Neonatal Emergencies
   1. Infections (e.g., neonatal sepsis)
   2. Hyperbilirubinemia
   3. Thermoregulation
   4. Fluid-electrolyte imbalance
   5. Newborn resuscitation
   6. Congenital conditions (e.g., ductal dependent lesions)
B. Behavioral Emergencies
   1. Self-injury (e.g., cutting, eating disorders)
   2. Mood disorders (e.g., depression, anxiety)
   3. Suicidal ideations/attempts
   4. Homicidal ideations
   5. Acute psychosis
   6. Aggressive behavior
   7. Substance abuse
   8. Post-traumatic stress disorder
   9. Pervasive developmental disorders
C. Maltreatment Emergencies
   1. Emotional abuse
   2. Physical abuse
   3. Sexual abuse or assault
   4. Neglect
   5. Human trafficking
D. Environmental
   1. Temperature-related emergencies (e.g., heat, cold)
   2. Envenomation emergencies (e.g., bites, stings)
   3. Chemical exposures (e.g., cleaning agents, organophosphates)
   4. Vector borne illnesses (e.g., rabies, ticks)
E. Toxicology
   1. Ingestion and poisoning (e.g., medications, alcohol)
   2. Carbon monoxide poisoning
   3. Drug interactions/withdrawal
F. Communicable diseases
   1. Childhood diseases (e.g., measles, mumps, pertussis, chicken pox)
   2. Multi-drug resistant organisms (e.g., MRSA, VRE)
   3. *C. Difficile*

5. Trauma Emergencies	25

A. Respiratory
   1. Upper airway trauma (e.g., tracheal disruption)
   2. Lower airway trauma (e.g., pneumothorax, hemothorax, pulmonary contusion)
B. Cardiovascular (e.g., tamponade, blunt cardiac injury)
C. Neurological (e.g., traumatic brain injury, intracranial bleeds, herniation syndrome, spinal cord injury)
D. Gastrointestinal (e.g., liver injury, spleen injury, bowel injury)
E. Genitourinary (e.g., straddle injury, renal contusion)
F. Environmental (e.g., submersion injuries, burns, electric injuries)
G. Maxillofacial (e.g., tooth avulsion, facial fracture)
H. Ocular (e.g., hyphema, corneal abrasions, globe rupture, ocular burns)
I. Musculoskeletal (e.g., fractures, joint dislocations, sprains, strains, amputations, compartment syndrome)
J. Integumentary (e.g., avulsions, abrasions, lacerations, degloving)

Total	150

* In addition to the 150 scored items, 25 unscored pretest items will be administered to each candidate.

© 2018. BCEN. All rights reserved.

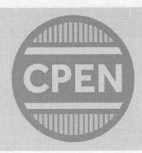

Recertify

Renewing your specialty certification demonstrates commitment to your patients and career through the lifelong learning required to keep the certification you worked so hard to achieve. Recertify... your way.

About Recertification

Health care is constantly changing. Staying on top of new information and best practices is more important than ever.

Maintaining your emergency nursing credentials reenergizes your passion for your profession, and puts you in the best position to bring new approaches to your team, your unit, your patients and your community.

Recertification for your CEN®, CFRN®, CPEN®, CTRN®, or TCRN® is required every four (4) years, and, while you are responsible for keeping track of your certification expiration date, BCEN® will communicate with you at just the right times during your four-year cycle to help keep you on track. Be sure to keep your contact information in your BCEN account current so you don't miss any messages from us!

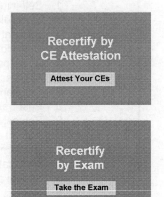

Option 1: Recertification by CE Attestation

Eligibility Requirements

- You must hold a current BCEN certification (CEN, CFRN, CPEN, CTRN, or TCRN) in the program you wish to recertify.

- You must have a current, unrestricted Registered Nurse license, or a nursing certificate that is equivalent to a Registered Nurse in the United States or its Territories.

- You must have completed 100 contact hours of nursing continuing education within your current 4-year recertification period.

- *Please Note: When you complete the CE attestation form for recertification, all 100 contact hours must have been obtained on or before the attestation date even if you are recertifying early. Should you be selected for an audit, BCEN cannot accept contact hours obtained past the date of attestation. You must successfully pass your audit to recertify. Should you fail the audit, BCEN does not issue refunds.*

Option 2: Recertification by Exam

Eligibility Requirements

- You must hold a current certification (CEN, CFRN, CPEN, CTRN, or TCRN).

- You must have a current, unrestricted Registered Nurse license or nursing certificate that is equivalent to a Registered Nurse in the United States or its Territories.

- Your exam application must be completed at least 91 days prior to your certification expiration date. (Your exam results must post to your account before your certification expires.)

Audit Information

BCEN's policy is to randomly audit 10% of Recertification by CE Attestation applications each year. View BCEN's policy on auditing of Recertification by CE Attestation applications (www.BCEN.org/recertify).

If randomly selected for an audit, you will receive audit instructions via email.

Understanding Continuing Education Required for Recertification

BCEN® developed the Continuing Education recertification program to emphasize the importance of life long learning to maintain knowledge and expertise.

BCEN no longer requires candidates to log their contact hours but to attest they meet the continuing education (CE) guidelines. It is important to keep a summary log of courses and original documentation in case of an audit. This information will be required to complete the audit.

Measurement of Continuing Education

Different terminology is used for continuing education credit. BCEN uses the measurement of contact hours in which one contact hour equals 60 minutes of instructional content.

The following qualify as one (1) contact hour:

- 1 Continuing Education Contact Hour (CECH)
- 1 Continuing Education Recognition Program (CERP)
- 1 Continuing Education Accredited Recognition Program (CEARP)
- 1 Continuing Medical Education (CME)

Continuing Education Guidelines

- Continuing education should have a clear and direct application to the practice of emergency, pediatric emergency, flight/transport, or trauma nursing.
- 100 completed contact hours earned within your 4-year recertification period;
    - 75 of the 100 contact hours must be of Clinical content specific to your specialty area of practice and up to 25 may be of Non-clinical content. It is acceptable to have more than 75 of the contact hours of clinical content.
    - 50 of the 100 contact hours must come from an accredited source (For example, American Association of Critical Care Nurses (AACN), American Nurses Credentialing Center (ANCC), Emergency Nurses Association (ENA), State Nurses Associations/State Boards of Nursing (SNA/SBN), and the Air and Surface Transport Nurses Association (ASTNA).

- All continuing education content must be at the nursing practice level.
    - BCEN cannot accept EMT or paramedic contact hours approved only by an EMS provider such as The Commission on Accreditation of Pre-Hospital Continuing Education (CAPCE).
    - If EMT or paramedic contact hours are also approved by a nursing provider, the contact hours will be accepted.
    - Advanced Medical Life Support (AMLS), Pre-Hospital Trauma Life Support (PHTLS), and International Trauma Life Support (ITLS) are NOT accepted.

Continuing Education Guidelines (continued)

- For continuing education to be eligible to use for recertification, it must have occurred during the four-year period of certification. For example, if your certification expired March 31, 2019, your four-year period of certification was from April 1, 2015 until March 31, 2019. Therefore, you could use contact hours that you accrued since April 1 of 2015.

- Certificants who successfully meet all program requirements will have their certification credential renewed for the following four years.

- Certificants who do not meet the program requirements must register and pass the appropriate certification exam to renew or reinstate their credential.

CE Certificate

Each time you participate in a continuing education activity, you should receive a certificate or letter of attendance indicating the following:

- Your name
- Date of Activity
- Title of Activity
- Name of provider of Activity
- Number of contact hours awarded
- Approver name or accreditor name of contact hours

Keep these certificates or letters of attendance, as you will be required to upload the documents if contacted by BCEN for an audit.

Please Note: Continuing education submitted without a certificate showing the number of contact hours awarded are not acceptable. Certificates of completion will not be accepted.

BCEN offers an optional easy to use CE tracker found in your BCEN account. It is an easy way to keep track of your activities. If contacted for an audit, those activities tracked will be automatically transferred over for you to review.

Clinical Content

Clinical content includes any educational offerings that primarily contain information applicable to direct practice in the clinical area. The program content must be primarily focused on knowledge the nurse can apply in providing direct care to an individual patient or community.

Examples include topics such as: "Care of the Patient with a Temporary Pacemaker," Flight Physiology," Teaching Diabetic Patients," "Management of the Trauma Patient," or "Toxicology."

Acceptable accredited college courses include educational offerings that have a clinical focus. Examples: Nursing 410: "Care of the Adult Patient," Nursing 601: "Trauma Nursing," or "Pathophysiology."

Non-Clinical Content

Non-clinical content includes any educational offerings related to the professional practice of nursing and the emergency (CEN®), pediatric emergency (CPEN®), flight/transport (CFRN®/CTRN®), or trauma (TCRN®) care system.

Examples include topics such as "Developing a Quality Improvement System," "Legal Aspects of Emergency or Flight Care," or "Public Relations in Healthcare."

Accredited college courses that focus on the nonclinical aspects of nursing may be used. Examples would include: "Medical Ethics," and "Leadership and Management."

BCEN recognizes there are accredited CE programs, which consist of multiple lectures, such as national/regional symposiums, or review courses.

Types of Continuing Education

CE Type & Description	Accredited	Non-Accredited
Continuing Education (CE), Continuing Nursing Education (CNE), or Continuing Medical Education (CME) AMA PRA Category 1 Credit™: Programs that have been provided or formally approved for contact hours by an accredited provider or approver of CE, CNE or CME. e.g. national/regional symposiums, review courses, formal continuing education offerings 60 minutes = 1 contact hour Note: Continuing education classes do not need to be formally approved and can be offered by hospitals, professional organization or independent education groups. The contact hours awarded from these types of classes will be considered a non-accredited source; however, no more than **50** contact hours can come from a non-accredited source.	X	
Provider Courses: These include, but are not limited to ACLS, PALS, ENPC, TNCC, Advanced Burn Life Support (ABLS), Advanced Trauma Care for Nurses (ATCN), Advanced Trauma Life Support (ATLS), Course in Advanced Trauma Nursing (CATN), Geriatric Emergency Nursing Education (GENE), Transport Professional Advanced Trauma Course (TPATC), and Neonatal Resuscitation Program (NRP). ***BLS / CPR is NOT accepted*** Only one (1) initial and one (1) renewal for each provider course will be accepted during your current recertification period. 60 minutes=1 contact hour If you are only able to submit your provider card as documentation, if audited, you will receive 8 contact hours for initial and 4 contact hours for renewal of ACLS and PALS.	X	
Teaching Activities: (e.g. presentation/lectures, teaching provider courses, etc...) The same presentation or lecture given to nurses, healthcare providers, or the public may only be counted once during your current recertification period. The presentation or lecture does not count if it was given as part of an educator or faculty expected job performance. 60 minutes = 1 contact hour	X If accredited contact hours were provided	X

Types of Continuing Education

CE Type & Description	Accredited	Non-Accredited
Academic Credit: Must have earned a "C" or higher and content must apply to emergency (CEN), pediatric emergency (CPEN), flight/transport (CFRN/CTRN), or trauma (TCRN) nursing from an accredited institution. 1 Semester course = 15 Contact Hours 1 Trimester course = 12 Contact Hours 1 Quarter course = 10 Contact Hours	X	
Preceptorship: In order to count preceptorship hours toward your recertification, the nurse(s) you precepted must have earned college credits for being precepted. A maximum of 15 contact hours will be accepted during your current recertification period. 1 Semester preceptorship = 15 Contact Hours 1 Trimester preceptorship = 12 Contact Hours 1 Quarter preceptorship = 10 Contact Hours	X	
Authoring: Publication must be peer-reviewed and content must be specific to emergency (CEN), pediatric emergency (CPEN), flight/transport (CFRN/CTRN), or trauma (TCRN) nursing. If co-authored, credit must be distributed evenly among authors. Article = 5 Contact Hours Chapter/module = 10 Contact Hours Textbook = 50 Contact Hours	X	

Types of Continuing Education

CE Type & Description	Accredited	Non-Accredited
Poster Presentation: 5 Contact Hours per poster developed. Each poster may only be counted once during your recertification period.	X If accredited contact hours were provided	X
Item Writing: 0.5 = 1 accepted exam item. A maximum of 5 Contact Hours may be counted per year.		X

© 2019 Board of Certification for Emergency Nursing (BCEN)

The information is subject to change without notice.
Please visit the BCEN website at BCEN.org for the most updated listings.

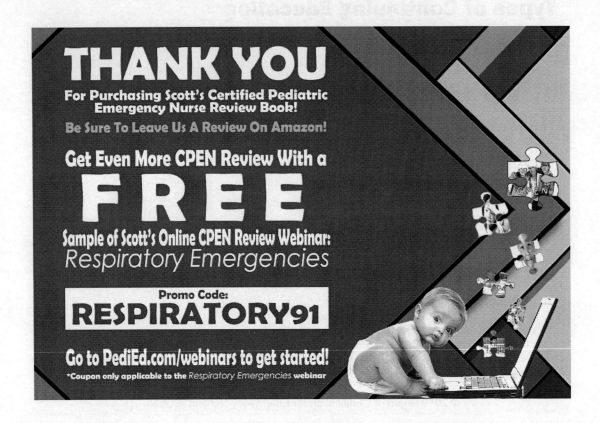

Your Prep For The CPEN Exam Just Got Even Easier!

8 Video Lectures
No death by PowerPoint! Scott works in funny videos, mnemonics and real-life case studies to help you stay engaged and retain the information!

Printable Course Handout
100+ pages of outlines and notes from the lecture! Print it out, download the PDF, or purchase a bound copy!

Continuing Education
Earn a certificate for (6) ENA/CAPCE-Approved CEUs at the completion of the full course!
This FREE Respiratory Module earns you (1) CEU!

Chapter 1
Emergency Assessment of Crashing Kids

Always be nice to your children, because they are the ones who will choose your nursing home.
-Phyllis Diller

Certified Pediatric Emergency Nurse (CPEN) Review IV

STUDY TIP..

Remove Sample Answer Sheet Page
... At the beginning of each chapter. Use it to cover the answer and rationale for each question until you mark your answer. No cheating!

Record Your Notes
... On the back side of the Sample Answer Sheet. Of course, the margins are good too, but we give you a mini notebook page for those major concepts you don't want to forget!

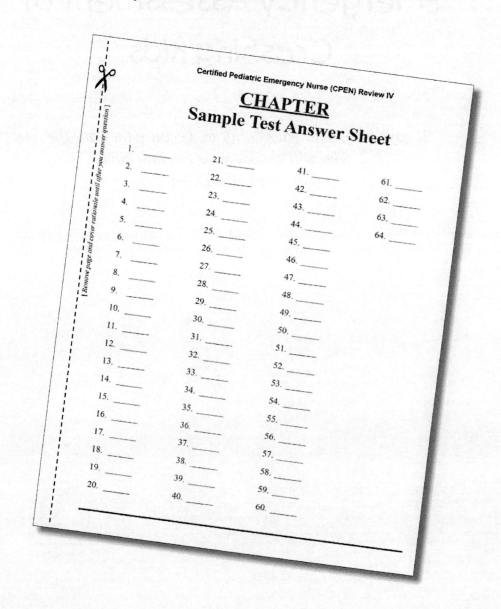

CHAPTER 1
Sample Test Answer Sheet

[Remove page and cover rationale until after you answer question]

1. _____
2. _____
3. _____
4. _____
5. _____
6. _____
7. _____
8. _____
9. _____
10. _____
11. _____
12. _____
13. _____
14. _____
15. _____
16. _____
17. _____
18. _____
19. _____
20. _____

21. _____
22. _____
23. _____
24. _____
25. _____
26. _____
27. _____
28. _____
29. _____
30. _____
31. _____
32. _____
33. _____
34. _____
35. _____
36. _____
37. _____
38. _____
39. _____
40. _____

41. _____
42. _____
43. _____
44. _____
45. _____
46. _____
47. _____
48. _____
49. _____
50. _____
51. _____
52. _____
53. _____
54. _____
55. _____
56. _____
57. _____
58. _____
59. _____
60. _____

61. _____
62. _____
63. _____
64. _____

Pertinent Pediatric Ponderings (NOTES)

Certified Pediatric Emergency Nurse (CPEN) Review IV

1) Infants are:

A) Obligate mouth breathers

B) Preferential mouth breathers

C) Obligate nose breathers

D) Preferential nose breathers

D - Infants and young children, especially those under 6 months of age, are preferential nose breathers. Many of us were taught that they are obligate nose breathers, meaning that they only breathe through their noses, but this is not accurate. Preferential nose breathers is a better description as they "prefer to breathe" through their nares. This concept is especially important to remember when they get upper respiratory infections (URIs) and the nares are clogged up with boogers. A bulb syringe goes a long way and can be a life saver.

2) Children, especially those under the age of six, have a natural anatomical condition which causes:

A) Neck extension when placed on a flat surface

B) Neck flexion when placed on a flat surface

C) Back extension when placed on a flat surface

D) Back flexion when placed on a flat surface

B - Small children have what might be referred to as "big head, little body syndrome," which results in neck flexion when they are placed on a flat surface. In real estate, the motto is location, location, location... and with little kids, the motto is positioning, positioning, and positioning. Think about a 2-year-old with a big head (aka Charlie Brown), flat on a spine board or sedated for a CT scan. What does their big head do to their airway? It shoves their chin on their chest and they don't breathe very well. Simply putting a diaper or towel behind their shoulders goes a long way to offset "big head, little body syndrome."

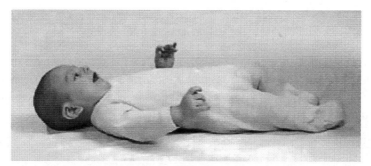

Chin on chest positioning

Photo courtesy of Ossur

www.ossur.com

Certified Pediatric Emergency Nurse (CPEN) Review IV

3) The narrowest part of a young child's upper airway is the:

A) Vocal cords

B) Thyroid cartilage

C) Cricoid cartilage

D) Articulating cartilage

C - The narrowest part of the airway in children is the cricoid cartilage (subglottic.) In adults, it is the vocal cords (glottis.) Children's airways are funnel shaped (big at the top and smaller at the bottom) versus adult airways which are tube shaped. This is an important consideration with intubation as passing the endotracheal tube (ETT) through the cords is only half of the battle. The ETT has to pass through the bottom of the funnel (cricoid cartilage) as well.

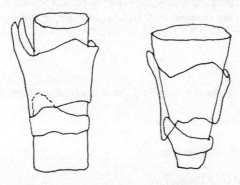

Adult vs. Pediatric Airways

Illustration by Nina DeBoer, then age 9 (my aspiring artist daughter, now aspiring baker daughter)

4) A 2-year-old child in severe respiratory distress initially was anxious and tachycardic with a heart rate (HR) of 184 and an O_2 sat of 92%. Now the heart rate has decreased to 92, the O_2 sat is 90% with no change in respiratory status, and the child is becoming sleepy. The nurse should realize that:

A) The heart rate is now approaching "normal" and this is a reassuring sign

B) The child is most likely going to arrest soon

C) The O_2 sat is still above 90% so "all is well"

D) The heart rate of 184 could be due to separation anxiety from parents

B – What looks like a "normal" heart rate is actually a low rate for a child this age. In a child who is getting sleepy with no improvement in their respiratory status, "normal" vital signs are an ominous, not reassuring, sign. This commonly means they can't compensate anymore and the respiratory distress may soon become respiratory arrest.

Certified Pediatric Emergency Nurse (CPEN) Review IV

5) A 5-day-old child is admitted to the ED as mom states he "looked yellow" at home. Beyond the skin on the palms and soles of the feet, other reliable areas to determine color changes include:

A) Sclera and conjunctiva

B) Nail beds

C) Tongue and oral mucosa

D) All of the above

D – Many of us commonly and appropriately look at the skin for color changes such as cyanosis, jaundice, etc. However, in children with naturally darker skin, and especially in African-American kids, skin color changes can be difficult to detect. Evaluating other areas such as the eyes, mouth, and nail beds can be very valuable.

6) How long is the normal capillary refill in children?

A) 1 second

B) 2 seconds

C) 3 seconds

D) 4 seconds

B – Capillary refill time of two seconds is now considered to be normal, as long as the child is in a nice, warm room. An easy way to remember this is for the nurse to say "capillary refill" at the same time you let go from pushing on the finger or toe. By the time you have finished saying "capillary refill," the finger or toe should be pink again. Remember, especially in "shocky or shocked" children, blood is shunted away from the extremities, so evaluating the fingers or toes, as well as a central circulation site such as the chest or forehead can be very helpful.

7) What is the normal minimum systolic blood pressure for a 2-year-old?

A) 54mm Hg

B) 64mm Hg

C) 74mm Hg

D) 84mm Hg

C - The formula *70 + (2 x age in years)* can be used to determine the <u>minimum</u> systolic mm Hg BP for a child 1-10 years of age. It is important to remember that this number is the bottom 5th percentile of systolic blood pressures. This formula only works if the "numbers match the child" and the correct size cuff is used.

Emergency Assessment

8) What is the normal blood pressure for a preterm or full term baby who delivers in the ED?

A) *70 + (2 x age in years)*

B) 60mm Hg

C) 70mm Hg

D) Mean arterial pressure (MAP) equal to or greater than the infant's gestational age

D – This is a neat trick a neonatologist taught me. For newborns, if you have the proper equipment to take an accurate BP, the minimum desired MAP is the gestational age in weeks. Systolic and diastolic pressures are way too many numbers to remember. So if mom delivers a "25-weeker" in the ED, the lowest desired, (i.e. it's under this and I should treat it), MAP is 25mm Hg. Concurrently you should consider treatment of a full-term, "40-weeker" with a MAP of less than 40mm Hg.

9) The leading cause of death among children is:

A) HIV

B) Cardiac disease

C) Trauma

D) Asthma

C – Though HIV, congenital heart disease, and respiratory failure are major factors; traumatic injuries are still the leading cause of death for kids.

10) In terms of the medical care of children, parents are:

A) A valuable source of information and guidance

B) Unreliably optimistic in terms of medical problems with their own children

C) Unreliably pessimistic in terms of medical problems with their own children

D) Often trying to hide poor parenting, Munchausen's, or even abuse

A – Parents, and especially those caring for technology dependent or special needs children, know their little ones much better than we ever will. If an infant is brought to the ED, especially during the first month of life, and even if the infant "just isn't looking right," it is appropriate to be concerned. Many times it may be common issues such as diaper rash or feeding intolerance. However, rare conditions such as sepsis, inborn errors of metabolism, or hypoglycemia can also be the culprit. In many cases, especially outside of major children's medical centers or with some very rare syndromes, parents are the regional experts on special needs diseases and devices. "Is this normal for your child?" should be a question asked of just about every parent. The idea of listening to the parents and using your gut, especially with infants in the ED is summarized in the following story from an experienced peds ED nurse:

"Sometimes it just involves watching a neonate. Many years ago, I picked up a chart to discharge a 14-day-old whose triage complaint was "vomiting." The discharge diagnosis was diaper rash. Mom was told to burp the baby frequently and follow up with her primary care provider in a week. The mother signed out at the desk, and I asked her to show me the infant being held by his Dad. As soon as my eyes made contact, I grabbed the discharge paper back from her, and asked if the baby had been given any Pedialyte or formula in the ED visit? She said no. I explained that usually for that complaint, we would try a small feeding to ensure it could be tolerated. But I told her I wanted to get the resident and peds ED fellow to come look at the baby before discharge one more time; all the while, trying not to alarm an already exhausted new mom. I took this baby to one of our resuscitation beds based on gut feelings and the facial expression of this infant all but screaming, "I have a surgical abdomen, please help me!" The story has a happy ending as he was in the OR about 90 minutes later, had his volvulus repaired, and I continued to watch him grow up during my years at the hospital, always amazed at how close that was. Sometimes I think we just try to move patients too quickly before we really get a handle on what made the parent come in that day."

Certified Pediatric Emergency Nurse (CPEN) Review IV

11) When performing an exam on a 2-year-old, the ER nurse should keep all of the following in mind **except**:

A) Evaluate uninjured and painless parts first

B) They may be scared of strangers at this age (stranger anxiety)

C) Toddlers prefer to be examined privately, away from the caregiver

D) Parents can be very helpful with undressing/redressing and eliciting a child's assistance

C – Two-year-olds are very aware and may be very leery of strangers, including nurses, medics, doctors and anyone who is not "Mommy." As exploratory as 2-year-olds are, they always want to make sure that mom or dad has "got their back!" As a rule, when examining children (and adults), start by talking to them, and if possible, evaluate something non-painful first. In addition, parents can be very helpful with preparing for and controlling anxiety during the exam.

12) Generally, children understand and respond to "No!" by age:

A) 1-3 months

B) 4-6 months

C) 7-9 months

D) 10-12 months

D – Telling an infant or 4-month-old child, "No!" is kind of like yelling at someone who is deaf. It doesn't make whole lot of sense. Most children don't begin understanding "No!" until 10-12 months of age. Having a basic overview of normal growth and development is very important for peds ED nurses. See the growth and development summaries at the end of this chapter for more information.

13) At which age does "body image become everything"?

A) 1-3 years

B) 3-5 years

C) 6-12 years

D) 13-18 years

D – You just have to go to the shopping mall to do "research" to answer this one. Teens and body image go hand in hand and hospital gowns are not the height of fashion. Body image is especially important with injury or trauma, (i.e. "Will this leave a scar?") and may also be a consideration with medications that can cause edema (i.e. "Will these steroids make me look fat?")

Certified Pediatric Emergency Nurse (CPEN) Review IV

14) The Pediatric Assessment Triangle (PAT) in EMS or the ED:

A) Is used to quickly determine if a child is "sick or not sick."

B) Is a detailed, comprehensive hands-on assessment

C) Is performed systematically from head to toe

D) Commonly takes 15-minutes to complete in its entirety

A – The PAT starts with the doorway assessment. You look at the kid from the door and say are they "sick or not sick"? Just about every child who comes to the ED is "sick," but "how sick"? Are they physiologically compensating for their illness or injury or are they beyond that point? How fast do we need to intervene? Is there time to get a full history first or are interventions needed immediately? It takes far less than 30 seconds and is a great triage and repeated assessment tool.

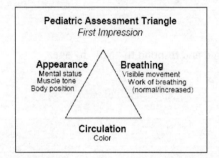

Gen. Appearance	Work of Breathing	Circulation to Skin	Pathophysiologic Category	Compensated?	Sick?
Good	Normal	Normal	No active compromise to vital functions	Yes	No
Good	Increased	Normal	Respiratory distress (varying degrees)	Yes	No
Poor	Increased or poor effort	Normal	Respiratory failure	No	YES!
Good	Normal	Abnormal	Peripheral vasoconstriction (medications, fever, hypothermia)	Yes	Probably not
Poor	Normal to mildly increased	Abnormal	Shock	No	YES!
Poor	Normal	Normal	Central nervous system dysfunction (postictal, head injury, intoxication)	No	YES!
Poor	Poor effort	Abnormal	Cardiopulmonary failure	No	YES!
Poor	None	None	Cardiopulmonary arrest	No	YES!

Pediatric Assessment Triangle (PAT) and Pathophysiology

Courtesy of Lou Romig MD, FAAP, FACEP

www.jumpstarttriage.com

Certified Pediatric Emergency Nurse (CPEN) Review IV

15) The mother of an 18-month-old child states her daughter has had a one-day history of a cough and runny nose. The child is watching your every move while mom is giving her a bottle. The respiratory rate (RR) is 32 and no retractions are noted. Chest expansion appears to be equal and her skin and nails are pink. Your initial assessment is:

A) The child is sick

B) The child is not sick

C) The respiratory rate is very high

D) The child is rapidly approaching respiratory failure

B - Not sick. Yes, the kid may have a runny nose and a cough, but she's alert, interactive, breathing fine and is pink. If it's December, it's probably RSV, and if it's not RSV, we'll both be amazed. Either way, the kid looks cute and cuddly. Sick or not sick? Urgent or non-urgent? It is essential to become well versed in recognizing "sick or not sick." This mother may need reassurance in dealing with symptom management of an upper respiratory infection. For the parent, such symptoms may result in lost days from work which adds to frustration in caring for a "non-urgent" illness. This scenario is mundane for the ED staff, but for the parent, it can be a colossal stressor.

16) When evaluating a 10-year-old child, it is generally best to do all of the following **except**:

A) Introduce yourself and maintain eye contact

B) Sit down and listen attentively while interviewing the child and the parent

C) Allow the parent to remain with the child during assessments or procedures

D) Restrain them before initiating any examination

D – Unless there is a clear safety issue, patients should not be restrained for an examination. 10-year-olds or "pre-teens" are in many cases both trying to act like teens and adults, but also are very much younger children at the same time. Treating them with respect, listening to the child and the parent, and allowing the parent to remain in the room during procedures or assessments are important techniques.

17) You are preparing to place an IV in a dehydrated 2-year-old child who is uncooperative with the procedure. It is reasonable to:

A) Ask the mother if she prefers to stay with her child during the procedure

B) Insist that the mother leave during the painful procedure

C) Insist that the mother remain to help restrain the child during the procedure

D) Send the mother to registration so you can do your job without her interference

A – Every patient is different and every parent is different. Some will want to stay; others will not. In either case, it is not appropriate to insist that they leave or stay, and certainly not appropriate to send a parent away under false pretenses. Family presence is for the support of the child, not of the nursing staff, and asking parents to help hold their child down, especially during painful procedures is not recommended.

Certified Pediatric Emergency Nurse (CPEN) Review IV

18) To take a blood pressure (BP) and actually believe the reading, all of the following are considerations are crucial **except**:

A) You have to use the right size cuff

B) You have to look at the child and the numbers

C) Rapid cuff deflation will make it more comfortable for the patient

D) You have to remember the limitations of automatic blood pressure machines

C – While an inflated blood pressure cuff may be uncomfortable, rapidly deflating it at the patient's request doesn't make for an accurate reading. Blood pressure is one of the least sensitive indicators of adequate circulation in children, so if you want the most believable results, remember the following: 1) Right size cuff – An adult cuff on a little kid will give BP results which are way too low. Don't believe the "something is better than nothing" line. Conversely, little cuffs on big kids will give you BP results that are way too high. 2) Numbers lie – kids don't. If the numbers you see appear to match the kid, great. If not, believe the kid that you see (Sick or not sick?) 3) Automatic blood pressure machines… Gotta love 'em. "Push the button and take a BP for me." But, remember a Cabbage Patch Kid doll's BP can be 110/70 with some machines! Blood pressures are still very important, especially if the kid is sick, obese, or has a history of hypertension. Use your gut and look at the kid, not just the numbers!

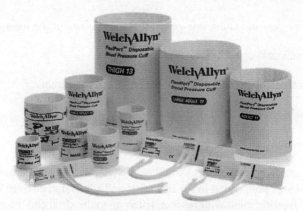

Range of BP Cuff Sizes

Photo courtesy of Welch Allyn

www.welchallyn.com

19) Placing a young trauma patient supine on a traditional spine or papoose board can result in cervical spinal:

A) Flexion

B) Extension

C) Hyperextension

D) Proper positioning

A – Remember the concept of "big head, little body syndrome" with infants and young children. Placing them flat on their backs pushes their chins onto their chests. This certainly does not result in optimal airway or cervical spine positioning. With this in mind, a little bit of padding beneath the shoulders, the pediatric "Peanut" papoose, or a pediatric spine board goes a long way to help maintain neutral cervical alignment.

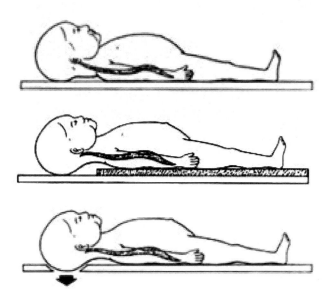

Pediatric Spinal Positioning

Photos courtesy of the

Journal of Bone and Joint Surgery

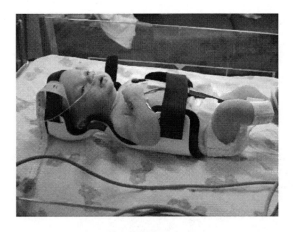

"Peanut" Papoose

Photo courtesy of Ossur

www.ossur.com

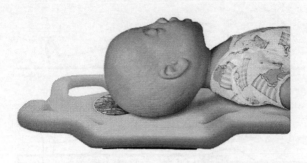

Pedi-Align Pediatric Spinal Board

Photo courtesy of Iron Duck

www.ironduck.com

20) The primary assessment in pediatric emergency care includes all of the following **except**:

A) Airway

B) Breathing

C) Circulation

D) Insurance information

D – Though it may seem that the "wallet biopsy" is a frequently a part of the medical examination, the delivery of emergency care does not involve verification of insurance.

21) When examining a sleeping infant, which portion of the assessment should be performed **last**?

A) Respiratory rate

B) Pulse

C) Rectal temperature

D) Pulse oximetry reading

C – Why wake the kid up until you really need to? Taking a rectal temp will certainly wake them up! Obtaining other items first is a much better option. And remember, it's pretty common for pulse ox readings to drop when children are deep in sleep.

22) Screening for suicidal ideations in children:

A) Is not needed as suicide only affects teens and adults

B) Should follow if any "red flags" appear in the history or presentation

C) Should be conducted only with a parent or guardian present for legal reasons

D) Should be limited to the referral to a competent child psychologist

B – Though horrible to consider, and thankfully quite rare, suicide is not limited to the adult population. Even school age children can become suicidal. If any "red flags" are raised during the initial history, specific questions about suicidal ideations should be asked. "Red flags" include suspicion of self inflicted injury, history of suicide attempts in the past, loss of interest in life, school, or work, giving away of possessions, and marked changes in personality or behavior.

Certified Pediatric Emergency Nurse (CPEN) Review IV

23) Abdominal assessments should be performed in which order:

A) Inspect, palpate, auscultate, and percussion

B) Inspect, auscultate, percussion, and palpation

C) Palpation, inspection, auscultate and percussion

D) Percussion, palpation, auscultate, and inspection

B – Look at them first while they are still calm and before you start pushing on things that hurt. After looking, listening next will avoid false bowel sounds induced by palpation. Percussion is next, then finally palpation. Especially if something hurts, push on it last as the rest of the exam will be difficult after you make them cry. Look, listen, tap, and touch.

24) Which of the following kinds of coughs suggest that the parents should have the child evaluated as soon as possible?

A) A cough that causes respiratory distress or cyanosis

B) Loud honking cough that disappears when the child is asleep

C) A cough that occurs after exercise in the known asthmatic

D) A nocturnal cough in a child that has been seen for sinusitis

A – As you can imagine, any cough that causes respiratory distress or even worse, visible cyanosis, should be evaluated as soon as possible.

25) When assessing an infant's abdomen, each of the statements below is true **except**:

A) The abdomen of a infant is naturally protuberant and may appear somewhat distended

B) It is not necessary to examine the rectum of an infant

C) Crying can result in significant abdominal distention

D) It may be necessary to evaluate the abdomen more than once for an accurate assessment

B – The abdominal exam in a child can be challenging. Deep palpation should be avoided during the initial exam. The examiner should approach the child with a calm demeanor and warm hands. Infant and young children who are stressed and crying will swallow large amounts of air (aerophagia.) Often, tenseness of the abdominal wall will disappear with decompression by a nasogastric or orogastric tube. Examination of the rectum should be accomplished in all children who demonstrate evidence of an intrabdominal or pelvic disorder, or those presenting with pooping problems or rectal bleeding.

26) A piece of good advice for parents is:

A) Starve a cold, feed a fever

B) Feed a cold, starve a fever

C) Starve a cold, starve a fever

D) Feed a cold, feed a fever

D - Parents should be instructed that regardless of what they have heard in the past about starving or feeding colds and fevers, feeding is always good. When children are given a nutritional, well-balanced diet, it helps fight infections and provides the nutrients that the body needs when dealing with fevers, colds, or any other ills. For children still on formula, that is always appropriate. Sick kids need increased caloric intake and lots of fluids.

27) Which of the following **best** describes toddlers?

A) Desires to please and likes choices

B) Has a short attention span and responds well to rewards

C) Desires privacy and attempts to gain control

D) Most concerned with the opinions of others, especially peers

B – Toddlers have a short attention span (some say they have the attention span of a door knob) and they do love rewards. That is why we have such a wide varieties of stickers and cartoons in the ED.

28) When taking the initial history at triage, which of the following statements is **true** regarding medications?

A) Only prescribed medications need to be documented

B) Social or recreational drugs aren't medications and don't need to be considered

C) Prescribed, over the counter, herbal, and alternative medications should all be documented

D) If a medication doesn't match up with the medical history, it doesn't need to be documented

C – It's important to ask not only about prescribed meds, but also over the counter meds, and other holistic, herbal, or alternative therapies. Also, the medications they *did* tell you about can clue you in as to diseases that they *forgot* to tell you about (and vice versa.)

29) The **best** way to communicate medical information to preschool children is to use:

A) Detailed anatomical models to better illustrate diseases or surgical procedures

B) Concrete, simple terminology

C) Word games like "taking your pulse" or "shooting an X-ray"

D) Cooperative decision making processes such as asking questions like "Can we start an IV now?"

B – Preschool children are concrete thinkers and respond well to simple, clear information. Keep it short and simple!

Certified Pediatric Emergency Nurse (CPEN) Review IV

30) A severely developmentally delayed toddler who is about to undergo peripheral IV placement is kicking the nursing staff despite repeated instructions from the mother to stop. The nurse aware of developmental concepts should:

A) Echo the mother's instructions to stop

B) Reason with the child concerning the need for the procedure

C) Try distractions with familiar objects

D) Kick the child to reinforce the consequences of his actions

C - This toddler is severely developmentally delayed and is more likely to respond to basic techniques as opposed to more advanced reasoning processes. In addition, toddlers seem to live to say "NO!" and they most likely hear "NO!" from various people countless times a day. Most toddlers, and certainly older children, are old enough to understand that kicking the nurse is not acceptable behavior. However, as this child is severely developmentally delayed, verbal instructions will probably not have the desired result.

31) A 1-year-old presents with respiratory distress. Upon auscultation, stridor is heard and can best be described as:

A) Rapid and deep breathing associated with diabetic ketoacidosis (DKA)

B) A high-pitched sound heard on inspiration associated with upper airway obstruction

C) A "whistling" sound produced by air moving through narrowed airway passages

D) An abnormal respiratory sound associated with liquid materials in the upper airway

B – Stridor commonly accompanies partial upper airway obstruction and may be present in kids with croup. Whistling and wheezing (think asthma) go together. Air moving through liquid/semi-solid materials that sounds like "rice-crispies" are rales (crackles.) Lastly, rapid/deep breathing with DKA is a pattern of breathing classically described as Kussmaul's respirations and is not an ausculatory finding.

32) A respiratory rate of >40 breaths per minute is normal for:

A) An infant

B) A preschool child

C) A teenage child

D) None of the above

A – The normal respiratory rate for an infant is 30-50. (See Appendix 1-A for more pediatric vital sign ranges.) This question is designed to remind you to have a good idea of normal and abnormal for children of different ages. In practice, remembering exact normal vital signs for each year of age is not critically important; there are lots of charts for such things. However, nurses need to have a basic idea as to what is "really abnormal." A respiratory rate of 40 is quite fast for a teenager, but it's perfectly normal for a newborn. A much more important consideration is to not only look not only at the numbers, but also the child. An infant breathing 40 times a minute sucking on a pacifier is very different from a child of any age breathing 40 times a minute working, wheezing, and retracting.

Certified Pediatric Emergency Nurse (CPEN) Review IV

33) When communicating with a preschooler about an upcoming procedure, it is **most** appropriate to:

A) Tell them about it hours in advance

B) Tell them it won't hurt a bit, even if it most likely will hurt because preschoolers won't remember

C) Tell them immediately before the procedure

D) Don't tell them at all, just do it

C – Telling the preschooler immediately prior to a procedure is when it's most appropriate. Telling the child hours before a nasty procedure means hours of screaming and worry. Why would you do that? If you think they won't remember, just offer a preschooler some sort of reward for doing something and you'll be amazed how well, and how long they remember. "Just do it" might work for Nike, but not for preschoolers in the emergency department.

34) Appropriate methods of comforting an infant before or after a procedure include all of the following **except**:

A) Rocking and relaxing

B) Swaddling and singing

C) Pacifiers and parents

D) Tossing and turning

D – Typically, tossing and turning should be avoided. All of the other methods mentioned above work well to help an infant calm down before or after any procedures.

35) Using the Pediatric Assessment Triangle (PAT), which patient should be seen **first**?

A) 10-month-old female: Complaint - 3 day hx of vomiting; General appearance – Listless; Work of Breathing - Moderate; Skin and Capillary Refill - Mottled, >3 seconds

B) 4-year-old female: Complaint - Cough; General appearance – Running around the waiting room; Work of Breathing - Normal; Skin and Capillary Refill - Pink, <2 seconds

C) 4-month-old female: Complaint – Fever; General appearance - Asleep in mother's arms; Work of Breathing – Normal; Skin and Capillary Refill – Pink, <2 seconds

D) 10-year-old male: Complaint – Wrist pain post-fall from skateboard: General appearance – Pain; Work of Breathing - Normal; Skin and Capillary Refill - Slightly pale, <2 seconds

A – This kid is sick. See patient "A" first, then patients "C and D." Patient "B" can wait a few days… Remember that the General Appearance is considered to be the most significant part of the PAT. Listless = "Danger Will Robinson… Danger"!

Certified Pediatric Emergency Nurse (CPEN) Review IV

36) For a critically ill appearing infant, the following information should always be completed at triage before placing the patient in the treatment area:

A) Age, birth weight and current weight (for drug and defibrillation calculations)

B) Full set of vital signs

C) Signed consent from parent or legal guardian

D) None of the above

D – This one should be easy. Before any of the above considerations, we need to "sort" the patient. Triage comes from the French word meaning to sort. Though the term was originally used to designate the quality of coffee beans, it is now much more commonly used to designate the process (not the place) of sorting patients for emergency medical care. If, at first glance, the child appears really ill or injured, immediate placement in a treatment area is most appropriate. Obtaining the rest of the information can be done later. Children very seldom have a "false positive" sick appearance at triage. In other words, if they look sick, they probably are sick.

37) The Pediatric Assessment Triangle (PAT) involves assessment of all of the following **except**:

A) Pulse at the arterialis temporalis

B) Work of breathing

C) Circulation to the skin

D) General appearance

A – Don't let the fancy terms fool you! The PAT utilizes the three assessments (appearance/breathing/circulation – yet another ABC to remember) to very quickly determine "sick or not sick." It does not involve any vital signs, fancy monitors, or equipment (not even a stethoscope); just your eyes, ears, hands, experience, and intuition.

38) Appropriate urine output for a 10kg child in the ED is:

A) 0.1ml/hour

B) 1-2ml/kg/hr

C) 30ml/hour

D) 100ml/hour

B – In the real world of most EDs, if they pee, we're happy. When kids are "shocky," we know that the blood goes to the core (heart/lungs/brain) and not to the "butt or the gut"! So if they are peeing (and perfusing their kidneys), we're happy. Unlike adults in the ICU, where 30ml/hr is the "magic number" for desired urine output, everything in children is "something per kg" and urine output is no different.

39) The greatest risk of sexual abuse to children comes from:

A) Total strangers

B) Family members

C) Teachers and school personnel

D) Religious leaders

B – Horrible, but true, statistics show that children are much more likely to be abused by family members or close relations, than by strangers or other acquaintances.

40) Early signs of shock in an infant include all of the following **except**:

A) Tachycardia

B) Hypotension

C) Deterioration in mental status

D) Tachypnea

B - Hypotension is a very late (and very scary) sign in pediatrics. It's the difference between compensated (early) and decompensated (late) shock. Children compensate until the very end and when their blood pressure drops, bad things are imminent. They've tried everything else to compensate first, it didn't work, and now profound badness is ensuing.

41) The ED nurse knows that many victims of child abuse exhibit which of the following behaviors:

A) Always wanting to know what will happen next

B) Still looking to adults for reassurance

C) Acting more "grown up" than other children of same age

D) All of the above

D – The abusers may physically hurt the children, but younger children perceive the abuse as attention, and bad attention is better than no attention in their eyes. In addition, these children are often told that the abuser is doing the act(s) because they love them so much. Younger abused children often still love the abusing family member and will look to them for comfort and reassurance. It doesn't make sense to us, but it does to them.

42) Which of the following factors increase a child's risk for abuse?

A) Physical disabilities

B) Developmental delay

C) Prematurity

D) All of the above

D – Anything that is "not normal" in children raises the potential for abuse. Many of these conditions result in children being fussy, difficult, or hyperactive; all of which are commonly associated with the occurrence of abuse because they stress out the caregivers.

43) The nurse should suspect child abuse if a 2-year-old child presents with:

A) Bruises on both knees

B) Bruises on the forehead

C) Bruises to the thighs

D) Bruises on both elbows

C – 2-year-olds who are in perpetual motion are seemingly always getting bruises. On their heads, arms, or legs; Absolutely. However, how does an active 2-year-old bruise both their posterior thighs? I don't know either. If anything in the history or physical doesn't fit, it's abuse until proven otherwise. Remember the "*Seven B's of Abuse*:" **B**umps, **B**ruises, **B**reaks, **B**urns, **B**ites, **B**athing suit (any injury in a "private area" that the bathing suit would cover), and anything that happens in the **B**athroom.

44) Which of the following is the **most** common cause of death from child abuse?

A) Chest and abdominal trauma

B) Burns

C) Head trauma

D) Asphyxiation

C - Head trauma. While rib/extremity fractures, especially old ones mixed with new ones, as well as burns in various stages of healing certainly can be found in abuse, head trauma is the most common cause of death in cases of child abuse. Unfortunately, many children have been seen in the ED several times for other issues/injuries, quite possibly from abuse, before they finally arrive for that final visit. A high index of suspicion is the key to saving these children from further and possibly fatal abuse. Remember the "*multiples rule*." **Multiple** bruises, **Multiple** burns, bumps, bruises, or breaks, **Multiple** visits, and **Multiple** different hospitals.

45) Which assessment findings are **most** suspicious of child abuse?

A) Forehead laceration in a 2-year-old

B) A sexually transmitted disease (STD) in a young child

C) Pregnancy in late adolescence

D) Anger by a teenage daughter toward her father

B – Anything involving STDs and young children is abuse. It's as simple as that.

Certified Pediatric Emergency Nurse (CPEN) Review IV

46) What should be the nurse's primary consideration when caring for a victim of child abuse?

A) The safety of the child while in the emergency department

B) The nurse's feelings regarding the alleged abuser

C) Shock as to how someone could do this to a child

D) Child's post-discharge needs and care

A – Though all of the above are certainly appropriate, ensuring and conveying the safety of the child while in the ED is crucial. Make sure that security is aware of possible issues involving unwanted removal of the child by caregivers. Treat alleged abusers with respect, as the concept of "innocent until proven guilty" applies even in the ED. But most importantly, care for the child and make sure your patient is safe while under your care.

47) Which nursing action is **most** appropriate in cases of suspected child abuse?

A) Assume that the physician caring for the child will suspect abuse and he/she will file a report with child protective services

B) Confront the parents directly and report findings to child protective services

C) Assume responsibility for reporting suspected abuse to child protective services

D) Assign responsibility for reporting suspected abuse to a social worker

C – Each state has mandatory abuse reporting laws. Never assume that other healthcare providers found/heard what you did. If you, as a nursing professional, feel that abuse is a possibility, you must make sure it is reported. Not only because it's the law, but because it's in the best interest of the child! If the parent, perpetrator, or victim says something directly to you, chart it verbatim and make it known to the professional investigator. Detailed charting, coupled with allowing professional investigators to "do the questioning" is vital to the future success of the court case. In the ED setting, it's appropriate for a formal report to be filed by one designated caregiver, usually the physician or social workers. Everyone who interviews/examines the child and their family doesn't have to personally report their suspicions to the authorities unless no one else is taking action. Everyone should do their part in documentation though.

48) A 15-year-old girl is complaining of stomach pain. The child's father says his daughter has had frequent vomiting and diarrhea for the past 72 hours. You find the child sitting in a chair with her hand over her stomach. She appears uncomfortable, but is aware of your presence. The child has listened intently to the conversation between you and her father. All of the following considerations should be followed concerning your interactions with a child of this age **except**:

A) Speak to the child in a respectful, friendly manner, as if speaking to an adult

B) When speaking with the caregiver, include the child

C) Tell the child's father that you suspect that his daughter has been sexually active

D) Obtain a history from the child without the caregiver in the room

C – Whether or not you suspect that the child has been sexually active, this is something that should be kept to yourself, especially with both the child and the father present. Teens, as a rule, appreciate when you treat them, and talk to them like adults. This concept should be applied to those in the ED as well. If they present with caregivers or friends, a history should be elicited with only the patient, the health professional, and an appropriate chaperonage in the room to protect both the patient and yourself.

Certified Pediatric Emergency Nurse (CPEN) Review IV

49) Your behavior has been bad and you've been banished to triage for your night shift in the ED. You walk in to find four patients waiting to be seen. Which of the following children should be seen **first**?

A) A child with hemophilia who fell in gym class and has a small hemarthrosis (bleeding into the joint) to his knee

B) A child with sickle cell disease (SCD) who reports joint pain 5/10 for eight hours

C) A child recovering from "a virus" who has unexplained bruising and intermittent epistaxis

D) A child who had chemotherapy 5-days ago who has a fever of 102°F (38.9°C)

D – In the ED there are several great guiding principles, such as "airway trumps everything" and "all women between 10 & 50 are pregnant until proven otherwise." Similarly, a hem-onc kid recently post-chemo is the first one to be seen because either they are already septic, possibly septic or thinking about becoming septic. The other patients with hemarthrosis, SCD pain, or unexplained bruising and intermittent epistaxis (most likely Idiopathic Thrombocytopenia Purpura or ITP) should certainly be seen as soon as possible; however, "hem-oncers" with a fever definitely trump the other three and should get pan-cultured, receive "boatloads" of IV antibiotics and be admitted to the appropriate unit (outside of the ED) ASAP to begin/continue the workup. Additional exposure to the bad bugs that play in the ED can be a death sentence for these patients.

50) A 12-year old male presents to triage with sudden, non-traumatic onset of severe (9/10) groin pain and active vomiting. As a testicular torsion certainly is a distinct possibility, on a 5-level triage scale, his triage category should be:

A) I

B) II

C) III

D) IV

B –This teen should be triaged as a level II (Emergent but Stable--to be seen ASAP/within 30 minutes). This for two reasons: 1) His pain is 9/10 and 2) Ask any teenage male if their testicles are vital organs and, of course, the answer is unquestionably, "YES!" In many cases, it takes a lot of pain over a long period of time before the patient will report it (and thus have his "parts" examined --so embarrassing!). Going beyond six hours from the first sudden onset of pain and the chance of saving the testicle begins to plummet. Remember, for myocardial infarctions, time = heart muscle and for strokes, time = brain tissue. With torsions, time = testicles (or ovaries, in the case of ovarian torsion--let's not be sexist)! For triage and "the test," it's crucial that you review "who's at what level" according to ENA and ENPC. Level I patients are just about dead or are dead but nobody's willing to admit it yet. Level V patients will do just fine in fast track. Level III patients are most of our patients who are a bit sick, but are most likely not going to die or lose a vital organ in the next 5 to 30 minutes. Of course, these are not the official ENA definitions, but should serve as a pretty good overview.

Two-level triage	Three-level triage	Four-level triage	Five-level triage
Emergent	Emergent	Critical	Resuscitation
Non-emergent	Urgent	Acute	Emergent
	Non-urgent	Urgent	Urgent
		Non-urgent	Semi-urgent
			Non-urgent

Overview of triage classifications
Adapted from Brecher, D. (2020). <u>Emergency Nursing Pediatric Course, 5th Edition</u>.
Emergency Nurses Association, Des Plaines, IL. 114

Certified Pediatric Emergency Nurse (CPEN) Review IV

51) The parent of a 2-year old toddler tells the nurse that she is frustrated with her child's behaviors. The child throws temper tantrum and says "no" every time she tries to help her. The nurse explains that toddlers are often negative and this expression is their normal desire to:

A) Increase their independence

B) Gratify oral fixation

C) Finish something they have started

D) Establish trust

A – The drive for independence is often expressed by the toddler opposing those bigger than them and in authority. From the perspective of the toddler, that is pretty much everyone! Establishing trust and oral gratification are developmental tasks of infants. The school-age child's developmental task is that of finishing projects. As many parents will tell you, this age is called "The Terrible Two's" for good reason.

52) The developmentally-appropriate strategy for the nurse to use when doing pre-procedure teaching with a 10-year old is to:

A) Keep explanations under one minute

B) Organize needed teaching points in order of what will happen and when it will happen

C) Use puppets to explain tests

D) Begin teaching hours before the procedure

B – The school-ager's developmental need is to know the order of information (what's going to happen, in what order, and when). Information should be shared close to when procedure will happen, as causing several hours or even minutes of anticipation is cruel to a child. Indeed, the anticipation of a procedure is often worse than any pain or discomfort caused by the procedure itself. Puppets and dolls are useful for preschoolers in the magical thinking period. A school-age child's attention span is hopefully at least a bit longer than one minute, so they should be able to process more complete explanations.

53) At what age would the nurse expect the child to be able to say "mama and dada"?

A) 4 months

B) 6 months

C) 10 months

D) 2 years

C – At 4 months, consonants like n, p, b, g, k are initially being verbalized. At 6 months, babbling (single syllables starting with consonants) should be expected. At 10 months, infants say short words with meaning. By 2 years, kids should speak in 2-3 word sentences, so "mama go" and "daddy sit here" would be considered appropriate. Amazingly, between the first and third birthdays, the number of words spoken increases from about less than 10 to over 300, and once they start talking, it seems that they never stop (unless they are really, really sick).

Certified Pediatric Emergency Nurse (CPEN) Review IV

54) The parents of a 5-month old complain to the nurse that their baby wakes up every 1-2 hours during the night. The mother indicates that when the baby wakes up, she (the mother) gets up and changes the diaper and nurses the baby. Which of the following is the **best** anticipatory guidance to tell the mother?

A) "Put the baby in bed with you."

B) "Try putting in the baby in her crib while she is still awake."

C) "Allow the baby to cry for 30 minutes and then rock the baby back to sleep before you put her back to bed."

D) "Give the baby formula instead of breast milk."

B - Parents need to develop bedtime rituals where the baby falls asleep somewhere other than in the parents' arms or in the presence of the parent. Discuss with parents how having the baby in bed with them can interfere with everybody's sleep and increases the risk for injuries to the baby. When putting babies to bed, crying episodes should be allowed in increasing five minute increments while regularly checking on the baby. This incremental increase allows the baby to learn to soothe themselves. Five-month old babies generally do not wake up every hour because they are hungry; it is generally to be soothed. When speaking of hunger, breast milk is almost always preferred over formula. Also, parents should never leave older babies in the crib with a bottle of milk or juice to suck on. Although you might think potential aspiration is a risk, the biggest problem is actually an increase in dental caries if the baby falls asleep with a bottle of milk or juice in their mouth.

55) Which of the following statements are **most** characteristic of a 2-year old child?

A) Toddlers walk alone, but fall down easily

B) Toddlers' activities are purposeful

C) Toddlers do not have a pincer grasp

D) Toddlers' language development includes no more than 15 words.

B – When you watch 2 year olds, you quickly notice that their movements are very purposeful. They can walk over to pick up (and often throw) a toy and can grasp every non-healthy/non-edible thing and place it in their mouth. Toddlers typically can walk very well, even up and down stairs, without falling. Pincer grasp should be developed during late infancy and, by age two; and the number of words children of that age can speak increases to over 300.

56) How does the onset of pubertal growth compare between girls and boys?

A) Pubertal growth is the same for both boys and girls

B) Pubertal growth occurs in boys two years earlier than girls

C) Pubertal growth occurs in girls two years earlier than boys

D) Pubertal growth occurs in girls two years later than boys

C – Statistically speaking, the average onset of puberty is 12 for girls and 14 for boys (though it sure seems like puberty is kicking in younger and younger these days).

57) While examining 13-year old David, you notice he has gynecomastia. You know that:

A) This is a sign of too much body fat and parents should be given dietary guidelines for teenagers

B) This is not necessarily abnormal at this age

C) This is a sign of hormonal imbalance and an immediate referral to an pediatric endocrinologist is in order

D) This is an indication of precocious puberty and should be watched for additional psychological sequela

B – Gynecomastia or enlargement of the breast tissue in males is common in about 1/3 of boys during onset of puberty. For most boys, this will disappear within two years. Should gynecomastia remain past two years post-puberty, it can be indicative of a hormonal imbalance and the patient and family should be referred to their pediatrician or an endocrinologist for follow-up. Precocious puberty (premature puberty) is the onset of puberty before age nine and is unrelated to gynecomastia.

58) A one-month old male presents to the emergency department with his mother. She explains that her son has been fussy and has not stopped crying for 4 days. She reports that today, just prior to coming to the ED, the child rolled over and off the bed and hit the floor. The nurse finds a boggy spot at the back of the baby's head. How should the nurse proceed?

A) Comfort the mother and remind her that "accidents happen"

B) Ask about the child's feeding habits and provide the mother with appropriate information concerning lactation and breast feeding since the child's fussiness and non-stop crying indicate that he is not feeding well

C) Provide safety for the child and consider the possibility that this case might involve child abuse

D) Immediately remove the child from the mother's arms, call security and child welfare and alert pastoral care for counseling

C – This question tests two important concepts: Child abuse and child development. One month olds are not able to roll over. Remember these general rules: Head (2 months), shoulders (4 months), knees (6 months) and toes (12 months). Shoulder (rolling) doesn't usually kick in until at least 4 months of age. The comment by the mother about the baby rolling off the bed should be a huge red flag. In addition, the mother says that the child has not stopped crying for 4 days. Non-stop screaming for 4 days + understandable parental stress + history that doesn't fit = high potential for child abuse. Last, but not least, if "safety" is part of the answer, that should be a big clue.

59) The pediatric assessment triangle (PAT) identifies patients who should have immediate intervention or treatment. Which triad below lists the components of the PAT?

A) Blood pressure, respiratory rate, temperature

B) General impression, work of breathing, circulation to skin

C) Pulse, temperature, respiratory rate

D) Pulse oximetry, blood pressure, temperature

B – The PAT is essentially a quick glance at the child using an auditory and visual assessment-- "look and listen, but don't touch." It is an "across the room" assessment of the child, with the ABCs being Appearance, Breathing, & Circulation.

Certified Pediatric Emergency Nurse (CPEN) Review IV

60) Paramedics arrive with a 1-month old infant with a suspected skull fracture. When the child's mother was asked about the circumstances of this injury, she stated the infant "sat up and rolled off the bed." This statement by the mother suggests the following course of action:

A) Provide the mother with the latest crib safety literature

B) Proceed with treatment and follow facility guidelines for suspected child abuse

C) Explain to the mother that the injury is most likely a result of Munchausen Syndrome by Proxy

D) Place the child in the protective custody of the emergency department using "Safe Haven/Safe Surrender" rules

B – The injury doesn't match the story, so while you treat the child, you should also follow procedures to report suspected child abuse. Even if all you can remember about growth and development is: "Head and shoulders, knees and toes," you know should be able to remember that at 2 months a child should start to lift up his/her head, followed by lifting shoulders and later with initiating movement with knees and toes. But rolling over and "rolling off the bed" is not something a 1-month old is capable of doing. Therefore, the mother's story cannot be how the child received this injury. This patient is a victim of abuse or another mechanism of unintentional injury that the mother isn't willing to admit. Providing crib safety literature would be appropriate if this had been a crib related injury, but it clearly wasn't. Munchausen Syndrome by Proxy may be a consideration in unusual reports of illness, but not typically in cases of injuries. Safe Haven, Safe Surrender and other safe drop-off programs are not considerations in the case where a parent brings in a child for treatment.

61) A 12-year old child presents to the ED with her mother who states that the child has been more agitated and irritable recently. The child has a history of cerebral palsy. What would be the **best** way to obtain pertinent information and a history?

A) Ignore the child and get the information from her mother to expedite care

B) Talk directly to the child and include her in the conversation as much as possible

C) Use puppets or dolls to facilitate communication with the child

D) Use sign language and slow, clear verbalizations with the child

B – Just because a child has cerebral palsy does not necessarily mean they have mental retardation. Talking directly to the child indicates that you are interested in them and view them as a person, and not just a sum of their disabilities. Ignoring this child might increase her agitation. Using puppets or dolls might be useful if she was 4-years old, but she's 12. There is no indication that she is deaf or hard of hearing, so sign language or exaggerated speech patterns would be inappropriate.

62) When palpating an infant's anterior fontanel to determine the presence of depression or bulging, the emergency nurse should place the infant:

A) In the mother's arms with his head upright

B) Prone on the examination table with his head to one side

C) Supine in the examiner's arms with his head turned to the right side

D) Lying across the mother's lap with his head dependent

A – It's all about the law of gravity. If the infant is in any position other than head upright, and especially if the head is dependent, the fontanel is more likely to bulge, potentially giving a false positive result. (The same is true if the infant is crying.) Sitting on mom's lap will not only lend itself to a much more accurate assessment, but it provides a source of comfort for the infant as well.

Certified Pediatric Emergency Nurse (CPEN) Review IV

Emergency Assessment

63) The AVPU score is used to quickly assess a patient's level of consciousness. AVPU stands for:

A) Alert, Violent, Pain, Unrecognizable

B) Artery, Vein, Pulse, Unilateral

C) Anxious, Verbal, Pressure, Unresponsive

D) Alert, Verbal, Pain, Unresponsive

D – The AVPU scale is a quick, down-and-dirty method of assessing level of consciousness. Is the child Alert? Does he respond to Verbal stimuli? Does he respond to Painful stimuli? Is he Unresponsive? Choose the most appropriate response.

64) It's very important to be able to perform a rapid assessment of your pediatric patient to determine how their illness or injury has affected their physiologic status. One of the tools commonly used to make this "snapshot" or "across the room" rapid assessment is the Pediatric Assessment Triangle (PAT). The three components of the PAT are:

A) Vital signs, color and general appearance

B) General appearance, work of breathing and circulation to skin

C) Respiratory rate, skin color and general appearance

D) Work of breathing, capillary refill and vital signs

B – The Pediatric Assessment Triangle uses three physiologic parameters that reflect how severely injured or ill the child is: 1) the child's general appearance, 2) work of breathing and
3) circulation to skin. The parameters can be assessed in any order. Work of breathing and circulation to the skin provide information as to which vital system(s) is/are most impacted, while the general appearance tells you how well the child's body is compensating for the insult. The PAT helps you answer the questions: "How sick?" (compensated or not compensated) and "How quick?" (urgency for intervention). Children with an acutely altered general appearance are assumed to be physiologically sick (decompensated) and require immediate intervention. With experience and practice, a triage nurse can use this technique to look into a room of children and very quickly sort out who needs to be triaged first.

Lundblom's Lessons

A 5-day old, born to a G1P1 mom was triaged with the chief complaint of "crying and diaper rash." At triage, the infant was noted to be afebrile with a respiratory rate of 60/min. The lungs were clear, O2 sat was 100% on room air, and HR and B/P were normal. Abnormal (persistent "I'm in pain") crying was noted during triage. The patient was carried by mom back to the treatment area and the physicians were informed of the initial assessment. Within about 15 minutes, I saw that the patient's chart was already in the "Discharge" slot with discharge instructions for diaper rash. I went to the Peds ED Fellow and explained my concerns (nursing gut feeling that this newborn was in pain and something was not right) and he agreed to go and evaluate the patient (smart physicians trust the experienced nurses!) I went back again 30 minutes later and again the chart was in the discharge slot; the ED Fellow stated that his exam and the CXR on this pt were "normal." I repeated a complete set of vital signs and they were still normal for the patient's age. I proceeded to provide extensive discharge teaching/education with this patient's father who stated "Mom had to go; she is in the car now. I'll tell her all this."

This infant presented back to our triage 48 hours later. This time the patient had a temp of 102.2°F (39.0°C) and a grossly distended abdomen. After a full sepsis work-up, fluids, and antibiotics in the ED, she was admitted to the PICU and then quickly taken to the OR for concerns of GI perforation. Operative findings were reported as "duplication of the sigmoid colon" or a sac in the colon which had ruptured, resulting in peritonitis and sepsis. This patient had a very, very stormy course, but did eventually recover and was discharged home from the children's hospital after 3 ½ months.

Certified Pediatric Emergency Nurse (CPEN) Review IV

Many years later, while I triaged another child, I looked the mom and said, "You look so familiar; do you have any other children?" When she said yes, and said that child's name, my knees buckled. The name of that child from 11 years earlier was still imbedded in my memory. Reminders of all the months spent calling the PICU each shift I worked, monitoring this baby's recovery and the tremendous guilt I felt in not more aggressively pursuing my nursing gut feeling came rushing back. I wondered if abdominal X-rays would have been helpful and if we might have noticed more if we had just kept this infant longer to observe feeding and activity. I wondered what might have been different if we had discharged her with instructions for a 24 hour follow up. I had a lengthy discussion with this mom about the discharge teaching I had done with the father and she said that she never was shown anything. In addition, apparently all he said to her was "I told you she was fine." Yes, Mom never got the printed or verbal instructions. More verbal discussion between mom and the physicians may have helped in that situation, but those types of delayed, but then rapidly deteriorating conditions (like the intestinal perforation) are notoriously hard to anticipate. Try as we might to be absolutely, perfectly thorough, sometimes the symptoms and signs are just not clear. Combined with situations where we are so packed with patients and have so many kids in the lobby waiting to get to an ED bed, it is possible that a tiny one like this falls through the cracks, especially when we are trying hard to move the patients though. All that being said, those "zebra" patients are important because they leave a lasting memory and effect on your nursing practice. This one reminds me to ask a lot more questions and try harder to do much more teaching during the ED stay; teaching and then re-teaching many times. Sometimes, making sure our parents/caregivers really "get it" is a real challenge. Standardized pre-determined discharge instructions are sometimes too general and just not adequate. If there are any teaching points that are especially important, we need to stress them ourselves, verbally and in additional, very specific writing, rather than relying on generalized instructions. Stressing the key points of what requires another look and what we consider worsening symptoms is never as easy as it seems. This is especially true for the many typical and not so typical illnesses pediatric patients present with.

The moral of this tale is to encourage ED nurses to go with your gut feelings, because many times, your gut is 100% correct! It's also safe to say that your good and bad experiences caring for little ones continue to affect your practice as you grow in your career. Try to consider them as opportunities to learn and evolve as an excellent nurse. For your own good and that of your future patients, try to turn any regrets for things you did or might have done into the energy and inspiration you need to do better every day.

Certified Pediatric Emergency Nurse (CPEN) Review IV

Appendix 1-A

Normal Pediatric Vital Signs

Adapted from Crash Cards - www.CrashCards.com

Age	Heart Rate/min	Respiratory Rate/min	Systolic Blood Pressure (mm Hg)
Full term newborn	80-160	30-50	60-90
6 months	80-150	30-50	87-105
7 months to 1 ½ years	80-150	30-50	87-105
2 to 3 ½ years	100-110	20-35	90 + (2 x years)
3 ½ to 5 years	70-110	20-35	90 + (2 x years)
5 ½ years to 7 years	70-100	15-25	90 + (2 x years)
7 ½ years to 9 ½ years	60-100	15-25	90 + (2 x years)
10 to 12 years	55-90	12-20	90 + (2 x years)

Appendix 1-B

Five-Level Triage

Title	Vital Signs and Resource Utilization	Examples
Resuscitation (I)	Unstable vitals and maximum use of resources "Definite threat to life"	Respiratory or cardiac arrest Major trauma Completely unconscious
Emergent (II)	Threatened vitals and high use of resources "Potential threat to life or limb"	"Not normal" level of consciousness Moderate-severe respiratory distress Fever in an infant under one month of age
Urgent (III)	Stable vitals and medium use of resources "Not likely to lose life or limb"	Belly pain Moderate pain Dehydration
Semi-urgent (IV)	Stable vitals and low use of resources "Really not likely to lose life or limb"	Bumps, bruises, and breaks Little kids with fevers
Non-urgent (V)	Stable vitals and no use of resources "They are not going to lose life or limb"	Fast track

Adapted from Brecher, D. (2020). Emergency Nursing Pediatric Course, 5th Edition.
Emergency Nurses Association, Des Plaines, IL. 114

APPENDIX 1-C
Triage Practice – What Level are These Patients?

Chief Complaint	Resuscitation (I)	Emergent (II)	Urgent (III)	Semi-Urgent (IV)	Non-Urgent (V)
Conjunctivitis					
Respiratory arrest					
Unresponsiveness					
Moderate respiratory distress					
Active seizure					
Dehydration					
Ear discomfort					
Unstable vital signs					
Simple laceration					
Altered mental status					
Cold or flu					
Intubated patient					
Fever in an infant <1 month of age					

I highly recommend *that those taking the CPEN exam review ENA's* <u>*Emergency Nursing Pediatric Course*</u>
*(ENPC) textbook, especially the section on triage, prior to taking the examination. (**<u>www.ena.org</u>**)*

APPENDIX 1-D

TICLS

TICLS	Questions to be answered
Tone	Is the child actively moving with good muscle tone, or is the child limp?
Interactivity	Is the child alert and attentive to what's going on, or is too sick to care? Will the child reach for a cool toy? Does the child respond to people, objects, and sounds?
Consolability	Does comforting the child help them chill out and stop crying?
Look/Gaze	Do the child's eyes follow your every move, or is the kid staring out into space?
Speech/Cry	Do they have a strong cry, or is it weak, muffled, or hoarse?

Adapted from Dieckmann, R. Editor. (2006). Pediatric Education for Prehospital Professionals, 2nd Edition. Jones and Bartlett: Sudbury, MA. 8

Appendix 1-E

CIAMPEDS

C	(C)hief complaint
I	(I)mmunizations and isolation
A	(A)llergies
M	(M)edications
P	(P)ast medical history and (P)arent's or caregiver's impression of the child
E	(E)vents surrounding the illness or injury
D	(D)iet and (D)iapers
S	(S)ymptoms associated with the illness or injury

Adapted from Hawkins, H. (Editor). 2004. Emergency Nursing Pediatric Course, 3rd Edition. Emergency Nurses Association: Des Plaines, IL. 51-52 - www.ena.org

Appendix 1-F

Common Indications of Non-Accidental Trauma (Child Abuse)

Family Behaviors	Child Behaviors	Historical Findings	Physical Findings	Radiographic Findings
Inappropriate parent-child interactions	Extreme behaviors, i.e. withdrawn or acting out	Story inconsistent with physical findings (doesn't fit)	Multiple injuries in various stages of healing	Multiple fractures
Hostile or unconcerned interactions with hospital staff	Doesn't oppose painful procedures	Story inconsistent with developmental stage (kids can't do that)	Injury and location of injury don't fit developmental stage	Fractures in different stages of healing
Unrealistic expectations of the child	Inappropriate sexual behavior	Delay in seeking medical care	Characteristic patterns (belt or bite marks)	Skull fractures
Parents deny any knowledge as to how injury occurred	Somatic complaints (i.e. chronic headaches, sleep disorders, bedwetting)	Child verbalizes abuse	Signs of poor overall care	Intracranial hemorrhage
Siblings blamed for injury	Suicidal threats or attempts	Multiple visits to the ED	Genital bleeding or discharge in pre-teen age children	
Parents over or under reacting to child's condition	Alcohol or drug abuse			

Adapted from Salassi-Scotter, M., Jardine, J., and Lawson, L. (1994). Child maltreatment. In Henderson, D. and Brownstein, D. Editors. Pediatric Emergency Manual. Springer: New York. 293-322.

Certified Pediatric Emergency Nurse (CPEN) Review IV

Appendix 1-G

Summary of Pediatric Developmental Milestones

Adapted from

Pediatric Nursing Certification

Review Course: Unlocking the Door to Success

Copyright 2011

Louise Jakubic PhD, CRNP, RN-BC

President and Chief Educational Officer - Nurse Builders

www.NurseBuilders.net

3 Months

Physical/Motor

—Starts coordinating movement of hands and eyes (notices own hands)

—Raises head and chest when lying on stomach

—Stretches legs out and kicks

—Posterior fontanel closes by 2 months

Language/Cognition

—Notices own hands

—Begins to babble

—Turns head toward sound

Social

—Beginnings of instinctual smile at six to eight weeks

—Social smile appears around three months

—More expressive with face

Vision

—Vision is poor at birth; black and white colors are seen best

—Watches faces

—By 3 months, follows objects with eyes 180 degrees

4-6 Months

Physical/Motor

—Reaches for objects

—Transfers objects from hand to hand

—Uses hands to rake objects

—Rolls both directions (front to back first, then back to front)

—When prone, the infant pushes up on knees and hands rocking back and forth and may begin to crawl

—Sits with support and may develop the ability to sit up without support

—Teething begins

Language/Cognition

—Finds partially hidden objects

—Explores hands and mouth

—Responds to own name

—Continuous babbling; babbles in response to sounds

Social

—Enjoys social play (smiles, laughs)

—Responsive to expressions of others

—Stranger anxiety appears

—Comforting habits begin such as thumb sucking or holding a favorite blanket

Vision

—Develops full color vision

—Distance vision improves

—Increased ability to track objects

Weight

—Birth weight doubles at 5 months technically; we teach that it doubles at 6 months because that it when the assessment of weight occurs (at the 6 month primary care visit)

Sleep

—Sleeps through the night with one or two naps per day

7-9 Months

Physical/Motor

—Pincer grasp develops

—Everything is placed in the mouth

—Feeds self bottle or cheerios/cracker

—Sits alone without assistance

—Crawls

—Stands up while holding onto an object for support (table, parent's hand)

Language/Cognition

—Develops object permanence and searches for objects out of view

—Understands "No" at 9 months

—The infant develops object permanence (a principle from Piaget's theory) where the infant searches for objects outside the visual field, knowing that even though the object cannot be seen it is still present. Therefore, if an object is hidden while the infant watches, the infant will look for it as the infant understands that the object is not gone just because it is out of site.

Social

—Imitates expressions of others

—Claps hands

—Enjoys games and play

—Weaning to a cup for fluid intake can begin

10-12 Months (1 Year)

Physical/Motor

—Puts objects into and takes objects out of a container

—Claps hands, waves bye-bye and enjoys rhythm games

—Gets into sitting position unassisted

—Crawls

—Pulls self up to stand

—Cruises (side steps while holding onto furniture) at 10 months

—Walks with support at 11 months

—Takes first steps (walks) beginning at 12 months with variability up until 15-16 months

Language/Cognition

—Finds hidden objects easily

—Looks at correct image when named

—Explores objects in a variety of ways (shaking, hitting, throwing)

—Responds to simple verbal requests

—Uses simple gestures (i.e. shakes head for "no" – shakes head when does not like/want food)

—Says about 5 words, but understands many more words

—Says "da-da" and "ma-ma"

—Tries to imitate words

Social

—Shy/anxious with strangers

—Cries when caregiver leaves

—Prefers certain people and toys (prefers mother over other caregivers)

—Tests parental responses to behavior (i.e. throws bottle or toy when in high chair)

—Repeats sounds and gestures

12-18 Months

Physical/Motor

—Anterior fontanel closes by 18 months

—Walks unassisted

—Climbs steps

—Stacks blocks

Language/Cognition

—Obeys simple commands

—Asserts independence

—Says "No"

—By 12 months, the toddler uses 5 words.

—By 18 months, the toddler use up to 50 words

—Points to objects when asked

Social

—Stranger anxiety decreases

—Extremely curious of environment

—Point to familiar objects when asked

—Demonstrates frustration

18-24 Months

Physical/Motor

—Feeds self with spoon/fork and cup without difficulty

—Turns pages in a book

—Climb stairs by 21 months

—Runs and jumps by 24 months

—Enjoys push and pull toys

—Beginning readiness for toilet training (shows interest)

Language/Cognition

—Puts 2 to 3 words together in a sentence

—Repeats words said by others

—Says own name

—Has understanding of routine and time

Social

—Exhibits temper tantrums

—Defiant behavior begins

—Has difficulty sharing

—Says "mine"

—Exhibits parallel play with other children

24-36 Months

Physical/Motor

—Walks up and down stairs

—Dresses self with assistance

—May begin to use cup without lid

—Rides a tricycle by 3 years

Language/Cognition

—Develops a full vocabulary

—Words are increasingly recognizable to adults other than parents/caregivers

—Speaks three to five word sentences

—By age 2, the toddler uses two-to-three-word sentences and comprehends many more words.

—At age 3, the toddler is a chatterbox, using about 11,000 words a day and three to four word sentences

—Knows first and last name

—Aware of gender and age

—Symbolic thought appears; exhibits pretend play

—Begins magical thinking where wishing, or thinking something will happen, make it happen

Social

—Transitions from parallel play to interactive play

—Imitates behavior of others

—May complete toilet training

—Does not like to share toys but is able to take turns

—Frustration decreases

—Decreased level of asserting independence in favor of more social conformity

3 Years

Physical/Motor

—Dresses and undresses self

—Walks backward up and down stairs

—Uses toilet

—Washes hands

—Draws

—Uses scissors

—Builds a tower of more than six blocks

Language/Cognition

—Develops a sense of body image

—Beginning understanding of causality, but still uses magical thinking

—Develops sexual curiosity

—Understands "mine" and "his/hers"

—Uses three to four-word sentences, but has trouble with pronouns

Social

—Exhibits fears of things such as the dark, etc.

—Has a full use of cooperative play; takes turns; plays in a group

—Develops self identity and family identity

—Plays make-believe with dolls, animals, and toys

4 Years

Physical/Motor

—Hops and stands on one foot for up to 5 seconds

—Throws overhand and catches ball

—Is increasingly agile in body movements

—Begins to copy letters

—Copies shapes

—Draws a person with 2 to 4 body parts

Language/Cognition

—Speaks in 4-5 word sentences

—Counts

—Names colors

Social

—Cooperates with others

—Increase in pretend play with dolls or other toys

—Negotiates solutions to problems

5 years

Physical/Motor

—Dresses and undresses self well; cannot tie shoes

—Runs, jumps, skips

—Hops, somersaults

Language/Cognition

—Speaks sentences of more than 5 words

—The 5 year-old uses sentences of more than five words and tells long stories.

—Preschoolers are concrete thinkers. Communication and explanations should provide concrete ideas and examples; preschoolers are often scared by health care lingo.

—Tells long stories

—Can distinguish fantasy from reality

Social

—Wants to please people, particularly friends

—Likes to play with and be like friends

—Enjoys singing and dancing

6 to 12 Years

Physical/Motor

—Permanent teeth begin at 6 years and are completed by age 12 years

—Vision is matured by age 6 years

Language/Cognition

—Language Development is completed

—The following develop:

—Concept of time and space

—Understanding of cause and effect

—Reversibility

—Conservation (permanence of mass and volume)

—Learns to read and spell

—Learns to do math and understand ratios

—Begins to enjoy games with strategy (cards, board games) and make-believe (video games, toys)

—Child understands rules (cheating in games is common).

—Engages in team play

Social

—School is the focal point of the child's activities shaping his/her cognitive and social development

--Teacher becomes a major non-parental influence

—Develops first true friend

—Morality develops (6-9 years: right or wrong; 10-12 years: sense of "shades of gray")

—Becomes aware of social roles

—Fantasy play and daydreaming emerge

13 to 18 Years

Physical/Motor

—Rapid increase in height and weight

—First pubescence changes are development of testicles in boys and breast in girls

Language/Cognition

-Changing body requires adaptation of self-image/concept

—Egocentric

—Can think hypothetically

—Uses past experiences when making decisions

Social

—Intense interest in peer group and perception of others

—Peer contact and involvement becomes increasingly important

—Sexuality emerges and dating begins

Appendix 1-H

If you remember nothing else about growth and development...

Remember these milestones

"Head and shoulders, knees, and toes..."
(Feel free to sing along)

2 months: (Head) Holds head up

4 months: (Shoulders) Rolls over

6 months: (Knees) sits unsupported

1 year: (Toes) walking

Or

3-6-9-12

3 months – Should be able to lift head

6 months – Should be able to sit up alone

9 months – Should be crawling and everything they find goes in their mouths

12-18 months – Should start walking and says/understands "No!"

Thanks to Kathleen Piotrowski-Walters BSN, RN, CCRN and Lynn Mohr PhD, APRN, PCNS-BC, CPN, FCNS for their help with these short and sweet summaries

Certified Pediatric Emergency Nurse (CPEN) Review IV

Appendix 1-I

"Baby Talk"
Communicating Effectively With Your Pediatric Patients (and other kids)

Lou E. Romig MD, FAAP, FACEP

Developmental Stages

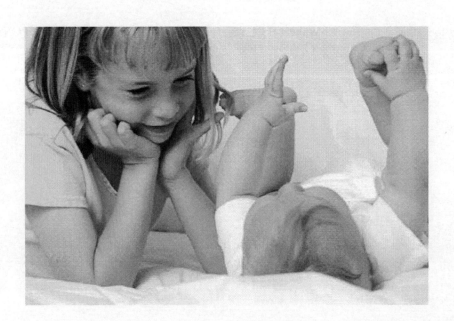

Birth to 6 months

- Infant is learning to regard the environment, especially faces.
- No stranger anxiety until late in this phase.
- Nonverbal communication is key
  - Facial expressions
  - Tone of voice
- Parents warm to medical personnel who treat their children as babies, not patients. Make faces and talk baby talk!

6 – 18 months

- Stranger anxiety! Try to keep the child with a caregiver.
- Communication is still mostly nonverbal, but talk to the child anyway.
- Development in motor skills is often faster than communication skills.
- Use stimulating objects to catch attention for distraction or assessment.
- Use toe to head approach.

18 months – 3 years

- More explorative, but still seek shelter with parents.
- Will understand more words than they can say.
- Constantly moving.
- Play and curiosity are big motivators.
- Use your tools and toys.
- Toe to head approach.
- Try not to hold them down, but don't wait forever for cooperation with exam.
- Toilet training often includes lessons about modesty and improper touching. Respect these lessons; uncover child selectively for exam.

3 to 6 years

- Usually a great age to work with.
- Learning to explore and be independent. Very curious!
- Can be very talkative and verbally enthusiastic.
- Are starting to understand about being hurt or sick and that people will try to help them.
- Are starting to understand the concept of "the future".
- May misinterpret words they hear.
- Have "magical thinking."
- Worry about being in trouble.
- Like to have choices.

3 to 6 years

- "This flashlight's DEAD."
- "I'm going to TAKE your pulse."
- "Don't CUT OFF the circulation with that strap."
- "We're going to have to TIE YOU DOWN on this board."
- "I didn't put my seatbelt on, so we got in a crash."
- "Put a bandaid on it!" (and the boo-boo goes away…)
- "I was bad in school so now I have to get a shot."

"Would you like your IV in this arm or that arm?"
NOT
"Where would you like your IV?"

6 – 12 years

- Fear failure & inferiority. Want to be treated as "big kids," but may feel "baby" insecurities.
- Want to be accepted and blend in.
- Body-conscious and modest.
- May feel pain intensely.
- Feel comfort with touching.
- Question the child directly and in simple, but not babyish terms.
- Use common interests to build trust.
  - Sports
  - TV and movie characters
- Treat them with respect.
- Offer limited choices.
- Don't embarrass them in front of peers.
- Don't tell them not to cry!
- OK to touch in comfort.
- Respect their modesty.

12 years and up

- Identity and peer relationships are the key issues at this age.
- Body image and future deformities and dysfunctions are very important.
- Reactions can be under- or over-exaggerated.
- Regressive behavior is common.
- Respect modesty and privacy.
- Avoid embarrassing the child.
- Direct yourself to the child as you might to an adult, with an adjustment in language.
- Make eye contact, but don't force it unless you need to make a point.
- Touch cautiously until you're sure touch is welcome.
- Don't lie & don't be condescending.

- Don't try to "be one of the group" unless you are. These guys can spot fakes a mile away.

- If drugs, pregnancy or other sensitive issues are involved, assure the child that your job is not to judge or enforce the law (unless it is.)

- Whenever possible, allow close friends to maintain support roles as socially-acceptable parent surrogates.

Cautions

- Don't ever intentionally lie to a child patient. If you're caught, it blows the credibility of all medical personnel.

- Always tell a child if something is going to hurt!

- Explain procedures in simple terms, but not until it's time to do it. Anticipation is often worse than the procedure.

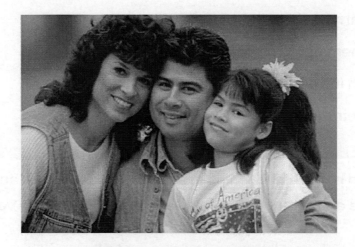

What parents like
The hardest part of taking care of kids is usually dealing with their parents and guardians.

What parents like and want

- Treat children as people.

    — Learn and use their preferred name.

    — At least get the sex right!

- Keep children as physically and emotionally comfortable as possible.

- Basic and advanced pain management is important.
- Try to relieve fear and anxiety as early and as much as possible.

• Treat every child as if they were the most special, beautiful, smartest child in the world. A compliment to a child is a compliment to their parents.
- Listen to what the child has to say, even if it sounds like nonsense.
- Every child has something you should honestly be able to compliment them on, even if it's just that they have such good lungs for them to be able to scream so loudly…

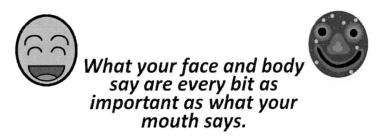

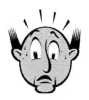

Nonverbal communication

• Get to the child's eye level.

• Try not to make the child look at you at an awkward angle.

• Make eye contact, but don't hold it in a challenging manner.

• Use your eyebrows to exaggerate your expressions, especially for babies through elementary-age kids.

• Use a soft voice with a moderate pace and interrupt only when necessary.

• Use noises like "um-hmm" and "I see" to encourage children to talk.

• For preverbal children, use a happy voice and bring the tone up at the ends of sentences (inviting a response from the patient.)

- Infants less than about 6 months can be touched anywhere first, but go to the most painful place last.

- For children with stranger anxiety, offer your hand or a tool for them to touch and explore first. Go for their heads and trunks and any painful parts last.

- Touch school-agers in a playful fashion. "High five" is often a good way to start.

- Tickling is good in young school-agers but don't do it until you've gotten your assessment done.

- Once a school-ager trusts your touch, try to maintain some contact while getting info from the parent.

- Touch teens only as needed for your exam, unless further touch is clearly welcome.

- Try to always have a witness when with a teen, especially a teen of the opposite sex, just in case one of your gestures is misinterpreted.

- Watch your facial expressions with teens! If you look like you don't believe them, you lose them.

Tools, Toys and Tricks

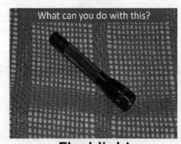

Flashlight

- Test range of motion of joints, mobility, and grip strength.

- Check pulmonary function ("blow out the candle!")

- Look in mom's throat or show the child your own.

- Look for Mickey Mouse, SpongeBob, etc. under clothes.

- Make an "ET finger."

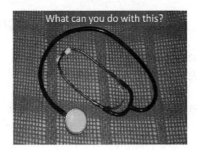

Stethoscope

- Check range of motion, etc…
- Let the child listen to somebody's heart and stomach.
- Make a "phone call" to the child.

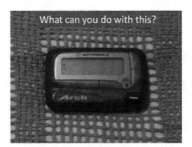

Pager/Cell Phone

- Check range of motion, etc…
- Get a page or call from Mickey, SpongeBob, etc.
- Play with the tones and/or vibration feature.
- Try to keep it from being thrown across the room…

Stuffed Animals

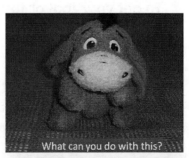
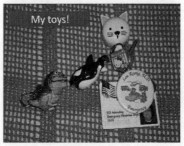

- Check range of motion, etc…
- Check cognition
    - Who/what is this?
    - What color is this?
    - What sound does he make?
- Check gait
    - Will you pick that up for me please?

Dr. Lou's Bag of Tricks

- Any toy or interesting tool can be used to check the motor exam and mental status of a child.

- If you don't have a toy and want to check neck flexion (nontraumatic,) ask the child to show you his/her belly button. They almost always look down as they pull up their shirt.

- If they don't look down, ask dubiously if they're sure that's their belly button.

- Demo what you want to do on mom or dad.

- If you want a young school-ager to do something, bet them that they can't do it as well as you can.

- To improve deep breathing for auscultation, ask the child to act like she's blowing up a balloon or blowing out a candle, but quietly.

- To check pulmonary function on a school-age or older child, have them see how far they can slowly count out loud on a single breath. Normally, they should get at least into the teens. Repeat to assess effectiveness of treatment.

- Tell a preschool child that you're going to give their arm a hug when you take their blood pressure.

- Have a child tilt their head back if checking their throat. You get a better view.

- To help palpate a ticklish abdomen, put the child's hand under yours and palpate with their hand.

- To get your tool or toy back, distract the child with something else while you or the parent retrieves it. Get it out of sight immediately!

Dr. Lou's Sure-Fire Laugh Lines

When a child's done a good job at deep breathing for you...
"Wow, you're a really good breather!
I'll bet you do it all the time, don't you?"

"Does your ... hurt?"
Mention normal painful body parts and then start throwing in others...
Hair, eyelashes, fingernails, toenails, freckles?

To a school-aged child:
"My goodness, you're so cute! How many girl(boy) friends do you have?"
OR
"Are you married? Have any kids?"

If no girlfriend, whisper loudly,
"You're supposed to say your mother's your girlfriend!"
OR
If horrified by the thought of a girlfriend,
"That's OK. Girls are yucky anyway."

Summary

- Getting along well with your pediatric patients often enhances your communication with their parents.

- Developmental stages influence your communication approach, but you should always talk to your pediatric patients, regardless of age.

- Tell the parents what they want to hear about their child. Then tell them about the medical stuff.

- Smiles are powerful communication tools.

- Sometimes it's not what you say, but how you say it; With your body as well as your words!

- Never lie.

- Shamelessly use any tools and tricks you have to enhance communications and build trust. This can only make your job easier.

- Make 'em laugh!

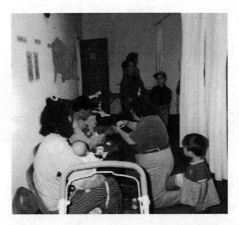

Thanks!
Lou Romig MD

This Baby Talk presentation and others are available for download at:
www.jumpstarttriage.com

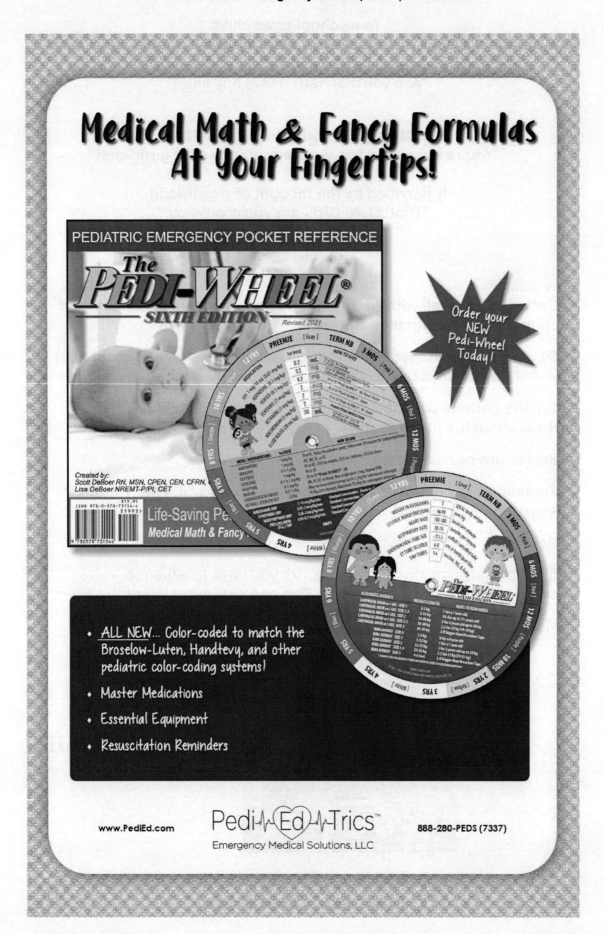

Chapter 2

Emergency Care of Crashing Kids

*Each generation has been an education for us in different ways.
The first child with a bloody nose was rushed to the emergency room.
The fifth child with a bloody nose was told to go to the yard immediately
and stop bleeding on the carpet.*
-Art Linkletter

Pertinent Pediatric Ponderings (NOTES)

CHAPTER 2
Sample Test Answer Sheet

[Remove page and cover rationale until after you answer question]

1. _____	21. _____	41. _____	61. _____
2. _____	22. _____	42. _____	62. _____
3. _____	23. _____	43. _____	63. _____
4. _____	24. _____	44. _____	64. _____
5. _____	25. _____	45. _____	65. _____
6. _____	26. _____	46. _____	66. _____
7. _____	27. _____	47. _____	67. _____
8. _____	28. _____	48. _____	68. _____
9. _____	29. _____	49. _____	69. _____
10. _____	30. _____	50. _____	70. _____
11. _____	31. _____	51. _____	71. _____
12. _____	32. _____	52. _____	72. _____
13. _____	33. _____	53. _____	73. _____
14. _____	34. _____	54. _____	
15. _____	35. _____	55. _____	
16. _____	36. _____	56. _____	
17. _____	37. _____	57. _____	
18. _____	38. _____	58. _____	
19. _____	39. _____	59. _____	
20. _____	40. _____	60. _____	

Pertinent Pediatric Ponderings (NOTES)

Certified Pediatric Emergency Nurse (CPEN) Review IV

1) Which of the following should be used to determine the correct uncuffed endotracheal tube (ETT) size in a child?

A) Age in years/2 + 12

B) 70 + (2 x age in years)

C) 90 + (2 x age in years)

D) Length-based resuscitation tape (Broselow Tape)

D – The classic formula of (age in years/4) + 4 has been taught for many years and works very well, unless the child is very sick and consequently you are really stressed. If this is the situation and your brain doesn't work right, doing formulas like this can lead to nutty tube sizes. Remember, if it looks like way too big of an endotracheal tube, chances are, it is way too big of an endotracheal tube. Other much more reliable "non-formula" methods to figure out pediatric ETT sizes include the Broselow-Luten tape/color coding system (www.ebroselow.com), "cheat sheets," and the little finger rule. The little finger rule says that if you find the endotracheal tube that is the size of the child's, not your, little finger, more or less, that is the size that is going to fit. It's not perfect, but in a crisis, it will get you close.

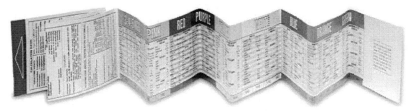

Broselow-Luten Pediatric Emergency Tape

Photo courtesy of Armstrong Medical

www.armstrongmedical.com

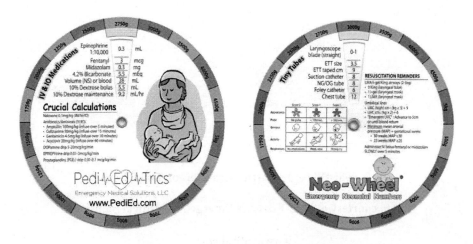

Neo Wheel: Emergency Neonatal Numbers

Photo courtesy of Pedi-Ed-Trics Emergency Medical Solutions

www.PediEd.com

Certified Pediatric Emergency Nurse (CPEN) Review IV

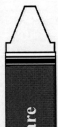

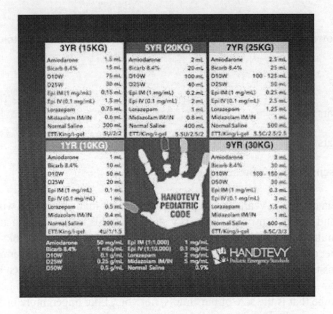

Handtevy Badge Buddy

Photo courtesy of Peter Antevy, MD

www.Handtevy.com

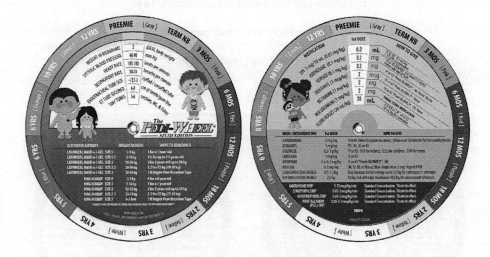

Pedi-Wheel Pediatric Resuscitation Guide

Photo courtesy of Pedi-Ed-Trics Emergency Medical Solutions

www.PediEd.com

Certified Pediatric Emergency Nurse (CPEN) Review IV

2) Parents run a 2-year-old near-drowning child into the ED in full arrest. CPR is initiated and the cardiac monitor reveals ventricular fibrillation (VF.) Which of the following should be performed immediately?

A) Establish vascular access and administer epinephrine

B) Defibrillate with 2j/kg

C) Perform synchronized cardioversion with 1j/kg

D) Establish vascular access and administer Amiodarone 5 mg/kg

B – The only cure for VF is "better living through electricity." Though administering epinephrine and possibly amiodarone are appropriate, the first intervention with witnessed VF is defibrillation using appropriate sized paddles or pads.

3) Each of the following statements is correct regarding pediatric defibrillation **except**:

A) The first defibrillation attempt should be at 1j/kg

B) The first defibrillation attempt should be at 2j/kg

C) The second and subsequent defibrillation attempts should be at 4j/kg

D) "Adult" paddles or pads should be used for children over 1-2 years of age

A – In the horrible event you need to defibrillate a child, the easiest way I've ever come across as to how to remember the essentials is to "pick up your paddles or pads and count them." If you are holding paddles or pads, how many should there be? Two. If there are anything but two, put them down, as another ED nurse should be defibrillating this child. If the child is one year of age (>10kg) or older, you should use the "big people" paddles or pads. Keeping with this idea in mind, everything in children is "something per kilo," so the first defibrillation attempt is 2j/kg. If that is unsuccessful, 2x2 is 4, so it's 4j/kg for the second and subsequent times. 4j/kg is as high as we go in most cases. Remember in the past with adults, we didn't go 200j, 300j, 360j, 720j, 1,440j, 2,880j… Pick up your paddles or pads and count them.

4) A 4-year-old arrives at the ED after being attacked by a pit bull. He has massive facial trauma and attempts at bag-mask ventilation and oral intubation have been unsuccessful. What is the suggested method of securing an airway in this child?

A) Supraglottic airway (King or laryngeal mask airway)

B) Surgical cricothyroidotomy

C) Surgical tracheotomy

D) Blind nasal intubation

A – In children, most importantly remember that if you can effectively bag-mask ventilate or "bag" the child, you've got time to get help! However, if you can't make air go in and out, the child is dead. So in this situation with massive facial trauma, a non-visualized supraglottic airway such as a King or laryngeal mask airway should be placed. In the rare event that these airways are unable to provide adequate ventilation, needle cricothyroidotomy or "cric" may be warranted. Place a 14-g IV catheter and the top of a 3.0 ETT together and begin bag-catheter ventilation. An alternative method is to attach a 3-way stopcock to the IV catheter. One port is attached to the catheter, one port is hooked up to oxygen flowing at 12-15 liters per minute, and the remaining one can be intermittently occluded to "give a breath." Surgical crics are for older teens and adults, and blind nasal intubation in this child is not going to be helpful. Children have a small, pliable, and mobile larynx and cricoid cartilage. This is coupled with the fact that the cricoid ring is the only circumferential support of the trachea in kids. If the cricoid cartilage is inadvertently sliced through, then the trachea may collapse. For these reasons, surgical cricothyroidotomy is generally contraindicated in patients less than 8 years of age. Though supraglottic airways and needle crics are not for long term use, they can keep a child alive long enough to get help, plan and prepare for a definitive airway, and are certainly better than the alternative of watching them die.

5) A 3-year-old who weighs 20kg arrives at the ED in full arrest. The appropriate volume of IV 1:10,000 epinephrine (1 mg/10 mL) should be:

A) 0.02ml

B) 0.20ml

C) 2ml

D) 20ml

C – Here's a really cool trick. When figuring out how much (volume) epinephrine to give and how much the recording nurse should document was given (mg), the rule is simply to move the decimal point one place. This child weighs 20kg, so you should administer 2ml of epinephrine, and the recording nurse should document that 0.2mg of epi was given. For an adult in full arrest weighing 100kg, you would give 10ml of epi and the chart should reflect that the patient received 1.0mg of epinephrine.

6) When giving epinephrine or other resuscitation medications IV during a full-arrest, you should follow the medications with:

A) A 1-10ml saline flush

B) A 1-10ml sterile water flush

C) A 10cc/kg saline bolus

D) A 20cc/kg saline bolus

A – Especially with little ones, the amount of medications actually given is incredibly small. Giving a little saline flush (1-10ml depending on the size of the child) gets the medications out of the IV tubing and into the heart.

7) Drugs which can be given via the endotracheal tube include:

A) NAVEL

B) LEAN

C) HEAVY

D) JUSTRIGHT

B – **L**idocaine, **E**pinephrine, **A**tropine, and **N**arcan (naloxone.) Though the absorption and efficacy of drugs administered via the endotracheal tube is questionable at best, it is still an option listed in many course manuals. The mnemonic used to be NAVEL with the "V" being Valium (diazepam) or Versed (midazolam), but recent texts have trimmed it to LEAN. With the introduction of newer intraosseous devices such as the EZ-IO (bone drill) and the NIO (bone gun), resuscitation medications are rarely, <u>if ever</u>, administered via the ETT anymore.

Certified Pediatric Emergency Nurse (CPEN) Review IV

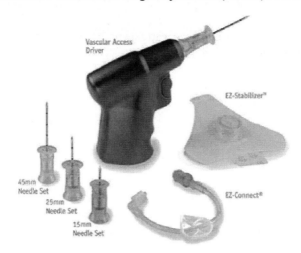

Arrow® EZ-IO Intraosseous Vascular Access System

Image courtesy of Teleflex

www.teleflex.com

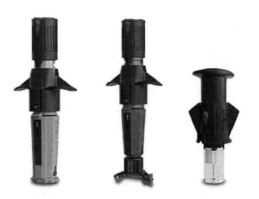

Adult, Pediatric, and Infant NIO Automatic Intraosseous Access Devices

Image courtesy of PerSys Medical

www.persysmedical.com

8) When administering epinephrine via the endotracheal tube (ETT), the dose should be:

A) The same as IV

B) Doubled that of IV

C) 10 times that of IV

D) 30 times that of IV

C – If epinephrine is going to be administered via the ETT, previous editions of PALS and ENPC recommended that you give 10X the dose and dilute the medication in 5-10ml of saline. (However, there are other research studies recommending that when giving ETT medications, you should give 20X and even 30X the dose). Moral of the story, intraosseous (IO) is the way to go!

9) A 2-month-old child arrives at the ED with a heart rate of 20. The ED nurse realizes that bradycardias in infants and young children are usually first treated with:

A) Epinephrine

B) Atropine

C) Transcutaneous pacing

D) Effective bag-mask ventilation with 100% oxygen

D – Almost everything bad that happens with babies and little ones is related to the respiratory system. With that in mind, before you push epinephrine or atropine (for which you will need IV or IO access), try bag-mask ventilation and starting chest compressions first!

10) Which of the following patients with palpable pulses should receive chest compressions?

A) A 1-year-old with a pulse rate of 100

B) A 16-year-old with a heart rate of 50

C) A 6-month-old child with a heart rate of 50

D) A 4-year old child with a heart rate of 80

C – While a heart rate of 50 can be normal in a healthy, athletic 16-year-old, it is certainly way too slow for a 6-month-old child. If ventilation with 100% oxygen doesn't quickly speed up the heart rate, even if there is a pulse with the heart rate of 50, this child should receive chest compressions. Though oxygen and ventilation will often fix the problem, if it doesn't make the child's hearts beat faster, you will have to assist them with chest compressions.

11) A 7-day-old infant arrives at the ED in mom's arms with a complaint of poor feeding. Initial assessment finds the child to be alert, pink, breathing 50 times a minute, and with a heart rate of 280/minute (SVT.) Oxygen saturation is 95% on room air and the temperature is 99.7F (37.6C.) With these findings, you should **first**:

A) Administer supplemental oxygen by blow-by or face mask

B) Immediately cardiovert the child at 1j/kg

C) Immediately defibrillate the child at 2j/kg

D) Establish IV or IO vascular access

A – Remember, almost everything bad that happens in little ones is seemingly respiratory in origin, and therefore "everybody sick in the ED gets oxygen," even children with cyanotic heart disease. Establishing an IV or IO is certainly appropriate, but providing supplemental oxygen while you are trying to get vascular access is absolutely appropriate. If the medications don't work once you have access, then you can think about sedation and cardioversion at 0.5-1j/kg.

Certified Pediatric Emergency Nurse (CPEN) Review IV

12) In the previous child, a 24-g IV was placed in the antecubital fossa. Anticipated next therapy:

A) Immediate cardioversion at 0.5-1j/kg

B) Immediate defibrillation at 2j/kg

C) Administering adenosine slow IV push over 10 minutes

D) Administering adenosine rapid IV push, followed by 10ml saline bolus

D – The child is alert, pink, and saturating well, so try meds first. Adenocard (adenosine) IV (0.1mg/kg, then 0.2mg/kg) is the treatment of choice for stable supraventricular tachycardia (SVT) and should be administered rapidly, followed by a saline bolus. If it is given slowly, it won't be effective. The heart rate is really, really fast so give adenosine really, really fast!

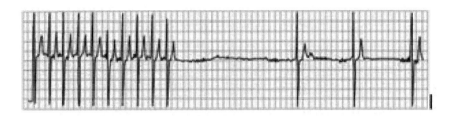

SVT and Adenosine

13) Synchronized cardioversion is appropriate for pediatric patients in:

A) Asystole

B) Supraventricular tachycardia (SVT)

C) Sinus tachycardia

D) Ventricular fibrillation (VF)

B – Of the rhythms listed above, supraventricular tachycardia is the only one for which synchronized cardioversion is appropriate. To achieve synchronized cardioversion, the machine tries to pick when the energy gets released, maximizing the chances of coming back with a rhythm that you like. Patients who are in VF have nothing for the monitor to sync onto, so defibrillation, not cardioversion, should be done. It might help to remember that Cardioversion begins with "C" and therefore you might use it if your patient is "C"onscious or "C"rashing (but still alive.) On the other hand, defibrillation starts with "D" and might be appropriate if the patient is (or is about to be) dead.

14) All of the following non-pharmacologic interventions can be used to possibly convert SVT **except**:

A) Valsalva "bear down" maneuvers

B) Carotid massage

C) Blowing through a straw

D) Applying a bag of ice to the face

B – Just as with adults, carotid massage is no longer recommended in children. There are lots of ways in stable (not crashing and needing cardioversion) children to slow their heart rates (at least temporarily.) If they are old enough, you can tell them to "act like you are pooping in the bed." However, up until age about 10 or so, they just laugh at you. An experienced pediatric ICU nurse taught me a trick I highly recommend. Have the child try to blow really hard through a small straw. It works just like blowing up a balloon, but without the latex/aspiration issues. And unlike the "bear down" maneuvers, you don't have to clean up the bed afterwards. Babies are not going to understand the straw thing, and while they do poop in the bed, they just don't typically do it on command and with sufficient pressure. So with infants, and this only works with infants, ice water facial immersion is commonly utilized. Remember, this does not mean you fill up a basin with ice water and plunge their faces into it. That's near-drowning (covered in another chapter.) Filling up a glove with ice water and placing it on their face for a few seconds can convert the rhythm and restore cardiac output.

15) A 4-year-old child is orally intubated with a 5.0 oral endotracheal tube. What size catheter should be used to suction the endotracheal tube?

A) 5Fr

B) 8Fr

C) 10Fr

D) 12Fr

C - Intubated adults are simple… everybody gets suctioned with a 14f. However, it's not that easy in children. The crash cart holds 5Fr, 6Fr, 8Fr, 10Fr, 12Fr, 14Fr, 16Fr, and 18Fr suction catheters. So, how do you remember which size to use in a child? Simply 2X the size of the ETT. The child is intubated with a 5.0 ETT, so suction with a 10Fr catheter.

16) Appropriate size NG and Foley (urinary catheter) for the child described in question 15 is:

A) 5Fr

B) 8Fr

C) 10Fr

D) 12Fr

C – The rule of 2X the ETT size equals the suction catheter, but it also equals the appropriate size NG and Foley catheter. 5.0 ETT = 10Fr suction, 10Fr NG, and 10Fr Foley. How cool is that!

17) For young children, which of the following types of airway adjuncts are **most** commonly used?

A) Cuffed endotracheal tubes

B) Uncuffed endotracheal tubes

C) Combi-tubes

D) Esophageal obturator airways (EOA's)

B – Outside of the operating room, uncuffed tubes are still most commonly used, especially those under 6 years of age. However, this is changing. Remember that pediatric airways are funnel shaped. They are big at the top and small at the bottom. That anatomical fact, coupled with concerns about cuff-induced tracheal necrosis, led us to use uncuffed endotracheal tubes in children. However, this is changing. In anesthesia for several years, and more recently in emergency medicine/critical care, cuffed tubes are now being used.

Certified Pediatric Emergency Nurse (CPEN) Review IV

The newer cuffed tubes do not have the same issues with tracheal necrosis, especially if cuff pressures are regularly measured. Also, consider a near-drowning child with ARDS and incredibly high airway pressures. In these cases, an uncuffed tube will probably leak and the tube will have to be changed for a cuffed tube. With these ideas in mind, more and more practitioners are placing cuffed tubes in children. *However, for the CPEN exam, remember the majority of practitioners still place uncuffed tubes in children.*

18) A 6-month-old is actively crying and in moderate respiratory distress. After supplemental oxygen is applied, further examination reveals the abdomen is distended and poor air exchange is heard. Suggested intervention:

A) Intubate the child

B) Place an NG/OG tube

C) Administer an albuterol nebulizer treatment because albuterol fixes everything in pediatrics

D) Place the child on BiPAP

B – The main muscle of respiration in little ones is the diaphragm. That's why gastric distension is such a problem. An actively crying child's stomach is easily distended as air is swallowed with the crying. The abdominal distension can easily compromise lung capacity. Placement of an NG/OG tube to decompress the belly can make a huge difference in their air exchange.

19) A 2-year-old has just been intubated and no breath sounds are heard on the right side of the chest. His oxygen saturation is 90% and the heart rate is 130. **First** intervention should be:

A) Needle decompression of the right chest

B) Chest tube placement in the right chest

C) Extubate and replace the endotracheal tube

D) Check how deep the ETT is and pull it back ½-1cm

D – Remember, whoever intubated the kid was probably so excited they saw 2-year-old vocal cords they couldn't stand it. So what do they do with the tube? Shove it down like it's going out of style. Many of us were taught that ETT's always go down the right main stem bronchi and in the vast majority of cases, this is true. However rare it might be, in infants and young children, the ETT can also go in the left. Before doing anything as dramatic as poking a needle into the child's chest or popping in a chest tube, consider moving the ETT. Generally speaking, the mark at which the ETT should be secured is 3X the size of the ETT. Example: a 5.0 ETT should be taped at 15cm at the lip. You should not wait for a chest X-ray to determine tube depth if there is only unilateral breath sounds and NEVER use a chest X-ray to determine esophageal versus endotracheal tube placement.

Certified Pediatric Emergency Nurse (CPEN) Review IV

20) You are doing "ride time" with local EMS. A call is received for a motor vehicle crash in which a 2-month-old is "blue and not breathing." Upon your arrival, the parents who are still trapped in the car are screaming "save my baby!" Your **first** intervention should be:

A) Ensure the infant's airway is patent

B) Perform a scene survey for scene safety

C) Assess the infant's mental status

D) Shake and shout, "Baby, baby, are you OK?"

B - In EMS, the first answer for everything is "scene safety." Though opening the airway and assessing mental status are certainly appropriate, in the uncontrolled prehospital environment, making sure that the "scene is safe" is always the first step.

21) Findings that suggest possible sudden infant death syndrome (SIDS) include:

A) Bloody drainage from the ears

B) Bulging fontanel

C) Blood-tinged fluid in the mouth

D) Multiple bruises on the extremities

C - A, B, and D are findings that suggest physical child abuse and it is important to differentiate between lividity and bruising. SIDS is suggested when other causes of death (including accidental or non-accidental trauma) have been eliminated. Though not always present, a common finding with SIDS is blood-tinged fluid in the mouth.

22) EMS arrives at the emergency department with a possible SIDS infant. An endotracheal tube and intraosseous line are in place and CPR has been ongoing for 20 minutes. Which of the following are signs that further resuscitation efforts are **not** indicated?

A) The infant is cold to the touch with dependent lividity (pooling of blood is evident where the patient was in contact with the bed)

B) Profound cyanosis

C) Cool extremities and torso

D) Apnea

A - Dependent lividity is a sign of being dead for a while. If lividity or other signs of extended post-mortem time (such as decomposition or rigor) are present, resuscitation should not be initiated. In the prehospital arena, SIDS cases are more often "worked" due to standing protocols, understandable hesitations with pronouncing death in an infant, and the wish to make it look like "everything was done." However, the fact that efforts by EMS have been unsuccessful, coupled with the associated physical findings, leads most practitioners to cease further resuscitation efforts.

Certified Pediatric Emergency Nurse (CPEN) Review IV

23) Causes of SIDS include:

A) Pneumonia

B) Non-accidental trauma, aka physical abuse

C) Sepsis

D) Unknown

D - Sudden infant death syndrome causes are unknown. Though there are many recommendations for decreasing the likelihood of SIDS, including the use of fans in the room and the American Academy of Pediatrics "Back to Sleep" campaign, the actual cause of SIDS still remains unknown.

24) Intraosseous (IO) placement should be considered in a critically ill child of what age?

A) Under 6

B) Under 8

C) Under 10

D) All ages

D – In the past, IO's were generally only considered for children under the age of 6; however, that thinking is no longer current. Now, "IO's for everyone" is the current mindset. If reliable IV access cannot be quickly obtained in a critically ill or injured patient of any age, intraosseous is the route of choice for fluid and medication administration.

25) Sites for intraosseous placement in a 2-year-old child include each of the following **except**:

A) Proximal tibia

B) Distal tibia

C) Distal femur

D) Sternum

D – Though the proximal tibia is the most common IO site in children, other options include the distal femur and distal tibia. In *adults*, the sternum, radius, ulna, and humerus are additional possible sites depending upon the particular IO device.

26) Proper placement and function of an intraosseous needle can be **most** reliably verified by:

A) X-ray

B) Fluid drip rate to gravity

C) Repeated palpation of the soft tissues near the needle

D) Aspiration of bone marrow

C – Though most pediatric IOs are placed in the tibia, the idea is the same wherever the IO is placed. Before you place the IO, feel the surrounding area to get a baseline. Make sure to move your hand and

DON'T support the area from below while placing the IO device. Should the needle exit the patient's extremity, you don't want it entering yours. (IO vs. palm = bad combo!) Once the IO is in place, feel the area for swelling. In addition, after and during any fluid or medication administration, reassess for swelling. It's a great, cheap, and effective way to detect early infiltration. Though X-ray may be used to verify placement, it is not a commonly used method. Fluids may drip to gravity, but most times an IV pump, pressure bag, or syringe bolus technique is needed to achieve adequate flow rates. Bone marrow may occasionally be aspirated with the initial placement of the device. This marrow can be used for blood cultures, as well as determination of electrolytes, coags, and blood type, but aspiration of marrow is not a reliable indication of proper placement.

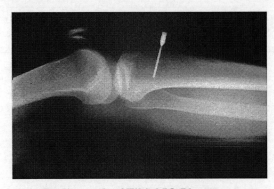

Radiograph of Tibial IO Placement

Photo courtesy of PerSys Medical

www.persysmedical.com

27) A 2-year-old, 10kg child is admitted with acute D and D (diarrhea and dehydration.) Appropriate fluid bolus amount:

A) A liter

B) 20ml

C) 200ml

D) 2,000ml

C – Remember that everything with kids is "something per kilo" and fluids are no exception. 20ml/kg is what we are taught in Pediatric Advanced Life Support (PALS) and the Emergency Nursing Pediatric Course (ENPC.) In a really sick kid, we will be on our knees praying we can find an IV somewhere between all the child's fingers and toes, so along the way, count them. How many fingers and toes are there? Hopefully 20. So, it's 20ml/kg. Remember, if it sounds like way too much fluid (i.e. 2 liters in a 10 kilo kid), it probably is way too much fluid. For dehydrated or shocky children, LR or 0.9NS, just like adults, are the fluids of choice. Glucose containing fluids, i.e. D5.2NS, D5.45NS, or "D5.anything" can be given later for maintenance.

28) The child weighing 10kg is to be admitted to pediatrics for IV antibiotic therapy. Anticipated maintenance fluid rate **(you really need to know this!)**:

A) 10ml/hr

B) 20ml/hr

C) 40ml/hr

D) 83ml/hr

C – 40ml/hr. 4/2/1 is the "rough guestimate" maintenance fluid rule. 4ml/kg/hour for the first 10kg, then add 2ml/kg/hour for each of the next 10kg, then add 1ml/kg/hour for each kg over 20. For example:

Maintenance fluids for a 6kg child: *4ml/kg/hour for the first up to 10kg* – The child weighs 6kg, so expect maintenance fluids around 24ml/hour.

Maintenance fluids for a 16kg child: *4ml/kg/hour for the first 10kg, then add 2ml/kg/hour for each kg up to the next 10kg.* The child weighs 16 kg, so 40ml/hour (1st 10kg) + 12ml/hour (next 6kg). Expect maintenance fluids around 52ml/hour.

Maintenance fluids for a 36kg child: *4ml/kg/hour for the first 10kg, then add 2ml/kg/hour for each kg of the next 10 kg, then add 1ml/kg/hour for each kg over 20.* The child weighs 36kg, so 40ml/hour (1st 10kg) + 20ml/hour (2nd 10kg) + 16ml/hour (remaining 16kg). Expect maintenance fluids around 76ml/hour.

29) Nasotracheal or endotracheal suctioning should be performed for no longer than ___ seconds per attempt:

A) 3-5

B) 5-10

C) 10-15

D) "As long as you can hold your breath"

A – Three to five seconds is more than enough to suction and in reality, the kid will let you know it's time to stop. If their heart rate was 130 and during suctioning it drops to 60, that should be a big clue. Stop! The previously taught idea to suction "as long as you can hold your breath" just doesn't make sense for little ones, and especially if you are a free diver who can hold your breath for 4 minutes or more!

30) Acceptable sites for peripheral IV placement in an 8-year-old pediatric trauma child include all of the following **except**:

A) Cephalic vein (wrist)

B) Saphenous vein (ankle)

C) Antecubital vein (arm)

D) Internal jugular vein (neck)

D – Internal jugular IV lines are considered central, not peripheral, access. Though the unwritten rule says that when the child can walk, you shouldn't put IVs in their feet anymore, with a critically ill child, all bets are off and any vein is a good vein. Anywhere you see a little blue line that's not pulsating, stick it!

31) Which of the following statement is **incorrect** about PICC lines?

A) Peripherally inserted central catheters (PICC) are associated with fewer complications than central venous catheters

B) PICC lines are single or double lumen catheters

C) PICC lines can be inserted at the bedside

D) A PICC line is inserted directly into a central vein, such as the femoral or subclavian vein

D – PICC lines, by definition, are inserted peripherally. This is a huge advantage over conventionally placed central lines in the neck, chest, or groin. Though not a good choice in an emergency, when the answers to where and when are "anywhere" and "right now;" for children who will require long-term IV infusions, early PICC line placement, even in the emergency department, should be considered.

32) When a child with a history of multiple medical problems and devastating neurologic delays presents in cardiac arrest, it is:

A) Not necessary to consult the parents about resuscitation preferences

B) Necessary to consult the parents about resuscitation preferences

C) Necessary to attempt all resuscitation measures as the child is a minor

D) Not necessary to attempt all resuscitation measures as the child is a minor

B - Even in the emergency department, asking parents about "how aggressive or not aggressive do you want us to be" is appropriate. Assuming that they will want "everything to be done" is not always appropriate. Remember what happens when you assume.

33) The majority of pediatric cardiac arrests are:

A) Cardiac in origin:

B) Traumatic in origin

C) Respiratory in origin

D) Neurologic in origin

C - Once again, just about everything that's bad that happens with kids is respiratory in nature or origin (or at least starts around the nose, mouth, or lungs.) Can children arrest due to cardiac conditions? Sure. But unlike adults who drop dead due to 50 years of bad habits, the majority of cardiac arrests in children are due to some sort of respiratory event first. The common scenario involves respiratory distress (bad), respiratory failure (really bad), bradycardia (really, really bad), then finally, cardiac arrest (the worst.)

34) What percentage of children survive neurologically intact following a respiratory arrest?

A) 20%

B) 30%

C) 40%

D) Over 50%

D - The key is getting children when "they are doing something." If they are in respiratory, but not full cardiac arrest, the chances of them being discharged neurologically intact are actually pretty good. If they arrive in cardiac arrest, i.e. "doing nothing," the outcomes are dismal. The notable exceptions to this rule generally involve cases of near-drowning in icy water and associated profound hypothermia

35) The mnemonic recommended when determining the cause of respiratory distress in children with ventilators is:

A) DOPE

B) HELP

C) OUCH

D) OHMYGOSH

A – DOPE – (D)isplacement – Is the ETT or trache tube in the right place? (O)xygen/Obstruction - 1) Is the oxygen hooked up and is it enough? Is there a natural or man-made obstruction? Check for a mucous plug or kinked tube. (P)neumothorax – Does your patient have one? (E)quipment – Is the vent itself broken? The moral of the story, is simple: If anything funky happens, check the tube/trache and bag (ventilate) until the cause of the problem is found and fixed.

36) Each of the following is true about SIDS **except**:

A) It is the most common cause of death for children from 1 month to 1 year of age

B) There is a higher risk if mother is a substance abuser

C) The highest occurrence is in the African-American and Native-American populations

D) It is the most common cause of death for children from 1 year to 10 years of age

D – SIDS is the most common cause of death between 1-month and 1-year, with most deaths occurring between 2 and 4 months of age. Risk factors such as maternal substance abuse and prematurity make sense; however, the reasons why African-Americans and Native-Americans are higher risk are still unknown.

37) Each of the following are desired features of a bag-valve-mask device **except**:

A) A clear, anatomically shaped face mask

B) The ability to give a maximum of 40% oxygen to prevent eye damage

C) Pop-off (pressure release) valve

D) Infant, pediatric, and adult sizes available

B – With the exception of limiting the oxygen delivered to a maximum of 40%, all of the above are desirable components for bag-mask-valve devices, especially for infants and children. Clear face masks let you assess for circumoral cyanosis and vomiting. Various sizes are needed as sometimes small children do better when ventilated with an "adult" bag. In addition, pressure release (pop-off) valves with infant devices can be very helpful to ensure that appropriate ventilator pressures are being used and to avoid potential barotrauma which can result in a pneumothorax. When working with sick kids who have really sick lungs, remember that the pop-off valves pop-off at a pre-set pressure, and that pressure may not be enough to adequately ventilate the child. In those cases, you may need to disengage the pop-off valve to allow enough pressure to be used.

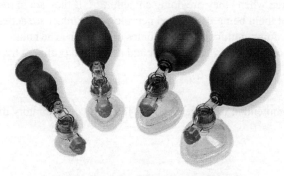

Size Range of Ventilation Bags

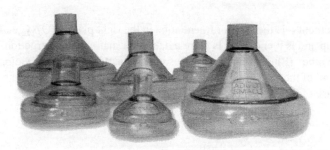

Size Range of Ventilation Masks

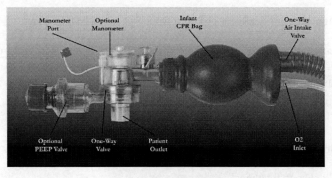

Infant Ventilation Bag

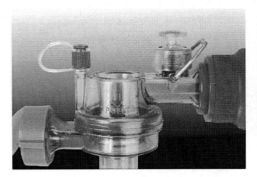
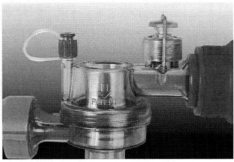

Infant Ventilation Bag with Pop-Off Valve

Photos courtesy of Mercury Medical

www.mercurymedical.com

38) A 2-year-old child with multiple traumatic injuries has been orally intubated. Which of the following would suggest a probable esophageal intubation?

A) "Fogging" in the endotracheal tube

B) Gold or yellow color on the colorimetric end-tidal CO_2 detector

C) Gurgling sounds heard over the stomach with "bagging"

D) Breath sounds only on the right side of the chest

C – If you hear sounds over the belly with "bagging," that's bad! Endotracheal tubes can only go to one of two places; the "right" place (i.e. trachea) or the "wrong" place (i.e. esophagus.) "Fogging or misting" in the endotracheal tube and gold or yellow color on the CO_2 detector are both suggestive of tracheal ETT placement. An easy way to remember the color change is that gold is good; it means the tube's probably in the right spot. However, if the detector turns purple, so might your patient! Breath sounds only on the right are suggestive of a right mainstem intubation, not an esophageal intubation.

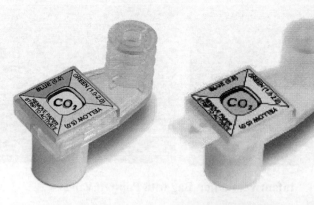

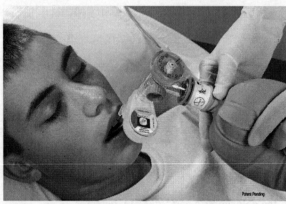

Colorimetric End-Tidal CO₂ Detectors

Photos courtesy of Mercury Medical

www.mercurymedical.com

39) A 4-year-old child with status asthmaticus is being emergently intubated, what type of laryngoscope blade should be used?

A) Straight

B) Curved

C) Whichever the physician/PA/NP/RT/EMT-P wants

D) It doesn't really matter in children

C – When intubating newborns, anesthesia/neonatology teaches that straight blades as a rule should be used. Infants have a big, floppy epiglottis and a tiny vallecula; conditions not conducive to intubation with a curved blade. However, outside of the neonatal NICU, simply ask the person putting in the tube, "Do you want a straight blade or a curved blade?" They will tell you.

40) The 4-year-old child with status asthmaticus is successfully orally intubated with a 5.0 ETT. The ER nurse would anticipate the ETT to be taped at approximately ___ cm at the teeth or gums?

A) 5cm

B) 10cm

C) 15cm

D) 20cm

C – Again, 2x the ETT size is a guide for suction/NG/Foley catheter size and 3x the ETT size is "more or guess" where you should tape it. So a 5.0 oral ETT should be taped at approximately 15cm at the teeth or gums.

41) To help confirm proper positioning of an endotracheal tube (ETT), you should **first** listen:

A) Over the stomach

B) Over the back of the chest

C) Over the left lateral chest in the axillae

D) Over the right lateral chest in the axillae

A – If you can only choose one place to listen on the first few breaths after placing an endotracheal tube, over the stomach should be your choice. Why? How much talent does it take to intubate the esophagus? None! So be pessimistic (or, if you prefer, cautious) and think about where would be the worst place for the ETT to be? In the belly. And if the tube is in the wrong place, when do you want to find out? Right away! So listen to the belly first. If you hear air going into the belly, what do you do? Pull the ETT and bag the child before trying again. Once you have confirmed the ETT is indeed in the lungs, anesthesia recommends listening first to the left chest near the axillae. Why? Remember, if the ETT goes too deep, which side is it most commonly going down? The right. So if you have no sounds over the epigastrium and good sounds over the left (and then right) axillae, chances are pretty good the ETT is in the correct place. But remember, the smaller the patient, the closer everything is together and the less you can depend on specific breath sound locations to assure tube placement. Once you've listened for breath sounds, it is appropriate to confirm placement through X-ray and capnography, as ETT placement should never be verified by only one method.

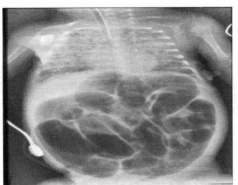

Massive abdominal distension

Courtesy of Christopher Straus MD - University of Chicago Hospitals

42) Which of the following statements is **incorrect** regarding the use of cricoid pressure?

A) Cricoid pressure occludes the trachea by displacing the cricoid cartilage posteriorly

B) Cricoid pressure is applied using one fingertip in infants and the thumb and index finger in older children

C) Cricoid pressure may result in tracheal obstruction in infants if excessive pressure is used

D) Cricoid pressure occludes the esophagus by displacing the cricoid cartilage posteriorly

A – Gentle cricoid pressure, at the discretion of the person performing the intubation, can be used to minimize the risk of vomiting and aspiration during intubation. The technique occludes the esophagus, not the trachea. Occluding the trachea at any point before, during, or after intubation, would be a really bad thing.

43) Even if performed carefully, bag-mask ventilation can easily result in all of the following **except**:

A) Distention of the stomach

B) Vomiting and aspiration

C) Simple or tension pneumothorax

D) Significant facial trauma

D - If performed carefully, manually ventilating or "bagging" a child should never result in significant facial trauma. Manually ventilating a child who has an endotracheal tube (ETT) in place isn't hard at all. You simply attach the bag and squeeze. However, without an ETT in place, proper bag-mask ventilation is not so easy on a PALS mannequin, and even tougher on real children. Anesthesia reminds us that "bagging" is an art." Using the "C" and "E" positions for your fingers as was taught in PALS & ENPC, allows for most children to be adequately ventilated until an endotracheal tube can be placed. Even with good placement and good technique, a good seal is difficult to maintain, and vomiting and aspiration certainly may occur.

44) A tight-fitting, non-rebreather mask can deliver up to what percent of oxygen at 10-15 liters per minute?

A) Up to 30%

B) 30-40%

C) 40-50%

D) 65-75%

D – Unlike what is commonly thought and taught, current research shows that with a properly sized, tight fitting mask, non-rebreather masks can theoretically deliver up to 75% oxygen, but the average is only 65%. However, for optimal delivery, the mask must fit tightly on the child's face and there must be enough oxygen flow for the rebreather bag to remain inflated. If you have a child who will let you put a non-rebreather mask on their face, they probably *need* to have a non-rebreather mask on their face!

45) A 2-year-old child arrives at the ED in cardiac arrest. She was orally intubated by EMS with a 4.5 ETT and bilateral breath sounds are present. The colorimetric CO_2 detector is not changing colors (from purple to gold.) The nurse knows that the lack of color change in the CO_2 detector is **most** likely due to:

A) Esophageal placement of the ETT

B) Right mainstem intubation

C) Poor perfusion associated with cardiac arrest

D) Malfunctioning CO_2 device

C – End-tidal CO_2 detectors change colors in the presence of expired CO_2. However, when a patient is in full arrest, little to no CO_2 is being produced and therefore exhaled. This frequently results in no color change on the CO_2 device and can result in removal of a properly placed ETT. If the patient is alive, the detectors work great. If the patient is dead, the devices don't work so well. Other techniques to verify placement such as looking to make sure the ETT is going through the cords or esophageal detection devices, in association with physical examination findings, are highly recommended.

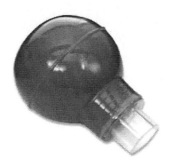 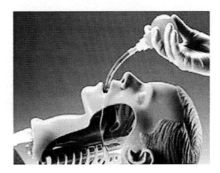

TubeChek Esophageal Intubation Detection Device

Photos courtesy of Ambu USA

www.ambuusa.com

46) In order to achieve the optimum flow rates, IV fluids connected to a pediatric intraosseous needle (IO) should be infused via:

A) 3-way stopcock

B) Gravity

C) Pressure bag, infusion pump or rapid infuser

D) Blood pressure cuff around the IV bag

C – To achieve "optimum" flow rates (which often means controlled, adequate flow), pressure bags or infusion pumps or even rapid infusers can overcome the inherent pressure inside of the bone (the medullary space). This "bone pressure" is present because bones have both arterial and venous blood vessels. While rapid infusers can be used with IOs to deliver large amounts of volume quickly, as may be needed in trauma cases, in other cases they are not necessarily required to achieve adequate flow rates. This can be achieved with pressure bags and or infusion pumps. Three-way stopcocks can be used with IV tubing connected to IO needles for administration of medications or fluid boluses, but they do not affect flow rates in and of themselves unless they accidently are closed. Gravity rarely creates enough pressure to overcome the inherent pressures found inside the bone. BP cuffs around the IV bag do not create consistent pressures and should only be used in a pinch.

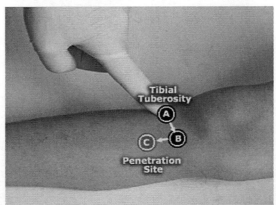

Consult individual intraosseous device manufacturers for their recommendations as to placement guidelines

Pediatric tibial intraosseous device placement landmarks

Photo courtesy of PerSys Medical - www.persysmedical.com

Certified Pediatric Emergency Nurse (CPEN) Review IV

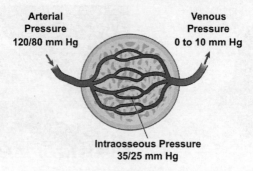

Arterial, venous, and intraosseous pressures
Image courtesy of Teleflex
www.teleflex.com

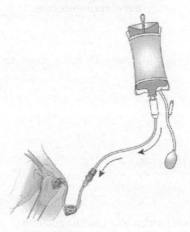

Intraosseous fluid administration with pressure bag
Image courtesy of Teleflex
www.teleflex.com

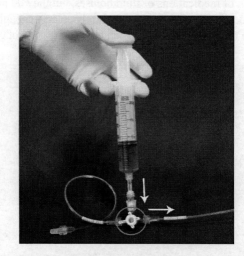

3-way stopcock review - "OFF" on stopcock means "OFF," i.e. no fluid will go that way
Photo courtesy of Medtronics
www.medtronics.com

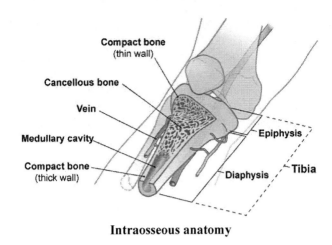

Intraosseous anatomy

Image courtesy of Teleflex

www.teleflex.com

47) A 3-year old comes in via ambulance with IO access in the tibia that is not infusing. The posterior calf is soft and EMS reports the IO access was running well in the ambulance. What should the health care professional do next?

A) Remove the IO access as it is most likely clotted

B) Immediately perform a moderately vigorous flush to the IO access and check for extravasation

C) Insert another IO access one centimeter proximal to the first IO access insertion

D) Inject tissue plasminogen activase (tPA) to lyse the clot in the IO access

B - Flushing the IO access and checking the site are the appropriate actions. If the flow rate through the IO access was not consistently high enough, the bone marrow can again move around the IO needle and occlude flow. A moderately vigorous flush displaces the bone marrow within the medullary space and helps create optimal flow rates when being infused with a pressure bag or infusion pump. The initial flush may be met with moderate resistance (similar to the feel of pushing an amp of 50% dextrose) as the thick fibrin network of the bone marrow is being displaced. The posterior calf should be assessed with initial IO access placement, flushing, and regularly thereafter for firmness and/or swelling which would indicate displacement or extravasation of the IO line. When an IO access is displaced, the fluid sinks into the posterior calf. Firmness of the calf is often the first sign of infiltration. There is no need to remove the IO access yet because, with a recent IO access insertion, it is more likely that the bone marrow itself is occluding the tip of the needle and thus affecting flow rates. Placing another IO access in the same bone is inappropriate because once there has been an IO access inserted into a bone, another IO access insertion into the same bone within 48-hours will typically result in the fluid taking the path of least resistance and exiting out the first hole, thus causing extravasation. TPA is not required, as flow can usually be re-established in a recently-inserted IO access by simply flushing with an age appropriate volume of 0.9NS. This is a whole lot easier, cheaper, and safer option.

48) The purpose of the saline flush immediately after IO access insertion and confirmation of patency is to:

A) Dilute the bone marrow so labs are not altered

B) To promote opening of the one way valves from the medullary space into the central circulation

C) Displace the thick fibrin network of the bone marrow to increase flow rates

D) To prevent medications from mixing in the medullary space

C - The medullary space (inside the bone) is filled with bone marrow that is made of a thick fibrin-like material. This thick substance makes fluid flow rates slow or non-existent. Providing a steady flush of 0.9NS displaces this thick material, creating a "pocket" in the bone marrow and allowing for much faster flow rates. It is not possible to "dilute" bone marrow and there are no "one-way valves" in the medullary space. Lastly, as this question is addressing the saline flush immediately after IO access insertion, there are no medications to become mixed. Certainly, if fluids are not flowing during drug administration, a saline flush should be given between medication administrations, as you would in a peripheral IV.

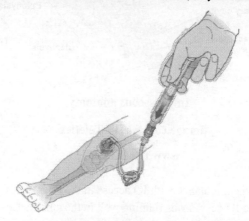

Syringe flush of intraosseous device

Image courtesy of Teleflex

www.teleflex.com

49) One rare complication of IO access is the delivery of a potentially life-threatening embolus into the central circulation. What possible form of life threatening embolus is possible?

A) Air

B) Bone marrow

C) Fat

D) Gas

A - Just like with a peripheral IV or central line, air emboli can be a risk if large amounts of air are injected through the line instead of fluid, medications or blood products. Microscopic amounts of fat can pass through the Volkman's canal in the bone, but are not clinically significant. Gas emboli are of concern with deep sea divers, not IO access placements.

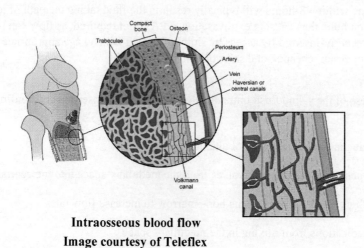

Intraosseous blood flow

Image courtesy of Teleflex

www.teleflex.com

Certified Pediatric Emergency Nurse (CPEN) Review IV

50) Prostigmin® (neostigmine) will reverse all of the following neuromuscular blockers (paralytics) used during emergency intubation **except**:

A) Succinylcholine ("sux," Anectine®)

B) Rocuronium ("rock," Zemuron®)

C) Vecuronium ("vec," Norcuron®)

D) Pancuronium ("pav," Pavulon®)

A – Succinylcholine, a commonly used depolarizing paralytic agent, will not be reversed with the administration of neostigmine. Test taking tip: look at answers. Remember "Sesame Street"… If one of those things doesn't look like the others…it might be the right answer. All of the "…roniums" are non-depolarizing neuromuscular blockers which ARE reversed by neostigmine. Remember from anatomy and physiology class that acetylcholine is the neurotransmitter your body uses to communicate between the nerves and the muscles. Non-depolarizing agents such as "Roc," "Vec," and "Pav" block the neurotransmitter receptors so acetylcholine can't pass the "message to move" in the neuromuscular system. Succinylcholine, on the other hand, essentially acts like acetylcholine at the receptor to cause muscle paralysis and sends a "moving message" to all the voluntary muscles and they all move (twitch) and then are exhausted after a few minutes. While "Sux" acts very quickly and has a relatively short half-life, it is important to remember the ONLY antidote/reversal agent for succinylcholine is time.

51) A 6-month old girl is in the emergency department with a ROSC (return of spontaneous circulation) after a prolonged cardiopulmonary arrest. As she arrests again, her mother arrives and asks to be at her bedside. It is a small ED and all the nurses are busy with the resuscitation. What is the **most** appropriate response in this case?

A) Have the unit secretary stay in the room with the mother as a support person

B) Have the unit secretary call the house supervisor, ICU or pediatric charge nurse to act as support

C) Tell the mother there is no one to act as a support person for her, she will need to wait outside and the nurse will update her as soon as possible

D) Allow the mother to be in the room without a support person

B – Guidelines from the ENA recommend a family presence facilitator or support person to provide for the needs of the family member, while others provide for direct patient care. The secretary (depending on his/her individual people skills, experience, and willingness), may be able to fill that role. However, the better choice would be someone with clinical and psychosocial experience in this type of situation. Seeking out these individuals in other areas of the hospital, such as the house supervisor or pediatric/ICU charge nurse, is a valid choice. Additionally, chaplains, social services, psych nurses or other psychosocial professionals could fill this role. The best choice is someone who is prepared for the role and has been assigned to it for the specified shift. A good way to ensure this takes place is to have the family presence facilitator position included in the hospital code policy. Neither having the mother at the bedside without support, nor asking her to wait until a nurse is free, is an optimal solution.

52) A 5-year old presents to the emergency department in full traumatic arrest. The father arrives a short time later and demands to see his son. Staff notices an odor of alcohol on his breath. The support person takes dad to the bedside, where he begins wailing and throwing his body over the child. How should the family presence facilitator handle this situation?

A) Call security and have him removed. Intoxication is a basis for automatic removal from the resuscitation room.

B) Escort the father to another room where he can compose himself

C) Take him aside and quickly negotiate a verbal contract outlining appropriate behavior for his ongoing presence

D) Have security on standby and insist the father be present by the door or foot of the bed

C – It is most appropriate to start with brief negotiations, explaining the need for the staff to have room to work and asking that he abide by those conditions for the sake of his son. This offers dad a choice and, in many cases, is a peaceful solution that will allow the parent to stay with his child without interfering with medical care. Using security as the first option may inflame, not enhance, the situation. Certainly it is appropriate for security to respond to all resuscitations, but their presence should be discrete unless they are needed to physically control a threat. The odor of alcohol does not automatically mean dad is intoxicated and unable to control his behavior. More information about his competence and self control should be obtained through your interaction with him and before making demands of the parent (and subtle threats with security "standing by"). Escorting the father to another room may ultimately be necessary if other interventions aren't successful in reducing his interference with the care of his child.

53) An 18-month old drowning victim arrives via EMS with CPR in progress. Parents arrive and ask to come to the bedside. All of the following are factors to consider **except**:

A) Ensure a staff person is available to remain with the family to explain procedures and provide emotional support during resuscitation

B) The family's state of emotional distress

C) Physical space available near resuscitation area

D) The availability of security personnel to accompany local law enforcement authorities

D – The Emergency Nurses Association (ENA) and the American Association of Critical Care Nurses (AACN) both endorse and support the option of allowing family at the bedside during pediatric resuscitation. Research confirms it decreases the family's anxiety and depression, and allows for more constructive grief behavior. If possible, a dedicated staff member needs to stay with the family, providing explanations, answering questions, and giving regular updates. Physical space in the resuscitation area needs to be adequate for the code team, but limitations in space should not be used as an excuse to have a family wait outside. The family's emotional state needs to be continuously assessed; screaming, hysterical, and/or out of control families may distract the staff working to resuscitate this patient. It is important to differentiate between expected expressions of grief (sobbing, crying loudly, clinging to each other or the family support staff member) and true interference with the team. While security personnel may be helpful in some circumstances, there is no indication that law enforcement authorities would be involved at this point.

54) Sam's mother has just suffered a cardiac arrest and died in the emergency department. The nurse is discussing with the father about what to expect when dealing with his grieving 10-year old son. Which one of the following statements by the father indicates that the discussions have been effective?

A) "I know it will be easy for Sam to talk about missing his mother."

B) "Since Sam is only 10, he will get over his grief more easily than we will."

C) "This is going to be tough because at age 10, Sam still believes that death is reversible."

D) "Sam may have low self-esteem and blame himself for some months."

D – Vulnerability to self-blame and low self-esteem is the correct answer because children of this age commonly feel that the parent abandoned them. As egocentric beings, they are focused on their part of the world and how what they do affects it (or so they believe). They often want to attribute everything to what they have done, or even thought. This is the age of "step on a crack and break your mother's back." School age children often blame themselves for family problems such as divorce, and want to believe that if they are "better" everything will be okay. As a rule, school-age children tend to avoid talking about their grief and often they do not have the verbal skills to adequately express what they are feeling. However it is crucial to remember that they suffer the same grief as an adult. We need to find alternative ways to allow them to express this, and art is often a useful tool. Developmentally, a child of ten has an understanding of death very much as adults do. Preschoolers think death is temporary or reversible, an example of "magical thinking" common at this age.

55) A young child arrives in the ED with a 2-day history of nausea, vomiting, and diarrhea. The paramedics successfully placed a 24g IV in the patient's right hand and administered an initial fluid bolus. Upon your re-examination, you determine the child would benefit from a second fluid bolus. Calculate the fluid bolus for this child who weighs 16kg.

A) 160ml

B) 180ml

C) 320ml

D) 360ml

C - IV fluid bolus amounts of 0.9NS or LR for children are 20ml/kg, which means this 16kg child should receive a 320ml bolus. Remember, count their fingers and toes and try like heck to find an IV somewhere between them. How many fingers and toes should there be? 20. So it's 20ml/kg for a fluid bolus. And boluses are like strikes in baseball, three is all you get. If the child still looks really sick after three boluses, which should be enough to "fill the tank" (blood vessels), then either a) they need some sort of vasopressor (dopamine, etc.), colloid (albumin), or packed red blood cells (if there's evidence of bleeding.) You really need to start thinking about other interventions if the child still looks really sick after two boluses, and while you are going into your third bolus. If you wait until the third bolus is done to prepare your next intervention, you're letting yourself get behind the eight-ball!

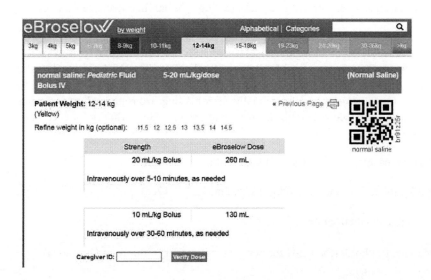

Color coded normal saline bolus

Courtesy of James Broselow MD & Robert Luten MD – www.eBroselow.com

56) After two fluid boluses have been administered to the above 16kg child, maintenance fluids are to be initiated. The attending physician has ordered D5 0.45%NS. What is the correct maintenance rate for this child?

A) 48 ml/hr

B) 52 ml/hr

C) 64 ml/hr

D) 96 ml/hr

B - To calculate maintenance IV rates for children:

Option 1) Go by the classic 4-2-1 rule:

> 0-10kg: 4ml/kg/hr
>
> 10-20kg: +2ml/kg/hr
>
> >20kg: +1ml/kg/hr

4ml/kg for first 10kg (10kg x 4ml/kg = 40ml)

+ 2ml/kg for the next 10kg (6kg x 2ml/kg = 12ml)

For a total maintenance rate of 52ml/hour

Option 2) Another way to remember the 4-2-1 rule is that the child hopefully has 4 extremities. So the first 10kg are 4ml/kg. Then ½ of 4 is 2. So the next 10kg are 2ml/kg. Then ½ of 2 is 1. So each of the remaining kg are 1ml/kg.

4 extremities (& 4ml/kg) for the first 10 kg (10kg x 4ml/kg = 40ml)

+ ½ of the 4 for the next 10kg (6kg x 2ml/kg = 12ml)

For a total maintenance rate of 52ml/hour

(Thanks to Julie Bacon RN, BA for her great keep cutting it in half maintenance fluid idea)

Option 3) You can just remember the idea of playing golf and drinking beer, which many of us would rather be doing than studying or taking the CPEN exam. So... when you play golf, what's the first thing you yell after teeing off? (before cursing) FORE! (4) So the first 10kg are 4ml/kg. Then if the weather is beautiful and life is good, you get to play two (2) rounds of golf. So... 4ml/kg for each of the first 10kg, and then 2ml/kg for each of the next 10kg. Finally, after playing two rounds of golf on a beautiful day, nothing would make the day complete like a frosty cold one (1)! So... 1ml/kg for each of the remaining kg. This child weighs 16kg, so it's

> 4ml/kg for each of the first 10kg (10kg x 4ml/kg =   40ml)
>
> + 2ml/kg for each of the next 10kg (6kg x 2ml/kg =   12cc)
>
> for a total maintenance rate of 52ml/hour.

(Thanks to Marlene Bokholdt RN, MSN for her great maintenance fluids and golf idea)

Certified Pediatric Emergency Nurse (CPEN) Review IV

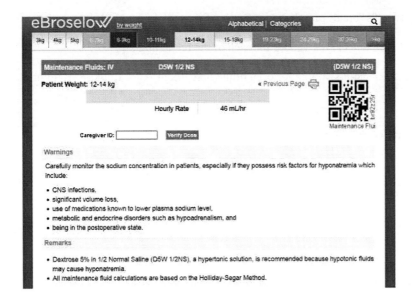

Color coded maintenance IV fluids

Courtesy of James Broselow MD & Robert Luten MD – www.eBroselow.com

57) What is the correct IV fluid maintenance rate for a 5kg child?

A) 5 ml/hr

B) 10 ml/hr

C) 15 ml/hr

D) 20 ml/hr

D - To calculate maintenance IV rates for children:

Option 1) Go by the classic the 4-2-1 rule:

    0-10kg: 4ml/kg/hr

    10-20kg: +2ml/kg/hr

    >20kg: +1ml/kg/hr

4ml/kg for first 10kg (5kg x 4ml/kg = 20ml)

For a total maintenance rate of 20ml/hour

Option 2) Another way to remember the 4-2-1 rule is the child hopefully has "4" extremities. So the first 10kg are 4ml/kg. Then ½ of 4 is 2. So the next 10kg are 2ml/kg. Then ½ of 2 is 1. So each of the remaining kg are 1ml/kg.

4 extremities (& 4ml/kg) for the first 10 kg (5kg x 4ml/kg = 20ml)

    For a total maintenance rate of 20ml/hour

Option 3) You can just remember the idea of playing golf…

Start the game with yelling "Fore" (4) so the first 10kg are 4ml/kg.

You get to play two (2) rounds of golf, so it's 2ml/kg for each of the next 10kg.

Post-game frosty cold one (1) It's 1ml/kg for each of the remaining kg.

This child weighs 5kg, so it's 4ml/kg for each of the first 10kg (5kg x 4ml/kg = 20ml/hr) as maintenance.

58) What is the correct IV fluid maintenance rate for a 22kg child?

A) 22 ml/hr

B) 42 ml/hr

C) 62 ml/hr

D) 82 ml/hr

C) - To calculate maintenance IV rates for children:

Option 1) Go by the classic the 4-2-1 rule:

0-10kg: 4ml/kg/hr

   10-20kg: +2ml/kg/hr

   >20kg: +1ml/kg/hr

4ml/kg for first 10kg (10kg x 4ml/kg = 40ml)

+ 2ml/kg for the next 10kg (10kg x 2ml/kg = 20ml)

+ 1ml/kg for the remaining kg (2kg x 1ml/kg = 2ml)

For a total maintenance rate of 62ml/hour

Option 2) Another way to remember the 4-2-1 rule is the child hopefully has "4" extremities. So the first 10kg are 4ml/kg. Then ½ of 4 is 2. So the next 10kg are 2ml/kg. Then ½ of 2 is 1. So each of the remaining kg are 1ml/kg.

4 extremities (& 4ml/kg) for the first 10 kg (10kg x 4ml/kg = 40ml)

+ ½ of the above for the next 10kg (10kg x 2ml/kg = 12ml)

+ ½ of the above for remaining kg (2kg x 1ml/kg= 2ml)

   For a total maintenance rate of 62ml/hour

Option 3) You can just remember the idea of playing golf...

Start the game with yelling "Fore" (4) so the first 10kg are ml/kg.

You get to play two (2) rounds of golf, so it's 2ml/kg for each of the next 10kg.

Post-game frosty cold (1) It's 1ml/kg for each of the remaining kg.

This child weighs 22kg, so it's

> 4ml/kg for each of the first 10kg (10kg x 4ml/kg =   40ml)
>
> + 2ml/kg for each of the next 10kg (10kg x 2ml/kg =   20ml)
>
> + 1ml/kg for each remaining kg (2kg x 1ml/kg =   2ml)
>
> for a total maintenance rate of   62cc/hour.

Play golf… Yell Fore (4), play 2 rounds, and enjoy (1) frosty cold one (after passing CPEN!)

59) A child with liver failure and active GI bleeding has received multiple units of packed red blood cells (PRBCs). The Pediatric ED nurse would also anticipate the administration of:

A) Fresh frozen plasma (FFP) and platelets

B) Albumin

C) Whole blood

D) Factor VIII

A – When patients bleed, they don't just bleed packed red blood cells. PRBCs will replenish just that-- red blood cells, but nothing else. Clotting factors (FFP) and platelets must also be replaced or the patient will become coagulopathic and continue to bleed. Colloids such as albumin are occasionally used for volume replacement and Factor VIII is for (you guessed it) Factor VIII replacement. Outside of the military, whole blood is just not used that often anymore, so we would not anticipate administering whole blood in this case.

60) A child is receiving 10ml/kg of packed red blood cells in the ED. Ten minutes into the transfusion, the child develops a fever of 101°F (38.3°C), chills and dyspnea, and complains that his lower back is hurting. Based on these symptoms, you suspect:

A) Acute hemolytic reaction

B) Febrile non-hemolytic reaction

C) Non-febrile, non-acute, non-hemolytic reaction

D) Graft vs. host disease

A – This child is showing signs and symptoms of an acute hemolytic reaction, usually caused by ABO incompatibility. This is the worst kind of transfusion reaction and can occur when a patient accidentally receives the wrong type of blood (for example, type A blood to a type B patient). Febrile non-hemolytic reactions, by definition, involve fever but would not commonly cause lower back pain or dyspnea, which is a serious reaction. Graft vs. host disease occurs in bone marrow transplant patients when the new grafted bone marrow cells (which have their own immune system) are transfused into an immune-compromised patient or host and the new (graft) cells attack the host cells as foreign invaders. (ED treatment = IV steroids.) As there was nothing in the question that indicates the patient was a recipient of a bone marrow transplant, this answer can be quickly eliminated. Lastly, since the patient is in fact febrile, and there is no such thing as a non-febrile, non-acute, non-hemolytic reaction, it should be easy to eliminate that as an option.

Certified Pediatric Emergency Nurse (CPEN) Review IV

61) Which of the following would be the priority intervention for the previously described patient?

A) Clamp off the blood and infuse normal saline wide open through the same tubing

B) Administer Tylenol® (acetaminophen, Panadol®) for the fever

C) Slow down the rate of the blood to a "keep vein open" rate

D) Stop the transfusion and cap the IV

D – The priority intervention is to immediately stop the transfusion. Infusing normal saline through the same tubing will just flush the remaining blood in the tubing into the patient, continuing on the same path. In the ED (and especially with sick kids), removing a perfectly good IV doesn't make a whole lot of sense, so just change the IV tubing at the hub and continue to use the IV (just with no blood and different tubing.) Tylenol® may be administered for fever, but it's not the priority in this situation. Slowing down the transfusion will only continue the symptoms, just at a slower rate. Remember the classic doctor joke:

Patient: Doc, it hurts when I do this. What should I do?

Doctor: Stop doing that!"

If the transfusion is making the patient worse, not better, stop doing it!

62) Sara is a 20kg, 8-year old girl who presents to the ED with nausea, vomiting and diarrhea. Vitals at triage: BP: 70/palp, HR 140, Temp 101.2°F (38.4°C.) She has dry mucous membranes, sunken eyes, and decreased skin turgor. The ED nurse practitioner orders a rapid fluid bolus to increase her perfusion. What is the appropriate technique and fluid to administer a rapid fluid bolus in this dehydrated pediatric patient?

A) 1 liter of D5LR on a pressure bag; give 400 ml

B) 1 liter of 0.9NS on a pressure bag; give 400 ml

C) 1 liter of 0.9NS with a 3-way stopcock and 20 ml syringe; give 400 ml

D) 400ml of 0.9NS given by counting drops

C – First, did you catch the fact that the appropriate amount of fluid for resuscitation on this patient is 400 ml? The formula is 20 ml/kg (20 x 20=400 ml). Although a rapid infuser and pressure bag certainly can provide rapid instillation of fluid, you won't be able to administer an accurate amount to the pediatric patient, and there is a huge potential for fluid overload. In addition, isotonic fluids such as 0.9NS or LR, but not D5LR, should be used for fluid resuscitation. Remember that a 20 ml/kg bolus of a D5-containing solution gives 0.5 gm/kg of glucose and will cause significant hyperglycemia, which is hardly ever good and can cause increased fluid losses through osmotic diuresis. Counting drops stopped being acceptable somewhere in the Stone Age! A stopcock attached to a 20 ml syringe is simple and quite effective. Push one filled syringe for every kilogram of weight. You can also use a larger syringe and adjust accordingly. Fluid can easily be pulled from the bag and infused without stopping to reconnect and infuse.

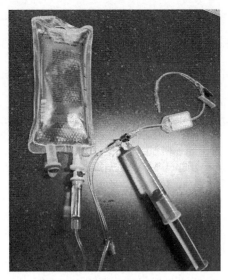

"Pull and push" fluid bolus technique

Photo courtesy of Joshua DeBoer, my then 14-year old aspiring computer genius son
Summit Studios Games

63) An 8-week old child presents in full arrest to the Pediatric ED. After successfully being resuscitated, a chest X-ray is performed, which reveals normal-appearing bones with numerous posterior rib fractures. These findings are **most** consistent with:

A) Vigorous chest compressions during CPR

B) Child abuse/Shaken Baby Syndrome

C) Falling out of the crib

D) Developmental brittle bone conditions

B – It is estimated that 85–100% of infant rib fractures are due to abuse and are particularly seen with Shaken Baby Syndrome. In this scenario, it is likely that the angry adult's hands encircled the baby's chest during the shaking, putting significant focused pressure on the posterior ribs near the costovertebral junction, resulting in fractures. Any time rib fractures are found in the absence of a clear mechanism of injury (such as a motor vehicle crash), this should be a huge red flag for the ED nurse to consider the possibility of abuse. Remember that kids are kind of like skin covered Nerfballs©. The immature bones are not fully calcified/mineralized, so the rib cage is very elastic. Rib fractures as a result of CPR on infants are very rare, occurring in ≤3% of cases. The vast majority of 8-week old babies are unable to roll over unassisted; therefore, they can't roll off of couches and changing tables, out of cribs, etc. It would be possible for an infant this young to roll off a supine parent's chest, but only if the parent's motion throws him/her off. Developmental brittle bone conditions can become evident very early in life; however, most show abnormal-looking bones on X-ray. Published case reports suggest that rib fractures due to CPR are uncommon, even in children with brittle bones.

64) EMS calls from a children's long-term care facility to give report on a 12-year old with a history of multiple chronic medical issues, including ventilator dependency and persistent vegetative state. The child is in severe respiratory distress, "about to code" and the medics are not sure of the child's Do Not Resuscitate (DNR) status. The ED physician designated to provide EMS medical control should:

A) Advise EMS to immediately begin treatment/ resuscitative efforts per local protocol

B) Advise EMS to not begin resuscitative efforts due to her neurological status and poor prognosis

C) Advise EMS to contact the child's parents before beginning resuscitative efforts

D) Advise EMS to ask facility staff about the patient's DNR status prior to beginning treatment

A – This child is not in full cardiorespiratory arrest, so this is not a decision as to whether or not to start CPR. This patient in respiratory distress/failure requires immediate treatment by EMS. A DNR order never means Do Not Treat, although such orders may specify to what degree emergent treatment may be carried out. (Note that intubation is probably not an issue for this patient, who most likely has a tracheostomy for chronic ventilation.) Ideally, any patient of any age in a long-term care facility should have their wishes and those of their family clearly (and officially) documented long before an acute episode of decompensation occurs. Staff at such facilities should be prepared not only to inform EMS of the patient's resuscitation status, but also to back up that information with copies of all documentation required by their state. In some states, EMS may comply with a DNR order only if a specific prehospital DNR order is presented to them. EMS providers must know their state laws and agency protocols in dealing not only with DNR orders (sometimes now called "Accept Natural Death" –AND orders), but also Living Will-type documents that specify treatments acceptable to the patient and family. It is always appropriate for EMS to ask facility staff or family members present with the child about the patient's DNR status and to request the appropriate documentation, but treatment should be initiated unless the documentation is immediately available. It is sound medical-legal practice to err on the side of treating, rather than not treating, when a patient's DNR status is not appropriately documented. Also, remember that one of the patient's legal guardians may verbally override a DNR order at any time.

65) In children who present directly to the Pediatric ED in full cardiopulmonary arrest, the decision to discontinue resuscitation efforts should consider all of the following **except**:

A) Mechanism of the cardiac arrest

B) Duration of the cardiac arrest ("downtime")

C) Treatment rendered before arrival, especially the performance of quality bystander CPR

D) The availability of a medical examiner

D – The availability of a medical examiner should not be a consideration in the termination of resuscitation efforts. Think about what is the longest you have attempted to resuscitate a child. Was it 15 minutes…45 minutes…1 hour and 45 minutes? It's a child and we understand that there will be so much emotion tied into a pediatric resuscitation. Even if you get the child back to a point of a spontaneous heart beat, that's only half the story. Getting a heart beating again, especially in a child, does not always equate with getting a functional brain back as well. Cases of cold-water near-drowning may be a completely different story, but those rarely occur. Really, really cold water (it must be ICE COLD water) can have a neuroprotective effect, and occasionally these patients have good outcomes even after prolonged exposure and subsequent resuscitation. The 2010 American Heart Association PALS guidelines state that there are no reliable predictors of outcome to guide practitioners as to when to terminate resuscitative efforts in children. This is especially the case for in-hospital cardiac arrest. Many factors, including all of the others (A, B, and C) listed above, must be taken into consideration when deciding to terminate resuscitation.

66) A 2-year old has been worked up for a fever in the ED and is about to be discharged home following an intramuscular (IM) injection of Rocephin® (ceftriaxone.) Which injection site would be the **most** appropriate for this child?

A) Dorsogluteal

B) Deltoid

C) Ventrogluteal

D) Vastus lateralis

D – The vastus lateralis is a large muscle mass in children and is a safe site. The dorsogluteal site is no longer recommended due to potential damage to the sciatic nerve. The ventrogluteal is not well developed in a two-year old and a 2-year old deltoid is just too small (and painful!) for a 2 ml injection.

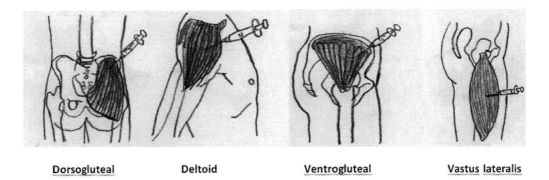

Intramuscular injection sites

Courtesy of Nina DeBoer, my then 12-year old aspiring artist/baker daughter

www.ninasbeliciousbakery.com

67) What is the proper way to restrain a 3-month old, 14 lb (6kg) infant in a vehicle?

A) Forward facing booster seat rated up to 65 lbs (30kg)

B) Forward facing convertible seat rated 30-65 lbs (14-30kg)

C) Rear facing infant seat/convertible seat rated up to at least 35 lbs (16kg)

D) Rear facing booster seat rated up to 65 lbs (30kg)

C – All children at this age should be in rear facing car seats, and as this child is only 14 pounds (6kg) and 3-months old, he's way to too small for just a booster seat, either in car or a restaurant. Plus, there is no such thing as a rear facing booster seat.

68) Your child, who is 2-years old and weighs 32 lbs (14kg), meets the height and weight requirements for your convertible car seat. All of the following are important points must you remember in order to correctly secure the child in the car seat **except**:

A) The car seat should be in an upright position according to the manufacturer's instructions

B) Harness straps must be at or above the child's shoulders and snug but comfortable, and the retainer clip should be at armpit level.

C) The child is now able to use a forward facing car seat

D) In order to ensure future seat belt compliance, the child should have enough freedom of movement to easily reach items on the floor of the vehicle.

D – If the child has enough freedom of movement to reach the floor, neither the child nor the car seat is properly secured. Otherwise, all of the other above considerations are correct.

Certified Pediatric Emergency Nurse (CPEN) Review IV

The factors surrounding the appropriate choice and placement of a child's car seat are associated with their height, weight, position in the vehicle, and the fact that "kids aren't just little adults!" So let's start with the reasons for rear-facing seats for children from birth to two years of age.

Why rear-facing for children under two years old?

The infant's head is larger and heavier in proportion to its body than that of an older child. The infant's shoulders are narrow and flexible. The pelvis is small, rounded and not fully developed.

Recommendations are based on the most common type of crash--a head-on collision. A rear-facing child seat supports the entire head, neck and back of an infant in a head-on collision and cradles and moves with the child, thereby reducing stress to the neck and spinal cord. The car seat shell absorbs the forces in a head-on crash.

Because the infant is placed rear-facing and the car seat rotates downwards in a crash, it is important to remember that the top of the child's head should be well-contained within the shell -more than 1 inch from the top. The harness needs to be snug enough to keep the infant from sliding up in a crash. The harness retaining clip, "pre-crash positioner", must be kept at the armpit level to help keep the child in the seat and minimize the possibility of being ejected from the seat during a crash. Harness straps are positioned at or below the infant's shoulders while rear-facing. "Pre-crash positioner" means the harness clip only serves to hold the harnesses together pre-crash. If you are ever at the scene with a child in a car seat, observe where the harness clip is after the crash. It will be below the armpit level. That is a normal position AFTER the crash.

Forward-facing

When the child reaches the highest weight allowed by the rear-facing restraint and the child is at least two years old, the child then graduates to a forward-facing child seat. Most convertible seats are for use by children from age two until they reach 40 pounds (18 kg), although there are more and more child seats rated for the internal harness up to 65 pounds (30 kg) or about 4 years old. The harness straps are positioned at or above the child's shoulders once they are placed forward-facing. The child's ears should not be above the top of the shell. The harness retaining clip must be kept at armpit level.

Booster seats

The next step in child passenger safety is a booster seat. Once the child outgrows his/her forward-facing seat (usually around 4 years old and 40 pounds (18 kg), a child should use a booster seat until the vehicle seat belt fits properly. Proper fitting seat belts mean that the lap belt should lie across the upper thighs and the shoulder belt across the chest (not the neck).

Booster seats serve as an important middle step between a restraint with harness and a vehicle lap/shoulder belt. Booster seats have weight ranges starting at 30-40 pounds (14-18 kg) with a maximum weight limit of 80-100 pounds (37-45 kg). High-back boosters must be used when the vehicle seat backs are low or do not have restraints to ensure that the child's head, neck and back are supported. Unlike infant and convertible seats, booster seats are not tightly installed in the vehicle. The child's weight and the vehicle's lap/shoulder belts hold the booster seat in place. When not in use, always keep the booster seat buckled to the vehicle. Otherwise it becomes a missile in the event of a crash.

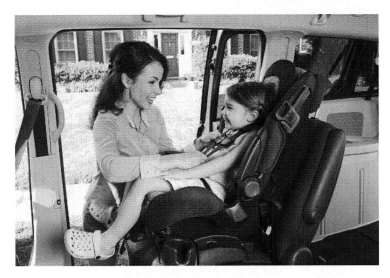

Car seat image 1 - Child in forward-facing convertible seat

- Child sitting upright
- Car seat's harness is flat and snug
- Harness retaining clip is at the armpit level (where it should be as this is a pre-crash position)
- Top of child's head well below top of car seat shell – (when the top of the child's ears are in line with the top of the car seat, the child will be too tall for the seat)

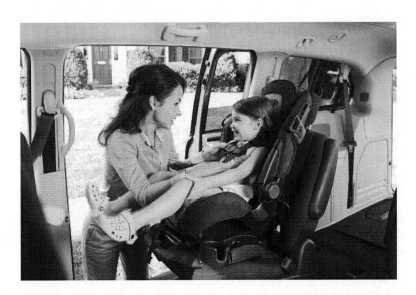

Car seat image 2 - Mother checking internal harness to make sure it is snug

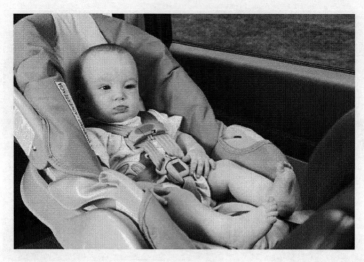

Car seat image 3 - Child in rear-facing infant seat with a 5-point harness

- Harness is laying flat and snug
- Harness retaining clip is at armpit level
- Seat appropriate for weight and height of child
- Top of head well below top of car seat shell

    (for infants the top of the head must be one inch below the top of the car seat shell)

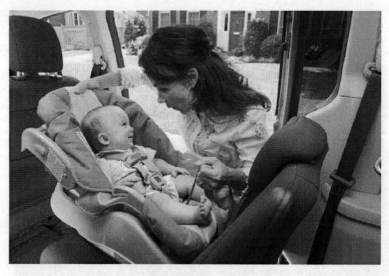

Car seat image 4 - Rear-facing

Mother is tightening internal harness so that it is snug on the baby

Certified Pediatric Emergency Nurse (CPEN) Review IV

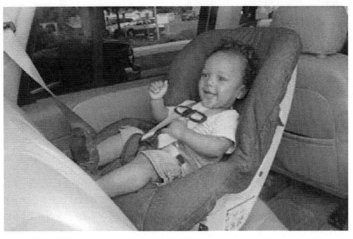

Car seat image 5 - Rear-facing convertible seat

Probably rated up to 35 pounds (16 kg)

- This can be used after an infant outgrows the infant seat, but must remain rear-facing until 2 years old (this is the new 2011 guideline from the AAP and NHTSA)

Car Seat Recommendations for Children

- Select a car seat based on your child's age and size, and choose a seat that fits in your vehicle and use it every time.
- Always refer to your specific car seat manufacturer's instructions; read the vehicle owner's manual on how to install the car seat using the seat belt or LATCH system; and check height and weight limits.
- To maximize safety, keep your child in the car seat for as long as possible, as long as the child fits within the manufacturer's height and weight requirements.
- Keep your child in the back seat at least through age 12.

NHTSA

AGE

Birth – 12 months
Your child under age 1 should always ride in a rear-facing car seat.
There are different types of rear-facing car seats: Infant-only seats can only be used rear-facing. Convertible and 3-in-1 car seats typically have higher height and weight limits for the rear-facing position, allowing you to keep your child rear-facing for a longer period of time.

1 – 3 years
Keep your child rear-facing as long as possible. It's the best way to keep him or her safe. Your child should remain in a rear-facing car seat until he or she reaches the top height or weight limit allowed by your car seat's manufacturer. Once your child outgrows the rear-facing car seat, your child is ready to travel in a forward-facing car seat with a harness.

4 – 7 years
Keep your child in a forward-facing car seat with a harness until he or she reaches the top height or weight limit allowed by your car seat's manufacturer. Once your child outgrows the forward-facing car seat with a harness, it's time to travel in a booster seat, but still in the back seat.

8 – 12 years
Keep your child in a booster seat until he or she is big enough to fit in a seat belt properly. For a seat belt to fit properly the lap belt must lie snugly across the upper thighs, not the stomach. The shoulder belt should lie snug across the shoulder and chest and not cross the neck or face. Remember: your child should still ride in the back seat because it's safer there.

DESCRIPTION (RESTRAINT TYPE)

A REAR-FACING CAR SEAT is the best seat for your young child to use. It has a harness and in a crash, cradles and moves with your child to reduce the stress to the child's fragile neck and spinal cord.

A FORWARD-FACING CAR SEAT has a harness and tether that limits your child's forward movement during a crash.

A BOOSTER SEAT positions the seat belt so that it fits properly over the stronger parts of your child's body.

A SEAT BELT should lie across the upper thighs and be snug across the shoulder and chest to restrain the child safely in a crash. It should not rest on the stomach area or across the neck.

 www.facebook.com/childpassengersafety   http://twitter.com/childseatsafety   March 21, 2011

Images courtesy of the National Highway Traffic Safety Administration

www.nhtsa.gov

69) The suggested maximum flow rate for supplemental oxygen via a conventional nasal cannula for a teen patient with pneumonia is:

A) 2 liters per minute

B) 6 liters per minute

C) 10 liters per minute

D) 15 liters per minute

B – Traditional nasal cannulas (as found in most emergency departments) allow for flow rates of up to 6 liters per minute (LPM), though there are now humidified high-flow nasal cannulas (such as Vapotherm™) which can deliver very high flow rates (up to 40 liters per minute for adults). If the patient requires more than 6 LPM per nasal cannula, they probably need some sort of an oxygen mask instead, unless a humidified high-flow system is available. Flow rates of more than 6 LPM via traditional nasal cannulas not only have issues with comfort and adequate humidification, but may actually induce the phenomenon where the cannula appears to launch itself out of the patient's nose.

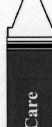

DEVICE	FLOW RATE	OXYGEN CONCENTRATION DELIVERED
Nasal cannula	1-6 LPM	24-44 Percent
Venturi mask	Varied depending on device and desired oxygen percentage	24-60 Percent
Partial rebreather mask	10-12 LPM	40-60 Percent
Non-rebreather mask	12-15 LPM	80-90 Percent

70) Oral airways in children should:

A) Extend from the lips to the tip of the tongue

B) Never be left in place after intubation

C) Be measured from the tip of the nose to the angle of the jaw

D) Only be used in children with no gag reflex

D – If the child has an active gag reflex, vomiting can occur as the oral airway, King airway or laryngeal mask airway hits the uvula and back of the throat. This will typically make the person gag and then barf (chuck), and barf and barf. Oral airways are measured from the corner of the mouth (nasal airways are measured from the nose--imagine that) to the tip of the earlobe or the angle of the jaw. Think about the story of Goldilocks and the Three Bears… If they are too big, they can push the tongue back into the retropharynx, causing airway obstruction. If they are too small, they may fail to keep the upper airway open, thus defeating the purpose of placing the oral airway. Oral airways may be placed before intubation to help open the airway for bag-mask ventilation or after intubation to help prevent the child from biting on the endotracheal tube. (Adequate sedation works great for that as well.) In adults, the airway is inserted into the person's mouth upside down, advanced to the back of the throat and then rotated 180 degrees. The method recommended for infant and pediatric oral airway insertion involves holding the tongue forward and down with a tongue depressor and inserting the airway with the concave curve following the curve of the tongue.

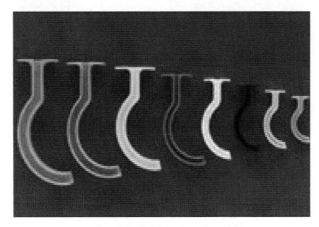

Size range of oral airways

Courtesy of Mercury Medical – www.mercurymedical.com

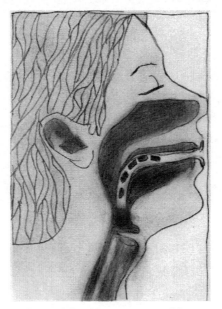

Oral airway in proper position

Courtesy of Nina DeBoer, my then 12-year old aspiring artist/baker daughter

www.ninasbeliciousbakery.com

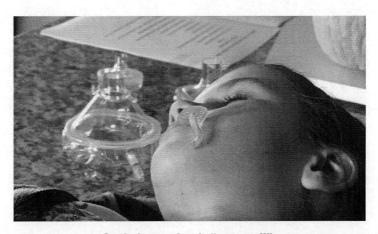

Oral airway that is "too small"

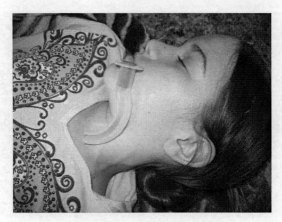

Oral airway that is "too big"

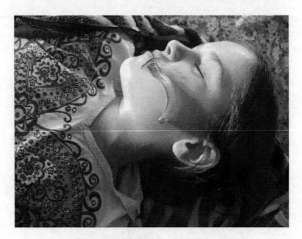

Oral airway that is "just right"

Photos courtesy of Joshua DeBoer, my then 14-year old aspiring computer genius son
Summit Studios Games

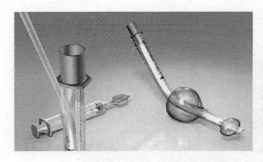
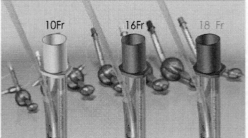

King Airways with gastric access port

Courtesy of Ambu USA

www.ambuusa.com

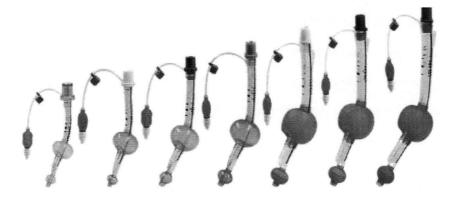

Range of King airway sizes

Courtesy of Ambu USA - www.ambuusa.com

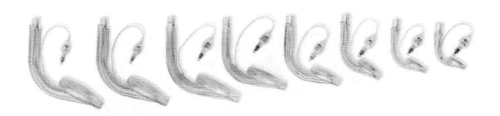

Range of Ambu Aura Gain Laryngeal Mask Airway Sizes

Courtesy of Ambu USA - www.ambuusa.com

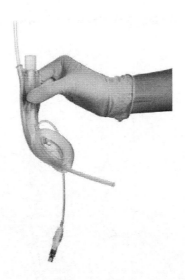

Ambu Aura Gain Laryngeal Mask Airway with gastric access port

Courtesy of Ambu USA - www.ambuusa.com

71) Nasal airways in children should:

A) Extend from the lips to the tip of the tongue

B) Never be placed before intubation

C) Be measured from the tip of the nose to the angle of the jaw

D) Only be used in children with no gag reflex

C – Nasal airways are measured from one of the nares to the tip of the earlobe or the angle of the jaw. Remember Goldilocks… If the nasal airway is too wide, bleeding can occur and if it is too small, it will not serve the purpose of maintaining the airway. Airways that are too long may end up in the esophagus and cause gagging. Nasal airways may be placed before intubation to help open the airway for bag-mask ventilation, but serve little purpose in an intubated patient, especially since an NG tube will probably be placed as well. In children, the airway is inserted into the nose with the bevel facing towards the septum and then gently advanced to the back of the throat. If the bevel is placed toward the outer part of the nose (opposite of the septum) it can function like a shovel and get clogged along the way with boogers, etc. Nasal airways, in conjunction with proper head positioning (something beneath the shoulders), are great for sick little children with an active gag reflex to allow for easier nasopharyngeal suctioning and airway patency.

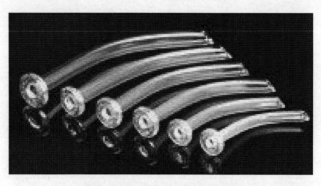

Size range of nasal airways

Courtesy of Med-Tech Resource - www.gomed-tech.com

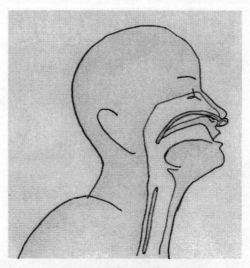

Nasal airway in proper position

Courtesy of Nina DeBoer, my then 12-year old aspiring artist/baker daughter

www.ninasbeliciousbakery.com

Certified Pediatric Emergency Nurse (CPEN) Review IV

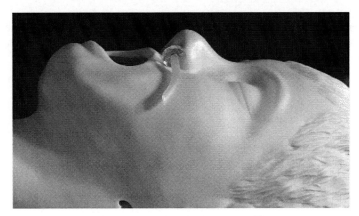

Nasal airway that is "too small"

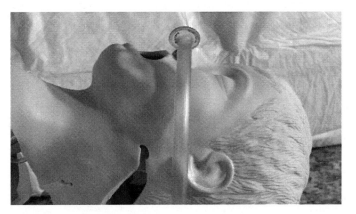

Nasal airway that is "too big"

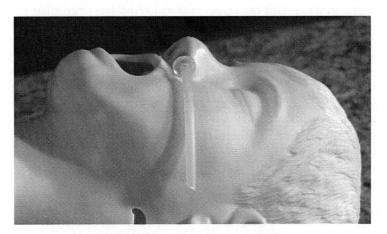

Nasal airway that is "just right"

Photos courtesy of Joshua DeBoer, my then 14-year old aspiring computer genius son

Summit Studios Games

Certified Pediatric Emergency Nurse (CPEN) Review IV

72) The mother of an intubated child asks the nurse to come to the room as "something is beeping." Upon entering the room, the nurse finds the low pressure alarm on the ventilator is the source of the alarm. This is **most** likely due to:

A) The child biting on the endotracheal tube

B) The child "bucking" the ventilator

C) The child being disconnected from the ventilator

D) The child's endotracheal tube being clogged with secretions

C – Low pressure alarms on a ventilator commonly mean one of two bad things: 1) The endotracheal tube or trach is no longer attached to the ventilator or, even worse, 2) The child's endotracheal tube or trach is no longer attached to the patient, i.e. they are extubated. Low pressure = you no longer have a closed system (something is disconnected somewhere). All of the other answers would result in high pressure alarms, indicating increased resistance to gas flow in and/or out from the ventilator. High pressure = your system is obstructed somewhere.

73) An 8-year old child with a double-lumen peripherally inserted central catheter (PICC) presents to the Pediatric ED with signs of gastroenteritis. The ED nurse knows that which of the following statements are correct regarding PICC lines?

A) A 10 ml or larger syringe should be used to flush the PICC line

B) Only continuous, non-turbulent, flush techniques should be used

C) Fluids must continuously be infusing in a PICC to prevent clotting

D) Placing the patient's arms over their head may create an internal line obstruction

A – For flushing PICC lines, the idea for syringe sizes is simply "Go big or go home." Though it may seem like you should use smaller syringes (1-5 ml) for smaller patients, the smaller the syringe, the higher the pounds per square inch (psi) and the higher the change of "popping" the PICC! Like peripheral IV lines, PICC lines certainly can be capped and patency maintained via intermittent flushes, preferably with the "push a little-stop-push a little" technique recommended to help remove build-ups in the catheter. Lastly, as with chest central lines or ports, if blood is not easily aspirated, then carefully changing the arm/patient position or having the patient perform a Valsalva maneuver can sometimes assist to remove, not create, internal catheter obstructions.

Lundblom's Lessons

The rescue phone rang in the ED to let us know that EMS would be arriving in 3 minutes with an unresponsive 2-year-old patient. Per family at the scene, the child has had a recent fever and cold.

Mom had been out shopping for about three hours and returned home to her live-in boyfriend and 2-year-old daughter. She found the child in bed, unresponsive and not breathing and called EMS, who immediately initiated bag-mask ventilation and chest compressions, placed an intraosseous line, and administered epinephrine. Upon arrival at the ED, the child was unresponsive, bradycardic and afebrile. She had a Glasgow Coma Scale (GCS) of 3 and fixed, dilated pupils. Per Mom, the history was that her daughter had a recent cold with fever that had resolved and stated she "was fine when I left to go to the store." We intubated the child because of her cardiopulmonary failure. The bradycardia and perfusion improved with oxygenation and ventilation. Labs (blood and urine) were unremarkable and the post-intubation chest X-ray was normal. Physical exam revealed no obvious injuries, but a brain CT scan showed cerebral edema, a skull fracture and intracranial bleeding due to a head injury unexplained by the mother or her boyfriend. The child died 2 days later in the Pediatric ICU without ever regaining consciousness.

Teaching points: The National Child Abuse and Neglect Data System (NCANDS) estimated almost 1800 children in the United States died from child abuse or neglect in 2008. During the past few years the numbers have been increasing without clearly identifiable causes. Many factors place a child at risk for non-accidental trauma (NAT). Children at increased risk of NAT include those who are very young, chronically irritable or demanding or have chronic medical or psychiatric conditions or developmental delay. Caregivers, who were abused themselves as children, are young or in a lower socioeconomic group (which increases the stress level of the family) may be more likely to abuse children under their care. Sadly, most experts believe that NAT is significantly under-reported.

Approximately 80% of children subjected to NAT are less than four years old. Infants constitute roughly 45% of abused children. Over 70% of all perpetrators are parents/caretakers. Fathers' and mothers' significant others are most commonly responsible for injuries resulting in death, while mothers are more often responsible for neglect, including failure to protect their children from their primary male caregivers.

Malnourishment/failure to thrive, poor hygiene, delays in emotional or intellectual development and failure to provide adequate medical and dental care are common forms of neglect. Common signs and symptoms of physical abuse include: bruises in unusual places or that resemble the shape of an item, multiple unusual bruises in various stages of healing, symmetrical burns or bruises, bite marks (are they really able to bite themselves in that spot?) and multiple fractures in different stages of healing. Ask yourself: Does this story make sense considering the injury? Are the caretakers/potential perpetrators changing the story either individually or jointly? Are they blaming a sibling? Has there been a delay in seeking care? Is this part of a "multiple" pattern (i.e., multiple bruises or breaks in multiple stages of healing, multiple visits to the ED, multiple hospitals used to lower suspicion, multiple stories)?

Remember that all charts will potentially become part of legal documentation/evidence, so chart accordingly! Facts, quotes from caregivers, witnesses and the children themselves, detailed descriptions of condition and injuries and an absence of conclusions or judgments on our part should be the rule. In addition, physical evidence such as blood, swabs, clothing and hair may need to be collected and maintained in a forensic chain of evidence, particularly in the case of sexual abuse. The best suggestion? Leave it to the experts! Whenever possible, utilize the skills and knowledge of a nurse examiner or law enforcement personnel trained in the investigation of child abuse. Our job is to stabilize immediate medical needs, ensure the child's safety in our ED, report to the appropriate agency or person and facilitate the preservation of evidence.

While the ED nurse will face many situations that are traumatic, one of the most difficult is a critical or fatal child abuse case. In our setting, we often are faced not only with taking care of the child, but also with dealing with a parent or caretaker that may be suspected of perpetrating the abuse. Due to the vulnerability of the patient, the often-horrific injuries and the frequent involvement of caregivers who should be trustworthy, a child abuse case can be a critical incident for the nurses and other staff involved with the child. Reactions to a critical incident vary from person to person, but can include physical and emotional symptoms such as: nightmares, changes in sleeping patterns, confusion, anxiety, difficulty breathing and many more. What is important is that we as health care providers don't neglect our own physical and mental health--talk to your supervisor, a counselor, a pastor--but don't let it take you out of the profession!

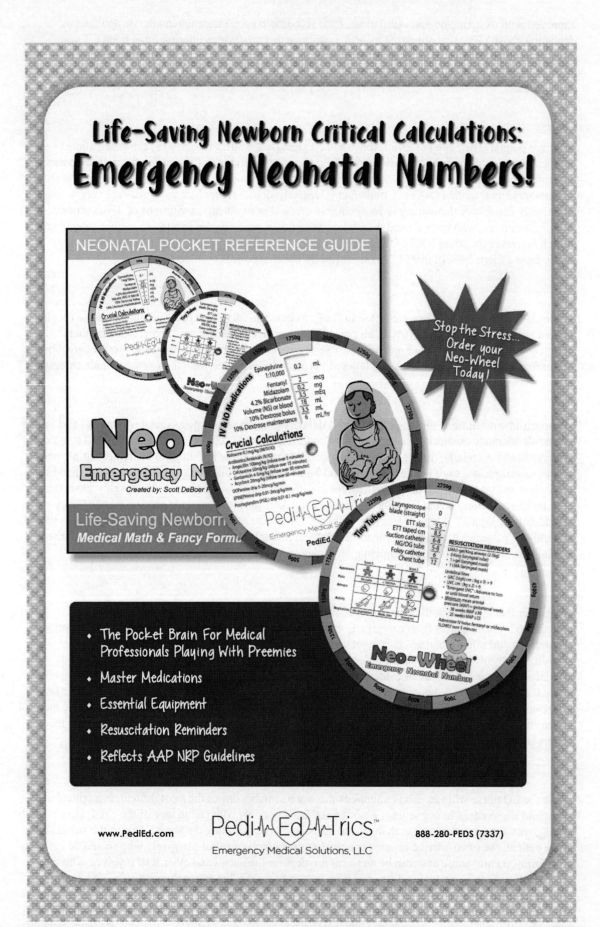

Chapter 3

Respiratory/EENT Emergencies
Working and Wheezing

Adam and Eve had many advantages, but the principal one was that they escaped teething.
-Mark Twain

Pertinent Pediatric Ponderings (NOTES)

CHAPTER 3
Sample Test Answer Sheet

1. _____	26. _____	51. _____	76. _____
2. _____	27. _____	52. _____	77. _____
3. _____	28. _____	53. _____	78. _____
4. _____	29. _____	54. _____	79. _____
5. _____	30. _____	55. _____	80. _____
6. _____	31. _____	56. _____	81. _____
7. _____	32. _____	57. _____	82. _____
8. _____	33. _____	58. _____	83. _____
9. _____	34. _____	59. _____	84. _____
10. _____	35. _____	60. _____	85. _____
11. _____	36. _____	61. _____	86. _____
12. _____	37. _____	62. _____	87. _____
13. _____	38. _____	63. _____	88. _____
14. _____	39. _____	64. _____	89. _____
15. _____	40. _____	65. _____	90. _____
16. _____	41. _____	66. _____	91. _____
17. _____	42. _____	67. _____	92. _____
18. _____	43. _____	68. _____	93. _____
19. _____	44. _____	69. _____	94. _____
20. _____	45. _____	70. _____	95. _____
21. _____	46. _____	71. _____	96. _____
22. _____	47. _____	72. _____	97. _____
23. _____	48. _____	73. _____	98. _____
24. _____	49. _____	74. _____	99. _____
25. _____	50. _____	75. _____	

[Remove page and cover rationale until after you answer question]

Pertinent Pediatric Ponderings (NOTES)

Certified Pediatric Emergency Nurse (CPEN) Review IV

1) Which of the following types of medications are **most** commonly used with asthmatic patients?

A) Bronchodilators and diuretics

B) Beta-blockers and bronchodilators

C) Corticosteroids and bronchodilators

D) Diuretics and beta-blockers

C – The mainstay of management for pediatric asthma remains bronchodilators i.e. Albuterol or Xopenex (levalbuterol), as well as steroids i.e. Prelone (truly awful tasting prednisolone), Pediapred (better tasting prednisolone), Orapred (best tasting prednisolone), and Solumedrol (IV methylprednisolone.) Asthma is characterized by three problems. First is smooth muscle bronchospasm, quickly followed by airway edema and finally the clogging of the airway by mucous. Bronchodilators take care of one problem, while steroids help with the other two. Beta blockers can induce bronchospasm and as such, are not recommended for asthmatic patients.

2) Bronchopulmonary dysplasia (BPD) is **most** commonly found in patients who:

A) Are ex-preemies

B) Have had multiple RSV infections

C) Have required multiple intubations for asthma

D) Have cystic fibrosis

A – Bronchopulmonary dysplasia (BPD) is also known as "Baby COPD." It is most commonly found in ex-preemies who required prolonged ventilation in the neonatal ICU and had their lungs beat up really bad in attempts to keep them alive. They, like many older "COPDers," are managed with albuterol, diuretics, and steroids.

3) A 6-week old child presents to the ED with persistent cough and is diagnosed with pertussis (whooping cough.) Which of the following orders should the ED nurse question?

A) Small, frequent feedings

B) Continuous cardiac/respiratory monitoring

C) Erythromycin PO q 6 hours for 14 days

D) No need for isolation precautions

D – Pertussis is a highly contagious respiratory tract infection and isolation is recommended for five days after initiation of appropriate antibiotics. Pertussis has made quite a comeback, in part because there is no such thing as lifelong immunity. Most adults who were immunized as children are no longer immune and can infect incompletely immunized babies. Small, frequent feedings are the answer for just about any dietary question and may help to alleviate the post-coughing emesis that frequently accompanies pertussis. Continuous monitoring is needed as the intense coughing spells can lead to hypoxia and apnea. Erythromycin is the first drug choice for pertussis.

EENT / Respiratory

Certified Pediatric Emergency Nurse (CPEN) Review IV

4) A 10-year-old patient presents to the ED with the following signs and symptoms: Fever of 102.6F (39.2C), sore throat, and difficulty swallowing. During the initial physical exam, the tonsils are noted to be reddened and swollen, with more swelling on the right and the uvula is deviated to the left. The **most** likely diagnosis is:

A) Epiglottitis

B) Peritonsillar abscess

C) Retropharyngeal abscess

D) Bacterial tracheitis

B – Peritonsillar abscesses can occur in all ages, but most frequently in those 10-40 years of age. All of the listed conditions would include fever, sore throat, difficulty swallowing, and perhaps decreased oral intake as symptoms. The hallmarks of epiglottitis are drooling and inability to handle secretions in the presence of fever, sore throat, and a really sick appearing child. Due to the success of the Hib vaccine, epiglottitis is very uncommon these days in young children. Retropharyngeal abscess occurs most frequently in children 3-5 years of age, following a bacterial infection such as strep throat or oropharyngeal trauma (recent intubation or toothbrush trauma.) In addition to fever and sore throat (with visible bulging posterior pharynx in 25% of cases), the child appears sick and has posterior neck pain, especially with flexion (meningismus.) This type of neck pain is a sign that all of the diseases above, as well as meningitis, should be considered. Bacterial tracheitis is best described as "between epiglottitis and croup." These previously healthy children have thick, purulent tracheal secretions and can quickly obstruct and crash, but are in as much danger of obstruction as with epiglottitis. Trached tracheitis kids commonly look better and are less sick than their previously healthy counterparts. Now that the other info is out of the way, what was the easiest way to get the correct answer on this question? The question specifically mentions tonsils, so chances are the answer involves tonsils.

5) Surgical cricothyroidotomy is a recommended procedure for children over:

A) 2 years of age

B) 4 years of age

C) 6 years of age

D) 8 years of age

D – Surgical cricothyroidotomy is generally contraindicated in patients less than 8 years of age. Remember that, if you can bag-mask ventilate the child and make air go in and out, you don't need to "cric" them emergently. Additionally, in small children who are unable to be intubated, and for whom placement of a non-visualized, supraglottic airway (laryngeal mask or King airway) does not result in adequate air exchange, a needle, not a surgical, "cric" is the recommended next step. Children have a small, pliable, and mobile larynx and cricoid cartilage. This is coupled with the fact that the cricoid ring is the only circumferential support of the trachea in kids. If the cricoid cartilage is inadvertently sliced through, then the trachea may collapse. Though needle crics are not ideal, they can keep a child alive long enough to get help and are certainly better than the alternative of watching them die.

EENT / Respiratory

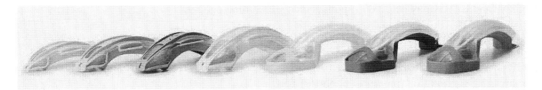

Range of i-gel Sizes

Photo courtesy of Intersurgical

www.intersurgical.com

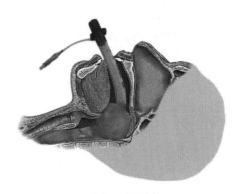

King Airway

Photo courtesy of Ambu USA

www.ambuusa.com

6) A 4-year-old child who fell from a three story window arrives at the ED with signs of a left sided tension pneumothorax. The ED nurse knows that emergent needle decompression with an IV catheter should be done at:

A) The fifth intercostal space, in the midclavicular line, just above the sixth rib

B) The fifth intercostal space, in the midclavicular line, just below the sixth rib

C) The second intercostal space, in the midclavicular line, just above the third rib

D) The second intercostal space, in the midclavicular line, just below the third rib

C – The first thing to remember is where to place the needle. Midclavicular – there are two breasts, so needle in the *second* intercostal space, between the second and third ribs. Midaxillary – You have five fingers, so needle just above the *fifth* rib (fourth intercostal space, between the fifth and sixth ribs.) The second important consideration is how to get into the place you've suggested. Always go **over** the lower rib, not under the upper rib. Routing the needle above the rib is suggested because important things like veins, arteries, and nerves (VAN) are under the ribs. An easy way to remember this is the VAN (vein, artery, and nerve) goes under the overpass (ribs.) If you stick a needle into the spots described in answers A and B, you will certainly decompress something; just not the lung, but the heart!

Certified Pediatric Emergency Nurse (CPEN) Review IV

7) Which of the following statements is **incorrect**?

A) CPAP and BiPAP may be used in spontaneously breathing patients

B) Use of CPAP or BiPAP does not require an endotracheal tube or tracheostomy

C) CPAP provides two levels of positive pressure; a higher level of pressure during inspiration and a lower pressure during expiration (pressure support/PEEP)

D) CPAP and BiPAP are used in the treatment of patients with acute and chronic respiratory failure

C – CPAP provides continuous positive airway pressure, while BiPAP provides Bi (two) levels of positive airway pressure; one for inspiration and a lower, second pressure for exhalation. Both are commonly used in emergency medicine and critical care areas with patients who are breathing on their own. Benefits of these modes of non-invasive ventilation include their use in non-intubated or non-trached patients and they can help avoid the need for intubation. BiPAP, by definition, uses two levels of pressure.

8) A 14-year-old male with a history of Marfan's syndrome arrives at your ED complaining of sudden onset of shortness of breath. Vitals: BP 85/54, HR 115, RR 40, Temp 98.9 F (37.2C), with only 86% oxygen saturation on room air. He is in moderate respiratory distress and has very diminished breath sounds on the left side. You suspect this patient has:

A) Aortic aneurysm

B) Spontaneous pneumothorax

C) Congestive heart failure

D) Pneumonia

B - This afebrile teen having sudden shortness of breath, decreased breath sounds, and hypoxia sounds like a pneumothorax, acts like a pneumothorax, and unless proven otherwise, has a pneumothorax. Marfan's syndrome is a genetic defect of the connective tissue which is commonly associated with tall children with unusually elongated faces, limbs, fingers and toes. The weaker connective tissues, coupled with slight deformities of the ribcage and sternum, can result in spontaneous pneumothoraces. Other feared complications that accompany these externally visible signs include 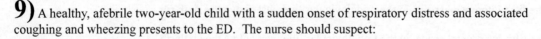 aortic aneurysms and congestive heart failure, but these set of symptoms do not point in those directions. The sudden onset and lack of fever make pneumonia a less likely diagnosis. When you hear Marfan's, think "bad things that can pop," i.e. pneumos and aortic aneurysms.

9) A healthy, afebrile two-year-old child with a sudden onset of respiratory distress and associated coughing and wheezing presents to the ED. The nurse should suspect:

A) RSV

B) Epiglottitis

C) Croup

D) Foreign body aspiration

D – As small children explore their surroundings, it is not uncommon for anything and everything to go into the mouth. Unfortunately, not everything belongs there and not everything leaves there easily. Foreign body airway aspiration should always be a prime consideration when the age and symptoms match the above situation. Children with epiglottitis tend to be acutely ill and febrile, while croup and RSV tend to be not as acute in their onset of symptoms.

EENT / Respiratory

10) A 4-year-old child who recently immigrated to the United States from a third world country presents to the ED with an oral temperature of 104F (40.0C), accompanied by respiratory distress, drooling, and severe sore throat. The ED nurse should suspect:

A) Epiglottitis

B) Croup

C) Pneumonia

D) Foreign body airway obstruction

A – This is classic epiglottitis. Though we don't see it that much anymore, due in great part to the widespread immunization with the H. Flu vaccine, epiglottitis is still out there. Classic signs of epiglottitis are: 1) Sitting up (they breathe better sitting up), 2) Drooling (they can't swallow spit as their throat is too swollen and tender), and 3) Acute fever of 103-104F (39.4-40C.) These children "tri-pod" so they can better align their airway, and they tip the lungs forward in the chest which results in better air exchange (like prone positioning for ARDS.) If someone mentions the "E" word, it's epiglottitis until proven otherwise.

11) The child in the above question continues to deteriorate and he is now in need of endotracheal intubation. This procedure should ideally be done in:

A) The emergency department

B) The operating room (OR, theatre)

C) The pediatric ICU

D) Radiology

B – Think about two things with this child's airway. First, who do you want to intubate this kid? The answer: Anesthesia. Second, where does anesthesia have all of their toys and like to play? The answer: In the OR. In addition, if anesthesia can't get this kid tubed, what is going to need to be done? The answer: A cric or trache, and honestly, where do we want to do a trache? The answer: In the OR. So if possible, the best place to put in the endotracheal tube is in the OR. This child was in need of endotracheal intubation from the time the diagnosis was recognized, as the goal is to intubate them *before* they deteriorate.

12) Which of the following is recommended when caring for a child with suspected epiglottitis?

A) Forcibly administer oxygen by tight-fitting, non-rebreather mask

B) Administer IM Rocephin (ceftriaxone)

C) Hold the child supine to examine the airway

D) Allowing the child to remain in her mother's arms

D – Allowing the child with possible epiglottitis to stay with her mother is one of the best actions that an ER nurse can take. All of the other choices can trigger the same consequence – Acute upper airway obstruction. This child is sitting up to try to breathe and if you hold him down, that only makes it more difficult for him to breathe. Soft tissue X-rays may still be requested by surgery to confirm the diagnosis as epiglottitis is so uncommon in the United States. Remember the "E" word and anesthesia should only take a peek at their airway in the operating room (theatre) when you have lots of help, the ability to do a peds surgical airway, and preferably a non-crying child due to general anesthesia.

Certified Pediatric Emergency Nurse (CPEN) Review IV

13) In January, a 6-month-old child arrives via parents to the ED with respiratory distress, cough, and runny nose for the past 12 hours. Vitals: RR 48, HR 138, and rectal temperature of 100.8F (38.2C.) Auscultation of the lungs reveals fine crackles and wheezing throughout, along with moderate subcostal retractions. The ED nurse should suspect a likely diagnosis in this child as being:

A) Asthma

B) RSV bronchiolitis

C) Epiglottitis

D) Pneumonia

B – Remember, all that wheezes is not asthma and most, but not all, bronchiolitis is caused by RSV. Most of the time, these symptoms would point to asthma. But in a 6-month-old child in the winter with a runny nose, it's most likely RSV. And if it's not RSV, it's because he's thinking about getting RSV or some other type of bronchiolitis.

14) Which of the following is one of the first signs of respiratory failure?

A) Decreased respiratory rate (RR)

B) An increase in heart rate (HR)

C) Circumoral cyanosis

D) A decrease in blood pressure

A – Patients in early respiratory failure have usually been tachycardic the whole time they've been in distress. Tachycardia is a very early sign of all kinds of stress in kids. Decreasing respiratory rates from failure must be distinguished from decreased respiratory rates from successful treatment. The way to differentiate is to look at the trending RR in the context of the whole patient. If the RR is dropping, but the mental status is deteriorating (or at least not improving), and the heart rate is remaining elevated or even rising (much less abruptly dropping), it's a BAD drop in RR. If the child is perking up, air exchange is improving, sats are going up, and the HR is staying about the same (due to nebs) or decreasing gradually with treatment, it's probably a GOOD drop in RR. Respiratory rates and mental status are much more sensitive indicators than tachycardia.

15) A common word used by parents to describe the cough that accompanies croup is:

A) "Whooping"

B) "Barking"

C) "Loose"

D) "Dry"

B – When parent's present to the ED with young children for evaluation of a cough, and describe the cough as sounding like "barking" or "like a seal," you can suspect croup. A "whooping" sound is associated with whooping cough (pertussis.) It never really left us, but as adult pertussis immunity wears out, we can now carry the bug and transmit it to children with inadequate vaccine coverage. With this in mind, adults with fragile respiratory conditions and healthcare providers are now being revaccinated to avoid getting the disease themselves and to cut down on transmission to our little patients. "Loose" or "dry" coughs can be found with various other conditions including pneumonia, RSV, and asthma.

EENT / Respiratory

Certified Pediatric Emergency Nurse (CPEN) Review IV

16) Croup is a:

A) Bacterial infection of the upper airway

B) Bacterial infection of the lower airway

C) Viral infection of the upper airway

D) Viral infection of the lower airway

C - Croup is a viral infection of the child's funnel-shaped upper airway. That means that at the bottom of the funnel, a little bit of edema quickly goes a long way. Current management of croup includes "cool-mist" via mask, hood, or blow-by, Vaponephrine (racemic epi), Heliox, and PO or IM steroids to minimize the airway edema. Antibiotics are not commonly indicated as most cases of croup are viral in origin.

17) Indications for endotracheal intubation include each of the following **except**:

A) Continued hypoxia despite the administration of O_2

B) Inadequate airway and/or loss of protective airway reflexes

C) Respiratory arrest or failure

D) Glasgow Coma Scale (GCS) of 10

D – The classic teaching regarding acute neuro-trauma and the Glasgow Coma Scale is: "If the GCS less than 8, then it's time to intubate!" Certainly if a child is in respiratory arrest, they should be bag-mask ventilated first, and then promptly intubated. However, if possible, the goal should be to intubate them before they stop breathing to prevent a possible secondary cardiac arrest. Airway protection, as it is a huge issue with head trauma patients, is another appropriate reason for intubation. Even if they are "breathing fine," if they can't protect their airway, aspiration and other complications of an unprotected airway are definite concerns.

18) Prior to chemical paralysis, children should receive each of the following **except**:

A) Neuromuscular blockers

B) Analgesics

C) Sedatives

D) Anxiolytics

A – Neuromuscular blockers are the medications used to induce chemical paralysis. Children, just like adults, should receive sedatives and analgesics prior to neuromuscular blockers (paralytics.) Anything else is simply inhumane. Unfortunately we still see this done and that is inappropriate, inhumane, and scary. I've had several transports involving pediatric trauma patients and asked "What did the child get for pain"? Answer. Norcuron (vecuronium.) "What did the child get for sedation"? Answer. Norcuron. "What did the child get to make him so wonderfully still"? Answer. Norcuron. One drug that does it all? Not the case! Paralytics, i.e. Norcuron, Pavulon (pancuronium), or Zemuron (rocuronium) begin with "P". They paralyze and that's all they do. The child is still awake, in pain, and scared out of their minds, but unable to do anything about it until the paralytic wears off. Remember, not only do you need to give the right medications (knowing what they will do,) you also need to know when to give them (knowing how long they will last.) Case in point: Versed (midazolam) lasts ½ hour. Sublimaze (fentanyl) lasts ½ hour. Pavulon (pancuronium) lasts 1 hour. That means that if your patient gets all three at about the same time, things are great for the first ½ hour. Your patient is asleep and pain free. But after about 30 minutes, your patient will wake up, trapped in a paralyzed body, and aware of things including the sensations of pain!

19) When caring for a child in ARDS (acute respiratory distress syndrome), suggested interventions include each of the following **except**:

A) Supporting optimal oxygen delivery

B) Supporting cardiac contractility

C) Maintaining an adequate hemoglobin

D) Never using positive end-expiratory pressure (PEEP)

D – We have all heard that to stay alive, blood needs to go round and round, and air needs to go in and out. The management of ARDS is no different. The goals are to maximize the ability of blood to go round and round (help the pump by supporting cardiac contractility), maximize the delivery of oxygen as the blood goes round and round (keep a good hemoglobin level and transfuse as needed) and help air go in and out. With ARDS, the biggest problem patients have is stiff lungs with non-cardiogenic pulmonary edema. PEEP is one of the mainstays of treatment for this condition. It allows for lower tidal volumes (6ml/kg) being used, resulting in lower risks of barotrauma (less beating up the lungs) and lower required amounts of supplemental oxygen, allowing the patient to be weaned down from 100%. Remember that PEEP is not without adverse effects such as hypotension, but when you think ARDS, think PEEP.

20) Classic clinical signs of a tension pneumothorax include:

A) Distended neck veins, tracheal deviation towards the affected side of the chest, and hyperresonance on the unaffected side

B) Flat neck veins, tracheal deviation towards the unaffected side of the chest, hyporesonance on the affected side

C) Distended neck veins, tracheal deviation away from the affected side of the chest, hyperresonance on the affected side

D) Flat neck veins, tracheal deviation away from the affected side of the chest, hyperresonance on the affected side of the chest

C – A tension pneumothorax, or a collapsed lung that is causing pressure on the heart and great vessels, can very possibly lead to death if not diagnosed promptly and if interventions are not performed quickly. Hopefully, it is diagnosed long before you get a chest X-ray to confirm the condition. Distended neck veins occur as the increased pressure in the chest causes the blood to back up. However, as with cardiac tamponade, this can be difficult to detect in little ones with virtually no necks. A very late finding can be tracheal deviation where the pressure on one side of the chest is so high that it actually pushes the trachea towards the unaffected side. This sign is occasionally found in adults in whom you can palpate the trachea from the suprasternal notch to the cricoid cartilage. Again, as little ones often appear to have no neck structures that we can easily distinguish, this sign may be hard to appreciate. Lastly, hyperresonance of the chest can be found with percussion. Air is trapped under pressure and upon tapping or percussing the chest may reveal that one side sounds are very different from the other. In addition to the classic symptoms listed above, the absence of breath sounds on one side, the look of impending doom, and compromised perfusion are signs that may indicate a tension pneumothorax, which should be treated as such until proven otherwise.

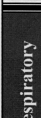

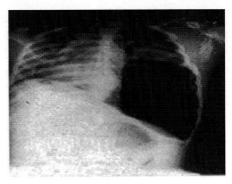

Tension pneumothorax

Image courtesy of Christopher Straus MD - University of Chicago Hospitals

21) The initial emergency treatment for the above child with a tension pneumothorax should be:

A) Placement of a pigtail chest tube

B) Admission to the pediatric ICU for observation

C) Needle decompression

D) Thoracoscopy

C – Though chest tube placement is certainly indicated in a child with a tension pneumothorax, in many cases, the child may well be dead by the time the chest tube tray is set up. Why wait? You can provide immediate relief with a needle decompression. Placing an IV catheter into the midclavicular or lateral chest allows the trapped air to be briefly released, and keeps the child alive long enough for someone to pop in a chest tube.

22) Which of the following does **not** cause tachypnea?

A) Diabetic ketoacidosis (DKA)

B) Metabolic acidosis

C) Respiratory alkalosis

D) Fever

C – Respiratory alkalosis does not cause tachypnea, but is actually caused by breathing way too fast (e.g. hyperventilating from anxiety.) DKA is associated with severe metabolic acidosis and children breathe faster to try to "blow off the acid." Children, like dogs who are way too hot, breathe fast to try to cool down.

23) Respiratory syncytial virus (RSV) is **most** common during:

A) Spring and summer

B) Summer and winter

C) Fall and winter

D) Year round

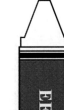

C – "RSV season," depending on where you are in the country, is most commonly from the late fall until early spring. Though patients can still get RSV during the summer, in most cases, summer is generally when we have time to recover from and prepare for the next RSV season. It is seen not only in "ex-preemies," but also in term babies whose siblings are playing with all the other supposedly healthy children in day care.

24) The **most** common reason(s) for cystic fibrosis (CF) patients coming to the ED involve:

A) Pulmonary exacerbations

B) Constipation

C) Congestive heart failure

D) A and B

D – Cystic fibrosis is a disease of the lungs, digestive system, or more commonly, both. It is a disease that is not well understood outside of the realm of the pediatric pulmonologist, gastroenterologist, or endocrinologist. Pediatric and adult ED nurses should become more knowledgeable about the disease, as CF patients now commonly live well into adulthood.

25) A 14-year-old CF patient presents to the ED with a complaint of constipation. What are the anticipated treatments?

A) Admit them directly to general pediatrics

B) Recommend stool softeners and discharge them to home

C) Deliver an enema and discharge them to home

D) Consider starting them on a stool softener, get sputum cultures, chest and abdominal X-rays, admit them to the hospital, and notify their primary CF physician

D – Ideally, CF patients should be followed in a CF center, but in many cases, that is not the reality in which they live. CF patients are prone to ileus formation, so with this complaint, abdominal X-rays should be done and the child should be admitted for further management. Just because they are complaining of constipation, doesn't mean we shouldn't be looking at the lungs as well, so we can help out the pulmonologist and get a sputum culture started while they are in the ED. It most likely took days for the constipation to get to the point that they came to the ED, and we are not going to fix it in a few hours with an enema or stool softeners. Here is another hint for getting correct answers on the test. "D" is the answer, not only because it is the correct answer, but also because it has the most things for you to assess or do for the patient. Perhaps the best thing to do for these children is to ask the parents and the patient what needed to be done the last time(s) this happened. Like it or not, they'll probably need the same thing again. It's important to utilize the caregivers of chronically ill kids to their best advantage and yours.

26) Cystic fibrosis (CF) should be suspected in infants and young children with each of the following **except**:

A) Congestive heart failure

B) Failure to thrive

C) Chronic cough

D) Meconium ileus

A – Congestive heart failure is not associated with cystic fibrosis. The earliest postnatal finding of CF is meconium ileus which occurs in up to 10% of newborns with the disease. CF is the most common organic cause of failure to thrive in infants and very young children because the condition interferes with the absorption of fats and fat-soluble nutrients. In the ED, when we think of CF patients, a child coughing up lots of nasty, thick mucus comes to mind and the same idea applies to the GI tract as they have chronic oily diarrhea. As the child with CF grows, the most constant medical feature is chronic cough with progressively increasing dyspnea. Way too much thick mucus in the lungs and GI tract is what seriously messes these kids up. In the neonatal ICUs of years ago, the down and dirty test for CF was the taste test. The nurses would literally lick the baby's skin and if it was really salty, then CF was probably the diagnosis. Happily, that technique has happily been replaced by formal sweat chloride testing. Generally speaking, in today's society, we tend to frown on the nurses licking the arms of the babies.

27) Emergency Department management of CF patients typically includes all of the following **except**:

A) Inhaled Pulmozyme (dornase alfa) and bronchodilators

B) Inhaled and/or intravenous antibiotics

C) Chest physiotherapy (CPT) and postural drainage

D) Intubation and positive pressure ventilation with 100% oxygen

D – Supplemental oxygen should be carefully administered, and as with "COPDers," non-invasive ventilation options to avoid the need intubation are preferred. As you can imagine, though gastrointestinal problems such as rectal prolapse (25% of CF cases), GE reflux, and constipation/obstruction can occur, respiratory problems are the reason for most ED presentations. With this in mind, continuing efforts to improve air exchange, remove the mucous that might be occluding, and quite possibly infecting, the airway, as well as treating the infections that might be present, are all very appropriate ED interventions.

28) Which of the following is an immediately life-threatening chest injury that should be identified and treated during the primary survey?

A) Tension pneumothorax

B) Pulmonary contusion

C) Myocardial contusion

D) Aortic transection

A – Tension pneumos and cardiac tamponades are the two chest injury conditions which present the most serious and most immediate threats to your patient. When these bad things occur, it is important to find them and fix them very quickly, before they kill the child. Pulmonary and myocardial contusions are serious situations, but like most contusions, we can worry about them a little later after the primary survey. Unfortunately, in most cases, children with true aortic transections are dead by the time they get to the ED.

29) A chest tube is placed in a child for a traumatic hemothorax. While the child is enroute to the pediatric ICU, the chest tube becomes completely dislodged from the chest. The initial nursing intervention should be to cover the wound with:

A) 4x4 gauze dressing

B) Vaseline gauze dressing

C) Tegaderm or Opsite dressing

D) Telfa dressing

B – Though conventional gauze dressings are helpful in catching the blood and keep the bed from getting dirty, they do little to stop the air from going in and out of what is now an open chest wound. With that in mind, tape an occlusive dressing such as Vaseline gauze on 3 sides (flutter valve effect) to stop the flow of air in and out of the wound. Suggestion: Keep an occlusive dressing handy, especially during transports, by taping the dressing to the chest drain system. That way, just like Mary's little lamb, everywhere the patient (and their chest tube go), the proper gauze dressing will surely follow.

30) In the above patient with a dislodged chest tube, what about if the tube is still in the chest, but the tubing becomes disconnected and is lying on the floor. Which nursing action should be undertaken?

A) Remove the entire chest tube immediately

B) Apply a clamp near the tube insertion site

C) Quickly pinch the chest tube and place the end of the tube in a bottle of sterile water or saline

D) Use the phone to order a new chest drain and do not do anything else with the chest tube

C – Placing the chest tube in a bottle of saline or water allows for some sort of a water seal to be maintained while someone else brings you a new chest drain set up. The old chest drain tubing is now dirty (it's lying on the floor and you know how nasty hospital floors can be), so it definitely should be replaced as soon as possible. Removing the entire chest tube makes no sense as it's still in the chest; just the tubing is disconnected. Clamping the tube can cause pressure to build up in the chest; a situation we would like to avoid. This is a serious situation, so just making a call and waiting doesn't really help your patient.

31) In 4-minutes, a 15-year-old child is going to arrive at the ED via EMS after sustaining a stab wound to the left lower chest. The ED nurse knows that this patient will most likely require workup for injuries to the:

A) Chest

B) Chest and abdomen

C) Chest, abdomen, and pelvis

D) Chest, abdomen, neck, and pelvis

B – Trauma surgeons still teach that penetrating gunshot or stab wounds anywhere below the nipples are injuries to the chest and abdomen until proven otherwise. The rationale is that you don't know at what point of the patient's respiratory cycle (inspiration or expiration) the injury occurred and you don't know where the bullet or knife went after the initial entry point.

32) Post-tonsillectomy bleeding is:

A) Expected and not a cause for concern

B) Most common 1-2 days after surgery

C) Most common 5-10 days after surgery

D) Most common 4-6 weeks after surgery

C – Though a small amount of bleeding after any surgical procedure may be expected, bleeding post-tonsillectomy can be life threatening. The bleeding can be just oozing or relatively brisk, but is rarely massive or continuous and rarely compromises the airway because these kids are usually awake, alert, and able to spit the blood and secretions out. Cumulative blood loss can be considerable, but it's rare to see a child bleed out in front of you. These are an ENT emergency, but usually nothing to get hysterical about. They tend to be pretty stable while in the ED, but you do have to watch their circulatory status pretty closely. This is one of the more common reasons a normal child might need a blood transfusion other than for major trauma or surgery.

33) A 5-year-old child who underwent a tonsillectomy one week ago is brought to the ED because of profuse bleeding from the nose and mouth. The child is pale, weak, tachycardic, and hypotensive. All of the following would be considered "primary interventions" **except**:

A) Clearing any blood clots from the nose and mouth

B) Administering 20cc/kg IV 0.9NS wide open

C) Drawing a blood sample for a CBC

D) Calculating the Glasgow Coma Scale (GCS)

D – Remember, it's all about the airway, but shock is a close second, and determining the GCS is not a priority intervention in this case. If the child can breathe around the clots, treat the shock. Obtain and maintain a patent airway and simultaneously treat for shock. Most children with post-tonsillectomy bleeding experience problems 5-10 days after the surgery when the eschar/scab at the surgical site falls off. As in the previous question, we have an airway problem! Airway management in these children can be difficult at best, as intubating a child with active airway hemorrhage is not fun by any means, but may be needed in conjunction with surgical repair. Remember your ABCs. If you don't have an Airway, you don't need to worry about Breathing or Circulation because without the "A," you won't have the "B or C" for very much longer. Here's another test tip: If any answer involves opening the airway, maintaining the airway, or asking the patient how they feel about having an airway, chances are that's the answer.

34) A 14-month-old child with a history of BPD has a tracheostomy and is ventilator dependent. While in the ED, the child develops increasing respiratory distress as evidenced by retractions and desaturations. The nurse's **first** action should be to:

A) Suction the trache

B) Replace the trache

C) Bag-ventilate the child with supplemental oxygen

D) Administer an albuterol treatment

A – Just as the unwritten law in the ED suggests that all women under the age of 90 are pregnant until proven otherwise, a similar idea applies to ventilator dependent children. With these patients, all problems are trache related until proven otherwise. This is especially true for the little ones whose traches are too small for an inner cannula. These small traches are easily clogged by even the smallest amount of, shall we say, boogers. Our first action should be to try to suction in an attempt to clear the trache and assess its patency. If you can't pass a suction catheter, then the trache must be changed, but this option should take place only after suctioning or finding out that you can't suction. Why remove a perfectly good trache if you don't need to? Administering supplemental oxygen, albuterol, and possibly bag-ventilating the child may be required, but try the easy stuff first.

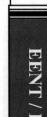

Certified Pediatric Emergency Nurse (CPEN) Review IV

35) A 16-year-old "frequent flyer" for sickle cell crisis presents to the ED with a fever, chest pain, and acute shortness of breath. In this child with a history of sickle cell disease (SCD), these symptoms are highly suggestive of:

A) Pneumonia

B) Acute myocardial infarction

C) Acute chest syndrome

D) Pneumothorax

C – Though most children in vasoocclusive or sickle cell crisis have pain in their extremities or abdomen, acute chest syndrome and stroke are two of the most feared complications of SCD. Acute chest, or acute occlusion of some of the smaller pulmonary arteries, is characterized by evidence of a new infiltrate on chest X-ray, fever, cough, chest pain, hypoxia, and respiratory distress. In most cases, it's virtually impossible to distinguish between pneumonia and noninfectious acute chest syndrome in the ED. So in most cases, these children are started on IV antibiotics assuming there's an infection present. As with more common vasoocclusive crises, management involves fluids, oxygen, and IV analgesics, however, children with acute chest may also require intubation, ventilator support, and emergency exchange transfusions.

36) Which of the following is **not** a suggested method for removing nasal foreign bodies?

A) Have parent blow into child's mouth while occluding non-affected nare

B) Using suction to remove object

C) Using alligator forceps to push object into the hypopharynx and then remove it from mouth

D) Using a catheter with balloon to facilitate removal

C – If it came in through the nose, then if at all possible, it should come out through the nose. Pushing the object back into the hypopharynx can be done, but is risky as it greatly increases the chance of aspiration into the airway.

37) A 12-year-old male arrives at the ED with his parents complaining of being awakened by a feeling of "something moving in his ear." The nurse notes a large, live cockroach in his external auditory canal. Anticipated initial treatment will most likely include:

A) Removing the live insect with forceps

B) Instilling mineral oil or lidocaine into the auditory canal

C) Irrigating the ear with warm water

D) Irrigating the ear with warm Raid ® cockroach spray

B - Mineral oil or lidocaine can drown or paralyze the insect and allows for a much easier removal. Until the insect stops moving, attempts to drown it or flush it out can result in the insect going deeper into the ear canal. Once it is chemically "neutralized," then removal with irrigation can be accomplished. Forceps removal is not recommended as lacerations of the ear canal and incomplete insect removal can occur.

EENT / Respiratory

38) An 8-year-old child is examined in the ED for complaints of ear pain. She is afebrile and has a 2-day history of itchiness in her left ear coupled with mild ear pain. Her mother informs the nurse that the child had been swimming in a public pool during the previous week. The ED nurse should suspect:

A) Otitis media

B) Otitis externa

C) Ruptured tympanic membrane

D) Mastoiditis

B – In an afebrile, well-appearing child, with a history of "itchy ear," otitis externa or "swimmers ear" is the most likely diagnosis. There is nothing in the history to suggest a ruptured tympanic membrane and children with otitis media are commonly in moderate to severe pain and frequently febrile.

39) All of the following are potential serious complications of untreated otitis media **except**:

A) Meningitis

B) Appendicitis

C) Mastoiditis

D) Permanent hearing loss

B – The expression, "You can't get there from here" applies in this case. Though rarely seen, otitis media can lead to meningitis, mastoiditis, and even permanent hearing loss. While analgesics and antibiotics are still commonly utilized for pediatric otitis media (OM) in the United States, times are changing. Current research is suggesting that in many cases, antibiotics may not be needed. With that in mind, the "wait and watch" approach is now recommended by the American Academy of Pediatrics and is increasingly being accepted by both pediatricians and families. With the "wait and watch" approach, the child is given analgesics and reevaluated in a few days. In many cases, the OM is found to be improving without antibiotics. Whichever treatment strategy is undertaken, it is important to remember that otitis media should not be ignored.

40) Which action is **inappropriate** for most pediatric patients with anterior epistaxis?

A) Having the patient or parent pinch the nose closed for 10 minutes

B) Alleviating patient and parental anxiety

C) Placing the patient in a semi-recumbent position with his head tilted forward

D) Administering IV fluids

D – Blood loss from anterior epistaxis (front of the nose nosebleeds) is rarely severe enough to warrant IV fluid administration. The majority of cases of anterior epistaxis stop completely on their own with sustained direct pressure. As with a cut on the arm, pressure must be held or it will start bleeding again. Alleviating anxiety (for the patient and the family) is always a good idea. Making sure the patient keeps his head tilted forward is appropriate and important because if the head is tipped back, the blood drips to the back of the nose and into the throat. If that happens, you can expect the patient to spit, cough, and even vomit if the blood is swallowed.

41) Despite sustained direct pressure, the previous patient continues to bleed through the nose. The nurse prepares a nasal tray by assembling all of the following **except**:

A) A catheter with a 30ml balloon

B) Sodium nitrate sticks and/or cautery

C) Gauze packing

D) Nasal cannula

D – A nasal cannula would not typically be used for packing. With continued bleeding, the physician, PA, or NP will commonly first try topical vasoconstrictors such as neosynephrine, as well as hemostatic dressings and agents to stop the bleeding. If that is unsuccessful, then gauze or balloon packing of the nares can be attempted.

42) The nurse informs the patient that the nasal packing will be removed after 24-48 hours. The purpose of removing the packing at that time would be to:

A) Assess the degree of edema

B) Prevent scar formation

C) Allow for further imaging studies

D) Minimize the chance of infection

D – Bacteria love blood and a bloody dressing left in a warm, moist place (like the nose) for a few days is a recipe for infection. Oral antibiotics are commonly prescribed for children who are discharged with nasal packing in place to help minimize the risk of infection.

43) A 16-year-old female arrives at the ED after being involved in a fight. She has obvious facial fractures and is evaluated by the ENT service. The physician informs the patient and her family that an open reduction of her facial fractures will be needed. Upon hearing this news, the patient becomes quite anxious. An appropriate nursing response would be to:

A) Obtain an order for Ativan (lorazepam)

B) Listen to the patient's concerns

C) Restrain the patient

D) Ask for a psychiatric consult

B – Remember, airway trumps just about every other answer. However, once the patient has no immediate airway concerns, then treatment of pain and "feelings" are the next "red flags" for answers. Before sedating (no matter how tempting it might be), calling psychiatry, or even restraining this patient, briefly finding out why she is so anxious and enlisting the help of the family members would be the correct answer.

EENT / Respiratory

Certified Pediatric Emergency Nurse (CPEN) Review IV

44) A 17-year-old presents to the ED with acute drooping of the right side of the face. The patient is previously healthy, has no history of trauma, and a negative head CT. The patient is diagnosed with Bell's palsy. As corneal abrasions can easily occur with this disease, the nurse should:

A) Apply "artificial tears" regularly to the affected eye

B) Place "steri-strips" to maintain closure of the affected eye

C) Rinse the affected eye regularly with an antibiotic solution

D) Apply eye patches bilaterally until the symptoms are completely resolved

A – The big ophthalmologic problem with Bell's palsy is corneal abrasions as the droopy eyelid does not completely close on its own. With this in mind, artificial tears to maintain the lubrication of the eye are regularly used. "Steri-stripping" the eye closed is not recommended and there is no indication for antibiotics in this patient as Bell's palsy is viral, not bacterial in origin. Lastly, patching both eyes closed, though indicated with eye trauma to prevent movement of both eyes, is unnecessary and would effectively leave this patient blind until the symptoms resolve (and that could be weeks or even months!)

45) A 17-year-old male apprentice carpenter arrives at triage complaining of severe eye pain and a feeling that "something is stuck in my eye." There are no obvious signs of penetrating injury to the globe. Which action would be **least** effective for relieving the patient's pain?

A) Instilling of fluoroscein stain

B) Instilling topical analgesics such as Tetracaine

C) Covering both eyes with gauze patches

D) Irrigating the eye with normal saline (NS) or Lactated Ringers (LR) solutions

A – Fluoroscein stain is commonly used prior to a slit lamp examination to help identify foreign bodies or corneal abrasions, but remember "the stain does nothing for pain!" After placement of an ophthalmic anesthetic such as Tetracaine, a Morgan Lens or similar device may be used to irrigate and hopefully remove the probable foreign body. Patching may be performed after the exam is completed.

46) A 15-year-old screaming male arrives at triage after an altercation in which unknown liquid chemicals were thrown into his eyes. Which nursing action has the **highest** priority for this patient?

A) Checking the pH of the patient's eyes with litmus paper

B) Instilling antibiotic drops

C) Flushing the eyes with a sodium bicarbonate solution

D) Continuously irrigating the eyes with normal saline (NS) or Lactated Ringers (LR) solutions

D – With few exceptions, irrigation with normal saline is the answer for most eye exposures. After a topical anesthetic is placed in the eyes, irrigation to remove the chemicals and checking the pH of the eyes is appropriate to determine the need for further irrigation. Irrigate first, do just about everything else, later. Just a quick side note, if the chemical had been in a powder form, the situation might be very different.

EENT / Respiratory

Certified Pediatric Emergency Nurse (CPEN) Review IV

47) Each of the following statements regarding chemical burns of the eye are true **except**:

A) Alkali burns are the most destructive

B) Acid burns are the most destructive

C) Alkaline chemicals continue to dissolve soft tissue in the eye until the chemicals are removed

D) The principles of management for alkali and acid burns to the eye are similar

B – Though certainly, neither acid nor alkali burns are desirable, alkali burns tend to be the worse of the two as they keep burning and dissolving tissue until the alkaline substance is completely removed. Irrigate, irrigate, irrigate... Pretty much whatever it is... Irrigate, irrigate, irrigate.

48) What is the **best** indication that treatment has been effective for the above alkali burn patient?

A) Evidence of corneal whitening

B) A pH value of 7.0 on a litmus paper reading

C) Intact extraocular movements (EOM's)

D) 20/200 visual acuity

B – While assessment of visual acuity and EOM's are certainly appropriate, when caring for patients with chemical burns to the eye, the goal in the acute phase is irrigation until a normal pH is restored.

49) A 16-year-old unrestrained driver presents to the ED with severe midfacial trauma. Because of the mechanism of injury, the nurse's **first** priority would be to:

A) Ensure an open airway

B) Notify the police about the crash

C) Perform a urine drug screen

D) Obtain facial x-rays

A – Again, airway trumps just about everything. If the answer involves airway, you should certainly read the other answers, but with few exceptions, the correct answer will be the airway one.

50) During the secondary survey, the nurse notes clear drainage from the patient's nose. The nurse should:

A) Order a head CT scan

B) Test the nasal drainage for cerebrospinal fluid (CSF)

C) Assume that the patient has an upper respiratory infection

D) Gently suction the nose with a 14f suction catheter

B – Though nasal drainage after a traumatic situation, could certainly be normal (especially with a crying child), far more serious is the possibility that the drainage is CSF. The trick is to be able to tell the difference. Is it treated with a tissue or is it treated with antibiotics and a neurosurgery consult? Most

148

of us remember the "Halo test" which involved taking blood mixed with CSF, placing it onto a gauze pad, and if you see a nice and pretty bulls eye pattern form, you've got CSF. Unfortunately, the Halo test only has a 50% sensitivity rate. This means that 50% of the time it works and 50% of the time it doesn't. That is the same as flipping a coin. But never fear; there is a better way. Test the drainage for glucose. There are a couple different ways to do this. 1) Taste it! (This is downright gross and understandably not recommended.) 2) "Dexi it." - Do an Accucheck, Glucometer, Dexi, Chem... Whatever you want to call it, check for glucose! If it tests positive for glucose, it's probably CSF. Here's an easy way to remember this for the test: Goobers have very little glucose and snot has very little sugar. If you have clear fluid dripping out of the ears or nose post-trauma and it tests positive for more than just a little bit of glucose, it's CSF until proven otherwise. Ordering a CT scan might be appropriate, especially if the drainage is positive for glucose, but can wait for the few seconds it takes to run the glucose test. We all know what happens when we assume something, and blind suctioning (beyond the opening of the nares) of nasal drainage of unknown origin, especially if it could be CSF, should never be chosen!

51) Le Fort fractures involve:

A) The facial bones

B) The cervical spine

C) The pelvic bones

D) The thoracic spine

A – Le Fort fractures are classified as Le Fort I, II, or III depending upon how badly the facial bones are messed up. What's much more important than memorizing Le Fort I fractures mean this is broken and Le Fort III fractures mean the face is completely broken, is looking at the big picture and saying "their face is broken… so what seriously bad things (i.e. airway) can potentially happen with a broken face."

52) A 12-year-old boy arrives at the ED with complaints of difficulty breathing. His parents state he has a long history of asthma with multiple ICU admissions and intubations. Initial ABG results on room air: pH 7.20, PCO_2 62, PO_2 65, and Bicarbonate 24. Interpretation of this ABG would be:

A) Metabolic acidosis

B) Metabolic alkalosis

C) Respiratory acidosis

D) Respiratory alkalosis

C – Respiratory acidosis. Answering ABG questions is easy when you remember three numbers and follow three basic steps. The numbers are 25 (Bicarb should be around 25) and 35-45 (CO_2 should be in this range and the pH as well (7.35-7.45.) 1) First, look at the pH. Is it normal (never on a test), down (acidotic) or up (alkalotic)? If the pH is less than 7.35, it is "something" acidosis. If the pH is above 7.45, it's "something" alkalosis. With just step one, you have narrowed the potential correct answers from 4 down to 2 (and you now have a 50/50 chance of getting it right.) 2) Look at the question. If the question mentions a patient with a respiratory problem, chances are the answer is respiratory "something." If the question mentions a patient with a metabolic or non-respiratory problem, chances are the answer is metabolic "something." 3) Lastly, once you have looked at the pH and the patient's complaint/history, then you can confirm the answer by figuring out which part is really messed up. Is the CO_2 (respiratory) out of whack (<35>) or is the bicarb (metabolic) out of whack (<22-26>)? Putting the acidotic pH (7.20) and history (asthma, a very respiratory history) together with an out of whack CO_2 (CO_2 of 62) reveals the correct answer of respiratory acidosis.

Certified Pediatric Emergency Nurse (CPEN) Review IV

53) Upon examination of the previous patient, which of the following findings would be the **most** concerning?

A) Pronounced wheezing and labored breathing

B) Productive cough with green sputum

C) "Silent chest"

D) Only able to speak two words between breaths

C – "Silent chest" is one of the scariest findings in an asthmatic. Wheezing, coughing, and speaking, even if only a few words at a time, means that the patient is still moving some air. Not wheezing and clear is very different than not wheezing and silent. Silence means that the patient is so clamped down, so mucous filled, and so edematous that he has a distinct potential of dying. The American Lung Association's current slogan summarizes it best. "If you can't breathe, nothing else matters!"

54) A 2-year-old near-drowning victim arrives via EMS at the ED in full arrest. He is intubated and ventilator support is begun. Initial pre-intubation ABG reveals pH 7.12, PCO_2 85, PO_2 33, Bicarbonate 12. In addition to intubation and ventilation, the patient is given a "big" bolus of sodium bicarbonate and a repeat ABG reveals pH 7.55, PCO_2 35, PO_2 425, Bicarbonate 36. The ED nurse interprets the latest ABG result as:

A) Metabolic acidosis

B) Metabolic alkalosis

C) Respiratory acidosis

D) Respiratory alkalosis

B – Remember those 3 steps to quick and easy ABG interpretation? 1) Look at the pH. It's alkalotic (above 7.45), so the answer is "something" alkalosis. 2) Look at the question. It specifically mentions the patient getting a bolus of bicarbonate. That's a clue that the answer is looking for something metabolic. 3) Still not sure… verify by checking which result is out of whack. The bicarbonate is way too high (36), so the answer is metabolic alkalosis.

55) A 16-year-old presents to the ED after doing crack cocaine reportedly for the first time. BP 150/70, RR40, HR130. He states he "feels like he's going to pass out" and has numbness in his hands and feet. ABG reveals pH 7.60, PCO_2 15, PO_2 140, Bicarbonate 22. The ED nurse interprets this ABG result as:

A) Metabolic acidosis

B) Metabolic alkalosis

C) Respiratory acidosis

D) Respiratory alkalosis

D – 3 steps to quick and easy ABG interpretation. 1) Look at the pH. It's alkalotic (above 7.45), so the answer is "something" alkalosis. 2) Look at the question. It specifically mentions the patient just did crack and now is hyperventilating (RR 40.) That's a clue that the answer is looking for something respiratory. 3) Still not sure… verify by checking which result is out of whack. The CO_2 is way too low (15), so the answer is respiratory alkalosis.

EENT / Respiratory

56) The goal of treatment for this patient would be to increase:

A) Oxygenation

B) Ventilation

C) Bicarbonate level

D) CO_2 level

D – This teen is oxygenating and ventilating just fine; in fact, probably too well. His hyperventilation is "blowing off" too much CO_2. Coaching the patient to help him restore a more normal respiratory rate in order to decrease the excess CO_2 excretion is the goal.

57) All of the following statements about the prior patient are correct **except**:

A) The patient will require follow-up counseling about substance abuse

B) The patient is having an anxiety "crack" attack

C) This patient's treatment will include rebreathing exhaled CO_2

D) This patient's treatment will include the administration of sodium bicarbonate

D – He is hyperventilating due to taking "crack," and the goal is to help him stop breathing so fast. Though medications such as Ativan (lorazepam) can be given, in many cases (especially with emotional teens), simple verbal reassurance and the placing a non-rebreather mask on the patient, but not hooking it up to oxygen can quickly resolve the symptoms. This technique forces the patient to rebreather his own CO_2 and his breathing should slow down (even without Ativan.) Of note, the "paper bag trick" is NOT recommended as the risk for hypoxia is very real.

58) The nurse appropriately suspects that the prior patient's symptoms are because of each of the following **except**:

A) Crack cocaine can cause these symptoms

B) Hypocarbia causes vasoconstriction of the blood vessels

C) Hypocarbia causes temporarily decreased calcium levels

D) Acidosis and hypercarbia

D – Hyperventilation results in alkalosis and hypocarbia. When the body starts playing with the pH (up or down), it affects other electrolytes as well, including calcium. Decreased serum calcium levels will result in the numbness or tingling sensations commonly found with hyperventilation, while the low CO_2 levels, associated alkalosis, and decreased cerebral perfusion from vasoconstriction will make the patient feel like he is going to pass out.

Certified Pediatric Emergency Nurse (CPEN) Review IV

59) A 16-year-old asthmatic has been successfully resuscitated from cardiac arrest and now is hemodynamically stable. An ABG is drawn and results are: pH 7.15, PCO_2 68, PO_2 50, Bicarbonate 18. The ED nurse interprets this ABG result as:

A) Metabolic acidosis

B) Mixed metabolic and respiratory acidosis

C) Respiratory alkalosis

D) Mixed metabolic and respiratory alkalosis

B – 3 steps to quick and easy ABG interpretation. 1) Look at the pH. It's acidotic (below 7.35), so the answer is "something" acidosis. 2) Look at the question. It specifically mentions the patient was in full arrest, but also is an asthmatic. That's a clue that the answer is probably looking both for something respiratory and/or metabolic. 3) Still not sure… verify by checking which result is out of whack. The CO_2 is way too high (68), but the bicarbonate is way too low as well (18), so the answer is mixed metabolic and respiratory acidosis.

60) The ED nurse would anticipate which of the following as the primary initial therapy for the above patient:

A) Improve oxygenation and ventilation

B) Administer IV fluid boluses

C) Administer sodium bicarbonate

D) Administer epinephrine

A – In this case, his asthma was severe enough to result in a cardiac arrest. Chances are if the oxygenation and ventilation improve, then the blood gas will normalize as well. Though bicarbonate may be given, the pH is low, but not "that low." More importantly, bicarbonate is frequently used to treat the numbers, but not the patient.

61) In late December, 4 children and 2 parents from the same family arrive at triage at noon complaining of headaches, nausea and vomiting for the past hour. Pulse oximetry at triage on all family members are >95%. The nurse suspects:

A) Carbon monoxide poisoning

B) Food poisoning

C) Viral syndrome

D) Lead poisoning

A – During the winter (and that was the big clue in the question), carbon monoxide (CO) poisoning should quickly be ruled out via arterial or venous blood gases determination of the CO level. There also are new pulse oximeters that not only display the pulse oximetry level, but also the CO level (www.masimo.com) and as such, do not require the child to get stuck. In traditional pulse oximeters, the sensor measures hemoglobin with "something on it." Usually that something is oxygen, but whether it is oxygen or carbon monoxide, most monitors don't care. They just read that something is attached to the hemoglobin. It is crucial to remember that a pulse ox of 100% paired with a CO level of 40, means that the "real" pulse ox is only 60%! That's why determining the CO level in cases such as this is so important. That being said, if several children in the same family present with similar symptoms present, could it be viral? Absolutely. But when all members of the family have the same story starting at the same time, viral syndrome is much less likely.

EENT / Respiratory

62) The nurse would anticipate the initial treatment for this family to include:

A) Breathing into an oxygen mask not hooked to oxygen

B) Administration of 100% O_2 via a nonrebreather mask

C) Albuterol nebulizers

D) Amyl and sodium nitrites

B – As carbon monoxide has a 230X greater affinity for hemoglobin than does oxygen, the immediate administration of high flow oxygen (via a non-rebreather mask) is indicated to try to even up the odds. If the symptoms continue, or the patients deteriorate, the use of hyperbaric oxygen therapy, though controversial, can be considered. Breathing into an unhooked oxygen mask will increase the carbon dioxide, and since the airway itself is not the problem, an albuterol treatment wouldn't be appropriate. Amyl and sodium nitrites are for cyanide, not carbon monoxide poisoning.

63) Which of the following is one of the **most** common causes of upper airway obstruction in unconscious children?

A) Food

B) Epiglottitis

C) Bronchospasm

D) Tongue

D – Little ones certainly put everything in their mouths and epiglottitis is still out there. However, in an unconscious child, as with adults, the tongue is the culprit in many cases of airway obstruction. Bronchospasm is a big word and might distract you, but remember we're talking about an upper airway obstruction.

64) Which of the following symptoms is compatible with complete upper airway obstruction?

A) Hoarseness

B) Inability to talk or cry

C) Forceful cough

D) Wheezing

B – If kids who are awake can't talk or cry, that is certainly not normal, and in a distressed child, is highly indicative of complete airway obstruction. Hoarseness, coughing, and wheezing mean than some air is going in and out, and are suggestive of a partial airway obstruction.

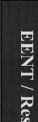

EENT / Respiratory

65) The nurse assesses a well known, "frequent flyer" asthmatic. All of the following are **late** signs of respiratory failure **except**:

A) Bradycardia

B) Tachycardia

C) Cyanosis

D) Loss of consciousness

B – The goal in treating asthmatics is to recognize that they are in trouble and intervene before the late signs of respiratory failure such as bradycardia, cyanosis, and unconsciousness are present. Remember, most of the treatments for asthma "jazz them up, not bring them down." So being tachycardic, jumpy, and alert, especially while on continuous albuterol nebs, is normal. Remember, subtle changes in mental status can signal the progression from respiratory distress to failure.

66) When reviewing the ABG on the above patient with acute respiratory failure, the nurse would initially expect to find:

A) Hypoxia

B) Hypoxia and hypercapnia

C) Hypercapnia

D) Hypocapnia

B – With asthma, air is having a hard time getting in, but more importantly, it can't get out. So, when really sick asthmatics get sleepy, the problem is not so much hypoxia (too little O_2), but hypercapnia (way too much CO_2.) This is different than a normal asthmatic that falls asleep because it's 3 A.M. Think about an angry young child who tells his mother, "I'm going to hold my breath until I pass out and die!" What should mom tell him? "Go for it!" What will happen? He will hold his breath and quite possibly pass out. Is he hypoxic? Probably not, but he's got way too much CO_2. As he passes out, his breathing changes from voluntary to involuntary, he blows off the extra CO_2, wakes up with a bad headache, and hopefully has learned not to try that tactic again. If an asthmatic gets sleepy, especially if his breathing is not a whole lot better, be prepared. This is not a reassuring sign!

67) Narcan (naloxone) is used to reverse respiratory depression associated with each of the following medications **except**:

A) Vicodin (acetaminophen and hydrocodone) and Tylenol #3 (acetaminophen with codeine)

B) Versed (midazolam)

C) Morphine and Sublimaze (fentanyl)

D) Heroin (smack)

B – There are two really good types of drugs that we play within the ED. Drugs to take away pain (opiates) and drugs to put people to sleep (benzodiazepines.) Opiates of the legal and illegal varieties are reversed with Narcan (naloxone), while "benzos" such as Valium (diazepam) or Versed (midazolam) are reversed with Romazicon (flumazenil, Anexate)

EENT / Respiratory

68) Which assessment finding is an **early** finding suggestive of hypoxia?

A) Change in level of consciousness

B) Peripheral cyanosis

C) Central cyanosis

D) Pulse oximetry reading of 85%

A – Remember, your brain only wants three things to be happy… blood, glucose, and oxygen. If a patient is becoming hypoxic, long before they turn purple (centrally or peripherally) or even desaturate, the astute nurse will notice changes in patient's level of consciousness. If a peds patient has an acute change in mental status, check for hypoxia, hypoventilation, and hypoglycemia before you start worrying about a problem with the brain itself.

69) The nurse would suspect a 15-year-old patient with a stab wound in the right upper abdominal quadrant is short of breath because of:

A) Pain and anxiety

B) Peritoneal irritation

C) Gastric injury

D) Associated chest injury

D – Pain and anxiety (after all, he was just stabbed), coupled with an unhappy peritoneum (i.e. one that was stabbed), certainly can result in shortness of breath. But… remember, with penetrating injuries, any injury below the nipples is chest and belly until proven otherwise. Gastric injuries are more common with left, than right sided injuries as the stomach is on the left side.

70) The above patient develops increasing shortness of breath and subcutaneous (SQ) emphysema in the right chest. This is **most** likely indicative of:

A) Pneumonia

B) Pneumothorax

C) Pericardial tamponade

D) Liver laceration

B – Whatever he was stabbed with probably hit not only the abdomen, but the lung as well. When air from the lung leaks out into the surrounding tissues, the result is subcutaneous (SQ) emphysema. SQ emphysema + shortness of breath = pneumothorax.

EENT / Respiratory

Certified Pediatric Emergency Nurse (CPEN) Review IV

71) The discharge instructions for a teenager with an isolated rib fracture should include information on the need to report fevers, shortness of breath on exertion, and abnormal sputum production. These symptoms are particularly suggestive of:

A) Pneumonia

B) Emphysema

C) Influenza

D) Pneumothorax

A – These are symptoms of pneumonia. Broken ribs hurt. In fact, they often hurt so much that people don't want to breathe as deeply as normally, and coughing (often the result of not breathing well) is especially painful with one or more broken ribs. Time for another formula: Shallow breathing + not coughing = pneumonia!

72) Autotransfusion is usually indicated for patients with which condition?

A) Left-sided hemothorax with hypotension

B) Hypotension secondary to bilateral femur fractures

C) Traumatic amputation of the right arm

D) Splenic trauma due to a motor vehicle crash

A – In the emergency department, autotransfusion involves using a chest tube and collection system (Pleurovac or similar device) to drain and temporarily store the patient's own blood from a hemothorax. This blood is then quickly re-infused into the patient through an IV. This is most commonly done in cases of massive chest trauma with significant hemothoraces. Blood from other sites, such as extremities or the abdomen, are not used for autotransfusion.

73) A flail chest is described as:

A) One rib broken in one place

B) One rib broken in two places

C) Two (or more) ribs broken in one place

D) Two (or more) ribs broken in two places

D – Flail chests are defined as having two or more ribs broken in two or more places (2x2.) This results in a "free floating" chest segment. The diagnosis is confirmed by radiography and is characterized by paradoxical chest wall motion (when most of the chest goes up, the flail segment goes down and vice versa, like a see-saw.) The problems with flail chests are not only the broken ribs, but also the associated pulmonary contusions under the flail segment. Remember flail chests are very uncommon in young children because their ribs tend to bend instead of breaking. Flail segments are seen more in older children and teens with significant blunt force trauma. Aggressive ventilator support may be appropriate, but the real key to managing a flail chest is to manage the pain associated with the condition. IV morphine works very well to take away the pain, but too much morphine can cause the patient to forget to breathe (never a good thing.) What many pediatric trauma centers are now doing for their patients with flails is really cool; they are placing epidural catheters for pain relief. When properly placed and maintained, epidural analgesia can allow for kids to get off a vent quicker; and if they are not on a vent, it helps keeps to them off a vent. The moral of the story is to treat the pain and allow the pulmonary contusions and the ribs to heal.

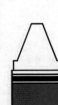

EENT / Respiratory

74) A 16-year-old with a clotting disorder arrives at the ED with left lower leg pain for two days. She relates learning that she was pregnant last week and was told to stop her Coumadin (warfarin) and start on Lovenox (enoxaparin.) However, she has not yet started the injections due to "insurance problems." Upon dorsiflexion of the foot, the patient complains of calf pain and the nurse correctly interprets this response as a positive:

A) Trousseau's sign

B) Homan's sign

C) Kehr's sign

D) Chvostek's sign

B – Homan's sign is pain with dorsiflexion (the opposite movement of push on the gas or brake pedal) and can be elicited when a patient has a deep vein thrombosis. Coumadin (warfarin) is contraindicated in pregnancy and starting this patient on Lovenox (enoxaparin) was an appropriate medication change. However, as she has a clotting disorder, is pregnant (hypercoaguable), and has not been on her anticoagulants for over a week, her leg pain screams "DVT!" Remember though, once the diagnosis has been confirmed via ultrasound, further testing for Homan's sign (that painful response) should no longer be done to avoid possibly causing a pulmonary embolus. As a side note, warfarin is commonly used as rodent poison. Something to remember when dealing with patients suspected to have ingested an overdose of this medication.

75) A 7-year old with cerebral palsy, a tracheostomy, and a home ventilator presents with upper respiratory symptoms. While the nurse is completing the initial assessment, the child experiences a severe coughing spasm and desaturates from 96% on room air with his vent to 78%, producing copious amounts of thick secretions from the tracheostomy tube, mouth, and nose. The nurse repeatedly suctions, alternating with ventilations with 100% oxygen via bag-valve device. The oxygen saturations do not rise above 86% and he becomes cyanotic and difficult to bag. What should the ED nurse anticipate to be the next step?

A) Continued suctioning, as the patient's oxygenation will not improve until the secretions are cleared from the airway

B) Asking the parent about the child's baseline saturations and pulmonary resistance to bag-valve ventilation

C) Removal of the tracheostomy tube, replacement with one a size smaller, and continued ventilation and suctioning

D) Removal of the tracheostomy tube, immediate bag-ventilation via the stoma or mouth/nose, and replacement of the trach tube with one of the same size

D – As with any emergency response, remember airway and breathing. In this case, we have an airway obstruction, so remove the obstruction and provide bag-mask ventilations. Replacement of the artificial airway can come after oxygenation has improved. Although asking the parent about their child's baseline is an important part of the assessment, especially with special needs children, the matter of immediate significance here is that the child is desaturating and has become/stayed cyanotic. This means that a saturation of 86% and being difficult to bag are not indicative of his usual status. Replacing the trach tube with a smaller size is a valid option when one cannot smoothly insert the same size into the stoma (why there should always be a smaller size trach available). But with thick copious secretions, downsizing the tracheostomy tube should only be done after the attempt with the same size tube has failed.

Additional Pediatric ED Attending Physician Insights: "I'd argue that it's unlikely you'll have a replacement tube right there during your initial assessment unless the family's got one in their "Go Bag." Frankly, I don't recall ever ordering a replacement tube to the bedside of a trached patient in the ED unless I suspected there were problems with the tube from the get-go. More realistically, the nurse doing the initial assessment needs to try bagging this child via the upper airways (conventional style) with the old tube still in place (although this will theoretically only work with an uncuffed tube or one in which the cuff isn't functioning,) OR remove the tube and try to bag through the stoma without a tube in place while a replacement tube is located. It's easy to forget that most kids with traches can be ventilated easily by the conventional route because they're not usually trached for abnormal upper airway anatomy, but for pulmonary toilet, prevention of aspiration or poor respiratory drive/effort. It's much better to gain control of airway and breathing outside of the trach tube. Then you can work on replacing the trach tube itself in a less-pressured, safer effort, with a stabilized patient. Think physiology instead of procedures or equipment. It's exactly the same as emphasizing bagging over immediate endotracheal intubation."

76) A 9-year old girl with sickle cell disease presents with complaints of chest and joint pain, fever and cough. Vital signs are an oral temperature of 102.1°F (38.9°C), HR 138, RR 40, BP 116/82 and SpO2 90% on room air. She rates her pain at 8 out of 10 on the numeric rating scale. Which of the following interventions represents the highest priority for her?

A) Obtain intravenous access and treat her pain with morphine, Sublimaze® (fentanyl) or Dilaudid® (hydromorphone)

B) Send blood to the blood bank for type and screen to prepare her for possible transfusion of packed red blood cells

C) Prepare her for a chest radiograph, send blood for CBC and culture, and begin intravenous antibiotic therapy

D) Apply high flow oxygen at 10-15 lpm via non-rebreather face mask and continue to monitor her oxygen saturation

D – It is important to remember to treat airway and breathing issues first when dealing with children with chronic illness, just like any other patient. All of the above interventions certainly should be done, but the order doesn't change in the face of chronic illness or pain. She is demonstrating signs of acute chest syndrome. Acute chest syndrome is a vaso-occlusive crisis affecting approximately 40% of patients with sickle cell disease and is the most common reason for early mortality. Younger children generally present with fever, cough and upper lobe disease. In sickle cell crisis, it is important to oxygenate the remaining (non-sickled) red cells capable of carrying oxygen. If you can't breathe... nothing else matters!

77) A ventilator-dependent child with a tracheostomy comes to the ED for a minor burn to the leg. As treatment is being completed, which of the following actions is appropriate?

A) The nurse should call child protective services because all injuries to children with special needs are reportable.

B) The nurse should ask the parents/guardians if the local EMS providers are aware that there is a technology dependent child in the community and recommend that they notify them if not already done.

C) The nurse should immediately advise EMS providers of the technology dependent child in the community because failure to do so would be considered to be endangerment of a minor.

D) The nurse and hospital administrator should call for a social service consult due the apparent inability to provide a safe environment for the child.

B - All too often, EMS providers are unaware of children (or adults) in their area with special medical needs. Many times their first encounter with a "trached" and/or ventilator dependent patient is in an emergency situation. These encounters are even more stressful for the EMS providers if the patient is a child. Many families are not aware of the benefits of making their situation known, not only to EMS, but also to the electric and phone companies. Utility companies commonly grant priority service for households with special needs patients. It is very appropriate for us to give the families this information. While we are especially vigilant about possible child abuse or unintentional endangerment, there is nothing in this scenario that should lead us to those concerns. Because of HIPAA, healthcare providers cannot take it upon themselves to inform EMS providers of potential patients in their area unless they have permission from the patient and/or family.

78) Emergency equipment that should be immediately accessible to a child with a trach includes all of the following **except**:

A) A back up trach of the same size

B) A back up trach one-half or one size smaller

C) An "Ambu™ bag" with the appropriate sized mask

D) A programmable defibrillator

D – Most children with traches will not require defibrillation, and if a defibrillator should be needed in an emergency, an AED (Automatic External Defibrillator) with pediatric pads would be preferable. All of the other equipment listed should be immediately accessible in case of emergency. In addition, children with tracheostomies who go on any sort of a "road trip" (whether it is to a physician's office, emergency department or vacation), should have a fully stocked "Go Bag" that includes:

- Two spare tracheostomy tubes with matching obturators (one the correct-size and another one-half or one-size smaller)
- Trach ties
- Gloves
- Correct size "Ambu bag" (infant/peds/adult)
- Correct size face mask
- Water-based lubricant
- Correct size suction catheters (2x the trach size) and a portable suction device
- Spare HMEs (heat-moisture exchange unit or "artificial nose")
- Trach dressings
- Hand sanitizer and alcohol wipes
- Stethoscope
- Scissors

Not all emergency departments stock a full range of trach supplies (especially supplies needed for children) and the "Go Bag" can be invaluable in pediatric emergency care.

79) Important information to gather from the caregiver about a child with a trach includes all of the following **except**:

A) The medical specialty of the patient's primary care provider

B) How long the child has had a trach and why do they have it

C) The degree of difficult (or easy) to replace the child's trach

D) If the child ever had a complication during a trach change and if so, what happened

A – The more you know about that child's trach, the better. You will want to know the answers to these questions to prepare for a decannulation emergency. Remember that the family/caregiver is often your best source of information regarding the "norm" for their child. Many times the parents/caregiver will be able to offer "tricks" for what works well in caring for and/or replacing their child's trach.

80) All of the following information is important when preparing to replace a trach tube **except**:

A) The "outside diameter" (OD)

B) The "inside diameter" (ID)

C) The "lip line" depth of the tube

D) The length in mm

C – This is a question to reinforce the need to really read the question, and hopefully everyone realizes that a trach tube doesn't pass through the lips. All of the other information is needed to order a comparable tracheostomy tube that will work as an emergent backup.

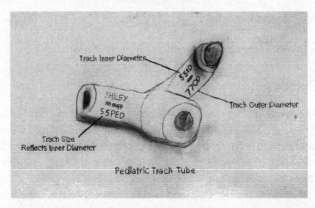

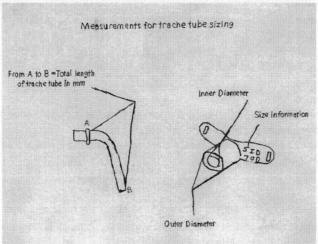

Tracheostomy tubes
Courtesy of Nina DeBoer, my then 12-year old aspiring artist/baker daughter
www.ninasbeliciousbakery.com

81) A ventilator-dependent child with a trach tube is in the emergency department and needs an emergent MRI for a possible acute spinal cord injury. Which of the following is the **most** significant concern for the staff?

A) Obtaining written, informed consent for the procedure from the legal guardian

B) There are no concerns with placing a trached patient into an MRI unless the trach tube is made of metal

C) Confirming the type of trach tube and preparing for recannulation if needed

D) Obtaining a non-metallic ventilator for the MRI

C – More and more tracheostomy tube manufacturers are making silicone tubes, and in some cases a metal coil is placed to add support to the silicone so it doesn't remain floppy. These types of traches (i.e. older Bivona®) will need to be swapped out prior to a MRI. Most respiratory therapy departments maintain a list of trach tube types that will indicate which tubes contain metal. If a patient needs a replacement, that list should tell you which trach tube is the best alternative. While obtaining consent is important, if the situation is emergent, written, informed consent may not be critical. Answer "B" is incorrect for the reason mentioned above and we are not familiar with any sort of non-metallic ventilator.

82) A 6-month old ventilator-dependent patient with a tracheostomy continues to be in severe respiratory distress despite suctioning. An obstructed trach is suspected because it is difficult to bag-ventilate the child. The pediatric ED nurse would anticipate which procedure to be performed next?

A) Chest percussion and repeat tracheal suctioning

B) Emergency tracheostomy tube change

C) Administration of an albuterol treatment

D) Oral intubation with a 4.0 endotracheal tube

B – The FIRST thing to do for a vent-dependent child in respiratory distress is to remove the child from the ventilator and bag-ventilate the child, even before suctioning or attempting to change airway equipment. In this situation, that step has already been taken. If respiratory distress continues and there is difficulty using bag to ventilate the patient, an emergency tracheostomy tube change should be performed as it is very likely that the tracheostomy tube has a mucous plug or other obstruction causing the sudden and rapidly increasing respiratory distress. Though the saying that "albuterol fixes everything" is prevalent in pediatric emergency care, it does not apply in this case. Chest percussion therapy and albuterol may be indicated, but only AFTER the child has a patent airway. If a replacement tracheostomy tube is not immediately available, an endotracheal tube (ETT) can be gently placed into the stoma. But it is crucial to remember that if used, the ETT does not need to go in very far before entering the mainstem bronchi and it is quite easily dislodged once it is in place.

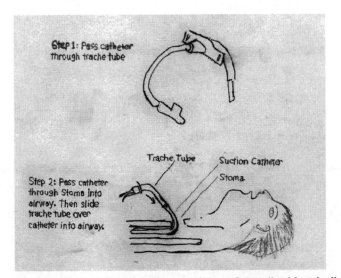

Replacing trach tubes with a suction catheter "guide wire"
Courtesy of Nina DeBoer, my then 12-year old aspiring artist/baker daughter
www.ninasbeliciousbakery.com

83) To emergently replace a tracheostomy tube, the child should be in what position?

A) Sitting up in the "tripod" position

B) Supine with a small towel roll under the shoulders

C) Lying on his left side

D) Reverse trendelenberg

B – A child requiring an emergency trach replacement should be positioned supine with a small towel roll under the shoulders. Remember the ever important "sniffing position" to optimize the pediatric airway. This position will ease the insertion of the trach back into the stoma. (Complications such as accidental decannulation occur at home in up to 58% of children with tracheostomies!) If the tracheostomy tube is partially or fully out of the stoma, don't panic. While a small percentage of children require the trach to keep their airway open, most children can breathe through the stoma for a short time. The aforementioned "small percentage" includes children with tracheomalacia (abnormal collapse of the tracheal wall) or tracheal stenosis, so the more you know about the reason for the trach, the better! After proper patient positioning, attempt insertion with the same size tracheostomy tube. If that is unsuccessful, quickly try again with another trach tube one-half to one full size smaller. As soon as the tracheostomy tube is replaced, placement should be confirmed much like oral or nasotracheal endotracheal tubes, using auscultation, observation of chest rise and documentation of pulse oximetry and capnography. In addition, watch and feel for the development of subcutaneous emphysema in the neck, the appearance of which might indicate the placement of the tube in a false soft tissue tract or tracheal perforation.

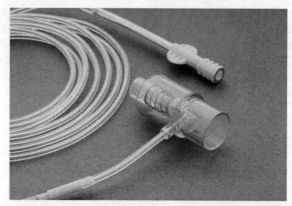

Endotracheal or tracheostomy tube capnography device
Courtesy of Oridion Medical - www.oridion.com

84) You have been unsuccessful with attempts to replace a dislodged tracheostomy tube in a child with both the appropriate size and one size smaller tubes. What is/are your other options?

A) Bag valve mask ventilation (BVM) over the mouth while occluding the stoma, or BVM over stoma while occluding mouth and nose

B) Use an endotracheal tube to intubate via the mouth or stoma

C) Attempt to place the trach using a suction catheter as a "guide wire"

D) Any or all of the above and call otorhinolaryngology (ENT) or surgery docs/nurse practititioners

D – Even when using an obturator, it can sometimes be difficult to get a trach back into the airway. Knowing one's options can help to relieve the anxiety of patients, parents and medical personnel alike. In patients with intact pharyngeal and laryngeal areas (basically the area from the mouth to the cricoid ring), bag valve mask ventilation on the face is possible using gentle occlusion of the stoma with your hand. In rare patients where the pharyngeal and/or laryngeal areas may be occluded (such as after surgery for tumors, scarring or even congenital abnormalities such as a very large tongue in a very small mouth), bag valve mask ventilation can be achieved by placing the mask over the stoma itself and gently bagging. There is also the option of obtaining an airway by passing an endotracheal tube thru the mouth (if there's no fixed high airway obstruction as listed above) or stoma. Sometimes helpful is the technique of passing a suction catheter through the stoma and into the patient's airway to act as a guide wire, then passing the trach over the catheter. The final option is to attempt another surgical airway. Elective tracheostomies are most commonly placed between the 2nd and 3rd or 3rd and 4th tracheal rings for best cosmetic results and to facilitate securing the tube. In these cases, the cricothyroid membrane is still intact and may be used in a true emergency. Remember, if the child is doing well and you are having trouble getting the trach back in, give supplemental oxygen as necessary and call ENT or Surgery (per hospital protocol). Continuing to try to replace the artificial airway may cause more harm than good. In the short term, the patient just needs an intact airway--it doesn't have to be plastic!

85) A 4-year old child presents to the ED complaining of cough, fever of 101.0°F (38.3°C), swollen glands, decreased appetite/activity, weight loss and night sweats. The mother tells you the child's fever and cough have been on and off for a couple weeks but have worsened over the last week. The child appears small for weight. The triage nurse should have a high index of suspicion for what disease?

A) Croup

B) Flu

C) Meningitis

D) Tuberculosis (TB)

D – This presentation virtually screams "possible TB!" Mycobacterium tuberculosis (TB) is spread through airborne particles when an infected person sneezes, coughs, speaks, or sings, yodels or raps. TB droplets can remain suspended in the air for several hours, so close quarters contact, such as in hospitals or homes, allows for the relatively easy spread of TB. Fortunately, TB is not generally transmitted through environmental surfaces (bedside tables, linens, etc.) or personal items (hairbrushes, etc.). Interestingly, most young children with TB are either minimally infectious or NOT infectious, as the TB bacteria are confined to the small air spaces. As the TB victim ages, the "tubercles" of bacteria grow around and rupture into the larger airways, making the bacteria much easier to expel.

Latent tuberculosis infection is when a person has a positive TB skin test, but has no symptoms of active TB and is not infectious. If the disease is going to develop into active TB, it will usually do so within the first two years following infection. Once the latent infection progresses to active disease, the classic symptoms (such as night sweats, weight loss--formerly "consumption"--and blood-tinged sputum) are present. TB is commonly initially treated with INH (isoniazid) and rifampin; however, multi-drug resistant TB (MDR-TB) which is resistant to INH/rifampin and, more recently, extensively-drug resistant TB (XDR-TB) which is resistant to INH, rifampin and fluoroquinolones (Cipro®, ciprofloxacin) have become a challenge. Of note, in 2009, the CDC reported that the average cost of hospitalization for one patient with XDR-TB was an astonishing $483,000!

Emergency department staff should have a high index of suspicion for possible TB cases and place patients in isolation with doors remaining closed until the absence of TB has been confirmed. In addition, staff in close contact with these patients must wear the N-95 masks to minimize the chance of becoming infected.

Certified Pediatric Emergency Nurse (CPEN) Review IV

86) Which of the following statements is **true** regarding chest tubes?

A) Chest tubes should always be routinely "stripped" or "milked" every 4 hours and as needed

B) Chest tubes are placed to "water seal" to overcome positive intrathoracic pressure

C) Chest tubes empty first into the water seal chamber, then the drainage chamber

D) The water seal chamber acts as a one-way valve, allowing air out of the chest

D – The water seal chamber acts as a one-way valve, allowing air in the pleural space to escape and not return.

False statement A – Stripping or milking can cause transient intrathoracic pressure changes which may injure the lung tissue. Stripping or milking of chest tubes should ONLY be done gently and as needed, per very specific physician or advanced practitioner's order.

False statement B – Chest tubes are placed to water seal to overcome negative intrathoracic pressures. The only way to get the bad stuff out of the pleural space is to suck on it harder than the patient's chest cavity is trying to keep it in there. Remember, we inhale by creating a negative pressure to suck air into the lungs. The main principle behind chest tubes is to create a negative pressure differential by using a greater negative pressure outside of the chest wall to pull the air, blood, pus or other fluid out. Any spot that is "negative" (i.e. lungs on inhalation, chest drain) is going to be sucking stuff into it!

False statement C – The drainage from the chest first goes into the drainage chamber (imagine that) and then to the suction collection device.

87) Which of the following statements is **true** regarding chest tubes?

A) Chest tubes can drain blood, air, pus, transudate fluid, and lymphatic fluid

B) Chest tubes may be unclogged by infusing 1:10,000 heparin into the tube

C) Chest tubes should have dependent loops in order to promote proper drainage and avoid back flow or regurgitation

D) Chest tubes should be clamped just before the collection chamber to assess for air leaks

A – Chest tubes are inserted to drain blood, air, pus, transudate fluid and lymphatic fluid.

False statement B – Heparin does not dissolve clots; it only prevents them from forming! Chest tubes may be unclogged with TPA (alteplase) or streptokinase, per your agency policies.

False statement C - Dependent loops can collect stagnant fluid, which then impedes drainage. This can cause a reaccumulation of air or blood, and serve as a breeding ground for bacteria.

False statement D – Tubing should be clamped as close as possible to the insertion site in the patient, in order to assess whether the leak is with the patient or with the collection system. If you clamp the tubing close to the patient's chest and still have an air leak, then the leak is in the system, not in the patient. There are really only three places that an air leak can occur with a chest drain system. Two leaks involve the patient and one is in the chest drain system itself.

EENT / Respiratory

1. A leak at the insertion site in the chest wall itself (inadequate dressing or sutures where the tube enters the chest)
2. A leak within the patient, meaning that the patient still has a pneumothorax
3. A leak in the system anywhere distal to the chest (the point of the chest tube insertion site). Simply put, something in the tubing/collection chambers has a leak

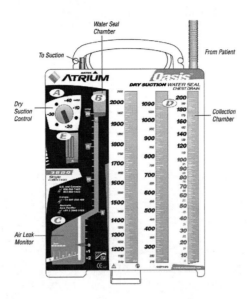

Overview of chest drain components 1

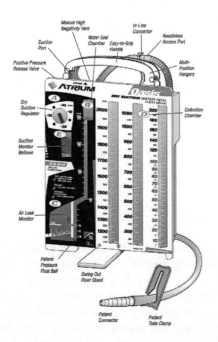

Overview of chest drain components 2

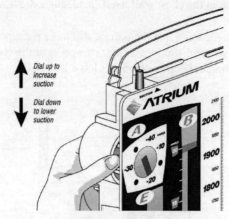

Suction control dial

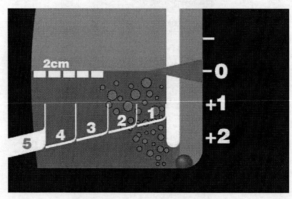

Bubbles in water seal chamber

Above chest drain components images courtesy of Atrium Medical
www.atriummed.com

88) A 3-year old child with H1N1 "swine flu" is being discharged from the ED. Which statement by the caregiver demonstrates correct understanding of the discharge instructions?

A) "I will give her 325mg of aspirin every four hours for fever."

B) "I will bring her back to the ED if her fever does not break or her breathing worsens."

C) "I will follow-up with our pediatrician in two weeks."

D) "It's OK to have her return to day care tomorrow."

B – Bacterial pneumonia is a very real complication of H1N1 and should be treated without delay. Worsening respiratory symptoms may signal that the child has pneumonia and should be considered a "red flag." Generally speaking, follow-up should be in a week or sooner, especially if the child remains febrile, gets new symptoms, or looks and/or acts sicker. Aspirin is no longer recommended to treat fever in children due to its association with Reye's syndrome. Day care is most likely where this child caught H1N1, so returning to the "scene of the crime" this early would definitely not benefit this child or the other children and staff. Remember that viral shedding continues for 5-10 days from the onset of symptoms, and even longer in young children. Kids with proven or strongly suspected influenza should generally be kept out of daycare/school for 1-2 weeks.

Certified Pediatric Emergency Nurse (CPEN) Review IV

89) A 6-year old child comes to the ED with complaint of a persistent fever. His mother states he was just diagnosed with H1N1 (swine flu) two days ago. The child is awake, alert and in no distress. What would the **priority** intervention be at this time?

A) Administer antipyretics for fever

B) Place the child in a private room

C) Place an isolation mask on the child

D) Obtain an accurate weight in kilograms

C – Safety questions can take many forms, and this is one of them. Based on the above presentation, it is obvious that this child is a "non-urgent" or stable patient. Considering that you really don't want an emergency department full of people exposed to H1N1, placing an isolation mask on the child will help to protect other patients, families, or staff members from potential infection. Even though all of the above interventions are appropriate, the first priority here is safety.

90) The mother of an intubated child asks the nurse to come to the room as "something is beeping." Upon entering the room, the nurse finds the high pressure alarm on the ventilator is the source of the alarm. This is most likely due to any of the following **except**:

A) The child biting on the endotracheal tube

B) The child "bucking" the ventilator

C) The child being disconnected from the ventilator

D) The child's endotracheal tube being clogged with secretions

C – Low pressure alarms on a ventilator commonly mean one of two bad things: 1) The endotracheal tube or trach is no longer attached to the ventilator or, even worse, 2) The child's endotracheal tube or trach is no longer attached to the patient, i.e. they are extubated. Low pressure = you no longer have a closed system (something is disconnected somewhere). All of the other answers would result in high pressure alarms, indicating increased resistance to gas flow in and/or out from the ventilator. High pressure = your system is obstructed somewhere.

91) Positive end-expiratory pressure (PEEP), especially at high levels, can cause:

A) Hypotension

B) Hypertension

C) Hyperventilation

D) Hypoventilation

A – To stay alive, two things have to happen. Blood needs to go round and round and air needs to go in and out. With cases of ARDS, pulmonary edema, etc., which result in stiff lungs and air having a really hard time going in and out, PEEP can be incredibly helpful to keep those noncompliant lungs open. However, the veins are the drains and if the pressure throughout the chest (where not only the lungs but also the heart and great vessels are located) is high (i.e. with lots of PEEP), blood has a hard time returning to the heart from the body. This can quickly result in hypotension. This demonstrates that it's a fine balance between flow in and out (air) and flow around and around (blood).

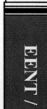

EENT / Respiratory

92) Heliox (a mixture of helium and oxygen) may be beneficial in the management of severe asthma because it is:

A) Less dense and less turbulent than O2 alone

B) More dense and more turbulent than O2 alone

C) Less dense but more turbulent than O2 alone

D) More dense but less turbulent than O2 alone

A – Heliox is less dense and less turbulent than oxygen alone, and this combination may help increase oxygen delivery and medication delivery to patients with a severe and acute respiratory problem, like a really bad asthma attack. The airway during a severe asthma attack could be described as a clogged up drinking straw; clogged due to edema, mucous, and bronchospasm. The patient may have no trouble breathing through the equivalent of a wide open pipe, but now he has to try to breathe through a clogged up straw. Albuterol nebulizer treatments work great to relieve the symptoms, but the problem is that the medicine has to make it from the mouth to the alveoli through the clogged up straw. Physics reminds us that dense or "heavy" gases get stuck and don't move as freely as lighter gases. Lighter gases are mellow and they just go with the flow. Helium is lighter than oxygen (that's why helium balloons float away) and heliox = helium + oxygen. This gas mixture (typically 60-70% helium/30-40% oxygen) is given in conjunction with continuous nebulized albuterol. It does a nice job of shepherding the albuterol and oxygen through the clogged up drinking straw, especially in really sick kids. Remember that heliox is NOT a treatment (it won't reverse the edema or bronchospasm), but it will allow for increased oxygenation and improved medication delivery while we are waiting for our bronchodilators to take effect.

93) Cultures for respiratory syncytial virus (RSV), influenza (flu) and pertussis (whooping cough) should be obtained using a swab inserted into the:

A) Posterior nasopharynx

B) Posterior oropharynx

C) Anterior nasopharynx

D) Anterior oropharynx

A – For icky/contagious things such as RSV, flu and pertussis in children, the posterior nasopharynx is the site of choice to obtain cultures. The anterior nasopharynx (front of the nose), anterior oropharynx (front of the mouth) and posterior oropharynx (back of the mouth) may, but are less likely to, yield positive results. Down the nose is where the swab goes!

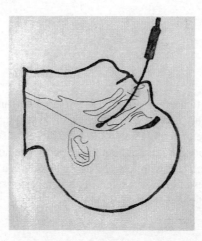

Nasopharyngeal RSV/pertussis/influenza swab technique
Courtesy of Nina DeBoer, my then 12-year old aspiring artist/baker daughter
www.ninasbeliciousbakery.com

94) A 14-year old presents to the ED after having an unknown substance splashed in his face earlier in the day. His eyes are visibly reddened and there is active tearing. A Morgan Lens® is to be inserted for irrigation. When placing the lens into position, it is important to remember to tell the patient to:

A) Look up while the superior part of the lens is inserted

B) Look down while the superior part of the lens is inserted

C) Look right while the lateral part of the lens is inserted

D) Look left while the lateral part of the lens is inserted

B – To insert the Morgan Lens®, ask the patient to look down while you retract the upper lid and insert the top of the lens. Next, have him look up while you retract the lower lid and insert the bottom part of the lens. (Note: There is no specified top or bottom of the lens. The part that you insert onto the upper part of the eye becomes the top by default.) If you know something nasty is going to happen, instinctively you look away and this concept applies to having something placed into your eye. Hopefully, looking down (away) when something is being placed up and looking up (away) when something is being placed down will minimize blinking. Removal is simple, just reverse the process. If available and not contraindicated, the use of ocular anesthetic drops (such as tetracaine or pontocaine) is advised prior to insertion of the lens. As with an IV line, the tubing and lens of the Morgan Lens® should be flushed prior to insertion. And you should continue running the fluid until it is time for removal of the Morgan Lens®.

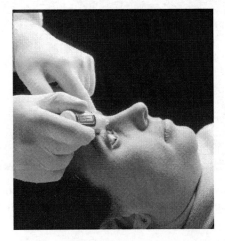

Morgan Lens® step 1 – Instill topical ocular anesthetic, if available.

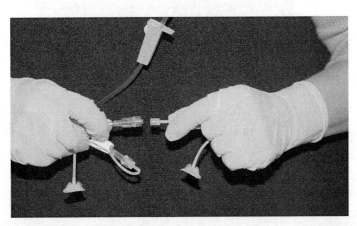

Morgan Lens® step 2 – Attach Morgan Lens® delivery set, IV set-up, or syringe using solution and rate of choice; Start flow.

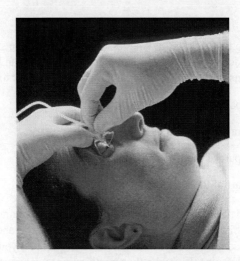

Morgan Lens® step 3 – Have patient look down, insert Morgan Lens® under upper lid. Have patient look up, retract lower lid, drop lens in place.

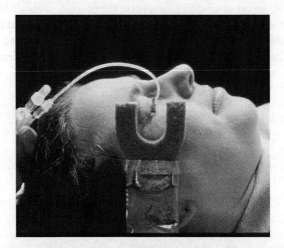

Morgan Lens® step 4 – Release the lower lid over Morgan Lens® and adjust flow. Tape tubing to patient's forehead to prevent accidental lens removal. Absorb outflow with the Medi-Duct®. Do not run dry.

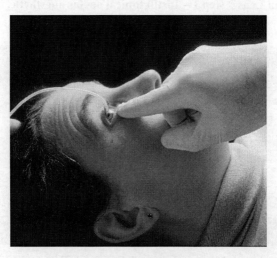

Morgan Lens® step 5 – Removal: Continue flow, have patient look up, retract lower lid – hold position.

Certified Pediatric Emergency Nurse (CPEN) Review IV

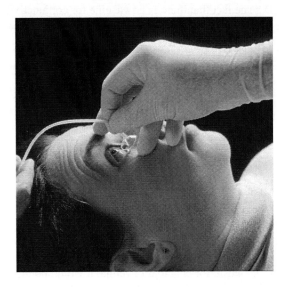

Morgan Lens® step 6 – Slide Morgan Lens® out; Terminate flow

Morgan Lens Uses	Solution	Mode with Morgan Lens	Rate	Frequency
Ocular injury due to acid burns or solvents, gasoline, detergents, etc.	Lactated Ringer's** I.V. Solution	Morgan Lens Delivery Set or I.V. set-up	500 ml rapid/free flow. Reassess and continue at slower rate.	Once. Repeat as necessary.
Alkali burns	Lactated Ringer's** I.V. Solution	Morgan Lens Delivery Set or I.V. set-up	2000 ml rapid/free flow. Reassess. Continue at 50 ml/hour or 15 drops/minute.	Continuous until pH of cul-de-sac is returned to neutrality.
Non-embedded foreign bodies	Lactated Ringer's** I.V. Solution	Morgan Lens Delivery Set or I.V. set-up	500 ml rapid/free flow. Reassess and continue at slower rate.	Once. Repeat as necessary.
Foreign body sensation with no visible foreign body	20 cc sterile solution	20 cc syringe	Slowly without force.	Once. Repeat once if necessary.
Routine pre-operative	10 cc of preferred ocular antiseptic	10 cc syringe	Slowly without force.	Once.
Eyelid surgery	Lactated Ringer's** I.V. Solution	Morgan Lens Delivery Set or I.V. set-up	4 drops/minute.	During entire procedure.
Severe infection	Lactated Ringer's** I.V. Solution with suitable antibiotic and steriod***	Morgan Lens Delivery Set or I.V. set-up	50 ml/hour or 15 drops/minute.	Continuous for 70 hours, then 10-hour intervals until marked improvement.

*Allows Lens to "float" over cornea and sclera.
**Recommendation based on pH: Tears approximately 7.1, Normal Saline 4.5 to 7.0, Lactated Ringers 6.0 to 7.5.
***Use only when indicated.

Quality Certified
ISO 9001 & 13485

The Morgan® Lens
MorTan Inc.

Morgan Lens® images courtesy of MorTan – www.mortan.com

95) In patients with conjunctivitis, which of the following statements is correct?

A) "I can stop taking the antibiotic eye drops in a few hours if my eye feels better"

B) "I don't need to take eye drops, as the internet says pink eye is only caused by viruses"

C) " I need to wash my hands very frequently"

D) "My little brother is not at risk for catching this because he's up to date on his shots"

C – Conjunctivitis (aka. "pink eye") can be either viral or bacterial in nature and is highly contagious. Antibiotic eye drops or ointment should be used as directed, and will most certainly be for longer than a few hours after leaving the ED. The fact that there is no vaccine for conjunctivitis (which can be caused by many different organisms), coupled with its highly contagious nature, means that hand washing is crucial to prevent other family members and staff members from acquiring and passing on pink eye.

96) Hyphema is a condition in which there is bleeding into the:

A) Posterior chamber of the eye

B) Anterior chamber of the eye

C) Retina

D) Cornea

B – Hyphemas most commonly occur as a result of ocular trauma and are a sign of bleeding into the anterior chamber of the eye. The easy way to remember that the bleeding is in the anterior "front" chamber is the fact that both the patient (while looking in the mirror) and you can see that there's blood in the front of the eye. If it was bleeding into the posterior chamber or retina, it would not be visible to the naked eye and an opthalmoscope would be required to visualize the hemorrhage. There is no condition known as corneal hemorrhage, so that answer should be ruled out pretty easily. Emergency management of patients with a hyphema is summarized as "P4." Pain--give them something for pain. Patching--it looks gross and they are freaking out looking at it, so cover it up. Positioning--sit them up to reduce intraocular pressure, thus minimizing edema and further bleeding (let gravity be your friend!). Also, in order to minimize intraocular pressure, it's often recommended to initially keep the patient mostly at bed rest, which is very hard to do with kids. And that leads to the final P for Patience--the vast majority of hyphemas resolve just fine on their own with time and the other "Ps" - but patience is the key.

97) A 2-year old child is brought to you in the triage room by her mother. You notice that she is sitting up and drooling, has a rapid respiratory rate and is pale. You should:

A) Allow her to stay in her mother's arms until an appropriate room is found for treatment

B) Immediately get a blood pressure, pulse, and oxygen saturation to determine triage acuity

C) Obtain a weight for medications she will receive

D) Start an IV quickly to prepare for possible intubation

A – Sitting up and drooling should be a huge red flag cluing you into the possibility of epiglottitis. The child should be allowed to maintain a position that optimizes her respiratory effort and reduces anxiety. No attempts should be made to perform invasive procedures unless absolutely necessary. Most patients with respiratory distress from suspected epiglottitis go directly to the OR for intubation or advanced airway management by anesthesia or ENT. Fortunately, because of the wide spread of use of the HIB (Hemophilus Influenza Type B) vaccine, classic epiglottitis is now rarely seen in the United States. Don't let that get you too comfortable though, because it can still be seen in unvaccinated or under-vaccinated children. The most likely scenario leading to this presentation in a fully vaccinated child is an esophageal or tracheal foreign body. Your approach should be the same as if she has epiglottitis - keep everyone calm and comfortable and prepare to take immediate control the child's airway if she deteriorates.

EENT / Respiratory

98) You are working the ED triage area when a 7-year old male presents with an avulsed permanent front incisor tooth after falling at school. You quickly treat the minor collateral damage (contusion and inner cheek laceration = ice pack and packed roller gauze). The parent then asks what he should do with the tooth. You work in a large teaching facility with a dental surgery clinic in-house that can immediately see the child for further work up and treatment. You should:

A) Consider reimplantation in the tooth socket

B) Consider placing the tooth in gauze moistened with 0.9NS

C) Consider placing the tooth in gauze moistened with milk

D) Advise the parent that the tooth will not be able to be reimplanted

A – Given that the child can be seen immediately, it is appropriate to consider reimplantation of the tooth in the tooth socket. Placing the tooth in moistened gauze (either 0.9NS or milk) are acceptable alternatives, but only if the physician or advanced provider is unable to reinsert the tooth. The key points are: 1) The longer the tooth is NOT reimplanted, the less likely it is that efforts will be successful and 2) If the tooth is not temporarily returned to its socket, it should be kept moist with milk, saline, or a commercially available tooth preservation product. This is a dental emergency as permanent retention of the lost tooth should ideally occur in less than 60 minutes. This tooth was totally avulsed and in one piece. If there was a dental fracture with pulp exposed instead of an avulsion, the portion of tooth remaining in the jaw can be sealed with Dycal® (calcium hydroxide) to protect the exposed nerves and vasculature from damage or infection until a dentist can evaluate the injury. Gauze packing, topical/oral analgesics and empiric antibiotics are also suggested.

Additional Pediatric ED Attending Physician Insights: Attempting reimplantation is unarguably the correct answer. It's not hard to put a tooth back in place if the anatomy isn't distorted. It doesn't even matter if you put the tooth into the socket backwards – as long as it's only for a short time. The dentist can reinsert the tooth in the correct direction if necessary. The absolute best place for that tooth is back in the socket! Barring any cognitive or behavioral problems, children who are old enough to have permanent teeth are generally old enough to understand they should leave the temporarily reimplanted tooth alone and to spit it out if it comes out again.

Adult and Pediatric Dentist Insights: Dental trauma cases can be tricky, especially in pediatric patients. A few things to keep in mind:

1) You must be sure it is a permanent tooth that is involved. If it is a deciduous (baby) tooth, do not try to reimplant it. A lot depends on the age of the patient as well.

2) The length of time the avulsed tooth has been out of the mouth (under 60 min. is critical). The odds of successful reimplantation dive rapidly after an hour.

3) Touching the root surface of the avulsed tooth is not advised. There are periodontal ligaments on the surface which should not be disturbed. Gentle saline irrigation is acceptable if there is debris on the tooth. Milk is fine as well. Hank's Balanced Salt Solution® (HBSS) is best, but seemingly nobody has that on hand. Saliva is always good. If age/aspiration risks are appropriate and ED staff can't put the tooth back into the socket, the patient can keep the tooth in his/her mouth (between the cheek and gum, like chewing tobacco) until a dentist can reimplant it. Soaking in water should be avoided.

4) If the tooth is broken off and only roots are left in the jawbone, it may not be able to be saved at all. A dentist or oral surgeon would have to extract it. The patient needs pain medication, a soft diet and a dental appointment ASAP.

5) In most situations of dental fracture, root canal treatment is recommended in approximately 7-10 days. Obviously, follow-up with a dentist is necessary.

6) You may want to consider antibiotic therapy and Tetanus booster (if indicated).

7) Overall, re-implanting the tooth is fairly easy. It only goes in one way. Make sure the tooth is pushed completely up or down into the socket and is not interfering with the patient's bite. They should feel that all of the teeth are touching evenly. If the tooth is fractured near or on the root, it is not recommended to reimplant it.

8) In any case, a good long-term prognosis for dental trauma is nothing that can be guaranteed. We can all certainly try our best!

99) A 12-year old male presents with frantic parents and a chief complaint of "one side of my face is paralyzed." He recently returned from a summer camping trip in the northeastern United States and is currently afebrile. The Pediatric ED nurse knows that possible causes of the facial nerve palsy include all of the following **except**:

A) Trauma

B) Genetic defect from birth

C) Bacteria

D) Viruses

B – There is no current evidence indicating that new onset facial nerve palsy is linked to genetic defects from birth. Most pediatric patients who present with facial nerve palsies have facial weakness or paralysis. However, in most cases, facial sensation is intact or just slightly reduced causing the patient to report that the area is "a little numb." The majority of cases are unilateral, and this is especially true with Lyme disease where only about 1% of cases involve bilateral symptoms. (Tip: The patient did just come back from camping in the northeast, which is considered a moderate risk state.). For children with facial nerve palsies, it is crucial to ascertain whether or not they can move the muscles of both sides of their forehead. It would seem to make sense that it would be worse if someone could only move half their forehead instead of the whole thing; however, as with many things in healthcare, nothing is that easy.

The forehead is innervated by ipsilateral (same side) neurons and the lower half of the face is controlled by contralateral (opposite side) motor neurons (cranial nerve VII.) If there was a stroke on ONE side of the brain, the person might likely exhibit mouth droop, slurring speech, and other symptoms unilaterally, but the forehead on that side would still maintain voluntary control because it would still receive innervation from the OTHER side of the brain. This means that if the child has had a stroke on one side of their brain, the nerves coming from the other side of their brain can "cover for them" and allow the forehead to still move normally. Therefore, patients with a brain (central) cause of facial nerve palsy can still move their whole forehead.

If the issue is between the brain and the face (a peripheral nerve palsy), such as with facial nerve injuries and most inflammatory or post-viral conditions (such as Bell's palsy), it's a different story. In this case, the forehead and mid/lower facial muscles all along one side don't work (patients can't close their eyes, ruffle their brow, or smile on the SAME side) because of a problem along the lower pathway. The other side of the brain can't cover for an affected peripheral facial nerve. So remember, patients with peripheral facial nerve palsy can only move the unaffected (contralateral) side of the forehead. In this case it's better to be able to move only one side of the forehead because having a problem with a single nerve is much better than having a problem with your brain!

Children whose top (forehead) and bottom (face) are both droopy most likely do not require CT scans, MRIs, etc. In most cases, it's probably a (usually temporary) peripheral nerve issue that can be managed with eye lubricants, possibly steroids, antibiotics if Lyme disease is suspected or antivirals if herpetic lesions (HSV) are suspected. And, most importantly, time and patience are needed.

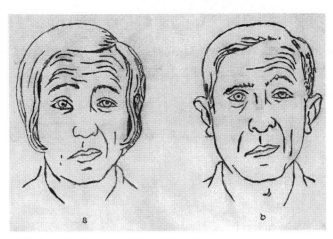

Peripheral nerves vs. brain issues and resulting facial droops
Courtesy of Nina DeBoer, my then 12-year old aspiring artist/baker daughter
www.ninasbeliciousbakery.com

Lundblom's Lessons

Mom signed in at triage, stating that all three of her children were sick with "colds and congestion." The two older siblings were alert and active in the waiting room. She then pointed down to her infant carrier on the floor and says "she has it bad." I removed the blanket Mom had used to cover the entire carrier and immediately took the baby out of the seat to optimize her airway when I noted her dusky color. The infant was 3 weeks old, full term and had no co-morbid conditions. I quickly placed her on the scale to get her weight and noted several periods of apnea, which responded to tactile stimulation. I took the family to a resuscitation bed and noted pulse oximetry readings quickly falling with each apneic event. We initially administered albuterol and oxygen for her wheezing but had to intubate the infant due to recurring apneic episodes with desaturation. It came as no surprise to the ED staff that the nasal swabs were positive for RSV. Happily, she was eventually discharged home fully recovered after her stay in PICU.

Teaching points: Always look at your patients on arrival! Mere minutes stood between our initial assessment of this baby and death. If neither our staff nor the mom had checked under that blanket at just the right time, we would have been working a possibly futile resuscitation. Remember that our first item of business is to optimize the patient's airway, which is NOT possible in an infant seat! Families of Neonatal ICU graduates should be made aware of the potential severity of illness due to RSV, as well as the recommendations for Synagis. Synagis (palivizumab) therapy is a monthly shot started before RSV season starts. It's given every 28-30 days for NICU preemie grads as well as term babies/infants/children with other co-morbid conditions (heart, HIV, heme-onc and pulmonary kids) who would be at risk for severe illness. Synagis is NOT an immunization, as many people think. It is a drug that blocks the RSV virus from attaching to lung tissue. After approximately one month, the Synagis is gone and another shot is needed to keep the patient from getting RSV, or at least from getting a severe case. Some RSV seasons seem to be much worse than others; this was the first of many intubations we did in a 1 month period for RSV that year.

Additional Pediatric ED Attending Physician Insights: Studies have demonstrated that there's no treatment that consistently helps patients with RSV (or any other viral type) bronchiolitis. It's been definitely proven that steroids are not effective, although it seems logical that they would be, based on the pathology. Beta agonists, racemic epi and nebulized NS or hypertonic saline are all inconsistent in their effectiveness and often do more to satisfy our urge to do something than they do for the disease itself. For the bronchiolitic wheezer in distress most of us will still try albuterol and then maybe switch to racemic epi if it doesn't work. We may try Atrovent® (ipratropium) too, in an effort to cut down on secretions, but it's also not a consistent aid. The point is to not continue a treatment that doesn't work. What seems to help our sicker (hypoxic) bronchiolitics these days is the Vapotherm®, which warms and humidifies oxygen so that it can be given at much higher flow rates/concentrations via nasal cannula. It can also help a bit with ventilation because the high flows create some PEEP but the primary task is to treat hypoxia. Ribavirin® (an aerosolized antiviral drug) may still be used very occasionally in the ICU setting but its cost alone is prohibitive, especially in view of its apparent limited benefits.

Appendix 3-A

The Modified Westley Clinical Scoring System for Croup

- **Inspiratory stridor:**
    - Not present - 0 points
    - When agitated / active - 1 point
    - At rest - 2 points

- **Intercostal recession:**
    - Mild - 1 point
    - Moderate - 2 points
    - Severe - 3 points

- **Air entry:**
    - Normal - 0 points
    - Mildly decreased - 1 point
    - Severely decreased - 2 points

- **Cyanosis:**
    - None - 0 points
    - With agitation / activity - 4 points
    - At rest - 5 points

- **Level of consciousness:**
    - Normal - 0 points
    - Altered - 5 points

Possible score 0-17
<4 = mild croup, 4-6 = moderate croup, >6 = severe croup

Chapter 4
Cardiovascular Emergencies
Congenital Hearts to CPR

I like children... Properly cooked.
-W.C. Fields

Pertinent Pediatric Ponderings (NOTES)

CHAPTER 4
Sample Test Answer Sheet

1. _____
2. _____
3. _____
4. _____
5. _____
6. _____
7. _____
8. _____
9. _____
10. _____
11. _____
12. _____
13. _____
14. _____
15. _____
16. _____
17. _____
18. _____
19. _____
20. _____

21. _____
22. _____
23. _____
24. _____
25. _____
26. _____
27. _____
28. _____
29. _____
30. _____
31. _____
32. _____
33. _____
34. _____
35. _____
36. _____
37. _____
38. _____
39. _____
40. _____

41. _____
42. _____
43. _____
44. _____
45. _____
46. _____
47. _____
48. _____
49. _____
50. _____
51. _____
52. _____
53. _____
54. _____
55. _____
56. _____
57. _____
58. _____
59. _____
60. _____

61. _____
62. _____
63. _____
64. _____
65. _____
66. _____
67. _____
68. _____
69. _____
70. _____
71. _____
72. _____
73. _____
74. _____
75. _____
76. _____

[Remove page and cover rationale until after you answer question]

Pertinent Pediatric Ponderings (NOTES)

Certified Pediatric Emergency Nurse (CPEN) Review IV

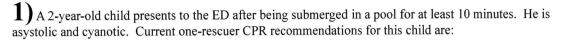

1) A 2-year-old child presents to the ED after being submerged in a pool for at least 10 minutes. He is asystolic and cyanotic. Current one-rescuer CPR recommendations for this child are:

A) 30 compressions and 2 ventilations

B) 15 compressions and 2 ventilations

C) 5 compressions and 1 ventilation

D) 3 compressions and 1 ventilation

A – 30 compressions and 2 ventilations. There are only two kinds of dead patients; newborns and everybody else. If the patient is a newborn, it's still 3 and 1. For everybody else, meaning it's not a newborn, it's now 30 and 2. There is now no differentiation between pediatric and adult patients. Either you are a newborn, or you're everybody else. (That makes it much easier for all of us to remember, until the next round of resuscitation revisions arrive…)

2) Early shock can be diagnosed by vital signs:

A – True

B - False

B – False - The textbook definition of shock is "a state of inadequate tissue perfusion." Notice that there is no mention of vital signs in the definition. No numbers, no formulas, no rules. So, if we can't diagnose shock by vital signs, what do we do? Simply put, shock is all those "red flags" that your patient is showing you saying "Hello… I'm about to die… and if you can do something to prevent this, I would really appreciate it!" Early shock or compensated shock means they are shocky, but the body is still able to deal with it (Hence the term compensated.) What would you see with early shock? You would typically see normal mentation, normal blood pressure, but prolonged capillary refill, tachycardia and decreased peripheral pulses. However, when they start having changes in their levels of consciousness, stop peeing, or even worse, drop their blood pressures; those are signs of very late or decompensated shock.

3) In pediatric emergency care, the **most** common type of shock is:

A) Septic

B) Hypovolemic

C) Cardiogenic

D) Anaphylactic

B – The most common cause of shock is hypovolemia, whether it is due to vomiting, diarrhea or trauma. Though pediatric patients may present with other types of shock, such as septic (especially in really young or chronically ill children), cardiogenic (in those with congenital heart disease), or anaphylactic (because children are likely to try anything once… or twice), these other types of shock are less common in the pediatric population.

Cardiovascular

4) The initial way that infants and young children primarily attempt to compensate for shock is:

A) Increasing cardiac contractility

B) Decreasing capillary refill time

C) Increasing the heart rate

D) Increasing urine output

C – While adults try to increase their perfusion by both increasing their heart rate (beating faster) and increasing cardiac contractility (beating harder), infants do not have the ability to increase contractility. Therefore, their primary method of compensation is for their hearts to beat faster. Tachycardia occurs long before other vital signs, laboratory results, or physical exam changes. Infants aren't capable of increasing contractility, but they definitely can vasoconstrict vigorously. That's why capillary refill, peripheral pulses, and skin temperature/color are better indicators of hemodynamic compromise in children versus adults. Decreased capillary refill or increased urinary output (without medication) would be the result of changes in perfusion as opposed to ways of correcting or compensating for shock.

5) A 13-month-old critically ill female is being treated in the ED with meningococcemia and septic shock as primary diagnoses. She initially was tachycardic with a heart rate of 210; however, the heart rate has now suddenly dropped to 70. The ED nurse interprets this to mean:

A) This is reassuring as the heart rate is now within normal limits

B) The drop in heart rate is a very ominous sign

C) The monitor has probably malfunctioned and is counting every third beat. Treat the patient, not the monitor

D) The medications being administered to treat the tachycardia are now taking effect and the patient is improving

B – When a sick child's heart rate drops significantly, and to a rate that is below normal for their age, this is indeed an ominous sign. To compensate for shock, little ones, just like big people, try to make their hearts beat faster. Their hearts can only beat really fast for so long, and then those little hearts poop out. When this happens and they become bradycardic, look out, as bad, bad things are going to be happening soon.

6) A 10kg child presents to the peds ED with fever, irritability, cool/mottled extremities, and 5-second capillary refill. The appropriate fluid bolus for this child is:

A) 200ml of 0.9NS over 30-60 minutes

B) 400 ml of D5W over 10-15 minutes

C) 400 ml of 0.9NS or LR over 30-60 minutes

D) 200 ml of 0.9NS or LR over 10-15 minutes

D - As evidenced by poor peripheral perfusion, this child is "shocky." In an attempt to restore circulating volume, 20ml/kg of LR or 0.9NS should be administered as fast as you can safely push it. After the bolus, the child should be re-evaluated regarding the need for a second, or possibly even a third, fluid bolus.

Certified Pediatric Emergency Nurse (CPEN) Review IV

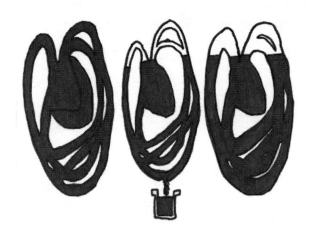

| Cardiogenic shock | Hypovolemic shock | Septic, neurogenic, or anaphylactic shock |

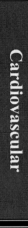

Illustration by Nina DeBoer, then age 9 (my aspiring artist daughter, now aspiring baker daughter)

7) What is the condition of the blood vessels in a child in septic, neurogenic, or anaphylactic shock?

A) Dilated

B) Normal

C) Constricted

D) Overloaded

A - The "pipes" (blood vessels) in septic, neurogenic (spinal) or anaphylactic shock are dilated. They are just way too big. Think of the following analogy. If blood vessels in a healthy patient are like a garden hose, the blood vessels in our patients with these types of shock are more like sewer pipes. If you have the same amount of fluid/blood in that big sewer pipe as you originally had in the garden hose, the pressure needed to distribute the fluid for adequate perfusion is going to suffer. So, treatment for these types of shock involves two steps: 1) First, fill up the pipes with fluids. 2) Second, try to make the pipes smaller with vasopressors such as Inotropin (dopamine), Levophed (norepinephrine), or Neo-Synephrine (phenylephrine.) The pipes are way too big, so fill 'em up and make 'em smaller.

8) What is the condition of the blood vessels in hypovolemic shock?

A) Dilated

B) Normal

C) Empty

D) Overloaded

C – The "pipes" (blood vessels) in hypovolemic shock are empty. Whether the child has gastroenteritis and subsequent vomiting and/or diarrhea or is a multiple trauma victim, the pipes are essentially empty so, once again, treatment for this type of shock involve two necessary steps: 1) Fill up the pipes with fluids and 2) "Plug the holes," either literally as with surgical intervention for a lacerated liver or spleen, or figuratively with medications to control the GI symptoms. Vasopressors are not indicated in hypovolemic shock because shrinking already empty pipes is not ideal. Either way, the pipes are empty, so fill them up and plug the holes.

Certified Pediatric Emergency Nurse (CPEN) Review IV

9) What is the condition of the blood vessels in cardiogenic shock?

A) Dilated

B) Normal

C) Constricted

D) Overloaded

D – In cardiogenic shock, the "pipes" (blood vessels) are overloaded. They are way too full because the pump (in this case a faulty heart) doesn't move fluid efficiently and the system is overfilled. Most children found to be in cardiogenic shock have a history of congenital heart disease or cardiomyopathy. Treatment again involves two steps: 1) Decrease the volume in the system with the use of diuretics and 2) Make the heart pump stronger with inotropes such as Dobutrex (dobutamine) or Lanoxin (digoxin) to move the fluid around better. Either way, both the volume and the pump are messed up, so fix both to fix the patient.

10) Common assessment findings with pediatric cardiogenic shock include all of the following **except**:

A) Low central venous pressure (CVP)

B) Jugular venous distention (JVD)

C) Pulmonary congestion, i.e. rales

D) S4 heart sound

A – Think about what's going in cardiogenic shock. The pump is failing and the system is way too full. So with those conditions, we commonly find funky extra heart sounds and blood backing up everywhere, including the lungs and jugular veins (especially visible in older kids who "have a neck.") If a central line is placed for hemodynamic monitoring, the CVP would be high, not low as there is too much fluid and hence too much pressure.

11) A 2-year-old presents to the ED in septic shock. The nurse would expect a patient in **"early"** septic shock to exhibit which of the following signs:

A) Weak, thready pulses and hypotension

B) Decreased urine output and elevated BUN/creatinine levels

C) Warm skin

D) Pulmonary and hepatic failure

C - In early septic shock, the child is still warm, or in many cases, really warm. Some believe this is one of the body's responses to an infection; an attempt by the body to make the environment for the infectious organism less hospitable. When the patient progresses into late or "cold" septic shock, they are going into total body failure as evidenced by organ systems shutting down, hypotension, and the skin getting cold and underperfused.

184

Certified Pediatric Emergency Nurse (CPEN) Review IV

12) The previous 2-year-old remains in septic shock. 0.9NS fluid boluses are given and the patient is becoming edematous. The ED nurse knows that many patients in septic shock are also hypovolemic due to all of the following factors **except**:

A) Leaky vessels leading to third spacing of fluid

B) Dehydration due to fever and sweating

C) Increased urinary output

D) Decreased intake of oral fluids

C – If anything, patients in shock will have decreased urinary output. The same "bugs" that dilate the blood vessels also make them leaky. While many patients appear puffy, remember that even though the tissues look full, the "pipes" (blood vessels) are both empty and way too big. Therefore, even with edema present, in addition to vasopressors to return the "pipes" back to their normal size, fluid resuscitation is frequently required.

13) Which assessment findings are commonly found with a teenage patient in neurogenic or "spinal" shock?

A) Hypotension and bradycardia

B) Hypotension and tachycardia

C) Hypertension and bradycardia

D) Hypertension and tachycardia

A – When someone is in neurogenic or "spinal" shock, the symptoms are typically hypotension and bradycardia. This is different from what we typically see in cases of hypovolemic shock where hypotension and compensatory tachycardia are commonly found. Hypovolemic trauma patients have a blood pressure of 50mm Hg and a heart rate of 150 to compensate. However, when one is in neurogenic or "spinal" shock, they become a member of a special club called the "50/50 club." That means that they may have a blood pressure of 50mm Hg, but with a heart rate of 50. This is due to the effects of the spinal cord injury and the resulting parasympathetic nervous system overdrive. The pipes (blood vessels) become way too big and the body doesn't compensate. Instead of becoming tachycardic, these patients go the other way and drop their heart rates. When you see hypotension and bradycardia, especially in an unconscious trauma child, think spinal shock.

14) An 8-year-old child is admitted in critical condition after a high-speed, rollover MVC. He has received three boluses of 20ml/kg 0.9NS and multiple packed red blood cell infusions. Which sign would the nurse anticipate seeing in a patient who has undergone multiple blood transfusions?

A) Brudzinski's sign

B) Chvostek's sign

C) Cullen's sign

D) Babinski's sign

B - Chvostek's sign can be elicited in patients with hypocalcemia. When patients get "boatloads of blood", the preservative in the blood can induce hypocalcemia. Chvostek's begins with "C" and tapping the "C"heek results in facial muscle spasm. Brudzinski's and Babinski's signs are associated with neurological issues, while "CU"llen's sign (bruising around the umbiliCUs) is found with retroperitoneal abdominal hemorrhage. Bonus item: Another good test question might involve Trousseau's sign, another sign of hypocalcemia. Trousseau's sign begins with "T" and if you "T"ake a blood pressure for "T"oo long, inflation of the BP cuff, can cause the hand/wrist to briefly spasm.

Certified Pediatric Emergency Nurse (CPEN) Review IV

15) Which statement is **not** correct regarding Kawasaki's Disease?

A) Kawasaki's Disease is known to start with a high fever (>104 F) for more than five days

B) The condition has no serious consequences and can be left untreated

C) Patients often present with swollen and peeling hands and feet, a purplish-red rash on the trunk of the body, and bilateral conjunctivitis without thick discharge

D) Kawasaki's Disease is most often seen in 2 years to 5 years old children

B - Kawasaki's Disease causes inflammation of several organs, including the coronary arteries, but rarely leads to death with proper treatment. Management includes high dose aspirin and IV immunoglobulin to reduce inflammation and prevent the development of coronary artery aneurysms. The first phase of the disease may include a high fever that is unresponsive to antipyretics. The child must also develop four or more of the following symptoms: 1) conjunctivitis without thick discharge 2) rash on trunk of body and genital area 3) red/dry cracked lips with a "strawberry" like tongue 4) edematous hands/feet 5) sore throat, or 6) swollen lymph nodes. In the second phase, the skin on the hands and feet may begin peeling, and joint pain, nausea, vomiting, and diarrhea may occur. In the third phase, signs and symptoms slowly go away unless complications develop.

16) A 10-year-old girl arrives in your ED post V-Fib arrest while playing soccer. She is currently intubated and sedated with stable vital signs. In interviewing her parents, you find that until recently she had no past medical history, but she had recently been experiencing fainting spells during sports. The parents state that she has been to a neurologist, but that all tests were negative. The father also states that he had a brother pass away at a very young age from what appeared to be a "bad heart." With this history and the patient's current condition the nurse expects:

A) Seizures

B) Dehydration

C) Severe asthma attack

D) Long Q-T Syndrome (LQTS)

D - Long Q-T Syndrome. After each heartbeat, the electrical system recharges itself to get ready for the next heartbeat. In Long Q-T Syndrome the heart takes longer than normal to recharge or re-polarize. This can lead to a rhythm disorder causing ventricular arrhythmias and may lead to fainting or even death. The disease can be hereditary, caused by some medications, or can be the result of other diseases such as congenital heart disease or anorexia nervosa and associated electrolyte imbalances. A patient with LQTS may be symptom free, until a significant physical or emotional stress causes the heart rhythm to spin out of control. In many children, the first indication of this condition is unexplained fainting in an otherwise healthy child or even seizures (due to oxygen deprivation during erratic heartbeats.) There is often a history of unexplained fainting, unexplained near-drowning or other accidents, unexplained seizures, or a history of cardiac arrest with the child or close family relative.

17) A 2-month-old child arrives at the ED in full arrest. Chest compressions should be administered at approximately how many times per minute?

A) 60

B) 80

C) 100

D) 200

C – The magic number for chest compressions in infants, children, and adults is 100.

Certified Pediatric Emergency Nurse (CPEN) Review IV

18) A 2-year-old with a history of asthma suffers a witnessed cardiac arrest. The next recommended interventions include?

A) 2 ventilations, followed by 30 chest compressions

B) 30 chest compressions, followed by 2 ventilations

C) 30 ventilations, followed by 2 chest compressions

D) 15 chest compressions, followed by 2 ventilations

B – CPR guidelines for infants and children are very much fair game on the exam. In the 2010 AHA PALS guidelines, the ABCs are no longer the ABCs... They are now the CABs. Compressions first, then airway and breathing later!

19) 6 month-old child is reported to be choking. You find the child awake and struggling, but unable to cry. Your next intervention should be:

A) Performing a blind finger sweep

B) Alternating 5 back blows with 5 chest thrusts

C) Performing direct laryngoscopy to visualize and remove the obstruction

D) Performing abdominal thrusts until the obstruction is relieved

B – This child is going to quickly die if you don't do something quickly to clear the airway obstruction. Basic CPR for awake choking infants involves alternating between back blows and chest thrusts, essentially flipping them over and back again until the obstruction is relieved. If the child loses consciousness, then 30 chest compressions and 2 ventilations should be performed as part of BLS resuscitation. Blind finger sweeps are not appropriate in this age because it can push the object or the tongue back down into the airway.

20) A 9-month-old child arrives via EMS in respiratory arrest. Initial attempts at bag-mask ventilation by the ED staff are unsuccessful. A foreign body airway obstruction is suspected. The next step should include performing a blind finger sweep to remove the foreign body:

A) True

B) False

B – False – Remember that it is very easy for children's airways to be malpositioned and that "bagging" a child is an art as well as a learned skill (not easily mastered.) Try repositioning the mask and head first before moving to more invasive maneuvers. If those two maneuvers are unsuccessful, then more invasive interventions can be undertaken, but none of these interventions involve a blind finger sweep. Blindly inserting your fingers into an infant's or child's mouth can not only displace the tongue, but a blind finger sweep can also shove a foreign body deeper into the airway. Before attempting ventilation, look in the mouth to see if a foreign body is visualized. If you see something in the back of their throat, certainly take it out, but otherwise, just say no to blind finger sweeps.

Certified Pediatric Emergency Nurse (CPEN) Review IV

21) A 16-year-old male is involved in a "car vs. tree" high-speed MVC with 60 minutes of extrication required on the scene. He presents to the ED with a heart rate of 150, profoundly cyanotic, and not moving. The nurse quickly checks for the presence of a perfusing pulse and finds none. The patient's cardiac rhythm appears to be sinus tachycardia and the ER nurse correctly interprets this to be PEA (pulseless electrical activity arrest.) Possible "reversible" causes of PEA arrest include:

A) 5 H's

B) 5 A's

C) 5 T's

D) A and C

D – PEA is characterized by a rhythm you can see, but not feel. The classic "possibly reversible" causes of PEA are known as the *5 Hs and 5 Ts*. The Hs include: **H**ypothermia, **H**ypovolemia, **H**ypoxia, **H**ydrogen ion (acidosis), and **H**yper/**H**ypo electrolytes (calcium, potassium, magnesium.) The Ts are: **T**ension pneumothorax, pericardial **T**amponade, **T**oxins, **T**rauma, and **T**hromboembolism.

22) The two types of congenital heart disease are:

A) Cyanotic and acyanotic

B) Hereditary and environmental

C) Distributive and peripheral

D) Conductive and mechanical

A – Congenital heart disease, or heart disease that infants are born with, is classified into two types, cyanotic (blue) or acyanotic (pink.)

23) A 3-day-old child presents to the ED with poor feeding, fussiness, lethargy, and central cyanosis. He is found to have a heart murmur and room air saturations of 80% on room air. A chest X-ray is obtained which reveals a "funny looking heart." He is diagnosed with possible congenital heart disease. The probable reason for this child's symptoms is:

A) Cardiac arrhythmia

B) Congestive heart failure

C) Inappropriate closure of the patent ductus arteriosus (PDA)

D) Pneumonia

C – Generally speaking, every truly sick baby who presents to the ED during the first month of life is septic until proven otherwise. However, hypoxia on room air, coupled with the other pieces of the history and exam findings, should lead the ER nurse to suspect that the very real possibility that this is a "heart kid" with a ductal (PDA) dependent lesion. While the baby is still inside of mom, the PDA, or structure between the aorta and pulmonary artery, allows for blood to go to where it's needed, instead of to the lungs. Mom takes care of oxygenating the blood before birth. Once born, breathing and oxygenation are the sole responsibility of the baby. The PDA normally closes a few hours after birth. However, for infants with congenital heart disease that depend on the ductus arteriosus for mixing of oxygenated and deoxygenated blood, the PDA keeps them alive. For these infants, when it does close, less and less mixing occurs and the child can become quite sick quite quickly.

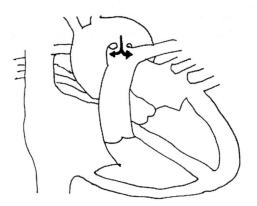

Patent Ductus Arteriosus (PDA)

Illustration by Nina DeBoer, then age 9 (my aspiring artist daughter, now aspiring baker daughter)

24) Anticipated medication for the previous "rule out heart disease" infant would be:

A) IV Lanoxin (digoxin)

B) IV Dobutrex (dobutamine)

C) IV Inotropin (dopamine)

D) IV prostaglandins (PGE_1)

D - Though digoxin, dobutamine, and dopamine can be used in patients with congenital heart disease and poor contractility or perfusion, in this child, prostaglandins are really what this child needs. PGE_1 is a smooth muscle relaxant and keeps the patent ductus arteriosus (PDA) open to allow ongoing mixing to occur. If the PDA has recently closed; it can actually help it to re-open. If your patient is only a few days old and if you are thinking about the possibility of congenital heart disease, think prostaglandins (and rule out sepsis.) If an echocardiogram shows that congenital heart disease is not the problem, you can always shut off the PGE_1, but the prompt delivery of this medication might very well save this child's life in the ED. Either way, the S.T.A.B.L.E. neonatal education program (www.stableprogram.org) recommends the following for any cyanotic infant who is suspected as having congenital heart disease: 1) ABCs, 2) 100% oxygen, and 3) Prostaglandin (PGE_1) infusion to maintain saturations (on right arm) above 75%. As a side note, the next time you are at work in the ED, I highly suggest you figure out where PGE_1 is kept. Is it in your medication refrigerator? Do you need to request it from pharmacy? This knowledge may save a baby's life!

25) Common side effects of initiating a prostaglandin infusion in a newborn include all of the following **except**:

A) Hypotension

B) Extremity rigidity

C) Skin flushing/fever

D) Apnea

B – Prostaglandins work by dilating or relaxing the smooth muscle of the patent ductus arteriosus, but they also tend to dilate and relax everything else. This means that the patient will become flushed as the peripheral vessels dilate, but also can become hypotensive as well. I recommend warding off the evil spirits by having a fluid bolus in a syringe ready to go when you are initiating PGE_1. In addition

Certified Pediatric Emergency Nurse (CPEN) Review IV

to hypotension, some babies like to go apneic during PGE_1 administration, especially within the first few hours of initiation. To ward off the evil spirits, consider the following suggestions when you are initiating PGE_1 therapy. 1) Have a fluid bolus in a syringe ready, and 2) Watch the patient really closely or prophylactically intubate. This works well if you have physicians or a PNP/NNP/RT readily available who can immediately intubate the child if needed. For transfers, we frequently sedate and intubate the infant prior to transport if PGE1. Intubating a neonate in the air or in an ambulance is not fun. Why be stressed if you don't need to.

26) An infant who was born at home presents to the ED with respiratory distress and mottled extremities. Physical exam reveals a definite decrease in the strength of the femoral pulses compared to the radial pulses and marked differences between the upper and lower extremity blood pressures. Based on the pulses, pressures, and perfusion, the ED nurse should suspect:

A) Coarctation of the aorta

B) Transposition of the great vessels

C) Tetralogy of Fallot

D) Pulmonary stenosis

A – Decreased femoral compared to radial pulses coupled with marked differences between the upper and lower extremity blood pressures should make the nurse consider the distinct possibility that this infant has coarctation, or narrowing of the aorta. This condition accounts for 10% of all cases of congenital heart defects. The coarctation typically takes place at or below the point where the aorta turns inferiorly, and this will result in higher BP's in the upper extremities (fed by arteries before the point of narrowing) and decreased pulses and prolonged capillary refill times in areas fed by the aorta after the narrowing.

27) A 16-year-old female presents to the ED with complaints of fever, body aches, and chills for 3 days. Her history is significant for having multiple body piercings done two weeks prior. In addition, she mentions that she had a "heart problem" at birth. Exam reveals a heart murmur and fever of 103F (39.4C.) The nurse should suspect which diagnosis in this patient?

A) Pneumonia

B) Influenza

C) Endocarditis

D) Meningitis

C – The combination of symptoms, past history of heart problems, and a recent history of multiple body piercings should place endocarditis (infection of the inner lining of the heart) right at the top of the list of likely suspects. While body aches, fever, and chills certainly can be symptoms of pneumonia, meningitis, or even the flu, the body piercings (or recent dental work) should be the big clue. When we think endocarditis, we often think about patients who are IV drug abusers. Recently however, there have been over 20 published cases of endocarditis after body art (tattooing/piercing) experiences, and one-half of those patients also had a history of congenital heart disease.

Certified Pediatric Emergency Nurse (CPEN) Review IV

28) EMS is in route to the ED with a 2-year-old who ingested an unknown number of Lanoxin (digoxin) tablets. They report his heart rate is "sinus bradycardia with a rate of 19," confirmed by auscultation and palpation. They are requesting permission to initiate external (transcutaneous) pacing. The ER nurse should deny the request as pacing is only indicated for adult patients:

A) True

B) False

B – False – In addition to oxygenating, ventilating, initiating chest compressions, and administering epinephrine, if a child's heart rate is extremely low, external pacing can be attempted. Pacing is not just for adults anymore. They do make pediatric pads, but in many cases, adult pacing pads work just fine. If the child is big enough to put a pad on their front and a pad on their back, the adult pads work just fine.

29) Methods for determining whether "pacing is working" in the above patient include:

A) Verification of pacing spikes on the ECG pattern

B) Verification of chest muscle movement with pacing

C) Verification of capture on the ECG pattern

D) Verification of a palpable/perfusing pulse with pacing

D – The rule for how much energy to use for pacing children is the same as for adults. You simply crank it up until it works. Looking at the ECG is good, but looking at the patient is better. If they have a pulse with pacing, it's working. If not, it doesn't matter what's on the ECG or if their chest muscles are jumping like crazy, it's not working.

30) Current age recommendations for adult automatic external defibrillator (AED) use in children are:

A) Over 1 minute of age

B) Over 4 years of age

C) Over 8 years of age

D) Over 12 years of age

A – It used to be that adult AEDs were only recommended for adults and understandably so. They were created for adults and tested on adults. However, pediatric pads are now available. They plug into the adult AED and decrease the energy delivered to a dose appropriate for children. If you have a set of pediatric pads and a pediatric patient, by all means, use the smaller pads. However, the American Heart Association (AHA) 2010 PALS guidelines removed the 1-year old and up age restriction, so if all you have is an adult AED, use it. Something is better than nothing, and it might actually make them better.

31) Which of the following statements are **true** regarding pediatric patients in sinus tachycardia?

A) Sinus tachycardia is a normal compensatory response to stress or increased physiological requirements

B) In sinus tachycardia, the heart rate is usually less than 200 beats per minute

C) Management of sinus tachycardia involves treating whatever is causing the tachycardia

D) All of the above

Certified Pediatric Emergency Nurse (CPEN) Review IV

D – Generally speaking, sinus tachycardia in children has rates of less than 200-220 (and slower as they get older.) When you have a child in sinus tach, it's important to look not only at the monitor, but also the child. Try to figure out why they are so tachy. Pain, anxiety, dehydration, and fevers are all common causes of sinus tachycardia.

32) While watching a middle school baseball game, the nurse sees the batter hit in the chest with the ball. He immediately collapses to the ground and appears lifeless. Which of the following is the likely cause?

A) Pericardial tamponade

B) Traumatic asphyxia

C) Beck's triad

D) Commotio cordis

D – Commotio cordis is when a sudden impact to the chest wall causes the heart to suddenly stop. You might see this in football or baseball players who get hit in the chest and drop dead on the field or during a martial arts exhibition or competition. If the impact hits at just the "wrong time" in the cardiac electrical cycle, it can result in cardiac arrest. This is an excellent example of why early CPR and the availability of AEDs are so important, even in pediatric cases. The longer they lay dead, the greater the chance of them remaining that way.

33) Which of the following is **not** part of Beck's triad (and **not** among the classic signs of pericardial tamponade)?

A) Jugular vein distension (JVD)

B) Muffled heart sounds

C) Narrowing pulse pressure

D) Nausea, vomiting, and diarrhea (NVD)

D – Pericardial tamponade can be the result of chest trauma or oncological emergencies and is characterized by Beck's triad. The triad, meaning three, has three (imagine that) classic symptoms. 1) JVD – The heart is squished so blood can't go round and round very well. This results in blood backing up and may be evidenced by JVD. Please remember that in infants and chubby young children with "no necks," JVD can be difficult to detect. 2) Muffled heart sounds – The heart is surrounded and squished by blood (or other fluid), putting a layer of sound insulation around the heart. This results in the heart sounds being muffled or distant sounding. 3) Narrowed pulse pressure – Since the blood doesn't go round and round very well and the patient is getting sicker and sicker, the diastolic pressure goes up and the systolic pressure goes down. If they meet in the middle, you are dead. They key is to suspect and detect a tamponade before this happens. The possibility of tamponade should be suspected in a shocky child who has no response to multiple fluid boluses and for whom the history is contributory (chest trauma or recent cardiac surgery.) It can be diagnosed by chest X-ray, the presence of Beck's triad, or more commonly, ED ultrasound. Bonus test question: While nausea, vomiting, and diarrhea are the "gastro triad," they are not Beck's triad. If you are asked about Cushing's triad, think head trauma and increased intracranial pressures (ICP.)

34) Effects of Lanoxin (digoxin) include:

A) Increased heart rate and increased contractility

B) Increased heart rate and decreased contractility

C) Decreased heart rate and increased contractility

D) Decreased heart rate and decreased contractility

C – Digoxin slows your heart rate down so it doesn't have to work so hard, and it also makes those beats stronger. Think about digoxin as giving you "more bang for your buck." Though not used in the ED as often as it used to be, is still very commonly utilized in children with cardiac disease.

35) The rapid response team is requested STAT to the pediatric floor where a 2-month-old with a "heart problem" was having blood drawn. The child is found to be crying and acutely cyanotic, but the lungs are clear and there is no respiratory distress. With this history and physical findings, the nurse suspects:

A) RSV pneumonia

B) "Tet spell"

C) Congestive heart failure

D) Reactive airway disease

B – This child with a "heart problem" is exhibiting classic signs of a "Tet spell." In children with yet unrepaired tetralogy of Fallot, unpleasant stimuli such as starting IV's, drawing blood, or immunizations can invoke this "spell." Profound cyanosis occurs from spasms of muscles around the pulmonary arteries and the significant decrease in pulmonary blood flow that results from the spasms. Treatment involves placing the child in a knee chest position (which increases pulmonary blood flow by decreasing circulation to the lower extremities), 100% oxygen by mask (they are profoundly purple after all), and administration of IM or IV morphine to chill out the child. In rare cases, IV Inderal (propanolol) or Neo-Synephrine (phenylephrine) may be administered, but in most cases, oxygen, positioning and relaxing will do the job. Of note, you would expect respiratory distress with any of the other answers.

36) Cardiomyopathy in children is managed with:

A) Diuretics and Lanoxin (digoxin)

B) Afterload reduction agents (beta blockers and/or ACE inhibitors)

C) Anticoagulants and an AICD (automatic implantable cardiovertor-defibrillators)

D) All of the above

D – Cardiomyopathy, whether it is defined as hypertrophic, restrictive, or dilated (the most common type found in children), simply means that the heart muscle can't pump as well as it should. Symptoms commonly include those associated with congestive heart failure; however, arrhythmias can result in sudden death as well, especially with hypertrophic cardiomyopathy. Management is primarily symptomatic in nature and may include medications and in the worst case, ventricular assist devices and/or heart transplant.

Certified Pediatric Emergency Nurse (CPEN) Review IV

Cardiovascular

37) The force against which the heart must pump to eject blood from the ventricles is called:

A) Preload

B) Afterload

C) Middle load

D) Wide load

B – Preload is "pre" or before the heart and refers to end-diastolic pressure and volume. It relates to the pressure associated with the amount of fluid and blood that is trying to enter the heart. Afterload is "after" the heart and describes the amount of pressure or force that the ventricle has to fight against to eject the blood.

38) Which of the following is most commonly the first drug administered in a pediatric cardiopulmonary arrest?

A) Amiodarone

B) Magnesium

C) Lidocaine

D) Epinephrine

D – In pediatric cardiac arrest, the initial drug of choice is epinephrine (and oxygen.) Amiodarone or lidocaine are frequently given for ventricular arrhythmias such as V-fib or V-tach, and magnesium is given for rare arrhythmias such as Torsades de Pointes (meaning the twisting of the points, seen as the fast, flipping, and funky looking V-tach.)

39) The peds ED rapid response team is summoned to the general pediatrics unit for a 2-year-old child in near-cardiac arrest. Oxygen via bag-valve mask is being administered, an IV is in place, and the cardiac monitor reveals a heart rate of 20. Amazingly you are able to palpate a weak central pulse. Your **first** intervention should be:

A) Give epinephrine and begin chest compressions

B) Administer atropine

C) Monitor the child closely

D) Administer Amiodarone

A - 0.1 ml/kg of 1:10,000 epinephrine (1 mg/10 mL) accompanied by chest compressions at a rate of 100 per minute are your first priorities. A number of important considerations are at play here. Often times, supplemental oxygen will bring a child's heart rate up without medications or other interventions. However, the oxygen in this scenario isn't helping, and if the heart rate remains at 20 despite oxygen being given, this child is going to die very, very soon. Atropine can be given if vagal stimulation (i.e. when adults "bear down") is suspected, but that isn't likely here. Amiodarone is used for ventricular arrhythmias, not bradycardia, and you will have plenty of time to closely monitor this child after you do what you need to do to keep her alive.

Certified Pediatric Emergency Nurse (CPEN) Review IV

40) If the peripheral IV in the previous patient is found to be infiltrated, which of the following methods of vascular access should be immediately attempted?

A) Intraosseous (IO) placement

B) Subclavian IV line placement

C) Saphenous vein cut down

D) Peripheral IV placement

A – IO placement is probably your fastest option for achieving vascular access. You don't have time to get a central line, do a cut down, or hunt for another peripheral IV as the child is nearly arresting.

41) An intraosseous line has successfully been placed in the child's right tibia. How many ml/kg of 0.9NS or LR should be given as a fluid bolus?

A) 10 ml/kg

B) 20 ml/kg

C) 30 ml/kg

D) 40 ml/kg

B – 20ml/kg – When giving isotonic fluids such as 0.9NS or LR as a bolus to children, 20ml/kg is the magic number.

42) Parents of a 4-year-old near-drowning victim run into triage and hand you their son. ECG monitor leads are placed and show ventricular fibrillation. Your **immediate** intervention should be:

A) Defibrillate at 4j/kg

B) Intubate, then defibrillate at 2j/kg

C) Cardiovert at 2j/kg

D) Defibrillate at 2j/kg

D – Before you intubate, you should defibrillate, but keep doing CPR until the machine is ready to shock. The first shock should be given at 2j/kg (Hint – it's the same number of the paddles you are holding)! If the first defibrillation attempt is unsuccessful, then while two minutes of CPR are being performed, the child can be bag-mask ventilated or intubated and intraosseous vascular access obtained. After two minutes of CPR, if the rhythm remains in V-fib, the child again can be defibrillated at 4j/kg (count your paddles and double them – 4j/kg.) Cardioversion is only appropriate for children who have a pulse; successful cardioversion of V-fib isn't going to happen.

43) You are caring for a two-year-old febrile child who the parents can't wake up. The possibility of meningitis should be considered:

A) True

B) False

Certified Pediatric Emergency Nurse (CPEN) Review IV

A – True – If a febrile child becomes difficult to arouse, increasingly irritable, or doesn't recognize her parents, these are very good reasons to be concerned and to consider something really bad, like meningitis, may be a factor. Certainly, with sick kids, it can be tough to tell if they are really sick or just really tired from feeling crummy and not sleeping well. When they stop recognizing their parents, this is a definite change in mental status and indicative of a serious condition. Using parents as a guide is always a good idea as they know their children better than we do.

44) What is the **earliest** clinical sign of shock in children?

A) Subtly altered level of consciousness

B) Hypotension

C) Tachycardia

D) Weak peripheral pulses

A – Not every tachycardic child is in shock. Pain, fever, fear, excitement, and exercise can certainly be other reasons for tachycardia. The most sensitive end organ to decreased perfusion is the brain and subtle changes in the level of consciousness are the earliest indication that hemodynamic compromise has tilted over into shock. The other answers listed are signs of late, not early shock.

45) Indications for the use of IV amiodarone in children include:

A) Asystole

B) Sinus bradycardia

C) Ventricular fibrillation (V-fib)

D) Sinus tachycardia

C – In cases of V-fib, after defibrillation and quality chest compressions are initiated, IV amiodarone can be administered. Though lidocaine is still administered in many institutions for ventricular arrhythmias, in the most recent versions of ACLS and PALS, amiodarone is considered the "drug of choice" for those nasty ventricular arrhythmias.

46) When giving atropine to a bradycardic child (> 5 kg), the <u>minimum</u> recommended dose is:

A) 0.1 mg/kg

B) 1 mg/kg

C) 0.1 mg

D) 1 mg

C - Whether atropine is given IM/IV to dry secretions or rapidly IV <u>for persistent bradycardia</u> (after trying oxygen first), the minimum recommended dose for kids > 5 kg is 0.1 mg. This is to prevent paradoxical bradycardia which can occur with smaller doses. Doses less than 0.1 mg can result in paradoxical bradycardia, meaning that the atropine actually reduces the heart rate instead of increasing it as intended. The crash cart box of atropine typically has 1 mg in 10 mL, so the minimum volume of atropine to give is 1ml. It should be noted that there is one very special population for whom atropine will not work. Atropine helps with bradycardias by blocking the effects of the vagus nerve, but in children who have had heart transplants, the vagus nerve is cut during the surgery, and therefore atropine will not work. Oxygen, epinephrine, or pacing should be utilized in these special children.

Certified Pediatric Emergency Nurse (CPEN) Review IV

47) A 6-month-old child with a history of congenital heart disease presents to the ED. She is pale, the liver size is normal, crackles are heard upon auscultation, and she becomes short of breath when she tries to feed. The nurse knows that these symptoms can be indicative of:

A) Left ventricular failure

B) Right ventricular failure

C) Left atrial failure

D) Right atrial failure

A – These are signs of left ventricular failure. Remember in basic cardiac anatomy, the left ventricle is responsible for pumping oxygenated blood from the lungs to the body. The right ventricle pumps blood from the body to the lungs. When the left side fails, blood backs up into the lungs and doesn't circulate well, hence the abnormal lung sounds and the pale skin. Left begins with "L" and blood backs up into the "L"ungs. Right heart failure causes blood to back up into the body, and might be evidenced by peripheral edema and liver congestion. Right begins with "R" and the blood backs up into the "R"est of the body. The atria feed the ventricles and are offered as answers to distract you.

48) The ED nurse understands that inotropic and vasodilative drugs are given to a child with congestive heart failure in order to:

A) Decrease preload, increase afterload, and decrease contractility

B) Decrease preload, decrease afterload, and increase contractility

C) Increase preload, decrease afterload, and increase contractility

D) Increase preload, increase afterload, and decrease contractility

B – The goals in CHF are three fold: 1) Decrease preload (what's coming into the heart), 2) decrease afterload (make it easier for the heart to pump out what just came in), and 3) increase contractility (make the heart able to pump stronger.) Just like adults, this is commonly done with a combination of therapies including diuretics, Lanoxin (digoxin), Dobutrex (dobutamine), and afterload reducers such as ACE inhibitors.

49) As with many cardiac medications, children receiving Lanoxin (digoxin) are at risk for developing toxicity. Which of the following is the most common **early** sign of possible toxicity?

A) Vomiting

B) Visual changes

C) Profound bradycardia

D) Hypotension

A – As is the case when the body has too much of just about anything, one of the earliest signs is vomiting. Vomiting is the body's way of saying: "Don't take any more of that stuff." If a child on Lanoxin (digoxin) is vomiting, checking a digoxin level is definitely warranted before ruling out the vomiting as just gastroenteritis. If the child is found to have a toxic level of digoxin, administration of Digibind (Digoxin Immune Fab) to bind digoxin should be considered. Though bradycardia, visual changes, and hypotension can occur with digoxin toxicity, vomiting may be the first sign.

Cardiovascular

50) A 2-year-old child, after successful resuscitation from cardiac arrest, is observed to have converted to a bradycardic rhythm with a rate of 22 and frequent premature ventricular contractions (PVCs.) The physician, noting the frequent PVCs, orders amiodarone to suppress the ventricular ectopy. Should the nurse question this order?

A) Yes

B) No

A – Absolutely yes! Stop everything and question the order. The child is having PVCs to try to compensate for having a heart rate of 22. If you give him amiodarone (or lidocaine) to stop the ectopy, he will still have a heart rate of 22 (or less if the monitor is counting the PVCs) and nobody wants that. Epinephrine, continued chest compressions, and external pacing to speed up the intrinsic heart rate are appropriate in this situation. Amiodarone is not.

51) While in the ED, an 11-year-old with an automatic implantable cardioverter/defibrillator (AICD) due to a history of Long Q-T Syndrome suddenly loses consciousness and is pulseless. VF is found on the monitor. The nurse should:

A) Defibrillate

B) Wait for the AICD to defibrillate

C) Begin CPR

D) Administer IV epinephrine

A – AICDs do a great job of keeping people who just went into a "really bad" rhythm from staying in that "really bad" rhythm. However, nothing is perfect, so if a child is in a rhythm not compatible with life, and the AICD didn't convert it, you have to try to convert it.

52) A 16-year-old male in shock is admitted to the ED after being extricated from a serious motor vehicle collision. He didn't wear his seat belt, and as a result, sustained significant chest trauma. A chest x-ray reveals fractures to the 3rd-6th ribs on the left side and a "big heart shadow." He is diagnosed with probable cardiac tamponade. In his initial resuscitation, IV fluid boluses:

A) Replace lost fluid volume

B) Increase preload and temporarily increase cardiac output

C) Increase afterload and temporarily increase blood pressure

D) Are contraindicated because of potential pulmonary contusions

B – Though fluids and blood products are typically given to help restore lost volume, in cases of pericardial tamponade, the primary rationale for fluid administration is to increase the preload. The heart is getting squished and giving extra fluids can help to temporarily "stretch" the heart, and hopefully this will help it pump more effectively (Remember Starling's curve and stretching/squeezing.) This intervention is done to help keep the patient alive until a pericardiocentesis, pericardial window, or thoracotomy can be done.

Certified Pediatric Emergency Nurse (CPEN) Review IV

53) All of the following can be complications of pericardiocentesis **except**?

A) Ventricular perforation

B) Pneumothorax

C) Ventricular fibrillation

D) Extravasation into the 4th ventricle

D – Don't be fooled by fancy sounding words, as the 4th ventricle is in the brain, not the chest. While ultrasound or fluoroscopy guided pericardiocentesis is becoming increasingly more common, this procedure is still largely a "blind" stick in which a big needle is inserted under the ribs and toward the heart. It can certainly have complications such as accidentally hitting the lung along the way or perforating the heart itself (and not just the pericardial sac.) Touching the heart with a sharp object (like a big needle) can easily induce V-fib.

54) During a pericardiocentesis, the ECG monitor should be closely watched for:

A) Premature ventricular contractions

B) ST-segment changes

C) Ventricular fibrillation

D) All of the above

D – All of the above are signs of an "unhappy" heart that can be caused by the pericardiocentesis needle going in too deep. Think about what's happening and bear in mind that the person doing the procedure is hoping to aspirate the blood from the pericardial sac and not from the ventricle. One easy way to know the needle has gone "too deep" is to watch for any of the above signs of an angry myocardium.

55) Which statement is **true** about Inotropin (dopamine) administered at doses greater than 10mcg/kg/min?

A) It causes peripheral vasodilatation

B) It causes peripheral vasoconstriction

C) It causes renal vessel dilation

D) It quickly causes cyanide toxicity

B – High-dose (10-20mcg/kg/min) dopamine infusions are given to vasoconstrict (clamp down the blood vessels) and help with hypotension. Middle dose, i.e. 5-10mcg/kg/min is administered to help boost cardiac output. Low or "renal" dose dopamine (3-5mcg/kg/min) was traditionally administered to dilate the renal vessels and help with poor urine output. However, current research shows that this technique is not nearly as effective as we once thought.

Certified Pediatric Emergency Nurse (CPEN) Review IV

56) A previously healthy 16-year old teen, the driver of a car involved in a head-on motor vehicle crash, is brought to the ED by ambulance. He is complaining of chest pain and shortness of breath. ECG monitoring reveals sinus tachycardia with frequent PVCs. Based on these findings, the ED nurse suspects:

A) An acute myocardial infarction

B) Fractured ribs

C) Pneumothorax

D) Cardiac contusion

D – The tachycardia and PVCs that this patient is exhibiting are classic signs of a cardiac contusion, sometimes referred to as blunt cardiac injury or a bruised heart. Echocardiography can show decreased cardiac wall motion and possibly decreased cardiac output. Treatment in the majority of cases is supportive. We watch them closely, and in most cases within about 24 hours, the PVCs are all better and anti-arrhythmics are rarely required. While fractured ribs and pneumothoraces (collapsed lungs) are not uncommon in this situation, and would be diagnosed by physical exam findings and chest radiography, the ECG findings are the big clue here as to what the best answer is. An acute myocardial infarction in a previously healthy teen is unlikely in this scenario.

57) A 6-month old infant with a history of a partially repaired HLHS (hypoplastic left heart syndrome, i.e. no left ventricle) and pectus excavatum ("sunken chest") presents to the pediatric ED with a chief complaint of recent onset of fever to 102.3F (39.1C) and vomiting three times today at home. He receives enteral feedings via a gastrostomy feeding tube and is usually on oxygen at ¼ L per nasal cannula with continuous pulse oximetry monitoring. Presenting vital signs are Temp 101.8°F (38.8°C) rectal, HR 164, RR 42, BP 82/60 mmHg and SpO2 82%. He is asleep, but opens his eyes to verbal stimulation, cries in response to pain and moves all extremities. He falls back to sleep when not examined. His skin is pale and diaphoretic, capillary refill and pedal pulses are normal, but there are severe sternal retractions. What would be the highest priority of the following nursing interventions?

A) Ask the mother about the child's baseline respiratory status, rate, skin color and oxygen saturation

B) Apply high flow oxygen via non-rebreather mask at 10 L

C) Begin bag-valve-mask ventilation and prepare for intubation

D) Obtain intravenous access and prepare to infuse a bolus of 20ml/kg normal saline

A – An infant who has not undergone complete repair of some congenital heart defects may have a low baseline oxygen saturation and may normally run a pulse oximeter in the low 80s. This is especially significant since the mother is likely to have a high level of knowledge and understanding regarding her son's condition and her chief complaint is not related to his respiratory status or his oxygenation levels. Additionally, pectus excavatum can present with an appearance of severe retractions. Since the mother is not alarmed by his respiratory status, it is reasonable to ask if this is normal for him and not assume the infant is experiencing acute respiratory distress. Because he has brisk capillary refill and good peripheral pulses, further examination is necessary before assuming dehydration and administration of a fluid bolus. This is especially true for children with certain cardiac defects who may be easily prone to fluid overload and are usually on some sort of diuretic to prevent heart failure.

Certified Pediatric Emergency Nurse (CPEN) Review IV

58) A 2-year-old is pulled from an icy pond and transferred in full cardiopulmonary arrest to your facility. The single **most** important factor influencing survival is:

A) Immediate defibrillation

B) Immediate cardioversion

C) Immediate re-warming victim to at least 86°F (30°C)

D) Immediate medication administration

C – Immediate and continuing attempts at re-warming are the single most important factors influencing survival for out-of-hospital arrest involving cold water submersion. Re-warming the patient to at least 86.0°F (30°C) is recommended before abandonment of CPR because the heart may be unresponsive to resuscitative efforts until a warmer core temperature is achieved. Defibrillation and anti-arrhythmia agents will most likely not be effective on the hypothermic patient until the patient is warmed to at least 86°F (30°C) as the heart is simply way too cold. Defibrillation is only indicated if the patient's cardiac rhythm is ventricular fibrillation and should be preceded and immediately followed by high quality CPR. Cardioversion works great for kids in SVT, but is not indicated for a patient in cardiopulmonary arrest. Remember, with cold-water drowning, "You're not dead until you're warm and dead!"

59) A 6-month old infant arrives at the Pediatric ED directly from his pediatrician's office. On exam, the infant was found to be in SVT (supraventricular tachycardia.) Vitals at triage are BP 78/52, HR 270, RR 28, SaO2 96% on room air. The infant is alert, has been feeding well, and is pink and well perfused. The ED staff has already placed him on 100% oxygen via face mask, attempted ice to the face, and adenosine IV x 2. The infant remains in SVT despite these efforts. The next intervention to expect is:

A) Defibrillation at 2J/kg

B) Start a Lidocaine (Xylocaine®, Lignocaine®) drip

C) Sedate and synchronized cardioversion at 0.5-1J/kg

D) Contact pediatric cardiology for additional medication recommendations

D – Many children tolerate SVT well, and this infant is in what's considered stable SVT. Why is it considered stable? He's alert and probably wondering why all these strange people are around him. He's feeding without any difficulty. His skin color indicates that he is adequately perfused, and he does not appear to be in any respiratory distress. To him, the biggest problem is who took away his "binky" (pacifier, dummy) and strapped that thing to his face? The patient may be stable, but he just can't hang out in SVT all day.

The ED staff appropriately tried vagal maneuvers initially, and then pharmacological treatments to bring the infant back to normal sinus rhythm. The cold immersion simulation (bag of crushed ice briefly applied to face) followed by adenosine (0.1 mg/kg x 1; can repeat to 0.2 mg/kg up to 12 mg rapid IV push/dose if no conversion) were unsuccessful, so the next step, (hopefully under the guidance of a pediatric cardiologist or pediatric referral center) is to try other medications (digoxin, beta-blockers, etc.) or consider synchronized cardioversion.

Defibrillation is for "Dead" people, and rhythms associated with death such as ventricular fibrillation and pulseless ventricular tachycardia. Defibrillation should only be used on a patient that has a disorganized, ineffective electrical impulse. This infant has a pulse and rhythm with a QRS complex; it's just REALLY fast. Defibrillating SVT can disrupt the QRS complexes and cause a full arrest in this patient. Lidocaine also can be used in "Dead" rhythms as mentioned above.

If he becomes unstable or with pediatric cardiology/referral center guidance, SEDATE FIRST as needed (Yes, babies feel pain and shooting electricity through the chest really does hurt!) and then synchronized cardioversion will hopefully convert the SVT into a NSR. Cardioversion starts at 0.5-1J/kg and then can be doubled to 2J/kg if there are no results – but no higher. It is crucial to remember to hit the "sync" button prior to each cardioversion attempt to ensure that cardioversion, not defibrillation, is done. Because the infant has a perfusing rhythm, you want the electricity delivered at the "right" point of the cardiac cycle so as not to knock the heart into V-Fib (as that would be a very bad thing). Remember this basic decision tree when it comes to the majority of cases of SVT:

1. Is the patient stable?

    Yes – Age appropriate vagal maneuvers and go to step 2

    No – Go to step 8

2. Recheck cardiac rhythm. Has the SVT resolved?

    Yes - It worked! – Great. Catch your breath and continue to care for the patient

    No - It didn't work. Go to step 3

3. Is the patient still stable?

    Yes. Go to step 4

    No – Go to step 8

4. Does the patient have IV or IO access?

    Yes – Give adenosine and go to step 5

    No – Get IV or IO access

    Give adenosine and go to step 5

5. Recheck cardiac rhythm. Has the SVT resolved?

    Yes - It worked! – Great. Catch your breath and continue to care for the patient

    No - It didn't work. – Go to step 6

6. Is the patient still stable?

    Yes – Go to step 7

    No – Go to step 8

7. Call peds cardiology or peds referral center, consider other medications vs. sedation and synchronized cardioversion

8. Give sedation if required and provide synchronized cardioversion as quickly as possible

60) A 13-year old child with a confirmed history of WPW (Wolff-Parkinson-White Syndrome) arrives in the ED with complaint of dizziness, mild shortness of breath, and a "racing heart." He is alert, pale, ambulatory, but "just not feeling right." BP is 102/54, RR 24, and SaO2 is 95% on room air. Quickly placing him on the cardiac monitor and supplemental oxygen, you notice that he has a rapid heart rate >200, and is in atrial fibrillation with a rapid ventricular response. What is the **most** likely intervention to be done for this patient?

A) Administer Cordarone® (amiodarone)

B) Administer Lanoxin® (digoxin)

C) Administer a calcium channel blocker

D) Defibrillation at 2J/kg

A - Amiodarone is the drug of choice for this patient since he is relatively stable. Dosing for amiodarone dosing is 5mg/kg IV over 20-60 minutes followed by a continuous infusion of 5-15mcg/kg/min IV. Since amiodarone has multiple mechanisms of action, it is less likely to cause a worsening of the arrhythmia (as will be explained below). Of course, if the patient was severely hypotensive, looking "shocky," generally unstable or unconscious, then the first course of action would be synchronized cardioversion at 0.5-1J/kg. WPW is a form of supraventricular tachycardia. In these patients, there is the normal electrical conduction pathway of the heart, as well as an extra pathway called an accessory pathway. In WPW, normal impulses take not just one, but both pathways, and go around the heart very, very quickly. This, in turn, causes the heart to beat very, very quickly and commonly presents as atrial flutter or atrial fibrillation (A-Fib.)

In most cases, when a patient presents with atrial fibrillation, the treatment is generally the administration of drugs that prolong the refractory period (time when the muscle fiber cannot be stimulated of the AV node--i.e. calcium channel blockers, beta blockers and Lanoxin® However, this patient is different. In addition to the A-Fib, he has a history of WPW Syndrome. Giving the above-mentioned medications to patients in A-Fib with the history of WPW will increase the rate of transmission through the accessory or alternative pathway. This will actually increase, not decrease, the ventricular rate. For WPW patients, calcium channel blockers, beta blockers and digoxin can cause the arrhythmia to deteriorate into ventricular fibrillation, and is one of the most common reasons for death from WPW.

61) EMS is en route to the pediatric ED with a 3-year old, previously healthy female who was found by the mother to be "very sleepy and breathing fast." EMS reports that the mother found an empty bottle of diet pills next to the patient. The initial assessment finds the child to have a Glasgow Coma Scale of 8, BP 48/22, RR 6, and SaO2 of 82% on 100% oxygen by face mask. ECG shows SVT with a rate of 290. Attempts x 2 for intraosseous (IO) access have been unsuccessful. Which intervention would you do **first**?

A) Administer 6mg of Adenocard® (adenosine) rapid IV push

B) Synchronized cardioversion the patient at 0.5-1J/kg

C) Have the patient blow through a straw

D) Defibrillate the patient at 2J/kg

B - Synchronized cardioversion is the appropriate and immediate intervention. The patient is in a really unstable SVT. She is nearly unresponsive, hypotensive, has ineffective respirations and needs to be stabilized as quickly as possible. Non-pharmacological vagal maneuvers such as ice to the face or forced exhalation through a straw have no place here when the child's condition is clearly critical. Adenosine (pediatric initial dose of 0.05 to 0.1 mg/kg) is indicated when patients are in stable tachyarrhythmias and when there is no great hurry to return the patient to normal sinus rhythm. Defibrillation is indicated when there is a lethal arrhythmia such as ventricular fibrillation or pulseless ventricular tachycardia. Remember: This child has a pulse, it's just REALLY fast and she obviously isn't tolerating it well. Immediate synchronized cardioversion, most likely quickly followed by intubation, is what this critically ill child requires.

62) Children with various ductal-dependent cardiac diseases may present with each of the following **except**:

A) Different preductal and postductal SaO2 readings

B) Markedly different upper and lower extremity blood pressures

C) Central cyanosis, tachypnea, and an audible murmur

D) Pyloric stenosis and projectile vomiting

Certified Pediatric Emergency Nurse (CPEN) Review IV

D – While pyloric stenosis and projectile vomiting do go together, they are not related to ductal-dependent cardiac diseases. Answers A and C are classic for cyanotic ductal-dependent lesions in general. Answer B is usually indicative of coarctation of the aorta, which is an acyanotic defect that is sometimes ductal-dependent. Additionally, signs and symptoms of CHF, as listed in answer C, are often observed. Cyanotic and acyanotic lesions are summarized in greater detail at www.congenitalheartdefects.com.

Additional Pediatric ED Attending Physician Insights: "It is important to determine whether the disease is cyanotic or acyanotic in the ED so you know: A) The patient's baseline (if they live at an oxygenation saturation of 84%, then 84% is just fine for them) and B) Whether the saturation isn't coming up because you're not doing enough or because it'll NEVER get above 84%! If a patient with acyanotic disease shows up cyanotic, that patient is in trouble. If a cyanotic disease patient is cyanotic, you may or may not have to improve his/her oxygenation.

63) During a softball game, the 12-year old shortstop suffered a witnessed sudden cardiac arrest. An automatic external defibrillator (AED) was promptly applied and revealed a "shockable" rhythm (assumed to be ventricular fibrillation). Defibrillation was successfully performed. Shortly thereafter, the child was alert and appropriate. The anticipated reason for her spontaneous ventricular fibrillation arrest:

A) Long QT syndrome

B) Spontaneous VF syndrome

C) Long PQRST syndrome

D) Short QT syndrome

A – Long QT syndrome is a hereditary condition in which the QT interval in the cardiac cycle is prolonged. This can result in an "R on T" phenomenon and predispose the child to spontaneous ventricular fibrillation. This condition is most often discovered in children who have a history of syncopal episodes or even unexplained near-drowning. Due to an increased awareness of the potentially-lethal consequences of this syndrome, it's more commonly being diagnosed during medical screenings prior to a child's participation in organized sports. If any patient is found to have long QT syndrome, all close family members should be screened for the same condition. The goal is to diagnose and treat the condition before significant dysrhythmias occurs. Once diagnosed, pediatric cardiologists will often prescribe anti-arrhythmic medications and may recommend the implantation of an automated internal cardioverter-defibrillator (AICD) to immediately convert any potentially lethal arrhythmias. It's important to remember that if a child or adult who has an AICD presents in a symptomatic "shockable" cardiac rhythm, you should NOT wait for the AICD to convert the rhythm. You should just "shock" them! If the AICD could have converted the rhythm, it would have. And since it didn't, you should! (Just don't place the defibrillator pads or paddles directly on top of the AICD.) Oh yeah, there is no such thing as spontaneous VF syndrome, long PQRST syndrome, or short QT syndrome.

64) A teenage patient with a history of intravenous drug abuse (IVDA) presents to the ED with complaints of "feeling crummy for a few days." He is alert with good perfusion, but is found to be febrile and have splinter hemorrhages (red/red-brown lines of blood beneath the nails that resemble splinters) under the fingernails and a new heart murmur. Specifically with his history of IVDA, which of the following is the likely cause of his "feeling crummy"?

A) Acute myocardial infarction

B) Kawasaki's disease

C) Cardiomyopathy

D) Subacute bacterial endocarditis

D – When assessing and caring for patients with a history of IVDA, the ED nurse should worry about overdoses, but must also be on the lookout for other serious complications, such as skin infections, hepatitis and HIV. One of the other feared complications is that of subacute bacterial endocarditis (SBE). This occurs when bacteria from contaminated drugs and needles lodge and grow on the heart valves, causing inflammation of the endocardium. The most commonly affected site is the tricuspid valve on the right side of the heart because the "icky" bacteria flow from the veins into the right side of the heart. The tricuspid valve is first convenient place for the bacteria to stop. The clues that endocarditis is the correct answer in this question include: the history of IVDA, the splinter hemorrhages (sometimes, but not always, occurring with endocarditis,) and, most importantly, a new heart murmur. Heart murmurs are found in about 90% of patients with infective endocarditis. Medical management for this teen will most likely involve multiple blood cultures, antipyretics and IV antibiotics in an attempt to avoid permanent damage to the heart valve and eventual surgical valve replacement.

65) A 6-year old male was kicked in the chest by a horse. The patient has equal bilateral lung sounds, muffled heart tones, JVD and a narrowing pulse pressure. Based on this assessment, the ED nurse should expect what condition and treatment?

A) Tension pneumothorax and a needle decompression

B) Pericardial tamponade and a pericardiocentesis

C) Tension pneumothorax and a chest tube

D) Pulmonary contusion and pain management

B – The three abnormal findings listed above are known as Beck's Triad: 1) Muffled heart sounds, 2) Jugular venous distention, and 3) Narrowing pulse pressure. Beck's Triad is indicative of a pericardial tamponade, which is a collection of fluid (likely blood in this case) in the pericardial sac. This causes obstructive shock by squeezing the heart, which prevents the normal pumping action. The treatment is a pericardiocentesis, otherwise known as placing a needle into the pericardial sac to drain the fluid that is collecting there. You probably recognized that two of these answers can be tossed aside right away. By carefully reading the question, you will note that the patient has equal bilateral breath sounds, so he does not have a tension pneumothorax and will not require a needle decompression or a chest tube. The assessment also clearly indicated that something more than a contusion and pain management was involved here.

66) A three day old infant presents to the pediatric ED in shock. He is afebrile and the ED physician suspects a ductal-dependent cardiac lesion. After assisting with intubation and intraosseous access, your next priority of care is:

A) Starting broad spectrum empiric antibiotics

B) Starting amiodarone

C) Obtaining a stat 12-lead ECG

D) Starting a prostaglandin drip (Prostin VR®, Alprostadil®, PGE1,)

D – In the ABC's of emergency care, after Airway and Breathing, the next priority is Circulation. In a three day old with distress, sepsis is certainly possible, or even probable, as the cause for shock. However, this infant has no fever and is therefore believed to have a ductal-dependent cardiac lesion. In the infant with possible cyanotic heart disease, emergency nurses usually see complications when the PDA CLOSES. This means that to take care of the "C"irculation, you have to reopen the ductus or keep a closing PDA OPEN with medications such as prostaglandins (PGE1). Some ductal-dependent cardiac lesions can present with abnormal ECGs and require inotropic infusions such as dopamine and/or dobutamine as their cardiogenic shock worsens, but the primary focus in a possible PDA closure is to maintain patency of the ductus arteriosus. Once the ductus arteriosus is reopened and remains open, hopefully the infant will start to stabilize and improve its cardiac function.

67) When caring for an infant that presents with complications from probable cyanotic heart disease, the emergency nurse should use an oxygenation/ventilation strategy revolving around:

A) Permissive hypercapnia

B) Titrating to SaO2 > 90%

C) Permissive hypotension

D) Titrating to SaO2 < 90%

D – One of the normal physiological triggers for a patent ductus arteriosus (PDA) to close is the increase in serum partial pressure of oxygen during the transition from fetal (baby is still inside of mom) to postnatal (baby is outside of mom) circulation. Remember that when babies are still inside of mom, mom is doing all the work of breathing. The baby's only job is to get strong to survive in the harsh outside world. Babies still in utero are what we would consider to be hypoxic and they do just fine being hypoxic because Mom is doing all the work.

However, when the baby needs to breathe on his or her own outside of Mom, the tables are turned and it is a different story indeed. At that point, the baby breathes and the oxygen saturation typically goes up to what we would consider to be "normal" levels. This increase in saturation stimulates the PDA to close, which is great in most cases. It's great unless the baby has "icky" heart disease in which the PDA being open and allowing blood to shunt from one side of the heart to the other or one vessel to the other is all that is keeping this baby alive. In this case, when the oxygen saturation hits "normal," the PDA says "time to close" and the baby quickly says "Something's wrong, I think I'm going to die!" Thus, one strategy used to keep the PDA open (patent) and supplying blood to the baby's lungs, body, and brain is to keep the oxygen sats < 90%. pCO2 should be kept approximately 35-45mm Hg, as the issue isn't CO2, it's O2. Especially with the infants with known or highly suspected "funky, flipped upside down, and backwards heart disease", be very careful with supplemental O2; they DON'T have to have "normal" sats!

68) Common side effects from intravenous prostaglandins include all of the following **except**:

A) Hypotension

B) Flushing

C) Hypertension

D) Apnea

C – Hypertension is not a common side effect of prostaglandin (PGE1) infusion. Prostaglandins don't just dilate the patent ductus arteriosus (PDA), they dilate all the vessels. This means that the child can appear red, flushed and certainly hypotensive (especially upon initiation), but not typically hypertensive. Many infants are intubated prior to the start of PGE1 just as a precaution. It is very important to remember that apnea may occur at the higher ends of the dose range. If you are titrating your PGE1 up (rarely needed, especially in the ED) you should be prepared to intubate and ventilate! As long as the patient is otherwise stable and improving clinically, apnea is NOT an indication to wean prostaglandins (PGE1!)

Certified Pediatric Emergency Nurse (CPEN) Review IV

69) An infant in distress with a suspected ductal-dependent cardiac lesion should receive IV prostaglandins (PGE1):

A) Only after a neonatology consult

B) Even prior to echocardiography

C) As an adjunct to CPR in the event of a lethal arrhythmia

D) After proper sedation has been achieved

B – In a suspected ductal-dependent cardiac lesion, you cannot go wrong if you start PGE1. All PGE1 can do is help after plain old oxygen fails to help! The adverse effects from PGE1 (such as apnea) occur in only approximately 10% of patients and can be appropriately managed with adequate preparation available in most emergency departments, i.e. intubation. There is no need to necessarily wait for a neonatology consult and we certainly don't want to wait until the infant has completely crashed. Sedation is not needed for prostaglandin infusion.

70) When administering IV prostaglandins (PGE1), which of the following statements are **true**?

A) It may be administered in the same IV line Nipride® (nitroprusside) or epinephrine

B) It may be administered in the same line as Inotropin® (dopamine) but not dobutamine

C) It needs to be administered through a fluid warmer to be brought up to the patient's core temperature

D) It should run separately

D – Just like any other drug that your patient is likely to be very sensitive to (e.g., nitroprusside, dopamine) PGE1 should be run separately. Your patient's life depends on smooth and continuous delivery of this drug. You do NOT want to piggyback PGE1 in a line that you are titrating and may inadvertently bolus or dilute.

71) You receive 14-year old pediatric patient who was hit by line drive to the chest during a baseball game. He presents to the ED with muffled heart sounds, jugular venous distension, a steadily narrowing pulse pressure and mild pulsus paradoxus (>10 mmHg drop in systolic BP during inspiration). He is rapidly becoming hypotensive. After continuous ECG monitoring and supplemental oxygen have been initiated, you would expect that the treatment for this condition would include "sticking a big 'ol needle" in the chest entering in what location?

A) 4th or 5th mid-axillary line at a 90 degree angle, aiming for left shoulder, patient sitting up 30 degrees

B) Xiphoid process at a 30 degree angle, aiming for left shoulder, patient supine

C) 2nd or 3rd mid-clavicular line at a 90 degree angle, aiming for left shoulder, patient sitting up 30 degrees

D) Just left of the xyphoid process at a 45 degree angle, aiming for the left shoulder, patient supine or slight reverse trendelenburg

D – This patient is presenting with classic signs of a cardiac tamponade (Beck's Triad--low arterial pressure, jugular venous distention and muffled distant heart sounds). The cardiac tamponade needs to be treated with pericardiocentesis, and the only correct description for performing needle pericardiocentesis is described in option "D." The most common site for insertion of the needle is the left sternocostal margin (next to the xiphoid). Monitor the EKG closely for arrhythmias and other changes (such as S-T segment elevation) that indicate direct contact with the myocardium. The other options will hit something, but probably not the pericardial sac. Pericardiocentesis is now commonly performed under ultrasound guidance, which takes a lot of the guesswork out of determining the proper positioning of the needle to hit the pericardium.

Certified Pediatric Emergency Nurse (CPEN) Review IV

72) The previously described patient with a cardiac tamponade and subsequent needle insertion for pericardiocentesis is noted to be rapidly deteriorating. Which of the following actions would you expect?

A) The needle should be attached to wall suction to assist with rapid pericardial fluid aspiration

B) Additional bloody pericardial fluid should be gently aspirated with a syringe

C) The original needle should be removed and another inserted to assure proper drainage

D) Place a second needle posteriorly to remove additional pericardial fluid

B – The bloody pericardial fluid should be gently aspirated with a syringe and NOT placed to wall suction. A syringe was used to indicate when the pericardial sac was entered, so simply use the same syringe to aspirate the fluid. In cases of large pericardial effusions it is helpful to place a three-way stopcock in-line with the needle and syringe so fluid can be ejected from the syringe prior to aspirating again. We don't even want to think about a posterior placement!

73) A teenage overdose patient suddenly becomes unresponsive and displays the following rhythm while connected to a cardiac monitor. After quickly ruling out artifact, determining absence of pulses and beginning CPR, your next correct intervention is:

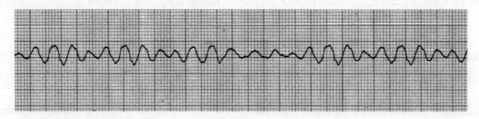

A) Unsynchronized shock at 0.5 to 1J/kg

B) Unsynchronized shock at 2J/kg

C) Synchronized shock at 0.5 to 1J/kg

D) Synchronized shock at 4J/kg

B - This patient is in witnessed V-Fib. The only correct option is to begin CPR while charging the defibrillator; administer an unsynchronized shock (defibrillation) at 2J/kg; and then immediately resume effective CPR. CPR continues for two minutes prior to the next rhythm check. Subsequent unsynchronized shocks are given at 4J/kg. Note: Many guidelines reiterate the 2J/kg, then 4J/kg defibrillation sequence that has been taught for many years; however, they remind us that if 4J/kg defibrillation attempts are unsuccessful, increasing the defibrillation energy sequentially up to 10J/kg may be considered.

74) A 2-year old patient is displaying SVT (supraventricular tachycardia) on the monitor with a rate of 260. She is hypotensive and has a decreased level of consciousness. An initial dose of adenosine (0.1 mg/kg) has been ineffective at breaking the rhythm. Your next correct intervention is:

A) Unsynchronized shock at 0.5 to 1J/kg

B) Unsynchronized shock at 2J/kg

C) Synchronized shock at 0.5 to 1J/kg

D) Synchronized shock at 4J/kg

C – This patient is in unstable SVT so the only correct option for the initial shock is SYNCHRONIZED shock (cardioversion) at 0.5 to 1J/kg. Subsequent synchronized shocks are at 2J/kg. Additional increased doses of adenosine may be considered, but not if they delay the administration of synchronized cardioversion.

75) You are performing a blood draw on a fussy 3-month old infant who presented to the Pediatric ED with persistent peripheral cyanosis. During the procedure he becomes tachypneic and very rapidly develops persistent central cyanosis. You suspect which of the following congenital defects?

A) Aortic stenosis

B) Tetralogy of Fallot

C) Coarctation of the aorta

D) Right ventricular hypertrophy (RVH)

B – The symptoms described are typical of a "tet spell" and this child most likely has Tetralogy of Fallot. Tetralogy of Fallot is the only option that decreases pulmonary artery flow and produces rapid-onset episodes of central cyanosis. Tetralogy of Fallot involves four defects, hence the "tetralogy" portion of the name: 1) A large ventricular septal defect (VSD), 2) An overriding aorta (meaning that the origin of the aorta straddles the VSD), 3) Right ventricular hypertrophy and 4) A right ventricular outflow obstruction (pulmonary artery either blocked or narrowed). The severity of the spell is directly related to how severe this pulmonary artery obstruction is – basically how bad the blockage is going from the heart to the lungs. A "tet spell" occurs when the blood going from the right ventricle to the lungs is shunted across the VSD and out the aorta (bypassing the lungs and causing a rapid onset of central cyanosis). There is no clear reason for this, although it has been suggested that the tract around the narrowed pulmonary artery may spasm. This may occur more commonly when the child has decreased systemic vascular resistance, as with moderate to severe dehydration or vagal stimulation (such as having a bowel movement or being extremely stressed). Aortic Stenosis and Coarctation of the aorta (conveniently labeled as options A and C) are acyanotic defects that reduce systemic (heart to body) blood flow. Isolated RVH also does not cause cyanosis.

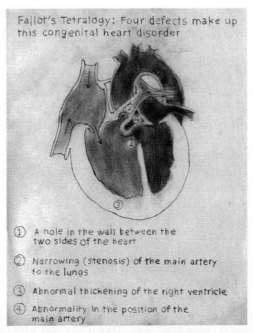

Tetralogy of Fallot 1

Courtesy of Nina DeBoer, my then 12-year old aspiring artist/baker daughter

www.ninasbeliciousbakery.com

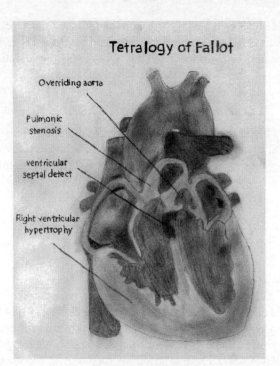

Tetralogy of Fallot 2

Courtesy of Nina DeBoer, my then 12-year old aspiring artist/baker daughter

www.ninasbeliciousbakery.com

76) Emergency treatment for the child with a "tet spell" includes:

A) Immediate cardiac echocardiogram and catheterization

B) Modified Blalock-Taussig shunt

C) Placing the knees to the chest and letting mother soothe

D) Placing 2 IVs or IOs and rapid sequence intubation

C – Staying calm yourself and calming the child are important, so placing the knees to the chest and letting mom chill the baby out is your best choice. As in epiglottitis, the mother's presence is soothing and may mitigate the existing triggering upset and reduce further pulmonary hypertension. Just as the exact mechanism of a tet spell is unknown, it's not certain why assuming a knee-chest position helps to resolve a tet spell. It's thought that the position increases the systemic vascular resistance in the lower extremities by squeezing the blood vessels (similar to the way it was thought MAST pants were supposed to work). When the systemic vascular resistance becomes higher than the resistance in the pulmonary outflow tract (caused by the fixed narrowing of the defect plus the spasm that's further cutting off flow), more blood goes to the lungs, following the path of least resistance. More flow to the lungs means better oxygenation. An echocardiogram is diagnostic, but not really an emergency treatment. A modified Blalock-Taussig shunt (a surgically inserted tube placed between the aorta or one of its branches and the pulmonary artery) is certainly not going to be done in the ED. The knees to chest positioning and calming the child will often keep us from progressing to the need for IVs or IOs and rapid sequence intubation.

Oxygen, knee-chest positioning (or squatting in older "tet kids,") and IV morphine are called for if the soothing/systemic resistance interventions don't work. We're not sure why morphine works either, but it might be that it relaxes the pulmonary vasculature enough to reduce resistance to flow. Tet spells are frightening to witness and can sometimes require intensive management but, fortunately, most resolve with little intervention.

Certified Pediatric Emergency Nurse (CPEN) Review IV

Lundblom's Lessons

A four-month old child was seen at the pediatrician's office for "congestion." She was afebrile with normal vital signs and was discharged home with instructions for treatment of an upper respiratory infection. The mom was 18-years old and this was her first baby.

The next day, the baby began having vomiting and diarrhea. When the symptoms continued for a second day, the mom called the grandmother. When the grandmother arrived at the home and saw the child, she was concerned at the infant's ill appearance and they all headed to the emergency department. When they arrived at triage, the baby was rushed to the resuscitation area due to the infant's altered mental status, sunken fontanel, and poor skin turgor. IV access was established and fluid resuscitation was started. The infant received a significant amount of fluid during her two hour peds ED stay as dehydration was estimated at 15-18%. Strict I/O was initiated - diapers weighed, stool losses replaced, etc. A stool culture was negative for bacterial infection, but was positive for rotavirus. The patient was discharged home after 5 days.

Mom indicated that she did not come in the first day because she had just seen the doctor who said the child was going to be fine.

I would stress to ED staff to always encourage parents to get their child reevaluated when symptoms change or worsen. It sounds pretty basic, but bears reinforcement.

Certified Pediatric Emergency Nurse (CPEN) Review IV

Appendix 4-A

Review of Common ECG Rhythms

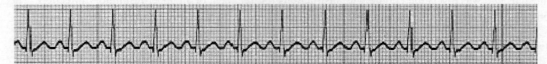

Normal Sinus Rhythm - Rate 60-100 (age dependent)

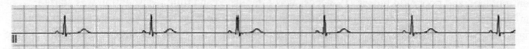

Sinus Bradycardia - Rate less than 60 (age dependent)

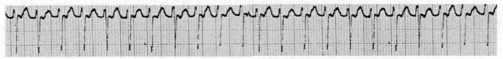

Sinus Tachycardia - Rate over 100 (age dependent)

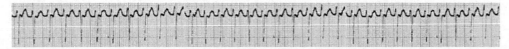

Supraventricular Tachycardia "SVT" (Fast and skinny (QRS)

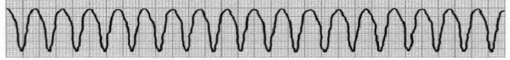

Ventricular Tachycardia (Fast and fat (QRS)

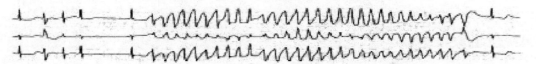

Torsades de Pointes (Fast, fat, funky, and flipping (QRS)

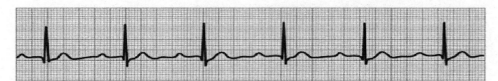

1st Degree AV block (PR >0.20)

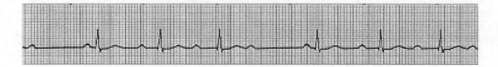

2nd Degree AV block - Type I (bad)
PR intervals getting longer and longer, then drop a QRS

Certified Pediatric Emergency Nurse (CPEN) Review IV

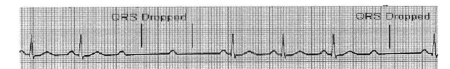

2nd Degree AV block - Type II (worse)
PR intervals OK, but drop a QRS

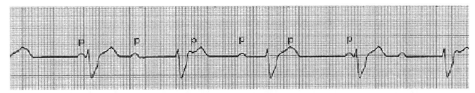

3rd Degree AV block (worst)
Atria (Ps) march out and ventricles (QRSs) march out;
But they are marching to different drummers and they are independent of each other

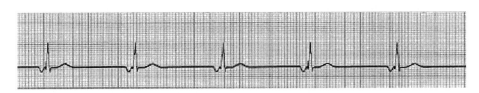

Junctional Rhythm – Slow and steady, but no P waves

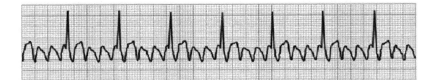

Atrial Flutter – Look for the saw tooth pattern

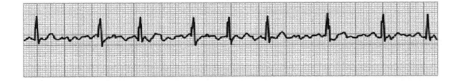

Atrial Fibrillation – No Ps and irregularly irregular

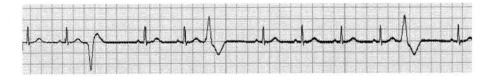

Multifocal PVC's – Simply PVC's that look different because they are different

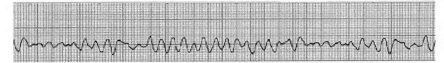

Ventricular Fibrillation – Imagine ECG leads on Jell-O

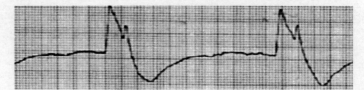

Agonal – About to be asystolic

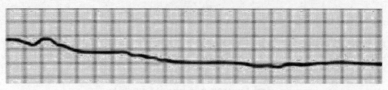

Asystole – If you can't identify this one, you probably shouldn't be taking the exam

Appendix 4-B

Summary of Common Congenital Heart Defects

Type of defect	Description	Pink or blue?	Blood flow	Medical or surgical management?
Atrial septal defect (ASD)	Hole between the right and left atriums	Pink	Increased pulmonary	Medical and either cardiac catheterization lab or surgical closure
Ventricular septal defect (VSD)	Hole between the right and left ventricles	Pink	Increased pulmonary	Medical and either cardiac catheterization lab or surgical closure
Patent ductus arteriosus (PDA)	Artery between the aorta and pulmonary artery that didn't close on its own	Pink	Increased pulmonary	Medical and either cardiac catheterization lab or surgical closure
Atrioventricular canal (AV canal)	ASD joined with a VSD	Pink	Increased pulmonary	Medical and surgical repair
Coarctation of the aorta (Coarc)	Narrowing of the aorta	Pink	Obstructed from ventricles	Medical and either cardiac catheterization or surgical repair
Tetralogy of Fallot (Tet)	Four defects: 1) VSD 2) Pulmonary stenosis (narrowing of artery) 3) Overriding aorta (aorta sits on top of both ventricles), and 4) Right ventricular hypertrophy (ventricle gets big trying to pump against the pulmonary stenosis)	Blue	Decreased pulmonary	Medical and surgical repair
Transposition of the great vessels (Transposition)	"Big vessels are switched." The pulmonary artery comes off of the left ventricle and the aorta comes off of the right ventricle	Blue	Decreased pulmonary	Medical, cardiac catheterization lab, and surgical repair
Hypoplastic left heart syndrome (Hypoplast)	Profound badness. Babies born with essentially no left ventricle.	Blue	Mixed	Medical and surgical repair vs. transplant vs. hospice

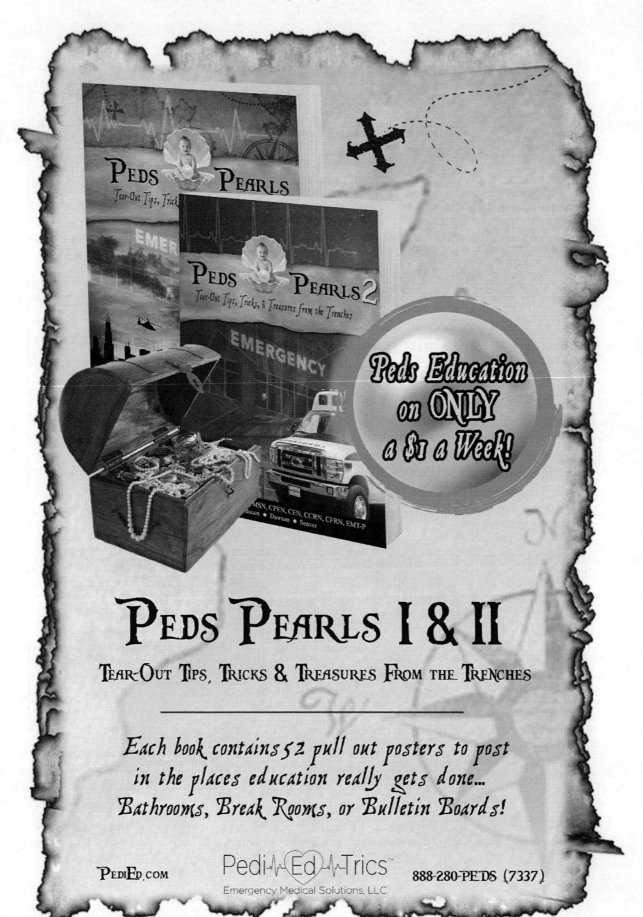

Chapter 5

Neurological/Psychiatric Emergencies
Neuro Nightmares and Dysfunctional Dilemmas

*I've been to war. I've raised twins.
If I had a choice, I'd rather go to war.*
-George W. Bush

Pertinent Pediatric Ponderings (NOTES)

CHAPTER 5
Sample Test Answer Sheet

1. _____	29. _____	57. _____	85. _____	113. _____
2. _____	30. _____	58. _____	86. _____	114. _____
3. _____	31. _____	59. _____	87. _____	115. _____
4. _____	32. _____	60. _____	88. _____	116. _____
5. _____	33. _____	61. _____	89. _____	117. _____
6. _____	34. _____	62. _____	90. _____	118. _____
7. _____	35. _____	63. _____	91. _____	119. _____
8. _____	36. _____	64. _____	92. _____	120. _____
9. _____	37. _____	65. _____	93. _____	121. _____
10. _____	38. _____	66. _____	94. _____	122. _____
11. _____	39. _____	67. _____	95. _____	123. _____
12. _____	40. _____	68. _____	96. _____	124. _____
13. _____	41. _____	69. _____	97. _____	125. _____
14. _____	42. _____	70. _____	98. _____	126. _____
15. _____	43. _____	71. _____	99. _____	127. _____
16. _____	44. _____	72. _____	100. _____	128. _____
17. _____	45. _____	73. _____	101. _____	129. _____
18. _____	46. _____	74. _____	102. _____	130. _____
19. _____	47. _____	75. _____	103. _____	131. _____
20. _____	48. _____	76. _____	104. _____	132. _____
21. _____	49. _____	77. _____	105. _____	133. _____
22. _____	50. _____	78. _____	106. _____	134. _____
23. _____	51. _____	79. _____	107. _____	135. _____
24. _____	52. _____	80. _____	108. _____	136. _____
25. _____	53. _____	81. _____	109. _____	137. _____
26. _____	54. _____	82. _____	110. _____	138. _____
27. _____	55. _____	83. _____	111. _____	139. _____
28. _____	56. _____	84. _____	112. _____	

[Remove page and cover rationale until after you answer question]

Pertinent Pediatric Ponderings (NOTES)

Certified Pediatric Emergency Nurse (CPEN) Review IV

1) The **most** common cause of death in children over 1 year of age is:

A) Motor vehicle crashes (MVC)

B) Drownings

C) Suicide/homicide

D) Abuse

A – In children older than one year, injury is the leading cause of death. Injury exceeds every other cause of death, combined. Motor vehicle accidents are the most common cause of death for one to nineteen year old children. The next most common cause of deaths are homicide or suicide (mostly with firearms), and then drowning.

2) The pattern of injury commonly found in cases of pediatric pedestrian vs. motor vehicles is called:

A) Cushing's Triad

B) Beck's Triad

C) Waddell's Triad

D) Trauma Triad

C – Waddell's Triad describes the pattern of injuries for pediatric pedestrians when they "Waddell" across the street and are struck by a moving vehicle. Considering the size of the child and the size of the vehicle, it's easy to understand what is likely to happen and what's going to hit what. The child's chest, abdomen, or lower extremities strike the car, quickly followed by the child flying through the air "with the greatest of ease," before the child lands, often head-first. Head, chest, abdominal, and lower extremity injuries should be anticipated in a child vs. motor vehicle scenario.

3) The <u>minimum</u> possible score on the pediatric Glasgow Coma Scale (GCS) is:

A) 0

B) 3

C) 10

D) 15

B – The Glasgow Coma Scale measures three things (motor, eye opening, and verbal response), and the lowest score on each is 1, so the minimum possible score is 3. Even a rock has a GCS of 3. A rock has no eye opening, no verbal response, and no motor response, so the GCS is 3.

Neuro / Psych

4) The <u>maximum</u> possible score on the pediatric Glasgow Coma Scale (GCS) is:

A) 0

B) 3

C) 10

D) 15

D) The maximum score on the GCS is 15. Since it measures three things, it would be nice if all three ranged from 1 to 5. But that's not how it works. One category is worth up to 4 points, another 5, and still another 6. So how do you remember what gets 4, what gets 5, and what gets 6? Try this little trick. The word "eyes" has 4 letters, so the maximum eye opening score is 4. "Voice" or "Vocal" has 5 letters, so the maximum vocal response is 5. The last one isn't quite as simple, but you might think of your motor being an engine. "Engine" has 6 letters so the maximum for motor response is 6. You now know the secret of figuring out the Glasgow Coma Scale.

Neuro / Psych

5) A 2-year-old falls from a shopping cart and briefly loses consciousness. Upon arrival to the ED, he is awake and alert, but even before a CT scan can be arranged, he quickly deteriorates. This situation is indicative of which type of intracranial hemorrhage?

A) Epidural

B) Subdural

C) Subarachnoid

D) Intracerebral

A – This child has classic symptoms associated with an epidural hematoma. These patients momentarily lose consciousness from the concussion, but then they quickly wake up as they recover from their concussion. Unfortunately, shortly thereafter, the child does the classic "crash and burn" due to the arterial blood squirting around the brain. These are often called the "smile and die bleeds" because at first, they are smiling, and then they are dying.

6) A 4-year-old with a clotting disorder requiring long-term anticoagulation with Coumadin (warfarin) presents to the ED after suffering a seizure at home. His mother reports that except for the clotting disorder, the child is healthy and states that he did fall off of the swing set a few days ago and bumped his head. There was no loss of consciousness at the time. This combination of history and symptoms is indicative of which type of intracranial hemorrhage?

A) Epidural

B) Subdural

C) Subarachnoid

D) Intracerebral

B – Subdural bleeds are venous in origin and for a child who is on anticoagulants, this type of bleed can just keep going and going and going. It's venous, so the symptoms can take a while to present, and that's why this child had a seizure. Note: Adults who have clotting problems from age, medication, or a long history of significant alcohol abuse are also at risk for the same situation.

7) Subarachnoid hemorrhages:

A) Occur primarily in adult patients and are often fatal if not treated promptly

B) Develop slowly over time

C) Are venous in nature like the subdural bleed

D) All of the above

A – Beware of the "All of the above" answers. Subarachnoid hemorrhages are more common in adults, but can occur in kids, especially after head trauma. Subarachnoid bleed symptoms commonly come on suddenly, often without warning, and symptoms may not last very long, because the patient may not last very long. The presentation typically involves a patient complaining of a sudden "worst headache of their life." This is what happens when the patient pops an aneurysm in their head and arterial blood is squirting where it shouldn't be. These patients are indeed downright sick. The thing to remember for the test is that if the question mentions "worst headache of their life," chances are the answer is subarachnoid hemorrhage.

8) Cerebral concussions are associated with which of the following?

A) Post-concussive Syndrome

B) Second-Impact Syndrome

C) Prolonged Loss of Consciousness Syndrome

D) A and B

D - Sports Related Concussion (SRC) is often defined as representing the immediate and transient symptoms of traumatic brain injury (TBI). In most patients, concussions are defined as amnesia or loss of consciousness after a head injury. The vast majority of patients with concussions do just fine. However, there are two relatively new syndromes associated with concussions. Post-concussive Syndrome means the head CT is fine, the MRI is fine, and the patient looks fine to everyone except for "Dr. Mom," who says "my kid's not the same." It's very real. Even after a minor head injury, neuropsychiatric changes can occur and parents need to know that in most cases, it will get better. But it can take weeks or even months for the little changes (that only mom/dad/friends notice) to resolve and the child returns to normal. Second-Impact Syndrome is described as a situation where a person sustains a second head injury before the first injury has completely healed or resolved. The second impact may be shortly after the initial insult, or may occur days later. If it occurs to a boxer or football player, the person may get hit on the head and be unconscious for a brief period of time. They "look fine" and return to the activity, only to be hit on the head again. The second-impact results in devastating cerebral edema and possible death.

In 2016, an international sports medicine consensus statement summarized the suspected diagnosis of Sports Related Concussion to include one or more of the following clinical domains:

1. Symptoms: somatic (eg, headache), cognitive (eg, feeling like in a fog) and/or emotional symptoms (eg, lability)
2. Physical signs (eg, loss of consciousness, amnesia, neurological deficit)
3. Balance impairment (eg, gait unsteadiness)
4. Behavioural changes (eg, irritability)
5. Cognitive impairment (eg, slowed reaction times)
6. Sleep/wake disturbance (eg, somnolence, drowsiness)

9) Shaken Baby Syndrome (SBS) is diagnosed by all of the following **except**:

A) Patient history

B) Diagnostic imaging findings

C) Retinal hemorrhages

D) Socio-economic and educational history

D – Socio-economic background and education are not factors in the diagnosis of Shaken Baby Syndrome. Currently, in court, if the patient has retinal hemorrhages (90% of SBS cases) and a CT scan (subdural bleeds) that doesn't fit the history provided, it's considered Shaken Baby Syndrome. If you ask physicians who work with child protective service agencies if more people shaking their babies, most don't really think so. They will tell you that we now just know what to look for so we're finding a whole lot more cases. Shaken Baby Syndrome is not caused by playing with children, rolling off the couch, or other commonly reported reasons for the child's status. Someone literally has to shake the child to death. That's an important clarification. As a point of reference, roller coasters produce 3-4 "G"s of force, fighter pilots experience 6 "G"s of force, and shaking causes linear and angular forces up to 9.3 "G"s. That means that shaken babies can experience more force than an adult Top Gun fighter pilots. Even worse, is as they are shaken, their head hits something solid, the forces *increase 50-fold*! Just remember that SBS kids need to be admitted. They need to be kept safe while the social "what's what" is figured out. If suspicions are there, do the CT right away, and then have ophthalmology take peek at the child.

10) Which of the following statements is **incorrect** regarding cerebrospinal fluid shunts?

A) The proximal catheter is usually inserted into one of the ventricles of the brain

B) The distal catheter is tunneled under the skin and is most often placed in the peritoneal cavity (ventriculoperitoneal (VP) shunt)

C) Shunts are named for the position of their proximal and distal catheters

D) Fever is a defining characteristic of a child with a malfunctioning shunt

D – Fever is not always present with a malfunctioning shunt due to obstruction, and shunt infections generally do not present with fever unless there is another concomitant infection. Symptoms such as irritability, headache, mental status changes, vomiting, and general malaise and are more common with VP shunt malfunction. Most infected shunts are not malfunctioning. The symptoms are caused by central nervous system infection, not the failure of the shunt to appropriately channel cerebral spinal fluid (CSF.) In children, ventriculoperitoneal (VP) shunts are commonly placed to drain CSF from the brain (ventricles) into the abdomen (peritoneum) where it will be reabsorbed. Though sometimes shunts are placed so CSF drains into the right atrium (VA), the majority of shunts are ventriculoperitoneal.

11) Which of the following statements are **correct** regarding Munchausen by Proxy Syndrome?

A) The child's father is typically the perpetrator

B) The child typically has a history of chronic illness or congenital defects

C) The caregiver denies knowledge as to the cause of the child's illness

D) The child usually establishes a much closer bond with the father than the mother

C – Munchausen's by Proxy Syndrome involves previously healthy children in whom caregivers induce illness or injury. It is actually a disorder of the caregiver who is using the child's condition as a way of seeking attention for themselves. The caregiver typically denies any knowledge as to the cause of the illness. Mothers are by far the most common perpetrators, though in rare cases, fathers have been involved as well. As mothers are the ones that spend the majority of time with young children, especially when the child is sick, strong bonding is expected. The child doesn't know that it is Mom (or Dad) who is making them sick; they just know they are sick, and that someone they trust is looking after them.

12) Which of the following is **true** concerning head injuries in children?

A) Vomiting within the first 30-60 minutes after a head injury is common

B) Vomiting persisting for several hours after a head injury is not a concern

C) Mental status change without headache is not a concern

D) Positive mental status change ("The kid got some sense knocked into him") should be appreciated, not evaluated

A – Vomiting "a couple of times" within the first hour after a head injury, neither is uncommon nor abnormal. However, if vomiting persists for more than an hour, is more than a "couple of times," or doesn't start until several hours after the injury, especially if there are any other symptoms present (headache, mental status changes), the child should be immediately evaluated.

13) A 6-month-old child with a history of hydrocephalus and VP shunt placement presents with irritability, fever, and vomiting. In this child, these symptoms are possibly caused by:

A) Influenza

B) Gastroenteritis

C) Central nervous system (CNS) infection

D) Any of the above

Neuro / Psych

D – Here is another truism for you. Just as "airway" is almost always your answer of choice when it is available, for a sick child with a VP shunt, ruling out shunt malfunction or CNS infections are the answers you should be looking for. If a little one is "just not acting right," or "has the flu," though it certainly could be viral (especially if there is a "gastro bug" going round), issues with the shunt and CNS must be ruled out as well.

14) Common concerns with intracranial shunts include all of the following **except**:

A) CSF ascites

B) Infection

C) Malfunction

D) Revision due to growth

A – While there has been rare documented cases of CSF ascites in children with a VP shunt, concerns about shunt malfunction (and rarely infection) are much more common. Depending on the age and growth of the patient, revisions may also be needed.

Certified Pediatric Emergency Nurse (CPEN) Review IV

15) A 10-year-old child presents with a knife impaled in his skull. You should expect to:

A) Secure the knife in place

B) Probe the wound to determine depth and apply a sterile occlusive dressing over the knife to preserve any trace evidence

C) Remove the knife immediately and apply direct pressure to the wound to minimize bleeding

D) Complete the primary survey, then remove the knife to assess the length of the blade and help determine possible injuries

A – Hopefully, the answer to this question didn't take a whole lot of thought. If impaled objects are still impaled, leave them in place until everyone and everything is in place to properly remove the object and repair whatever damage it created.

16) Which of the following describes Cushing's triad?

A) Hypertension, bradycardia, and bradypnea

B) Hypertension, tachycardia, and tachypnea

C) Hypotension, bradycardia, and bradypnea

D) Hypotension, tachycardia, and tachypnea

A – Cushing's triad describes the signs associated with greatly increased intracranial pressure. With Cushing's triad, the systolic blood pressure goes progressively up, while the diastolic pressure drops (widened pulse pressure.) The heart rate and respiratory rate plummet both reflexively and due to acute brain/brainstem compression associated with impending herniation. Cushing sounds like pushing, and that's what is happening inside the head.

Neuro / Psych

17) In pediatric patients, which of the following is the **most** common type of skull fracture?

A) Linear

B) Depressed

C) Basilar

D) Open

A – Linear skull fractures are a simple skull fracture (not depressed/multiple pieces) seen on X-ray or CT. While it may not look like much, the problem is not the skull fracture, but the fact that the energy it took to break the skull doesn't stop at the skull. Intracranial injury is 10-20 times more common with a skull fracture than without one. Depressed skull fractures are when the skull is depressed into the brain and the patient is very depressed because their skull is fractured. Raccoon eyes (periorbital bruising), Battle's sign (bruising behind the ear), hemotympanum (bleeding behind the ear drum), and CSF leaks from the ear or nose are associated with basilar skull fractures. Open skull fractures are just bad.

18) All of the following are priorities during status epilepticus (SE) **except**:

A) Respiratory status

B) Detailed psychiatric history

C) Glucose level determination

D) Anticonvulsant administration

B – Seriously, the detailed psychiatric history can wait. Patient safety is our priority, and the things that will do the most harm to the patient include airway problems, hypoglycemia, and continued seizures. Status epilepticus is defined as a continuous seizure activity lasting more than 5 minutes or 2 or more seizures occurring without restoration of normal level of consciousness between the seizures.

19) For a small child with a suspected cervical spine injury, the ED nurse should:

A) Apply traction to the neck

B) Place the child directly onto a regular long spine board

C) Maintain neutral spinal alignment

D) Place a pillow under the head to protect against "Floppy Neck" syndrome

C - If a child has a suspected spinal injury, simply maintaining "neutral spinal alignment" with an appropriately sized hard cervical collar and a pediatric spine board is recommended. Traction without neurosurgery guidance is not recommended, and placement on a spine board without proper padding or a pillow behind the head won't even come close to neutral alignment. Remember, kids have big heads and little bodies!

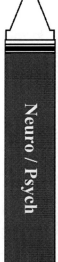

Neuro / Psych

20) Children presenting to the ED with a first time seizure should:

A) Be given Tylenol (acetaminophen, Panadol) since pediatric seizures are febrile in nature

B) Be discharged home with fever instructions and advice on how to tell shivers from seizures

C) Have a CT and a seizure work-up unless the seizure is presumed to be febrile

D) Be considered a low priority because only subsequent seizures cause damage

C– Not all seizures in children are febrile in nature. Unless the seizure is presumed to be febrile in origin, as long as the child recovers quickly and had no focal characteristics, most facilities recommend a non-emergent MRI of the head, in addition to the other customary portions of the "why did they have a seizure" workup.

21) A 3-month-old child with a history of hydrocephalus and VP shunt presents to the ED with symptoms of acutely increased intracranial pressure. Which of the following nursing interventions is **not** recommended?

A) Regularly monitor neurologic status

B) Keep head of bed elevated to 30 degrees

C) Keep head in midline position

D) Allow and encourage the infant to cry because doing so helps to decrease ICP through hyperventilation

D – Crying increases, not decreases the ICP. As the history mentions hydrocephalus and a shunt, assessing neurologic status is always a good thing to do, and just as with head trauma, 30 degree head elevation and midline head position are easy methods to help manage increased intracranial pressure.

22) Many children with a history of spinal bifida frequently are allergic to:

A) Latex

B) Penicillin

C) Morphine

D) Peanuts

A – When you hear spinal bifida, not only should you think neural tube defect, but also latex allergies. The Spinal Bifida Association reports that latex could be a problem for up to 73% of children with spinal bifida. With this in mind, many children's medical centers have gone latex free.

23) Reye's syndrome is associated with exposure to which of the following?

A) Tylenol (acetaminophen, Panadol)

B) Aspirin (aspirin)

C) Penicillin

D) Morphine

B – When the question involves Reye's syndrome, chances are the answer involves aspirin if it is medication related, or viral exposure (especially influenza or chicken pox) if it is history related.

24) If a properly fitting hard cervical collar is your first choice for immobilizing the cervical spine of a pediatric patient, which of the following would be your **last** choice?

A) Towels

B) Blanket rolls

C) Wash cloths

D) Sand bags or IV bags

D – Sandbags or IV bags may have been recommended many years ago, but, as we know, times are changing. The weight, size, and shifting nature of these bags make them a poor choice for pediatric cervical spinal immobilization. There are pediatric sized hard cervical collars, including those sold by Ossur, formerly Jerome Medical, which are made in sizes to fit babies and children. A nice feature of those collars is that they are color-coded to the Broselow-Luten Color Coding Kids system. If you don't have a collar that fits, the tried and true second choice is towels and tape.

Neuro / Psych

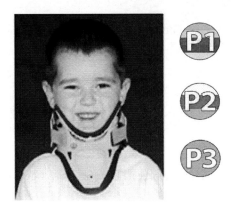

"Color-Coded" Cervical Collars

Photo courtesy of Ossur - www.ossur.com

25) Antibiotics should never be given to an infant or child with suspected meningitis until:

A) CSF cultures have been obtained

B) Blood cultures (ideally two sets) have been obtained

C) Urine cultures have been obtained

D) None of the above

D – Definitely none of the above. If the child truly has bacterial meningitis, their chance of dying or being neurologically devastated for life is really good. Ideally, CSF, blood, and urine cultures should be obtained prior to antibiotics. However, if the child is really sick, or there is a delay in obtaining the cultures (like going for a CT scan or the LP is going to be done in the pediatric ICU), then give the IV antibiotics (and steroids) first, and get the cultures later. Cultures still will be able to reveal the "culprit" even up to a few hours after the first dose of antibiotics; but if you wait to give the medications, the child very well might die.

26) A 14-year-old has been diagnosed with probable viral meningitis and is awaiting admission. While in the ED, which nursing action would **not** be appropriate for this patient?

A) Provide a quiet, restful environment

B) Admission of the patient to a non-private room

C) Frequent temperature monitoring with fever control measures

D) Encourage fluid intake

B – Until the diagnosis of viral meningitis has been confirmed, patients should be in isolation for 48 hours after the first dose of antibiotics and antivirals have been administered. Treatment for viral meningitis typically includes rest, fluids, and medications for fever and headaches.

27) Which of the following is a common sign of meningococcal disease?

A) Petechiae

B) Hypothermia

C) Ipsilateral pupil dilation

D) Hypertension

A – Petechiae (multiple purple, non-blanching, >2mm lesions all over the body) are a common sign of meningococcal meningitis, so much so that it is often called the "meningococcal rash." Most children with meningitis are febrile and often in the late stages of septic shock, so they would be hypotensive, not hypertensive. Ipsilateral pupil dilation can be indicative of direct eye trauma or cerebral herniation. Remember that most petechial rashes are not meningococcal, but they are all meningococcal until proven otherwise!

28) Kernig's sign is:

A) Flexion of the hips and knees as a result of flexion of the neck and supports the suspicion of meningitis

B) Flexion of the hips and knees as a result of flexion of the neck and may rule out meningitis

C) Pain and resistance when extending the knees while the hip is flexed at 90 degrees and supports the suspicion of meningitis

D) Pain and resistance when extending the knees while the hip is flexed at 90 degrees and may rule out meningitis

C – A positive Kernig's sign is pain when extending the knee while the hip is flexed and supports a diagnosis of meningitis. The other sign described above is Brudzinski's sign, and is also supportive of the diagnosis of meningitis. Both Kernig's sign and Brudzinski's sign are associated with meningeal irritation, most commonly, but not exclusively meningitis. Knowing which is which may be helped by remembering that Kernig's sign begins with "K" and is when the patient screams or resists when you straighten his "K"nees. Brudzinski's sign begins with "B" and is when the patient "B"ends their hips and knees after you "B"end her neck. Though neither sign is 100% diagnostic for meningitis, if either or both are present, your suspicion for possible meningitis should be much higher.

29) In pediatric patients, which of the following statements is **not** correct?

A) The infant skull is thin and pliable

B) The softer skull absorbs the impact from trauma protecting the brain from significant damage

C) The non-fused sutures and fontanels allow for intracranial expansion

D) They have large heads and weak neck musculature

B – The thin and flexible skulls of infants and young children do not absorb and protect the brain, as the energy from trauma (MVCs, falls, etc.) doesn't stop with their skulls. And even though soft, kids can break their skulls. Much more concerning, however, is the damage that's done underneath as the energy continues almost full force into the brain. Adults, as opposed to children, are "hard headed" (physically and psychologically) and this means that while there is more protection, there is also less room for brain swelling. Lastly, remember that the "big head, little body syndrome" comes into play again as the analogy of a bowling ball sitting on top of pencil is pretty descriptive and can help us to understand pediatric head and spinal cord trauma.

30) Which of the following is **not** true about febrile seizures?

A) They usually last less than 5 minutes

B) They usually end by age 5

C) The rapid rise of temperature is thought to be the cause

D) Febrile seizures are the precursors of epilepsy in 1 of 5 children

D – There is no link between febrile seizures and epilepsy. Statistically, 1 in 25 children over 6-months-old will experience a febrile seizure. These seizures are accompanied by a fever, typically last less than 5 minutes, and children generally grow out of them by age 5. These seizures are most likely to occur during the first 24 hours of a fever.

31) A fixed/dilated or "blown" pupil is:

A) An early sign of increased intracranial pressure (ICP)

B) A late sign of increased ICP

C) An early sign of decreased ICP

D) A late sign of decreased ICP

B – The "blown pupil" is a late and very ominous sign of increased ICP. Another late sign is Cushing's triad of hypertension, bradycardia, and bradypnea or apnea. In most cases, signs such as tachypnea (they are trying to decrease their pCO_2) and other neurologic indicators, such as progressive changes in the level of consciousness were present long before Cushing's triad and blown pupils.

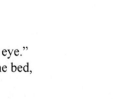

Neuro / Psych

32) An 8-year-old presents after an altercation with another student at school in which he was "poked in the eye." Physical examination reveals a hyphema. You can expect to give the parents and the child each of the following instructions **except**:

A) Avoid contact with others while he has the "pink eye"

B) Avoid excessive moving and jumping around

C) Avoid laying flat

D) Avoid rubbing the eye

A - Hyphemas are an injury to the eye, not a disease, and is certainly not the very contagious "pink eye." Treatment for hyphemas varies considerably, but all seem to agree that rest, elevating the head of the bed, and protecting the eye are important.

33) Which of the following **best** describes simple febrile seizures?

A) They last over 15 minutes

B) Multiple seizures are likely throughout the course of the fever

C) They are usually caused by a central nervous infection such as meningitis

D) They are often associated with a rapid rise in core temperature

D – Simple febrile seizures are exactly that, simple and febrile in origin and can recur in 50% of otherwise healthy kids. They are thought to occur not due to the actual fever, but from the rapid rise in the temperature. In most cases, the seizure will only occur during the first day of the fever, and they are not related to a CNS infection (CNS infections have their own seizures.) Motrin (ibuprofen, Brufen), if the child is over 6 months, and Tylenol (acetaminophen) are recommended for fever control and comfort.

34) During the clonic phase of a tonic-clonic seizure:

A) The child suddenly senses an unusual taste, change in vision, or odor

B) The child experiences continuous motor tension or rigidity

C) The child experiences rhythmic contractions alternating with relaxation of major muscle groups

D) The child slowly awakens post-seizure, but is often sleepy and confused

C – The "Clonic" phase of the seizure is when the muscles rhythmically "C"ontract and relax, or "C"onvulse (The "C" words may help you remember.) The "Tonic" phase is when the major muscle groups become rigid, or "T"ighten, which conveniently starts with a "T." Tonic-clonic or grand-mal seizures are the most common type of seizures we see in pediatric emergency care. Pre-seizure auras are experienced by some children and are described as sudden changes in taste, hearing, smell, or vision. The slow awakening after seizure activity has stopped is called the postictal phase and is very common after generalized tonic-clonic seizures.

35) Which of the following medications are typically given in the initial management of seizures?

A) Barbiturates

B) Benzodiazepines

C) Neuromuscular blockers

D) Dilantin (phenytoin) or fosphenytoin

B – Benzodiazepines (Benzo's) such as Valium (diazepam), Versed (midazolam), or Ativan (lorazepam), are the mainstay of initial treatment for most seizures in the emergency department. If those types of medications are unsuccessful in terminating the seizure activity, then other types of drugs such as fosphenytoin, or more rarely, Dilantin (phenytoin) or Phenobarbital are used in an attempt to stop the seizures and prevent them from recurring. If the second line of drugs is not successful, then drugs such as Diprivan (propofol), lidocaine, pentobarbital, and even general anesthesia can be used. If the situation has progressed to this point, the child is usually in the pediatric ICU. Neuromuscular blockers (paralytics) such as Norcuron (vecuronium) do NOTHING to stop seizure activity. They stop the muscles from moving, but the patient is still seizing; we just don't see it any more. That's why neurology and neurosurgery get so unhappy if neuromuscular blockers are given to head injury or status epilepticus patients, because unless continuous EEG monitoring is available and initiated, we really have no good way to know if they are still seizing.

36) Which statement is **true** concerning generalized tonic-clonic seizures?

A) They involve an isolated section of the temporal-parietal region

B) The entire brain is commonly involved

C) They are characterized by the slow relaxation of major muscle groups

D) "To"xic levels of "nic"otine are thought to be the cause of the seizure

B - In most cases of generalized seizure activity, one small portion of the brain is responsible for instigating the seizure, but then it spreads to the rest of the brain and brainstem.

37) The emergency nurses **first** action when caring for a postictal pediatric patient should be to:

A) Obtain a complete medical history

B) Start an IV of D5W

C) Ensure an open airway

D) Immediately notify the physician

C – Always look for the airway related answer, and in this case, airway is specifically mentioned in the answer. In some cases, airway positioning and possibly inserting a naso-pharyngeal airway may be required, and always have suction available. Obtaining a history, notifying the physician or nurse practitioner, and initiating an IV of 0.9NS (not D5W) are certainly appropriate actions, but after airway.

38) Dilantin (phenytoin) should be administered through an IV of:

A) 0.9NS

B) D5W

C) D5.45NS or D5.2NS in children under 5

D) All of the above

A – Dilantin should only be administered in a solution of normal saline. Easy reminder… "D"ilantin + "D"extrose equals "D"isaster. 0.9NS is the fluid of choice with seizures because benzodiazepines, Dilantin, fosphenytoin, or phenobarbital can all be safely administered through the IV (just not all at the same time)!

39) A 12-year-old with a history of seizures is brought to the ED because of recurrent seizures. While in the ED, he develops tonic-clonic movements starting at the fingers of the right hand and moving up the arm. The nurse identifies this patient as exhibiting which type of seizures?

A) Generalized or grand mal seizure

B) Absence or petit mal seizure

C) Focal seizure

D) Hemiparetic seizure

C – This child is having a focal seizure. It is caused by abnormal electrical activity in a localized area of the brain, and may manifest a wide variety of signs including head or eye movements, lip smacking, or rhythmic movements in specific areas. Generalized seizures involve all four extremities, while absence seizures are when the child briefly "spaces out," without loss of bowel or bladder control. A hemiparetic seizure is described as hemiparesis being a manifestation of focal seizures.

40) In the previous patient, what should the emergency nurse anticipate after the initial seizure activity ceases?

A) Recollection of the event in simple Jacksonian or partial seizures

B) Loss of consciousness

C) Incontinence of bowel and/or bladder

D) Subsequent left sided seizure activity

A – Patients experiencing simple partial/focal/Jacksonian seizures typically do not experience any change in awareness or alertness.

41) Which statement is **correct** regarding absence or petit mal seizures?

A) Absence seizures are associated with loss of bowel and/or bladder control

B) Absence seizures are associated with a transient loss of awareness of surroundings without loss of motor tone

C) Absence seizures typically last over 10 minutes

D) Absence seizures are followed by a postictal state

B – Absence or petit mal seizures involve a transient loss of awareness without motor involvement. Often the child appears to be "spacing out" or "staring out into space" for a few moments, and then returns to "normal" with no physical manifestations. These seizures do not involve a postictal period or incontinence.

42) A 15-year-old female presents via EMS to the ED after "flying through the windshield" in a high-speed motor vehicle crash (MVC.) She has clear fluid dripping from her left ear and mid-face instability. Rapid-sequence intubation is performed and she is successfully orally intubated. The ED nurse knows that to decompress the stomach, which type of gastric tube should be placed in this patient?

A) Nasogastric

B) Orogastric

C) Percutaneous (PEG)

D) None of the above

B – This patient is exhibiting two of the cardinal "NO NG TUBE" signs. First, clear fluid dripping from the ear. In a patient with head trauma, fluid dripping from the ear is CSF until proven otherwise and CSF fluid leakage is suggestive of a basilar skull fracture. The other sign is the mid-face instability, which indicates a disruption of some of the bony structures that help protect the brain. Pushing an NG tube into the nose, and then into the brain because of a basilar skull fracture or mid-face instability would just be bad form.

43) When assessing the level of consciousness in a patient, AVPU stands for:

A) Arousable, Visually responsive, Pupils responsive, Unable to determine

B) Alert, Verbal, Pain/Physical, Unresponsive

C) Awake, Verbally responsive, Positionally appropriate, Understands instructions

D) Asymptomatic, Vocalizes, PERRLA, Unconscious

B– Remember the AVPU scale stands for: (A)lert, responds to (V)erbal stimulus, responds to (P)ain/Physical stimulus, or (U)nresponsive. Essentially the scale ranges from needing no stimulation to unresponsive to nasty stimuli. If the patient is awake and alert, that's a very reassuring sign.

44) The Pediatric Glasgow Coma Scale is intended for:

A) Children under 2 years of age

B) Children under 5 years of age

C) Children under 12 years of age

D) Children under 16 years of age

A – The Pediatric Glasgow Coma Scale is intended for children under 2-years old.

45) Which of the following is the **best** way of determining a child's neurological status in the ED?

A) Glasgow Coma Scale (GCS)

B) Response to painful stimuli

C) Testing finger to nose coordination

D) Checking for pupillary reaction to light

A – Unless the patient is chemically paralyzed, the Glasgow Coma Scale is the most appropriate way to assess a child's neurological status. It is more specific than the "AVPU" scale which only reports the patient's alertness or responsiveness. (Alert, responds to Verbal stimulus, responds to Painful/Physical stimulus, or Unresponsive.) Pupil assessment may be your only option with patients who are chemically paralyzed, and finger to nose coordination works well, but only in older children. Generally speaking, assessing and trending GCS scores are your best bet.

Neuro / Psych

46) An unconscious 12-year-old is brought to the ED by ambulance after hitting his head while diving into a river. Which would hold the **highest** priority after the initial assessment has been completed?

A) Computed tomography (CT) of the head and cervical spine

B) Plain films of the cervical spine

C) Arterial blood gas (ABG) measurements

D) Routine "trauma labs"

235

A–Since the initial assessment would cover the "ABCs," we don't have an airway answer to choose. Given the history and mechanism of injury, we should have a high index of suspicion for a possible head and cervical spine injury. Many institutions are now forgoing plain films of the cervical spine in favor of CT scans, especially if a head CT is also being obtained.

47) The previous trauma patient suddenly deteriorates and his arms are now bilaterally reaching toward his mid-chest. The ED nurse knows this is described as which type of posturing?

A) Decorticate

B) Decerebrate

C) Delicious

D) Diving

A – This is decorticate posturing. And yes, unless you play with really sick neuro patients every day, it can be quite easy to forget which is which. An easy way to remember the difference between decorticate and decerebrate (the other two were just made up) is that decorticate (abnormal flexion) is when the arms reach toward the spinal CORD or the core of the body. Decerebrate (abnormal extension) is simply the other one (in which the arms straighten and the wrists turn down and out.) So which is worse? Decerebrate, as you are "down and out." In reality, both of them mean the brain is seriously messed up.

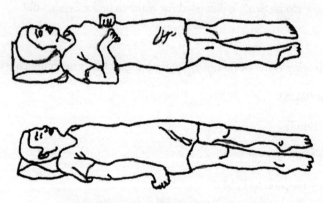

Decorticate and Decerebrate Posturing

Illustration by Nina DeBoer, then age 9 (my aspiring artist daughter, now aspiring baker daughter)

48) A 15-year-old arrives at the ED via ambulance after sustaining a stab wound to the upper mid back. He is unable to move his left extremities, but can move his right extremities. On further examination, he also has lost pain and temperature sensations on the right side. The emergency nurse knows that this syndrome is called:

A) Brown-Sequard syndrome

B) Anterior cord syndrome

C) Half cord syndrome

D) Central cord syndrome

A – Brown-Sequard syndrome is a rare, but very real, spinal cord syndrome occurring when the spinal cord is hemisected or partially (versus completely) transected. It is important to assess not only movement, but also sensation with suspected spinal cord injuries. Different parts of the spinal cord are responsible for different neuromuscular functions. Test help note: Brown-Sequard syndrome is the only spinal cord syndrome whose name is divided with a hyphen (Brown-Sequard.) So, this syndrome describes spinal cords that are divided as well.

49) An 8-year-old arrives at the ED via EMS after attempting to fly out of a window like Superman. The medics report that the patient has neck pain, diminished movement and sensation of his legs, but he can't move or feel his arms. The emergency nurse knows that this syndrome is called:

A) Brown-Sequard syndrome

B) Anterior cord syndrome

C) Half cord syndrome

D) Central cord syndrome

D – Central cord syndrome is an incomplete spinal cord injury characterized by a greater impairment to the upper extremities and lesser (or no) impairment to the lower extremities.

50) Each of the interventions below are indicated to help manage increased ICP **except**?

A) Maintaining neutral neck alignment

B) Administering supplemental oxygen

C) Administering diuretics such as Osmitrol (mannitol)

D) Hyperventilation to a pCO_2 of 20

D – Each of the interventions mentioned above are routinely utilized to manage increased intracranial pressure, except "extreme" hyperventilation. Hyperventilation to this level can result in cerebral ischemia and severely decreased cerebral perfusion.

51) Osmitrol (mannitol) for increased ICP post-traumatic brain injury should be administered via:

A) IV bolus

B) IV infusion over 1 hour

C) IV infusion over 4 hours

D) IV infusion over 24 hours

A – Mannitol, an osmotic diuretic, should be given as an IV bolus, not as a continuous infusion. In the same manner, hypertonic 3% saline is also now being given with increasing frequency to assist with management of increased ICP.

52) Stimulation of the sympathetic division of the autonomic nervous system results in all of the following **except**:

A) Pupillary dilation

B) An increase in blood pressure

C) An increase in heart rate

D) Increased saliva production

D – Stimulation of the sympathetic division of the autonomic nervous system decreases, rather than increases, saliva production. If we get nervous, we get a dry mouth. The sympathetic nervous system is responsible for the "fight or flight" response. If you are about to get shot, you have two options. Fight (stupid) or flight (smart.) Your heart rate goes up and your blood vessels constrict, directing blood flow to the important internal organs and away from the periphery. Cold hands go right along with the dry mouth and the feeling that your heart is racing. The pupils dilate so you can see where to fight or run away to and your blood sugar goes up so you have energy for either option. What does your bladder do? If you've even been so scared that you've had to change pants, you know the answer to that one!

53) An 11-year-old patient with multiple traumatic injuries is brought to the ED by EMS after being an unrestrained passenger in a high-speed MVC. Cervical spinal radiographs confirm a fracture at the C3 level. The nurse should anticipate the need for:

A) ICP monitoring

B) Intubation and ventilator support

C) Cardioversion

D) A police report detailing the extent of the injuries and prognosis

B – A fracture above the level of C5 typically means intubation and ventilator support, even if only prophylactically. The saying goes: "C5 keeps your diaphragm alive" and without the diaphragm working, it's hard to breathe. ICP monitoring might be needed, but this scenario didn't mention a head or brain injury. Likewise, cardioversion is not part of this scenario. The police report will be completed by someone else, so don't worry about that. Other important spinal cord areas include C7-T1 for arm movements, T12-L1 for leg movements, and S2-S4 for bowel and bladder control.

54) While in the ED, the patient develops spinal shock. Symptoms with this type of shock include all of the following **except**:

A) Hypotension

B) Bradycardia

C) Hyperreflexia

D) Urinary retention

C – Acute spinal shock often results in the depression or temporary loss of spinal reflex activity, particularly below the level of the injury. Other hallmark characteristics of spinal shock are the combination of hypotension, bradycardia, and urinary retention.

55) In the above patient with a cervical spinal cord injury, early respiratory failure is best diagnosed by:

A) Poor air exchange

B) Cyanosis

C) Shortness of breath while talking

D) CO_2 retention on ABG

C – While all of the above are signs and symptoms associated with respiratory failure, with a cervical spinal cord injury, the problem is most likely related to the muscles used for breathing as opposed to the functioning of the lungs. Therefore, one of the easiest ways to detect early respiratory failure with a SCI patient is simply to talk to the child. If they can only speak a few words between breaths or actually complain of being short of breath, these are ominous signs. The other signs will follow shortly.

56) In the pediatric ED, one of the **most** reliable techniques for testing upper extremity motor function is to:

A) Watch for spontaneous movement

B) Test the deep tendon reflexes

C) Ask the patient to squeeze the nurse's hands

D) Ask the patient to close her eyes and to raise her arms straight up in front of her

D – It is important to differentiate between reflexive movement and deliberate movement. With her eyes closed, you can evaluate the actual movement and whether or not both arms move equally well. The other techniques, even asking the patient to squeeze your fingers, do not necessarily indicate intentional versus reflexive movement.

57) In the pediatric ED, one of the **most** reliable techniques for testing lower extremity motor function is to:

A) Watch for spontaneous movement

B) Test the deep tendon reflexes

C) Ask the patient to wiggle their toes

D) Ask the patient to, one at a time, raise and hold their legs off the bed

D – As with upper extremity testing, it is important to differentiate between reflexive movement and deliberate movement. With his eyes closed, you can evaluate the actual movement and whether or not both legs move equally well. The other techniques, even asking the patient to wiggle his toes, do not necessarily indicate intentional versus reflexive movement. Wiggling of toes is good, but babies wiggle their toes, and comatose people move their toes. Better is the "push down on the gas pedal" technique, but even if they can move their ankle, we don't know if they can move their leg. One of the best techniques is to have them raise and hold their legs off the bed. It takes a fair amount of brain function and strength to perform this maneuver and gives the nurse a much better idea as to how much help you will need to have when you try to stand this child up for the first time. However, in patients with musculoskeletal leg, back, or hip pain, or those with any kind of peritoneal irritation, this technique may not be completely reflective of motor function.

58) Which statement about pediatric brain death is **true**?

A) It is defined as the irreversible cessation of brain and brain stem functions

B) A patient in a deep coma is considered brain-dead

C) A patient in a persistent vegetative state is considered brain dead

D) Due to anatomical differences, brain death cannot be declared in children

A – Brain death, the irreversible cessation of both brain and brain stem function, is not commonly diagnosed in the pediatric emergency department because most medical centers require a defined observation time period before the formal brain death examinations can occur. Brain dead patients are not comatose or vegetative as that implies there is still some cerebral function.

59) In cases of organ donation, the legal time of brain death may be recorded as when:

A) Examinations by the organ/tissue coordinator confirm brain death

B) The ventilator is turned off in the operating room or pediatric ICU

C) The donor's heart is removed during organ retrieval

D) None of the above

D – Even though the heart very well may still be beating, the time of death is usually listed as when a second attending/consultant physician confirms the presence of brain death. The examinations to confirm brain death include the following and can only be done when there are no drug levels (i.e. sedatives or neuromuscular blockers) or hypothermia which can impair the examination.

- Fixed and dilated pupils

- No corneal, gag, or cough reflexes

- Absent doll's eye reflex (If the cervical spine is cleared, the child's head is quickly rotated to one side and then the other. When the brainstem centers for eye movement are intact, the eyes move opposite to the rotation.)

- No response to cold water calorics (The external ear canal is irrigated with 10ml of ice water over 20 seconds. In non-brain dead patients, the eyes move towards the cold water.)

- No response to painful stimuli

- No spontaneous movements (may still note spinal reflexes)

- Apnea test to confirm lack of brain stem respiratory drive

- Additional confirmatory tests such as EEG or cerebral blood flow studies may be done as well

If the patient is a donor, the ventilator is discontinued in the operating room. If the patient's family chooses against donation, then the ventilator is discontinued in the pediatric ICU. Either way, the time of death is usually when the second attending/consultant physician examination confirms brain death.

60) A pediatric patient with a significant head injury and urine output far greater than the IV fluid intake may have what condition?

A) Fluid overload

B) Diabetes insipidus (DI)

C) Polyuric phase of renal failure

D) Diabetic ketoacidosis

B – Head injuries are among the causes of diabetes insipidus and DI is characterized by the body's inability to conserve water. Therefore, bad head injury + lots and lots and lots of urine output = diabetes insipidus. This is not uncommon after a severe head injury, so the peds ED nurse should definitely be "on the lookout" for this serious complication.

61) When caring for a potential organ donor, the nurse should keep in mind that if possible, the use of vasopressors such as Inotropin (dopamine) or Levophed (norepinephrine) should be avoided because they:

A) Are extremely potent vasoconstrictors and may cause kidney and liver damage

B) Cannot adequately be metabolized by a brain dead patient

C) Are ineffective in a brain-dead patient

D) Cause donor-recipient reactions

A – We know that Inotropin (dopamine) and Levophed (norepinephrine) are potent vasoconstrictors, but that same vasoconstriction may also cause kidney and liver damage. Some of the worst words that an organ procurement coordinator can hear are hypotension, dopamine, and/or Levophed. With this in mind, vasopressors lower the chance of recovering viable organs, so hemodynamic monitoring and fluid management, not vasopressors, are commonly recommended for potential organ donor patients.

62) When should the organ procurement agency be notified about a potential pediatric organ or tissue donor?

A) After consent for organ retrieval is obtained

B) When the operating room is ready

C) As soon as a potential donor is identified

D) When the attending physician confirms brain death

C – As soon as brain death is being entertained as a prognosis for the child, the procurement agency should be notified. This process has definitely evolved over the years. Currently, most organ procurement agencies prefer that one of their representatives be the first medical professional to address and discuss the idea of organ donation with the family. This allows for their staff to review the records and discuss the case with the staff before any brain death/organ donation discussions are initiated with the family.

Certified Pediatric Emergency Nurse (CPEN) Review IV

63) Children who present with acute psychiatric emergencies must have all of the following **except**:

A) Chemical and behavioral restraints applied immediately for the safety of the patient and the staff

B) Evaluation for substance abuse

C) Evaluation for suicidal ideations

D) Medical evaluation and clearance

A – While patient and staff safety are always a prime concern, we don't automatically restrain patients. Even though a child may have a "psych" history, they still must be medically evaluated and cleared prior to transfer/admission to a psychiatric facility or discharge to home. In children older than 5 years of age, this includes evaluation for possible substance or alcohol use, as well as suicidal ideations.

64) Common signs and symptoms of autism spectrum disorders include all of the following **except**:

A) Dislike of being touched

B) Impairments in social communication

C) Narcissism

D) Restrictive, repetitive, and stereotyped behaviors

C – Narcissism would not be considered a common sign or symptom of autism spectrum disorders. Autism is best described as a "spectrum" in which symptoms can range from non-verbal, hand-flapping and head banging children to those that are "just a little different." Parents or regular caregivers are truly lifesavers in the ED when caring for these children as they know the best ways to introduce medications, procedures, and the like. For more information, The American Psychiatric Association defines the criteria for autism spectrum disorders in the <u>Diagnostic and Statistical Manual of Mental Disorders</u> (DSM-V).

65) Suicide threats made by adolescents:

A) Are rare because most kids get everything they want

B) Should always be taken seriously

C) Are usually an attention seeking behavior and rarely serious

D) Are the results of playing too many video games where the players can reset the game and get extra "lives"

B – Each and every suicide threat and attempt must be taken seriously. Though many threats and even attempts are indeed "cries for attention," they are also typically "cries for help." If not responded to appropriately, a threat may become a reality, and the next attempt may be successful. Remember, it's better to be prepared a thousand times, than to die once!

66) Current management of pediatric attention deficit hyperactivity disorder (ADHD) includes:

A) Stimulants

B) Sedatives

C) Behavioral therapy

D) A and C

D - Though the idea of giving a stimulant to an already "over stimulated" child seems to not make a whole lot of sense, in conjunction with behavioral therapy, they are the current drug therapy of choice for pediatric patients. Stimulants in children with ADHD can have a paradoxical effect, actually calming them down, not "jazzing" them up. We should also be aware that ADHD medications such as Ritalin (methylphenidate) are now becoming a common drug of abuse by non-ADHD teens and some experts have recommended that children with ADHD not be given stimulants because it could lead to future drug addiction. Most research studies, however, demonstrate that children who were appropriately on these medications were much less likely to abuse illegal substances later in life. It is thought that children with ADHD who are not on medications, later turn to street drugs to "self-medicate."

67) A 15-year-old, accompanied by multiple police officers, is escorted (walked/dragged) to the peds ED in handcuffs. He had been standing on the school roof screaming profanities and yelling "I'm going to kill all of you!" The **priority** nursing intervention at this time would be to evaluate the patient's:

A) Orientation to time, place, and person

B) Vital signs

C) Threat to the safety of self and others

D) History of psychiatric illness

C – Though airway trumps just about everything, if he's able to walk and scream, chances are his airway is just fine. In this case, he appears to pose a definite threat to others and quite possibly himself, and that is the priority for interventions. Once the patient and staff are safe, then vital signs, additional history and a detailed neurological examination can be obtained.

68) The previous teen patient has calmed down, is evaluated by the nurse, and the handcuffs are replaced with other restraints. Which statement would be **most** appropriate at this time?

A) "If you promise to be good, we won't have to restrain you anymore."

B) "We will remove the restraints now and you will not be restrained as long as you can control yourself."

C) "I know that the restraints are uncomfortable, so we will take them off now."

D) "As you have calmed down, we will gradually remove the restraints."

D – Telling the patient that continued calm behavior can result in removed restraints lets them know what is expected and the consequences of "good" or "bad" behavior. In conjunction with close observation and repeated assessments of limb circulation, etc., removing one restraint at a time is appropriate to ensure patient and staff safety. Restraints are uncomfortable. But so is getting wailed on by a psychotic patient. The promise of "being good" might work when dealing with Santa, but not for psychiatric patients in an emergency department. Ideally, other interventions to avoid physical or chemical restraints should be tried first; however, in this situation, hard restraints and lots of security are certainly justified.

69) The patient appears anxious and guarded during the interview. The nurse knows that such anxiety may be minimized by:

A) A detailed explanation of the entire emergency department evaluation process

B) Approaching the patient confidently and offering simple, direct explanations

C) Focusing on silent physical assessments, rather than conversation

D) Having a warm attitude and the frequent use of touch to demonstrate caring

B – Short and sweet is appropriate for agitated patients. Detailed descriptions will most likely not be heard or remembered by this patient. Silent assessments in an already agitated patient would probably just make things worse. Lastly, frequent touching can be very frightening to a person in this situation, and certainly if the person has stated that he "wants to kill everyone," it just doesn't make a whole lot of sense.

70) A 15-year-old female with a history of bipolar disorder is brought to the ED by parents who report that she has not eaten or slept in 3 days and that she has become "more manic" over the past week. While waiting to be examined, the patient begins singing loudly to "sing the babies to sleep." The ED nurse's best intervention at this time would be:

A) Request that security physically restrain the patient

B) Recognize that this behavior is an expected characteristic of bipolar disorder

C) Lead the patient to a quiet, private room

D) Obtain an order for sedative medication to control her activity

C – Attempting to de-escalate the manic patient by placing her in a quiet, private room is an appropriate initial action before considering physical or chemical restraints. While this behavior may be an expected characteristic of bipolar disease, something must still be done. And finally, while some ED nurses, if they are honest, might vote for answer D (Ativan (lorazepam) for everyone), for the purpose of the test and in real life as well, this is not the best initial choice.

71) Accompanied by his father, a 16-year-old teen walks into the ED asking: "Can someone please take the I-Pod out of my brain?" While waiting for the triage nurse to complete an assessment of another patient, the patient begins screaming "Somebody has to help me. I have to change the song!" Which nursing action is **most** appropriate at this time?

A) Alert the security team that the patient has become agitated and ask them to please watch him closely while you triage the other patients

B) Approach the patient with 2 other staff nurses, and ask, "What brought you to the ED today?"

C) Walk over to the patient and say, "There really isn't an I-Pod in your brain. How could it get in there? Should we get an X-ray to prove that you're wrong?"

D) Sit next to the patient and say, "I'm a nurse and we're going to do our best to help you."

D – "Therapeutic conversation," once the patient is safe in a private room, is the correct test answer for these situations. What the patient is "feeling" is very real to him, and it is important to explore those feelings. Threatening behaviors or arguing with the patient probably won't help resolve the situation. For the purpose of the test, airway trumps everything, but if mental health is an issue, then "feelings" are a close second (in addition to a drug screen.) I, like many ED nurses, would love to ask, "How did the I-Pod get in there?" as it's probably a fascinating story, but in this case, feelings (with security in close proximity) is the correct answer.

72) Which nursing action would be **most** appropriate if the previous patient were to become uncontrollable and aggressive toward nursing staff members?

A) Address and touch the patient in a warm, reassuring manner

B) Administer IM sedative medication while the patient is being restrained by two security guards

C) Restrain the patient with the help of at least three other trained personnel

D) Administer sedative medications to avoid the need physical restraints

C – Safety first... If possible, the "takedown" of an uncontrollable patient requires at least 4 trained personnel. In some cases, this "show of force" can result in the patient calming down enough to make the restraint application easier. But if not, increasing the odds is certainly to your benefit (and the patient's too), as unintentional injury is less likely with adequately trained personnel in adequate numbers. Sedative medications can be given in a warm and reassuring manner if physical restraints are not needed. However, these medications are not instantaneous in action, and in this situation, should be used in conjunction with, not instead of, physical restraints.

73) A 17-year-old presents to the ED stating the CIA and FBI are following him and the doctors are out to get him. Assuming the drug screen is negative, the **most** likely diagnosis is:

A) Bipolar disorder

B) Depression

C) Multiple personality disorder

D) Paranoid schizophrenia

D – Incoherent speech, grossly disorganized actions, delusions, and auditory/visual hallucinations are the hallmark signs and symptoms associated with paranoid schizophrenia.

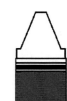

74) Most mental health laws are specific about the conditions under which and length of time for which a patient may be restrained, commonly stipulating that restraints:

A) Cannot be used for longer than 24 hours

B) Cannot be used if the patient has cardiac or respiratory disease

C) Can be used only after the patient is evaluated by a psychiatrist

D) May be applied if the patient poses a danger to himself or others, provided the risk of danger is reevaluated according to hospital policy

D – Restraints can be applied to protect the patient or others, but if possible, other non-chemical or physical options should be attempted first. Although psychiatry does not have to evaluate the patient first, they do require a physician order, and the patient must be reevaluated on a regular basis to determine the need for continued restraints or less "restraining" physical options. Remember, restraints are not a therapeutic intervention, but rather a security procedure.

75) A mother brings her 12-year-old son to the ED on the way to school. She states that for several days, he has woken up with a headache and vomiting, but didn't feel nauseated. He now "feels OK except for a bad headache." This morning, he reportedly tripped over the bathroom rug and complains that his vision is blurry. This presentation should make the ED nurse suspicious of:

A) Epidural hematoma

B) Intracranial tumor

C) Diabetic ketoacidosis

D) Vestibulocochlear disorder

B – This child has classic symptoms of a brain tumor or some other space occupying lesion in the brain causing increased intracranial pressure. General signs of increased intracranial pressure include headache, vomiting, seizures, as well as ataxia, visual problems, and changes in level of consciousness. Headaches, especially upon waking, combined with vomiting without nausea, should make the nurse particularly suspicious of the possibility of an intracranial tumor.

76) A 6-year-old child is brought to the ED by EMS. His parents state that he usually is healthy, but he had "the flu" several days ago. For past two days, he has been complaining of pain and a "prickly" feeling in both legs, but this morning, he started to have trouble walking as well. The nurse finds his gait to be unsteady, and he has noticeable bilateral foot drop. There is no history of trauma. The ED nurse should suspect:

A) Guillain-Barre Syndrome

B) Myasthenia gravis (MG)

C) Tetanus

D) Botulism

A – Flu-like symptoms are not only common to many diseases, but may present as precursors of many other, more serious conditions. Guillain-Barre is just such a condition. This syndrome may occur after several types of bacterial or viral illnesses or even after the administration of certain vaccines. Guillain-Barre Syndrome involves inflammation and demyelination of the spinal and cranial nerves. What this means is that the child becomes acutely and progressively weaker, then paralyzed; but still awake. It only affects the nerves, not consciousness. Starting in the lower extremities, it can quickly move up to the point that the child requires intubation and ventilator support. The progression may take up to 4 weeks before the plateau phase begins, which can last days to weeks. Recovery with the aid of plasmapheresis or IV immunoglobulin (IVIG) and steroids can take weeks to months. The muscles regain full strength in the reverse order of paralysis (the chest muscles come back before the leg muscles.) In most cases, especially in children, full recovery can be expected; it just takes time.

Myasthenia gravis is a disease that affects the neuromuscular junctions and acetylcholine receptors. Symptoms initially include optic and facial muscle weakness (droopy eyes, double vision, difficulty swallowing or speaking), and later weakness of all skeletal muscles, which gets worse as the day goes on. MG can be diagnosed in the ED by the "Tensilon Test" in which a dose of IV Tensilon (edrophonium) results in an immediate, though short lasting improvement in symptoms. For long term management of MG, medications such as Mestinon (pyridostigmine), thymectomy, steroids, IVIG, and plasmapheresis may be used.

In healthy, fully immunized children, we just don't see tetanus or "lock jaw" that often any more, but in non-immunized children and underdeveloped countries, it is definitely still out there. Tetanus, like Guillain-Barre, only affects the nerves and the patient remains fully awake unless sedatives and analgesics are given. When you see a question that mentions botulism, think honey, improper canning, or biowarfare, as these are three of the prime culprits causing botulism in children.

Certified Pediatric Emergency Nurse (CPEN) Review IV

77) A 14-year old teen with no significant past medical history presents to the Pediatric ED with acute slurred speech and weakness on the right side. He is being worked up to rule out an acute ischemic stroke. The initial head CT, tox screen, and alcohol level is negative and the electrolytes are normal. What might you suspect is the etiology of a stroke in this 14-year old?

A) Thrombosis

B) Trauma

C) Embolism

D) Intracranial aneurysm

C – The most common cause of childhood stroke, which is defined as a cerebrovascular event occurring in patients between the ages of 30 days and 18 years, is ischemia due to an embolism. Childhood strokes may also be hemorrhagic in nature, though these are far less common. Neonatal strokes (occurring in patients between 28 weeks gestation and 28 days of age) are most commonly due to a cardiac congenital abnormality such as an atrial septal defect (ASD) or patent foramen ovale (PFO) that results in hemorrhagic events (mostly seen in preemies) or hypoxic/ischemic events. Trauma is the most significant risk factor for intracranial hemorrhage in children with hemophilia. Intracranial aneurysm is also a risk factor for hemorrhagic stroke. In this question, there is nothing to suggest an intracranial hemorrhage because the CT is negative.

78) A 7-year old boy with autism spectrum disorder presents with a 1.5 cm laceration on his forehead from a trip and fall. The child becomes agitated, crying and hitting his head with his fist whenever the nurse enters the room. Which of the following options demonstrates the **best** choice in approaching the child to repair the laceration?

A) Provide distraction in the form of a video and have the parent apply a topical anesthetic to prepare him for the procedure

B) Explain to his parents that the team will try to gain his cooperation, but it will likely require restraint with a papoose board

C) Obtain intravenous access and prepare for procedural sedation using Versed® (midazolam) and ketamine. Explain to his parents that the chosen medications will provide amnesia of the procedure

D) Ask the parents what has worked in the past in dealing with situations that produce anxiety in the child and try to incorporate those techniques for this procedure

D – Children with autism spectrum disorder can become agitated in situations where they feel a loss of control, and can experience high levels of anxiety. An injury requiring a laceration repair is an excellent example of just such a situation. Unless the child is in a critical state (cyanotic, bradycardic, signs of respiratory failure), asking the parents for additional information will often be the best answer. In addition, the nurse should always integrate the parents into the planning of care and should understand that there is no single method that works well with all autistic children. While all of the first three options might represent valid choices, the parents are likely to have experienced difficult situations previously and should have insight into what conditions provoke increasing agitation and what actions might lessen said agitation. Distraction may work and having the parent apply the anesthetic may be a successful strategy. This is especially true in cases of children with autism. Procedural sedation (answer C) may provoke additional agitation, as it often requires the insertion of an intravenous line. Even though midazolam produces amnesia, the child may still remember events prior to the sedation.

Certified Pediatric Emergency Nurse (CPEN) Review IV

Autism Emergency Contact Form

Autism Risk & Safety Management
© Debbaudt Legacy Productions
www.autismriskmanagement.com

Name of child or adult with autism: _____
Nickname if any: _____ Date of birth: _____ Height: _____
Weight: _____ Eye color: _____ Hair color: _____
Scars or identifying marks: _____
Medical conditions: _____
Address: _____ City: _____ State: _____
Zip: _____ Home phone: _____ Other phone: _____
Method of communication, if non verbal: sign language, picture boards, written word, etc: _____

Identification worn: ex: jewelry/Medic Alert®, clothing tags, ID card, tracking monitor, etc: _____

Current prescriptions (include dosage): _____

Sensory, medical, or dietary issues and requirements, if any: _____

Inclination for wandering behaviors or characteristics that may attract attention: _____

Favorite attractions and locations where person may be found if missing: _____

Likes and dislikes (include approach and de-escalation techniques): _____

Attach map and address guide to nearby properties with water sources and dangerous locations highlighted.

Attach blueprint or drawing of home, with bedrooms of individual highlighted.

Medical Care Providers:
Name: _____ Phone: _____
Name: _____ Phone: _____
Name: _____ Phone: _____

Parents/Caregiver name: _____ Home phone: _____
Address: _____ City: _____
State: _____ Zip: _____ Cell phone: _____
Other contact info: _____
Emergency contact name: _____ Home phone: _____
Address: _____ City: _____
State: _____ Zip: _____ Cell phone: _____

Please attach any additional information, use extra paper if necessary.

Autism Emergency Contact Form

Courtesy of Autism Risk & Safety Management - www.autismriskmanagement.com

79) A 22-month old child was brought to the ED by his mother after he reportedly tumbled head first down several wooden steps approximately 6-hours ago. The child did not lose consciousness after the fall, was initially upset (understandable after falling down four wooden steps) but then seemed completely normal. The mother now reports the child has become difficult to keep awake, vomited twice and is developing some bruising around his eyes. The pediatric ED nurse correctly suspects the child might have a:

A) Subdural hematoma

B) Temporal skull fracture

C) Basilar skull fracture

D) Subarachnoid hemorrhage

C – Periorbital ecchymosis or "raccoon eyes" is a classic sign of a basilar skull fracture involving the anterior cranial fossa. This sign will usually appear several hours to a few days after the injury. It is very important for ED nurses to remember that "raccoon eyes," like all bruising, takes time to become visible; therefore, they may not be present in the initial ED visit. Other classic signs of a basilar skull fracture include "Battle's sign" (bruising behind the ear) and a cerebral spinal fluid (CSF) leak from the nose or ears.

80) The pediatric ED nurse anticipates the child with a possible basilar skull fracture will need further testing to determine the extent of the injury. The most likely diagnostic test for this child would be:

A) Lumbar puncture

B) CT scan

C) Skull X-ray

D) MRI

B – Basilar skull fractures are not often seen on plain skull radiographs. CT scans (including bone windows) are the standard for the diagnosis of skull fracture. CT scans are also able to show intracranial hemorrhages, cerebral contusions, and signs of increased intracranial pressure.

81) Basilar skull fractures commonly have associated leakage of cerebral spinal fluid (CSF) from the nose (rhinorrhea), ears (otorrhea) or both. This is most commonly due to a tear in the dura. CSF leaks can increase the potential for infection. This risk can be minimized by:

A) Having the patient blow his nose to keep CSF from pooling in the sinus cavity

B) Packing the nares or ear canals with sterile cotton

C) Administer oxygen via nasal cannula at 2 L per minute

D) Lightly tape a "moustache dressing" under the patient's nose and monitor the frequency of dressing changes

D - Simply taping a sterile gauze pad on the outside of the ear or creating a "mustache dressing" under the nose are the current recommended techniques of ED CSF leak management. In addition, this patient should be maintained on bed rest in a semi-fowler position. Nothing should be placed into the nose or ears of a patient with rhinorrhea. Doing so might introduce bacteria into the nasal cavity or ear and may impede the flow of CSF, thus increasing the chance for infection. Sneezing and nose blowing are discouraged, as they will raise the intracranial pressure and likely increase the amount of drainage.

82) A 17-year old with a history of schizophrenia presents to triage stating that he hears God telling him to kill his parents. He says that he really doesn't want to, but states "You have to obey God, don't you?" The emergency nurse would correctly describe hearing voices as a(n):

A) Hallucination

B) Illusion

C) Personalization

D) Delusion

A – Hallucinations are sensory perceptions without a stimulus in the environment. Hearing is one of our senses, so hearing voices, or seeing, smelling, or tasting things that aren't present are also hallucinations. Illusions are also sensory in nature, but have a real stimulus in the environment. An example of an illusion would be thinking that the IV pole is really a praying mantis. The thought process where one thinks that everything that occurs in the environment is related to them (it's all about me) is personalization. Delusions are fixed false beliefs whether they are paranoid, grandiose, or religious in nature.

83) The primary ED nurse notices small, circular burn marks on a teenage patient's arms that were not noted in the triage note. When questioned about the marks, the patient responds with, "Oh, sometimes I accidentally burn myself with my cigarette." The nurse asks, "How does that happen?" The patient smiles and says, "Well, maybe it really wasn't an accident." Pediatric ED nurses should realize that the significance of the patient's statement is:

A) The patient is telling the nurse that these are intentional acts used to help cope with stress

B) The patient wants the nurse to know that the burns are "no big deal"

C) The patient believes she has no control over the impulses to self-injury

D) The patient is expressing suicidal intentions

A - Self-mutilation is the deliberate destruction of body tissue without conscious intent of suicide. While some acts of self-mutilation, such as cigarette burns or cutting or tearing the skin are spontaneous, this patient's acts are clearly premeditated and she is admitting that the behavior is not accidental, but rather, it is purposeful in nature. Although over half of self-mutilators have attempted suicide at least once, the mutilation isn't part of the suicide attempt. These are two different behaviors with a common goal–escape from the stress.

84) Which of the following would indicate that your pediatric patient has a much higher risk for suicide? The patient:

A) Is giving away personal items

B) Is actively receiving ongoing pharmacologic and behavioral treatment for depression

C) Has had several angry outbursts in the last few days

D) Is very active in his religious organization

A - Giving away personal possessions is a common pre-suicide gesture and should be a "red flag" to the pediatric emergency nurse. This young patient is at high risk for suicide. Patients with a history of depression are at risk for suicide, but if the patient is specifically noted as actively under mental health care, he would be having regular assessments for suicidal ideations on an ongoing basis. Anger is not a specific risk for suicide, and since most religious organizations are generally considered to be supportive, this may actually be a protective factor.

85) The ED nurse is assessing a teen whose family is concerned that the patient may be at risk for suicide. The **best** initial question that the nurse should ask the patient is:

A) "Have you ever had these thoughts before?"

B) "Are you having any thoughts of wanting to kill yourself?"

C) "How are you planning to kill yourself?"

D) "How did you try to harm yourself?"

B – "Are you having any thoughts of wanting to kill yourself?" is the best initial question for the nurse to ask. Contrary to popular belief, asking patients this question will not "put the idea in their head" and lead them to consider suicide. Being straightforward and asking the patient specifically about suicidal ideations is the correct approach. If the patient is having suicidal thoughts, asking about a "plan" is an appropriate follow-up question. Questions regarding previous suicidal thoughts, attempts and/or plans are important, but can be addressed later in the assessment process. If the patient admits to current suicidal thoughts, then the patient's safety and protection from self-harm are the priorities. Just like the ABCs of airway, breathing and circulation are always foremost with medical/trauma patients, your patient's safety is the key for the emergency department treatment of psych patients. After clearing medical concerns, keeping the patient SAFE involves paying close attention to Security, Affect, Feelings and Emotions.

86) The nurse is caring for a child who is at high risk for suicide. The ED nurse knows the **priority** intervention is to:

A) Lecture the patient on the negative consequences of suicide

B) Have a medical professional remain with the patient at all times until the patient can be moved to a safe place outside of the emergency department

C) Develop a no-harm contract

D) Check the patient's whereabouts and safety every 10-15 minutes

B - Continuous supervision by a staff member is necessary until the patient is in a safe environment outside of the emergency department. When the patient is no longer acutely suicidal and on an inpatient mental health unit, an irregular schedule of observation every 10-15 minutes is appropriate. As a rule, ED nurses shouldn't be "lecturing" patients, and especially about the negative consequences of suicide. No-harm contracts can be created with the assistance of mental health staff, but are not commonly done in the emergency department setting and therefore are not a priority intervention.

87) You are caring for the family of a teen who has just committed suicide. What is the **best** initial intervention in the emergency department?

A) Help them make up an acceptable story to tell casual friends

B) Explain to them that their anger just complicates the grieving process

C) Point out the warning signs of suicide that they missed

D) Provide opportunities to discuss the death

D – What the family needs is to be able to have the opportunity to discuss the suicide as part of an ongoing process of coming to terms with the death. The family will decide how to discuss the death with relatives and friends, and we may be able to assist by contacting hospital social work, chaplain, mental health or the family's own religious support. Making up acceptable stories for families of any patient is not an appropriate emergency nursing intervention and hopefully should be easy to rule out as an obviously incorrect answer. There is no suggestion in the question that the family is angry, but if they were exhibiting non-harmful anger, we should recognize this as a normal part of the grieving process. Pointing out missed warning signs would probably only serve to magnify the guilt the family is probably already feeling should also be seen as an incorrect answer.

Certified Pediatric Emergency Nurse (CPEN) Review IV

88) Sam's mother has just suffered a cardiac arrest and died in the emergency department. The nurse is discussing with the father about what to expect when dealing with his grieving 10-year old son. Which one of the following statements by the father indicates that the discussions have been effective?

A) "I know it will be easy for Sam to talk about missing his mother."

B) "Since Sam is only 10, he will get over his grief more easily than we will."

C) "This is going to be tough because at age 10, Sam still believes that death is reversible."

D) "Sam may have low self-esteem and blame himself for some months."

D – Vulnerability to self-blame and low self-esteem is the correct answer because children of this age commonly feel that the parent abandoned them. As egocentric beings, they are focused on their part of the world and how what they do affects it (or so they believe). They often want to attribute everything to what they have done, or even thought. This is the age of "step on a crack and break your mother's back." School age children often blame themselves for family problems such as divorce, and want to believe that if they are "better" everything will be okay. As a rule, school-age children tend to avoid talking about their grief and often they do not have the verbal skills to adequately express what they are feeling. However it is crucial to remember that they suffer the same grief as an adult. We need to find alternative ways to allow them to express this, and art is often a useful tool. Developmentally, a child of ten has an understanding of death very much as adults do. Preschoolers think death is temporary or reversible, an example of "magical thinking" common at this age.

89) A 14-year old is in the emergency department for treatment of hypokalemia related to vomiting and use of laxatives to purge after binge eating. Which of the following symptoms indicates this electrolyte imbalance?

A) Muscle weakness and cardiac arrhythmias

B) Hypothermia

C) Elevated serum creatinine and peripheral edema

D) Esophagitis and a "cathartic colon"

A – The most common electrolyte imbalance resulting from eating disorders involving loss of fluid is hypokalemia. Muscle weakness and cardiac arrhythmias, specifically premature ventricular complexes (PVCs), are common clinical signs of low potassium levels. Temperature regulation has nothing to do with hypokalemia, and serum creatinine is related to kidney function. While purging from "above and below" can result in esophagitis and "cathartic colon," these are signs of the eating disorder, not specifically of hypokalemia.

90) A 16-year old patient who is in the manic state of bipolar disease is unable to sit still and answer questions during an initial assessment. Which action would be **best** for the nurse to take?

A) Confront the patient with the inappropriateness of the behavior

B) Contact the physician to request an order for a sedative

C) Set firm limits and insist the patient provide the information

D) Involve the family in the interview

D – Though your initial inclination might be to select answer "B" (sedation), the correct answer really is "D." Patients with acute hyperactive behavior (ADHD, bipolar-manic,) are often unable to control the

252

hyperactive behavior. Direct confrontation or insisting that information be provided will not work. The patient is simply unable to comply with your request. In cases such as this, as with young preverbal patients or those with cognitive or expressive disorders, the family is often an invaluable resource in the process of obtaining the desired information.

91) The pediatric ED nurse is speaking with a young patient who is exhibiting flight of ideas (describing her experiences in school, her trip to the Grand Canyon, how her big toe hurts, and her memory of being stuck at an airport-- all within 30 seconds.) What is the **best** response on the part of the nurse?

A) The nurse should speak loudly and rapidly to keep the patient's attention

B) The nurse should focus on the theme and feelings being conveyed by the patient

C) The nurse should tell the patient that she can only talk about one subject at a time.

D) The nurse should allow the patient to talk freely to discover what is on the patient's mind

B – The big clue here is the word "feelings." Since the logic of flight of ideas is incomprehensible, noting the patient's feelings may be the only way you will understand what the patient is trying to communicate. Speaking loudly and rapidly will only escalate the situation and possibly be agitating. The patient with flight of ideas is, by definition, unable to talk about only one subject and ED nurses are way too busy to allow most patients to talk freely to discover what is on the patient's mind. We need to find out what is happening acutely with the patient in order to keep them safe. Remember that with psych patients, keeping them SAFE means focusing on Security, Affect, Feelings, and Emotions.

92) A six-year old female is brought to the emergency department two days after she was involved in a minor motor vehicle crash (MVC.) During the MVC, the patient was appropriately restrained and suffered no apparent injuries. After a day of complaints, her primary care physician ordered an outpatient head CT. The results of the CT indicate that she has a small arteriovenous malformation (AVM) that was leaking and causing an intracranial hemorrhage (ICH.) During your assessment of this patient, you would expect to find all of the following symptoms except:

A) Nausea and vomiting

B) Contralateral facial paralysis

C) Headache with light sensitivity

D) Decrease in extremity strength

B – Facial paralysis would not be a likely finding in this situation. The patient was noted to have a small intracranial hemorrhage, so you would expect to find typical symptoms as you would with any ICH or lesion that causes increased intracranial pressure. Arteriovenous malformations are congenital defects involving abnormal connections (snarled tangles of vessels) between cerebral arteries and veins. These malformations most commonly involve branches of the middle cerebral artery. Instead of the arteries and veins interconnecting by capillaries (which slow the flow of blood and allow for O2/CO2 exchange,) they connect with large abnormal fistulas. Arteries typically have a higher pressure and flow rate than veins, so blood therefore will follow the path of least resistance and will shunt the blood across the fistula to the vein, without oxygen delivery to the brain tissues. The high-volume, high-pressure flow of blood from the cerebral artery to the vein results in dilation of the vein. Over time, the cerebral vein can rupture if it becomes dilated and frail, often resulting in a fatal intracranial hemorrhage. The fact that this patient experienced an event that led to a small bleed is a blessing in disguise. If left with no symptoms, most AVMs continue to dilate and may end up eventually rupturing, causing sudden death. Treating an ICH is the same whether it's caused from trauma, anticoagulation, or an arteriovenous malformation. Treat the ABCs and other signs and symptoms (pain, nausea/vomiting, vital signs, coags) until neurosurgery can fix the cause by clipping or coiling the source of the bleed.

Certified Pediatric Emergency Nurse (CPEN) Review IV

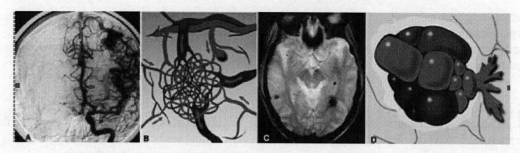

Vascular malformations of the brain

A) Cerebral angiogram showing AVM cluster of abnormal blood vessels

B) Artist diagram of AVM with shunting between arteries and veins

C) Magnetic resonance scan showing dark spots characteristic of cerebral cavernous malformations or cavernous angiomas

D) Artist diagram illustrating mulberry-like vascular structure

Courtesy of Professor Issam Awad MD, MSc, FACS, MA (hon)

Neurovascular Surgery Program, University of Chicago Hospitals, www.issamawad.com

93) Appropriate nursing interventions with a violent or potentially violent teenage patient might include:

A) Standing sideways to the patient

B) Keep both hands deeply in your scrub pockets

C) Standing facing the patient

D) Shutting the door to the patient's room

A – Standing sideways is less visibly threatening to the patient and presents a smaller potential target for the patient. Standing and facing the patient makes you appear more threatening and can provide a much bigger target. It is recommended that caregivers always keep both hands visible, both for balance and also so that it's obvious no weapons are being concealed. Lastly, NEVER shut yourself into a room with a potentially violent patient. Always maintain unobstructed access to the patient (as well as an unobstructed escape route for yourself) and get help as quickly as possible. Remember, psych SAFEty... Security, Affect, Feelings, and Emotions!

94) While driving home after a very long shift in the ED, you see a car fly past you and crash into another car. After you make sure that all traffic is clear and that it is safe to approach the vehicles, you hear a small baby crying and see a baby strapped into a child safety seat. The paramedics arrive and you would anticipate they will **first**:

A) Remove the baby from the car seat and place him on the abdomen of the mother, above the level of the heart

B) Place a cervical collar on the patient, remove the baby from the car seat, and place him on a back board

C) Leave the baby in the car seat and ask law enforcement to place the child in protective custody

D) Leave the baby in the car seat and secure the car seat to a long spine board

B – Optimally, we would like the child secured appropriately on a backboard, with a correctly sized cervical collar. This offers the most protection to the child, and allows us the best access in an emergent situation. That being said, let's talk about some of the real-life challenges that we may encounter. Although there are cervical collars and spinal motion restriction devices that are made for and actually fit infants and small children, many prehospital services and emergency departments do not have them immediately available. Assuming that the child was properly secured into the car seat and the car seat was properly secured into the car, we have a good starting point. At that point, two issues really come into play. The first is whether or not to remove the child from the car seat. Experts are divided on this issue. On one side are the providers who follow the NHTSA (National Highway Traffic Safety Authority) guidelines, teaching that car seats are not made to immobilize a child's spine and that the structural integrity of the car seat must be verified after a major collision. The opposing side suggests that if the child survived the crash in the car seat, don't mess with it! In the prehospital setting, EMS protocols should dictate the preferred method of spinal motion restriction for these patients. The other issue involves cervical collar sizing. If you have a collar that truly fits a little one of this size, wonderful; we suggest that you use it. However, placing a collar that is too large on a child can cause not only airway compromise, but also improper cervical spine alignment. So if there is not an appropriately sized collar immediately available, what do ED nurses do so very well? Improvise! A towel roll can be used "like a horseshoe" to minimize lateral motion of the head, and a washcloth or towel under the chin can be used to prevent flexion of the neck. Just like for adults, a board and collar (or towel rolls and tape) are where it's at for spinal motion restriction until the spine has been clinically cleared, with or without radiographic studies.

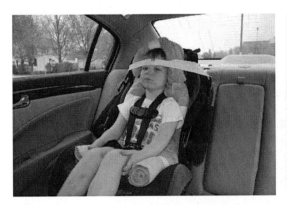
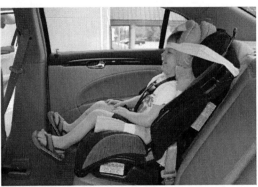

Horseshoe towel / car seat spinal immobilization technique

Courtesy of William Justice NREMT-P, TEMS-I and Sara House EMT-P

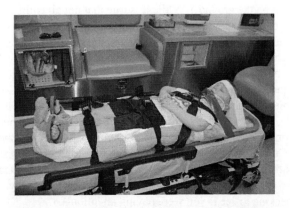

Proper post-removal from car seat spinal immobilization technique

Courtesy of William Justice NREMT-P, TEMS-I and Sara House EMT-P

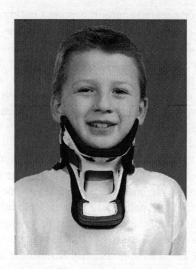

Miami-Jr. pediatric cervical collars (that actually fit kids)

Courtesy of Ossur - www.ossur.com

95) As you are passing the nursing station, you hear an ambulance crew calling in a radio report on a 7-year old patient. Another nurse acknowledges the call and says to you "sounds like Waddell's triad." Based on this comment, what kind of patient would you expect?

A) A little league baseball player hit in the chest with a fast pitch

B) A child struck by a car

C) A little league baseball player hit in the head with a baseball bat

D) A child with an upper respiratory infection

B - When young children waddle into the street and are hit by a car, the ensuing injuries are sometimes described as Waddell's triad. (Seriously, we didn't make this up!) Typically presentation of Waddell's triad is: 1) Femur fracture (contact with the bumper) 2) Intra-thoracic and/or intra-abdominal injuries (impact from the car grill and/or hood,) and 3) Head injuries (being thrown into the air by the car and the eventual impact of the head landing on the ground.) While it is true that not all children struck by a car will present with all of these injuries, or even with these specific injuries, it is important to remember that children involved in high-energy impact will rarely display isolated injuries. It is much more likely to see multiple traumas from multiple secondary impacts (car vs. body, body vs. street, etc.). Waddle's triad actually was initially used to describe adult, not pediatric, injuries associated with pedestrian vs. automobile collisions. Though a frequent test question, as kids and cars come in all different shapes and sizes, research has shown this triad not to be reliable in predicting pediatric injuries. An impact to the chest, as in answer A, may cause cardiac tamponade, which would present with Beck's triad (distended neck veins (JVD), distant heart sounds, hypotension) or commotio cordis. Head trauma patients with severely increased intracranial pressure would display Cushing's triad (hypertension with widening pulse pressure, bradycardia, agonal respirations.) A child with an upper respiratory infection might present with Dayquil's triad (cough, nasal congestion and a sore throat) and really shouldn't be in an ambulance anyway. (Okay, we made up the Dayquil® triad. Just checking to see if you were paying attention!)

96) The **best** approach to assessing suicide risk in an adolescent with a history of depression would be to:

A) Ask the parents

B) Assume a suicide risk based on the history of depression

C) Ask the patient

D) Let the ED physician question the patient

C – If you want a direct answer, you have to go directly to the source, i.e. the patient. This is an important answer to get as part of the initial triage assessment. Parents may not give you all the information you need and there may be opposing views and different stories between the different parties (parent vs. parent and child vs. parent). Although the ED physician will hopefully ask questions about suicidal ideation during the history, the physician will probably not be the first person the patient encounters in the ED. As far as assuming anything without evidence, well that's just not a good idea. You know what they say about assume… it makes an ass out of u and me!

97) A 15-year old male is brought to the ED by his parents, who state he has been "violent and out of control" for the past week. During triage, the patient screams, "I'm going to kill you for bringing me here!" to his parents. The **priority** intervention at this time would be to:

A) Ensure the safety of the parents, other patients and staff in the immediate area

B) Insist that the patient and family move to a closed room away from the triage area so any further outburst won't disturb others in the waiting room

C) Tell the patient not to speak to his parents that way

D) Get an order for restraints

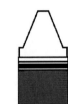

A – The safety of yourself and others should be the immediate priority in any situation. Confronting a potentially violent patient at triage is never a good idea and will just add fuel to the fire. Never get into an enclosed space with the patient without having backup and assure that you have a clear path to the door and a way to call for help. In this case, you might need to separate the patient and his parents. You'll also want to get this patient into a gown (probably not easy) as soon as possible and otherwise assure he's weapon-free (physical search by security and/or metal detector). Lastly, remember for psych questions, safety is always a primary consideration and look for ways to avoid physical or chemical restraints.

98) Patients in physical restraints should be reassessed by the ED nurse:

A) Every hour

B) Every 30 minutes

C) Every 15 minutes

D) As per the institution's policy and guidelines

D – While reassessments every 15 minutes may be the most common policy and may be the policy at your institution, test questions are written to address everyone, and not every institution's policies and procedures are alike. Therefore, choosing an answer suggestion that indicates following your institution's guidelines, especially for monitoring of patients in restraints, is a safe bet.

99) A 14-year old male is brought to the ED with his parents who state he has been "acting out" and "behaving strangely" for the past 3 days. At triage, the patient seems agitated and frequently interrupts the triage process with questions. The **priority** plan for this patient should include:

A) A psych consult

B) An order for a sedative

C) A thorough history and physical exam including tox screen and alcohol level

D) Placing him in a room away from the nurse's station so as not to disturb the other patients

C – A thorough history and physical is the priority in this situation. Though his issues very well may be psychiatric in origin, the ED should always try to rule out an organic cause of behavior changes first. A psych consult certainly may be ordered, but not until after non-psychiatric causes are ruled out. Administering a sedative (such as a "B-52" cocktail – they need to "B"ehave, so they get "5"mg of Haldol® (haldoperidol) and "2"mg of Ativan® (lorazepam) before a history and physical is completed could potentially prove harmful and certainly will diminish one's ability to get an appropriate verbal history from the patient. Agitated patients with changes in behavior should be placed close to the nurses' station so that they may be monitored closely. It can also be helpful to reduce environmental stimuli, so minimize sound intrusions (equipment alarms, etc.), the coming and going of extraneous personnel and visitors, and monitor the patient's reactions to TV or video programs that might be available in the room for entertainment.

100) Common signs and symptoms of lithium toxicity would include:

A) Confusion, nausea, vomiting, and tremors

B) Neck spasms, difficulty swallowing, and protruding tongue

C) Hyperthermia, muscle rigidity, delirium, labile pulse and blood pressure

D) Tachycardia, dilated pupils, chest pain, and tachyarrhythmias

A – Confusion, nausea, vomiting and tremors are classic symptoms of lithium toxicity, although symptoms and signs do not always correlate with levels. Lithium, commonly used to treat bipolar disorder, has a relatively narrow therapeutic index (i.e. it's easy to get too much or too little). Serum lithium levels can quickly change due to alterations in lifestyle, medications or diet. Answer "B" describes a dystonic reaction (extrapyramidal symptoms) associated with certain antipsychotic medications, especially the phenothiazines (i.e. Thorazine® (chlorpromazine) or Compazine® (prochlorperazine). If you have ever given IV Compazine® too fast, you might remember what the patient looked like -- their faces and necks would twitch and spasm until you frantically pushed Benadryl® (diphenhydramine) or Cogentin® (benztropine mesylate) to make it stop. Answer "C" describes the symptoms of neuroleptic malignant syndrome, an even worse reaction, and one of the most-feared sequelae of antipsychotic drug toxicity. Lastly, answer "D" describes the classic presenting symptoms of cocaine abuse (HR up, BP up, heart pounding, clutching of the chest). So what's the clue as to the correct answer? Since lithium is a psych drug, think about which of the answers includes something "psych" sounding. Confusion and tremors sounds like a possible psych thing, so that's a clue that "A" is the correct answer. In addition, remember that nausea and vomiting are early signs and symptoms of toxicity for just about every drug and that toxicity means having too much of the substance in the system. So look for an answer that mentions nausea and vomiting, your body's way of saying "don't take any more!"

Certified Pediatric Emergency Nurse (CPEN) Review IV

101) A 16-year old female is brought to the ED by police after she was found dancing in the street in the middle of the afternoon. At triage, she states "Please help me. I've missed my tryout for 'Dancing With The Stars!" The **best** approach at this point would be to:

A) Get an order for Haldol® (haldoperidol)

B) Speak calmly, focusing on the "here and now"

C) Apply restraints

D) Offer to be her dance partner

B – This patient is presenting with symptoms of acute psychosis (disorganized thoughts and words.) She needs to be calmly but firmly addressed, focusing on what's happening "right here and right now" (great song by Jesus Jones). Getting an order for Haldol® or other sedative may be eventually warranted, but not before the patient has been medically evaluated. Restraints, whether physical or chemical (think Haldol®), require an order from a licensed independent practitioner and should only be used as a last resort or in the event that the patient poses a clear threat to self or others. Although it might be lots of fun to dance with her (certainly more fun than playing in a busy ED), feeding in to her delusions does not help you or her, so answer "D" shouldn't be too difficult to identify as an incorrect answer.

102) A teenage patient with possible suicidal ideation is being discharged home from the ED in the care of her parents. Which of the following statements would indicate the need for further teaching for the parents?

A) "We will make sure she gets her medication as prescribed."

B) "We will follow up next week at the adolescent psychiatric clinic."

C) "Both of us are going out of town this weekend, so we will have her twin brother watch her while we're gone."

D) "We will remove all our guns from the house and secure all medications and alcohol."

C – This patient needs appropriate adult supervision while at home. A sibling (the patient is a teenager; therefore, her twin brother is a teenager) cannot and should not be given that responsibility. Making sure all medications are correctly given is certainly appropriate, and scheduled follow-up is paramount in any psychiatric discharge situation. While Guns and Roses was a great 80's metal band, guns and alcohol, separately or in any combination, should never be a good answer when dealing with suicidal patient. Don't forget that ALL medications should also be carefully secured because even over-the-counter medications can kill! Also, the patient should not have unsupervised access to cutting implements.

103) Munchausen Syndrome by Proxy is typically considered a psychiatric disorder of the:

A) Sibling

B) Patient

C) Aunt

D) Mother

D – The key word is psychiatric disorder. Munchausen Syndrome by Proxy is when a caregiver (usually the mother) gets personal satisfaction and gratification by having her child undergo medical evaluations and treatment. In most cases, the mother actually induces illness or injury to her child in order to get the needed attention. This differentiates her from the "hypochondriac" mother. Other family members, such as siblings, fathers, aunts and uncles can occasionally be associated with Munchausen's but, in most cases, the culprit is Mom. The patient is more likely the victim in these cases.

Certified Pediatric Emergency Nurse (CPEN) Review IV

104) Common symptoms and signs of anorexia nervosa include:

A) Weight gain

B) Euphoria

C) Amenorrhea

D) Binging and purging

C – Loss of menses (amenorrhea) is a common finding in girls with anorexia nervosa. Weight loss (not gain) and extreme fatigue and depression (rather than euphoria) are other typically encountered signs and symptoms. Binging and purging are associated with bulemia (binging and bulemia both begin with "b"). Practice note: When assessing teens with suspected anorexia or bulemia, check their knuckles and fingernails. Since they often induce vomiting by putting their fingers down their throats, bruises or scars on their knuckles (from contact with teeth) can be a clue, as can pitting of the fingernails, which can be caused by chronic exposure to gastric acids.

Neuro / Psych

105) Children with attention deficit hyperactivity disorder (ADHD) are often managed with:

A) Hospitalization and stimulants

B) Stimulants and behavior management

C) Hospitalization and sedatives

D) Sedatives and behavior management

B – The key to this question is the knowledge that Ritalin® (methylphenidate), the most commonly prescribed AHD medication, is actually a stimulant. It appears that in cases of ADHD, a kind of paradoxical effect occurs with stimulants such as Ritalin®. In conjunction with behavioral therapy, it is the treatment of choice in many cases. It's thought that the stimulants provoke an increased production of dopamine by the brain, which in turn calms the patient and helps them focus. Hospitalization is rarely required unless the child presents a danger to themselves or others. Sedatives are not commonly indicated in the treatment of ADHD.

106) EMS arrives to find a 13-year old male who was struck in the face with a baseball and then fell to the ground. He had a Glasgow Coma Scale (GCS) of 6 on the scene and was orally intubated by the paramedics. The primary survey has been completed, and during the secondary assessment the nurse notices clear drainage from the ears. It's clinically evident that the patient has several fractures of his mid-face, as well as a basilar skull fracture. As the primary nurse, you would expect orders for each of the following **except**:

A) IV antibiotics

B) Placement of an NG tube and Foley urinary catheter

C) Chest X-ray to confirm endotracheal tube placement

D) Maintenance of full spinal precautions

B – This question can be tricky at a first glance. They all seem to be appropriate; however, it is contraindicated to place anything blindly in the nose of a patient with suspected mid-face or basilar skull fractures. Remember, in a multiple choice exam, the answer must be 100% correct. Although a Foley urinary catheter may be appropriate, placing a NG tube in a patient with a mushy face is not.

107) Autoregulation controls cerebral blood flow by all of the following mechanisms **except**:

A) Vasodilation and vasoconstriction of the cerebral arteries in response to increases or decreases in systemic blood pressure

B) Vasodilation of the cerebral arteries when pCO2 is high and vasoconstriction of the cerebral arteries when pCO2 is low

C) Cerebral vasoconstriction when pCO2 is below 45 mm Hg

D) Cerebral vasodilation with acidosis and cerebral vasoconstriction with alkalosis

C – This question asks about cerebral blood flow autoregulation, but finding the correct answer also involves a review of ABG values, and since 45 mm Hg is in the normal range for pCO2, there is no need for auto regulatory vasoconstriction at this level. So you get a 2-for-1 on this question! Now it's time for a quick review of cerebral blood flow. You have to get blood to your head, otherwise you are dead. It's as simple as that. The fancy medical term for the big part of your brain is cerebrum which begins with "C" and "C"O2 is the key factor in determining "C"erebral blood flow. While hypoxia is certainly a bad thing, the level of CO2 has a greater effect on blood flow to the brain. We used to automatically hyperventilate many head injury patients in order to constrict the cerebral blood vessels and reduce the blood pressure in the brain to help prevent swelling. It's now been discovered that we were probably often going too far, constricting the cerebral vessels so much that there wasn't enough blood getting to the brain. Too much lowering of CO2 (hyperventilating) = cerebral vasoconstriction = less blood to the brain, which is why we don't routinely hyperventilate patients anymore. When we do intentionally hyperventilate patients, usually because of impending cerebral herniation, we avoid taking the CO2 beyond the low to mid-30s. More CO2 = more blood to the brain, which sounds like a good thing, but remember, too much of a good thing can actually be bad for you. For the majority of head injuries, "normal ventilation," i.e. a normal pCO2 of 35-45, is what most neurosurgeons now recommend. This allows blood to go round and round, to the body and the brain.

108) Cerebral perfusion pressure (CPP) is calculated according to which of the following formulas?

A) SBP – ICP

B) MAP – ICP

C) ICP + CBF

D) MAP + ICP

B – Mean arterial pressure (MAP) is a measure of the body's blood pressure. Intracranial pressure (ICP) is a measure of the pressure of the brain (normal being less than 15 mm Hg) and is measured by placing a catheter (bolt) into the child's (cerebral, not cardiac) ventricles. You must have enough blood pressure to push the blood (supplying oxygen and glucose) into the brain. However, if the intracranial pressure is rising, or if the child is hypotensive, the MAP may not be adequate to push blood into the brain. Cerebral perfusion pressure (CPP) is the number representing this important relationship. Body pressure minus brain pressure = how effectively the blood is getting to the brain tissue. In a child, studies have shown that sustained CPP < 40 mm Hg is a predictor of impending brain death. Systolic blood pressure (SBP) is not a direct factor in the equation. Cerebral blood flow (CBF) is a measurement of volume (ml/min) and is also not a direct factor in the equation.

109) Which of the following is an **early** sign of increased intracranial pressure?

A) Bradycardia

B) Dilated pupils

C) Changes in level of consciousness

D) Respiratory depression

C – Long before they have pupillary changes, neuro patients have changes in their level of consciousness-- short and to the point. No tools needed!

110) The primary goal in the acute management of a severe traumatic brain injury is to prevent a secondary brain injury due to all of the following **except**:

A) Hypotension, intracranial hypertension, hypercarbia

B) Electrolyte abnormalities, coagulopathy, seizures, hyperthermia

C) Hypoxemia, hypertension, hyperglycemia, hyperthermia

D) Normoventilation, normotension, & normothermia

D – Primary brain injury is what happens at the moment of the event, i.e. when the head hit the windshield, the skin lacerated, the skull fractured, and the brain tissue sheared, causing neuronal injury. Prevention of primary head injuries is the key here. However, if the child presents to us with a primary head injury, our goal in the acute management phase is to prevent it from getting any worse via a secondary brain injury (such as pressure from a hematoma, hypotension, etc.). Normal blood pressure, normal blood gases, normal temperature, normal blood sugars and electrolytes, normal coags, and normal intracranial pressures are all goals in controlling secondary brain injury.

111) In the first 24-hours after a traumatic head injury, what is the **most** significant factor in poor outcomes and increased morbidity (death)?

A) Hypertension

B) Hypotension

C) Hypercarbia

D) Hypoglycemia

B – Though hypertension, hypercarbia, and hypoglycemia are certainly bad, of the four answers, hypotension is the worst thing for an acutely injured brain. Remember: Cerebral perfusion pressure = body pressure (MAP) minus brain pressure (ICP). If the brain pressure is high and the body pressure is low, no blood gets to the brain. No blood to brain = dead or dying brain and, as you can imagine, a really, really bad outcome.

Certified Pediatric Emergency Nurse (CPEN) Review IV

112) What is the purpose of inducing hypothermia in a patient with a traumatic brain injury?

A) Hypothermia vasodilates cerebral blood vessels, increasing CPP

B) Hypothermia augments the post-traumatic inflammatory response

C) Hypothermia decreases cerebral metabolism and cerebral O2 consumption

D) Hypothermia will increase cerebral metabolism and cerebral O2 consumption

C – Think about what happens when bears hibernate. Everything slows way down. Therapeutic hypothermia works the same way. The technique of allowing the brain to hibernate, and thus allowing the cerebral metabolism and oxygen consumption to slow down for a while to let the brain heal, is now being trialed in the pediatric ED and ICU settings for pediatric post-cardiac arrest and with traumatic brain injuries.

113) What is the definition of intracranial hypertension?

A) It is the spontaneous elevation of ICP to ≥5 mm Hg for more than 5 minutes

B) Is the spontaneous elevation of ICP to ≥ 10 mm Hg for more than 5 minutes

C) It is the spontaneous elevation of ICP to ≥ 20 mm Hg for more than 5 minutes

D) It is the elevation of ICP to ≥ 25 mm Hg with noxious stimuli (i.e. suctioning) regardless of length of time

C – Normal intracranial pressure (ICP) in most patients is 0-15 mm Hg; however, depending on the situation and age of the child, ICPs up to 20 mm Hg can be accepted. When the ICP is above 20 mm Hg for more than five minutes, that's a problem and treatment is recommended. If you've ever had the pleasure of suctioning a patient with an ICP monitor in place, you will never forget the spikes it temporarily induces in their brain pressures. If the ICP spontaneously remains above 20 mm Hg, that's the definition of intracranial hypertension.

Neuro / Psych

114) Osmitrol® (mannitol) given for the treatment of head injuries because:

A) It is an osmotic diuretic that will decrease ICP by decreasing intracellular volume

B) It is an osmotic diuretic that will decrease ICP by increasing intracellular volume

C) It is an osmotic diuretic that will increase CPP by decreasing intracellular volume and increasing vascular volume

D) It is an osmotic diuretic that will increase CPP by increasing MAP

C – Lasix® (furosemide) is a loop diuretic which means it works in the kidney and says "pee." Mannitol works in a different way; it is an osmotic diuretic (a "big, clunky molecule"). The blood stream doesn't like having "big, clunky molecules" floating around it, so it shifts fluid from the tissues (i.e. brain) into the bloodstream to dilute the "big, clunky molecules." In other words, it shifts "edema fluid" from the brain cells into the vascular space. When all of this extra fluid hits the kidneys, they recognize there's way too much fluid in the blood stream, and it's time to pee, pee, and pee some more. Having more fluid in the toilet than you do in your swollen brain is the rationale for mannitol use in head injuries.

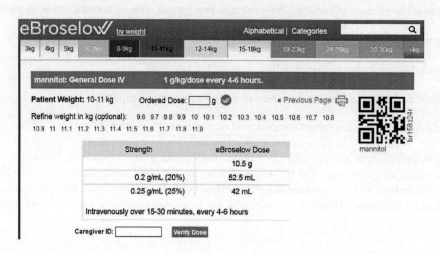

Color coded mannitol administration
Courtesy of James Broselow MD & Robert Luten MD – www.eBroselow.com

115) The use of hyperventilation (measured by pCO2 ≤ 35 mm Hg) to treat increased ICP is indicated in which of the following situations?

A) During brief periods when signs of significant neurological deterioration are present with increased ICP

B) Any time ICP increases to ≥ 20 mm Hg

C) Continuously for the first 48-hours after injury to prevent increases in ICP as swelling peaks

D) Hyperventilation should never be used in traumatic brain injury patients

A – Some nurses remember when we used to hyperventilate every head injury. Blowing off CO2 seemed like it must work! But then, several years back, the research showed that hyperventilation can actually make people worse. So, currently, hyperventilation is recommended for one and only one kind of pediatric or adult patient- -those who are neurologically "crashing and burning" in front of your eyes with impending herniation. Neurologically "crashing and burning" means: 1) They "blow" a pupil, 2) They acutely stop moving one side of their body, or 3) They acutely start posturing. Whenever one of these three occur, it means that something really, really bad is going on inside of the child's head and you are watching it happen. If you can briefly hyperventilate them long enough to get a CT and a neurosurgeon to fix the problem, great! Remember, the current emphasis is on brief hyperventilation.

116) Which of the following are measures that would improve the cerebral perfusion pressure?

A) Increase the MAP (mean arterial pressure)

B) Decrease the MAP (mean arterial pressure)

C) Increase the heart rate

D) Decrease the heart rate

A – In order for the brain pressure to go up, the blood pressure must go up. Otherwise there will be no blood going to the head, and from previous questions, you know what that means…

117) What measure will decrease ICP by promoting venous outflow from the head and neck?

A) Placing the patient in Trendelenburg position

B) Keeping the head of the bed ≥ 45 degrees

C) Keeping the head midline

D) Placing the patient in a prone position

C – Head elevation over 45 degrees, prone positioning, and Trendelenburg positioning can all contribute to decreased cerebral blood flow (not a good thing.) Keeping the head and the body facing the same way (midline) to allow the "veins to drain the brain" is the correct answer for the test and real life.

118) Which of the following pharmacologic interventions is a hyperosmolar therapy helpful in the management of increased ICP?

A) Maintaining adequate sedation

B) Pentobarbital infusion

C) Neosynephrine infusion

D) 3% saline infusion

D – The questions specifically mentions "hyperosmolar therapy" and, of the answers, the only one that involves a hyperosmolar therapy is 3% (hypertonic) saline. Sedation and "sedation to the extreme" (i.e. pentobarbital coma) can be used to decrease ICP, but are not hyperosmolar therapies. Neosynephrine is a vasopressor that helps increase the body pressure, but does nothing to decrease the ICP. Normal saline is 0.9%, while hypertonic saline (much more concentrated saline) can be 3%, 5% or 7.5%. Think about how mannitol works and the body's response in efforts to dilute the "big, clunky molecule." Hypertonic saline works in a similar way. The body doesn't like having really concentrated things floating around the bloodstream (it likes everything to be balanced or equal), so the fluids shift from the tissues (i.e. brain) into the bloodstream to dilute the blood. When all that extra fluid hits the kidneys, the patients pee, pee, and then pee some more.

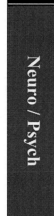

Neuro / Psych

119) Which of the following interventions will affect the mean arterial pressure (MAP) and lead to an increased cerebral perfusion pressure (CPP)?

A) Pentobarbital infusion

B) Isotonic fluid administration

C) Maintaining adequate sedation

D) Administration of Osmitrol® (mannitol)

B – Intravenous fluids such as 0.9NS or lactated Ringers (LR) are isotonic ("equal pressure") fluids, meaning they are supposed to stay in the blood vessels. This extra fluid in the blood vessels will commonly result in an increased blood pressure (MAP). Mannitol promotes diuresis (more fluid in the toilet than in the blood stream) and is typically administered in order to reduce intracranial pressure (ICP). Sedation and sedation to the extreme (inducing a pentobarbital coma) can result in hypotension if not managed carefully. Decreased blood pressure (MAP) = decreased cerebral perfusion pressure (CPP). If the blood pressure drops, the patient's prognosis drops!

Certified Pediatric Emergency Nurse (CPEN) Review IV

120) If a teenage football player suffers a concussion during a game, when should he be allowed to return to play?

A) If he is alert without neurological deficits after 5 minutes

B) If he is alert without neurological deficits after 15 minutes

C) If he is alert without neurological deficits after 60 minutes

D) After evaluation by a health professional trained in concussion assessment

D – If a concussion has occurred or is highly suspected, the injured player should not be allowed to return to the game until after evaluation by a health professional formally trained in concussion assessment and management. The time is not a factor. Even if a CT scan does not provide conclusive evidence of a brain injury, a concussion should be suspected if there has been a blow to the head (possibly followed by vomiting and/or loss of consciousness) and things just don't seem quite right. Signs include alterations in vision, speech, hearing, balance, memory, etc. Concussions are finally getting the attention that they deserve and have become an injury of increased interest for health professionals, coaches, parents and even the government. Although the neurosurgeons, neurologists and sports medicine physicians have had formal guidelines in place for several years as to when a concussed player should return to play, there are now at least seven states that have passed laws dictating conditions relative to the return to play as well. Moral of the story: When in doubt… sit them out!

Neuro / Psych

121) The AVPU score is used to quickly assess a patient's level of consciousness. AVPU stands for:

A) Alert, Violent, Pain, Unrecognizable

B) Artery, Vein, Pulse, Unilateral

C) Anxious, Verbal, Pressure, Unresponsive

D) Alert, Verbal, Pain, Unresponsive

D – The AVPU scale is a quick, down-and-dirty method of assessing level of consciousness. Is the child Alert? Does he respond to Verbal stimuli? Does he respond to Painful stimuli? Is he Unresponsive? Choose the most appropriate response.

122) According to the Centers for Disease Control (CDC), Down syndrome is the most common genetic birth defect in the United States today. It is caused by:

A) Alcohol consumption by a mother in her 2nd trimester

B) Lack of prenatal care in the 1st trimester

C) An extra copy of chromosome 21

D) Poor socio-economic conditions for the mother

C – What causes Down syndrome? Remember from nursing school that we are a mix of 23 chromosomes from both our mother and father--for a total of 46 (23 pairs). In chromosomal abnormalities, something happens to alter this count. In the case of Down syndrome, there is not just a pair of chromosome 21, but an extra chromosome or piece of chromosome. This is referred to as Trisomy 21.

There is currently no evidence that alcohol consumption, lack of prenatal care, or socio-economic conditions have any relevance or bearing on a child having or not having Down syndrome. There is evidence that increased maternal age (over 35) carries an increased risk of having a child with Down syndrome.

Certified Pediatric Emergency Nurse (CPEN) Review IV

123) Children with Down syndrome sometimes have a condition known as AAI (atlanto-axial instability). Due to this condition, it is important to have a high index of suspicion for what type of injury when treating a Down syndrome patient who has been in a traumatic incident?

A) Dislocated hip

B) Fractured patella

C) Greenstick fractures

D) Cervical spine injury

D – At the top of the spine, the occiput, atlas (C1) and axis (C2) form one unit, called the occipito-cervical articulation. It is very mobile, supported primarily by strong but elastic ligaments and has little bony support. These joints (the atlanto-occipital joints) allow movement of extension and flexion. If these joints are displaced, which can happen in pathological conditions such as Down syndrome, the dislocated bones can compress the spinal cord. It is estimated that 10–30% of all people with Down syndrome have AAI. In these cases, AAI (confirmed by radiograph) may be asymptomatic. If there are symptoms, they progress slowly and difficulties are primarily motor related, such as gait problems and weakness. Torticollis (stiff neck with muscle spasm) is considered a positive sign of atlanto-axial displacement until proven otherwise. It has been recommended that any child with Down syndrome considering sports activity have lateral cervical spine films.

Additional Pediatric ED Attending Insights: The AAI is asymptomatic until the unstable ligaments allow the spinal bones to move and impinge on nerve roots or the cord. The AAI doesn't cause the symptoms; it's the movement allowed by the AAI that causes them.

124) Which of the following statements is **true** regarding individuals with Down syndrome?

A) Most people with Down syndrome will be institutionalized

B) Children with Down syndrome must be segregated from other students at all levels of public or private education

C) Due to their disability, people with Down syndrome cannot hold a job or be gainfully employed

D) All individuals with Down syndrome have some degree of intellectual disability (formerly known as "retardation") ranging from mild to profound

D – This is one of the rare cases where the word "all" is in the correct answer. While it is true that all individuals with Down syndrome have some degree of intellectual disability, many are able to actively participate in educational, social, recreational and employment activities.

Let's clear up some common misconceptions regarding Down (or Down's) Syndrome.

Myth: People with Down syndrome are severely "retarded."

Truth: The majority of people who have Down syndrome have IQs that are in the mildly to moderately compromised range. This range refers to level of intellectual disability (formerly known as "retardation").

Myth: Most people with Down syndrome are institutionalized.

Truth: People with Down syndrome may live at home with their families or in assisted living facilities. They are active participants in all facets of society, including educational, vocational, social and recreational activities in their community.

Myth: Children with Down syndrome must be placed in segregated special education programs.

Truth: A child with Down syndrome should be included in regular academic classrooms in schools whenever possible. In some cases, they may be integrated into specific courses while being provided with special services for other areas. The most recent trend in education is for the student with Down syndrome to be fully included in the social and educational life of the community as much as able.

Myth: Adults with Down syndrome are unemployable.

Truth: Businesses quite often look for young adults with Down syndrome for a variety of jobs, tasks, and positions. They may be employed in multiple types of positions depending on their skills, abilities and intellectual functioning. People with Down syndrome may bring many special attitudes and attributes to their jobs, including extraordinary enthusiasm, dedication and reliability.

125) You are assessing a stable 9-year-old male in your ED who has Down syndrome. He was brought in by his parents with a complaint of right ankle pain. They state he was playing quarterback on his pee-wee football team when he was tackled. They are unsure of how he hurt his ankle. To gain a better history of the injury, you should:

A) First put on gloves, a gown and a mask

B) Disregard any answers the child gives because he has an intellectual disability

C) Speak directly to the child in clear, concise language and allow him time to answer

D) Speak only to the parents since they are the only ones who can understand you and answer your questions correctly

C – When you verbally interact with people with disabilities it is best to speak directly to them, and not solely to their family, aides, companions or interpreters. When you verbally interact with someone who has a cognitive disability, speak in clear, simple sentences. Try to use concrete examples as opposed to using euphemisms and abstract phrases such as "butterflies in your stomach" or "This IV will feel like a bee sting." You must also be patient with them and give them time to communicate back to you, as they may not process the question/answer as quickly as someone without a disability. We MUST make an effort to refer to individuals with a syndrome or disability as people first! Rather than referring to a child as "a Down syndrome child," we should make every effort to use "a child with Down syndrome." This places the child first and the syndrome second, not the other way around. Last, but certainly not least, donning gloves, gown and mask is not necessary when obtaining a history from this patient. Down syndrome is not contagious but, rather, a congenital chromosomal abnormality involving the presence of all or part of an extra 21st chromosome (trisomy 21.)

126) Which of the following represents the **earliest** sign of impending cerebral herniation due to increased intracranial pressure (ICP)?

A) Altered mental status

B) Projectile vomiting

C) Altered breathing pattern

D) Unilateral dilated pupil

D – The presence of a unilateral dilated pupil is the classic sign of early transtentorial herniation. The other three can be indicative of increased intracranial pressure (ICP) but, of the four choices, a single dilated pupil, on the same side (ipsilateral) of the side of injury/pressure, is the earliest specific indicator of impending herniation. If the increasing ICP is not addressed, it will eventually lead to full cerebral herniation and death.

127) Your two-week old patient presents with a fixed stare, lip smacking and "swimming" motions of the extremities. When you gently restrain the patient's extremities, then release them, the arm and leg waving starts right back up. This patient is **most** likely:

A) Hungry

B) In pain

C) Seizing

D) Soiled

C – This patient is probably seizing. In addition to classic seizure presentations such as focal or tonic/clonic movements, seizing neonates often present with the characteristics described in the above question. Other signs might be drooling, bicycling motions of the legs or unexplained tachycardia accompanied by mental status changes. How do you differentiate between seizing and jitteriness? If you are presented with jitteriness as an answer choice, those children typically do NOT have a fixed gaze and their motions will stop with gentle restraint. Jitteriness is most often associated with hypoglycemia in the neonate. Whether caring for jittery or seizing infants, remember to obtain oxygen saturation and finger/heel stick glucose at the bedside and send a stat electrolyte panel as soon as possible. Hypoxia, hypoglycemia, hypocalcemia, hyponatremia and hypomagnesemia can all cause infant seizures. These seizures are usually controlled by fixing any electrolyte imbalance, benzodiazepines and other anticonvulsants.

128) A 6-week old presents with lethargy and generalized seizures. The fontanelles are soft and flat, urine output is adequate and bedside blood glucose is normal. There is no history of trauma and this is the very young mother's first child. The infant has no significant prior medical history and has been taking formula very well. The mother tells you that the infant eats so much that she has begun to use less powdered formula when mixing the bottles in order to make the formula last longer. You immediately suspect which of the following electrolyte imbalances?

A) Hypermagnesemia

B) Hypocalcemia

C) Hyperchloremia

D) Hyponatremia

D – Hyponatremia is the most likely imbalance. This patient presentation points to severe hyponatremia from excess free water intake. In this case, a classic example, there has been too much water in the formula and not enough powder in the mix. Another cause of hyponatremia is when parents add bottles of water as substitutes for feeds during the day. They often believe it is a safe and effective way to stretch their resources. This is very similar to the classic case of the "Kool-Aid® kid" in which Kool-Aid® is substituted for formula because formula is expensive, but "Kool-Aid® is cheap". But remember, what is Kool-Aid®? Sugar + Water! All of this extra free water leads to decreased serum osmolarity (thin and dilute), seizures and cerebral edema. Possible risk factors for hyponatremic seizures are young parents, lower socioeconomic status and lack of parenting experience.

129) To no surprise, the above hyponatremic patient's serum sodium comes back at 120 mEq/L (normal is 135-145 mEq/L). To reverse cerebral edema and minimize brain damage, the sodium should be corrected:

A) Rapidly

B) Slowly

C) Initially rapidly then slowly

D) Initially slowly then rapidly

B – The management of hyponatremic seizures due to increased free water intake is similar to the management of diabetic ketoacidosis. The child didn't get a sodium level of 120 mEq/L (or go into DKA) in a matter of minutes or a few hours, so it is crucial not to try to correct the imbalance in a matter of minutes or a few hours. It will require a lot of fluid shifting and should be done carefully. Even an increase of 9mEq/L over a short period of time has been shown to cause demyelinating brain lesions. With the goal of achieving a rate of correction of less than 8mEq/L/day, correction of the sodium level over 24+ hours is commonly done to minimize the risk of brain damage. Slow and steady wins this race!

130) You are assessing two teen brothers at triage. They both present complaining of headaches, lethargy, fever, photophobia and stiff necks. In addition, one has a petechial rash. Their recent histories differ only in that while they were at the same summer camp on a large freshwater lake, one avidly participated in water sports, while the other did not, due to a recent severe "cold." Other than the "cold" that one brother had, both were reportedly completely healthy while sharing a room at camp. You recognize that both patients should be immediately placed on what kind of isolation precautions?

A) Standard/Universal

B) Contact

C) Airborne

D) Droplet

D – Both patients should be placed on droplet precautions because both teens are presenting with classic symptoms of meningitis. The mode of transmission for most of the organisms that cause meningitis is respiratory droplets that are larger than 5 micrometers in diameter. Because the brothers were in the same cabin, they should BOTH be on empiric droplet precautions for 48 hours after antibiotic therapy has been initiated. They may be cohabited in the ED if no other option is available, but ideally, they should be placed in separate rooms. There is no guarantee that they are currently BOTH infected, just a really high probability. Droplet precautions incorporate standard or universal precautions with the addition of a mask. Standard precautions alone are inadequate. Airborne precautions involve negative pressure rooms and are for particles less than 5 micrometers (TB, chicken pox, measles, etc.).

131) The lumbar puncture in the ED of the "non-swimmer" quickly shows Gram negative intracellular diplococci. Both brothers and all household/camp members who have been in close contact with the patient over the past week should begin an immediate prophylactic course of:

A) Gentamicin

B) Amphotericin B

C) Vancomycin

D) Rocephin® (ceftriaxone) or Rifampin

D – Potentially sick patients, like potentially sick nurses (i.e. those who have been exposed to patients with icky things like meningococcal meningitis) need R & R, (aka Rocephin® IM or Rifampin PO). Ciprofloxacin PO can also be used for prophylaxis of meningococcal disease, but that wasn't listed as an option. Gentamicin and vancomycin are IV antibiotics and amphotericin B is an antifungal, none of which are commonly administered for prophylaxis of any kind.

132) Treatment for bacterial meningitis, due to N. meningitidis includes:

A) Gentamicin

B) Amphotericin B

C) Vancomycin

D) Penicillin-G

D – Penicillin-G is the "G"old standard for treatment of N. meningitidis once the infection is confirmed by culture. In fact, that is exactly what the "G" stands for--Gold standard! Ampicillin may also be used. Rocephin® (ceftriaxone) is used when the infection does not respond to Penicillin-G or Ampicillin.

133) Patients with Reye's syndrome typically present afebrile, with an acute altered mental status, protracted vomiting and elevated liver function tests. It is commonly associated with which of the following:

A) Aspirin (ASA)

B) Monoamine Oxidase Inhibitors (MAO inhibitors)

C) Selective serotonin receptor inhibitors (SSRIs)

D) Tricyclic antidepressants (TCA's)

A – Although aspirin has NOT been identified as a definite cause of Reye's syndrome, research has identified aspirin as a major preventable risk for developing Reye's syndrome. Since the use of aspirin in children was actively discouraged, Reye's syndrome has virtually disappeared. Aspirin is NOT recommended for use in children under the age of 19 without expert consultation. Remember that aspirin is an ingredient in many over-the-counter medications used to treat viral symptoms, so be meticulous in taking history from parents. In the past, Reye's syndrome occurred in children during recovery from a viral infection. Reye's syndrome is characterized by encephalopathy and fatty liver disease (also called hepatic lipidosis or hepatic steatosis). If you see Reye's syndrome in a test question, chances are the answer is something involving aspirin.

134) When attempting to interact with a child with cerebral palsy (CP), if the child does not respond, you should:

A) Assume he/she doesn't understand and direct your attention only to the caregiver

B) Continue to address the child as you would any other child of that age group

C) Pay no attention to the noises made by the child, as they will be random and have no meaning

D) Do not be concerned about what you say about the child to the caregiver. You will not scare the child, as they will not understand what you are saying.

B – Cerebral palsy is an umbrella term for a variety of neurological disorders that affect body movement or muscle coordination. Difficulty in speaking and communication due to the muscle disorders is a common occurrence and may occur in conjunction with other developmental delays. Approximately half of kids with CP have associated mild to severe cognitive disabilities, but just because a child has CP does not mean they are unable to understand you. Although many cases are present from birth, symptoms are often not seen until several months of age or older. There is no definitive reason for CP, although risk factors may include premature birth, maternal infection, intrauterine hypoxia and low birth weight. It may also result from illness such as encephalitis in the early years of life. There is no cure. Symptoms involving the muscles range across the spectrum from muscle tightness and spasms to severe hypotonia.

135) Cerebral palsy is a condition that refers to a variety of neuromuscular disorders in infants and children. All of the following statements are true about cerebral palsy **except**:

A) Though the term cerebral palsy covers several neuromuscular conditions, all children with cerebral palsy are born with it. These neuromuscular disorders will get worse as the child grows older.

B) Premature birth and low birth weight children are more likely than full term babies to have problems that might lead to cerebral palsy. However, even children who are full term and normal birth weight can develop cerebral palsy.

C) Some forms of cerebral palsy can be prevented by avoiding head trauma. Examples of this would be wearing a helmet while riding a bicycle or properly securing a child in a car seat.

D) Cerebral palsy can be caused by jaundice. Kernicterus happens when a newborn baby has too much bilirubin and commonly causes cerebral palsy as well as hearing loss.

A – Not all cases of cerebral palsy are present from birth. There are many possible causes of the brain damage associated with cerebral palsy. Genetic conditions and problems with the blood supply to the brain can affect how the child's brain develops during the first months of pregnancy. Other causes of cerebral palsy occur after the fetal brain has developed later in pregnancy, during delivery or in the first years of the child's life. These can include meningitis and other infections, bleeding in the brain, lack of oxygen (such as from near drowning, a prolonged seizure or any other cause of prolonged hypoxia), severe jaundice, and head injuries.

136) A child with a left sided ventriculoperitoneal (VP) shunt malfunction is in your ED. The neurosurgeons are preparing to emergently remove the shunt and place an external ventricular drain (EVD). In addition to somnolence and unilateral neuro/neuromuscular deficits (e.g. fixed and dilated left pupil or right-sided weakness), you might expect to see all of the following clinical findings except:

A) Hypertension

B) Bradycardia

C) Hypotension

D) Respiratory depression

C – You would not expect to see hypotension in a patient with a malfunctioning VP shunt. A VP (cerebral ventricle to peritoneum) shunt may be placed when the patient no longer can adequately drain the cerebral spinal fluid (CSF) from the brain. The resulting increase in CSF volume (and pressure) in the brain can lead to many different effects on a child.

Symptoms can be as subtle as nausea, vomiting and mild headache. Though rare, more severe symptoms such as unresponsiveness and Cushing's triad (bradycardia, hypertension and apnea or irregular breathing) may occur. In the most severe cases, completely uncontrolled cerebral hypertension from pressure overload can result in brain herniation and death. Remember that the severe signs are late and truly ominous signs of impending doom for the child. In this case, the VP shunt would need to be removed and an externalized system (EVD) must be rapidly placed to decrease the fluid on the brain/brain stem to prevent increasing intracranial pressures and eventual herniation. In addition, this patient would be placed on antibiotics and monitored in a Pediatric ICU.

Additional Pediatric ED Attending Physician Insights: The vast majority of shunt malfunction kids are minimally to moderately symptomatic and very stable. It's not uncommon for them to be scheduled for surgery the next day unless they present during "regular working hours" and can be fitted into the OR schedule.

137) A 9-year old known oncology patient arrives in your Pediatric ED with complaints of vomiting, headache and vision changes. The triage history finds that he completed a course of radiation and chemotherapy about a month ago for an aggressive brain tumor. The brain CT reveals that the child has significant fluid in the ventricles and a dramatic increase in the size of his tumor. Plans are made to admit the child to the Pediatric ICU (PICU) and place an EVD (external ventricular drain) when a bed is available. While waiting for the bed, the child becomes difficult to arouse and has unequal and sluggish pupils. After contacting neurosurgery, what would you expect to do next?

A) Prepare the child for a head CT

B) Draw emergency labs

C) Admit child to the floor in anticipation of a PICU bed

D) Prepare the child for emergency EVD placement

D - This child will need an emergency EVD placement. The child has already had his head scanned and the medical team knows what the problem is. There is no need to rescan. Since he has been in the ED for a while, we all know labs have already been done. As far as admitting to the floor, that would be an unacceptable change in the level of care needed for this patient. The child shows signs of increasing intracranial pressure. Symptoms such as headache, vomiting, weakness and lethargy are early signs of increased ICP. As ICP increases, more ominous signs are: further decrease in LOC, pupil changes (dilation, slow or no reaction), increased BP, agonal respirations and decreased HR (the classic Cushing's Triad). Findings such as these require immediate/emergent intervention to decrease ICP before further and permanent damage to the brain, or death, results. Neurosurgeons may choose to place the ventricular drain in the ED if they can't get this child to the PICU or the OR expeditiously.

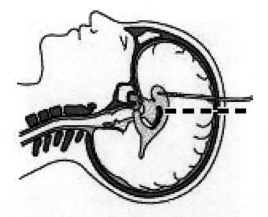

External ventricular drain (EVD) in ventricular space

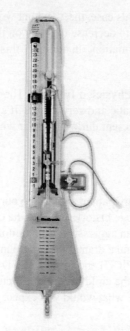

Duet™ external ventricular drain

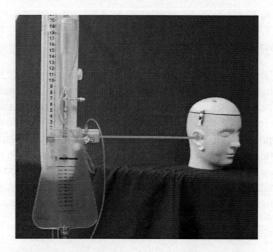

Correct level of EVD (ear) for drainage and pressure reading (Upright patient)

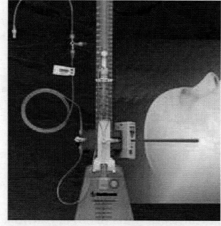

Correct level of EVD (ear) for drainage and pressure reading (Supine patient)

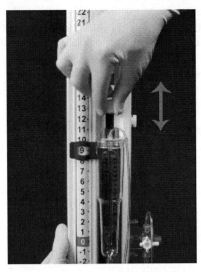

Adjusting the desired CSF drainage level

External ventricular drain images courtesy of Medtronics – www.medtronics.com

138) The PICU is trying to make a bed available for your 10-year old patient in the ED. The child has a history of acute hydrocephalus and had an EVD (external ventricular device) placed in the ED on the previous shift. He is now alert and has asked to go to the bathroom. As the patient's nurse, what must be done PRIOR to letting the patient get up and out of bed?

A) Disconnect the EVD tubing from the drainage system

B) Increase the height of the drainage system to where it needs to be when the patient is standing

C) Clamp off the EVD tubing so that it is OFF to the patient

D) Decrease the height of the drainage system to where it needs to be when the patient is sitting

C – The patient's drainage system should ALWAYS be clamped during any position change, (lying patient flat, raising head of bed, standing up, etc.). Once the child is in the desired position, you can then re-zero, level the pressure scale with the patients ear/temple area (with 0 cm's being the estimated zero point) and then, finally, UNCLAMP to resume drainage at the prescribed pressure level. An EVD drainage system is a closed STERILE system and, therefore, at no time should it ever be disconnected from the drainage system. (The only exception would be when accessing the system to obtain a CSF culture, but this is done under sterile technique, usually by a physician or nurse practitioner.) The EVD system is a FREE FLOWING system without back valves and is based on pressure and gravity. Remember gravity is one law that must be obeyed and because it will always win! If the patient stands up with an open drainage system, their head will now be higher than the drain and CSF will just take the path of least resistance and free flow right down the tubing into the drainage system. As a result, you, the nurse, will now be picking up your patient after he has collapsed to the floor. Vice versa, if you raise an open drainage system higher than the patient's head (remember gravity), all the CSF in the tubing will flow right back into the ventricles of the brain and quickly increase the ICP. (Obviously something we are trying to avoid!) The prescribed height of the drip chamber determines how high the pressure (and amount of fluid) in the brain needs to reach before excess fluid drips into the drainage chamber. If the drain is placed higher than the patient's head, then the brain needs to reach a much higher level (ICP) to overcome the set pressure and drain off the extra CSF.

139) A two week old, actively seizing infant is brought to the ED by EMS. The baby appears pale pink, but has no localized response to pain. What should the Pediatric ED nurse do **first**?

A) Administer rectal Valium® (diazepam)

B) Do a bedside glucose check

C) Administer supplemental oxygen

D) Get more information from the child's mother

C – Remember… airway and breathing trumps just about everything! Although hypoglycemia is easily detected and treatable, supporting oxygenation and ventilation would still be the first priority. Neonatal and pediatric research studies have found that visual observation alone is an unreliable way to assess cyanosis in babies and children. It is certainly appropriate to keep mom close to obtain additional history, but take care of the child's airway first. Rectal drug administration, while very convenient and not so repugnant to give to a small child, is no longer the route of choice for treatment of an actively seizing child because of the erratic and unpredictable drug absorption rate. IV or IO routes are preferred. Nasal administration of benzodiazepines is gaining rapid acceptance as well. Rectal administration isn't completely out of consideration, but if you can get a quick IV/IO line (or if EMS already got one), use it instead.

Lundblom's Lessons

The rescue phone rang in the ED and we were told that EMS was 3 minutes out with a 15-year-old male with "a bad allergic reaction." The medic stated the patient had been on a hunting trip and, after returning home, had developed a rash and a headache and felt warm. The patient's mother said he got some medicine during the night that he may be reacting to. The paramedics placed a large bore IV, started fluids and stated he was alert, but tachycardic. When the doors opened and we glanced at the patient covered with petechiae and purpura, we grabbed our masks and noted the puzzled looks on the faces of the EMS providers. We placed the patient in a treatment area and immediately began further assessment. The teen was alert and able to answer questions appropriately, but was very ill/toxic looking. He was tachycardic but normotensive. We sent labs, began aggressive IV fluid therapy and gave meningitic doses of antibiotics. Despite these interventions, his perfusion and capillary refill remained abnormal and the petechiae and purpura continued to spread. We quickly transferred our patient to the Pediatric ICU, where he was intubated one hour after arrival due to hypotension and deteriorating mental status. Despite multiple pressors at high doses, ventilatory support and aggressive antibiotic treatment, sadly, this adolescent died 10 hours after arrival from his fulminant meningococcal disease.

Teaching points: Meningococcal disease can present as meningitis, sepsis or both. A purple non-blanching rash in a sick-appearing patient is meningoccoal disease until proven otherwise. Patients with sepsis need prompt antibiotic treatment and aggressive circulatory and ventilatory support. Patients with meningococcal disease should be in respiratory isolation for 48 hours after antibiotics are started to avoid transmitting the infection to others. Antibiotic prophylaxis with Cipro® (ciprofloxacin) or "Doxy" (doxycycline) or Rocephin® (ceftriaxone) is indicated for staff with a significant exposure. A not-so-obvious teaching point for us is that we should stress discharge teaching to all ED patients about infections that can be prevented by recommended immunizations. Sadly, this illness can still occur in immunized patients since most, but not all, the different serotypes are covered by the meningococcal vaccine.

Overall mortality for all forms of meningococcal disease is 5-10%. Interestingly, the outcome for patients with meningococcal meningitis without meningococcemia (bacteremia) is much better than for those with bacteremia without meningitis. Once a patient with meningococcal sepsis develops septic shock and disseminated intravascular coagulopathy (DIC), the mortality rate is 90%.

Again, what we expected and what we got were very different. Subsequent education regarding this type of illness was conducted for EMS, including the need for prophylaxis and follow-up for the EMS providers themselves.

Appendix 5-A

Pediatric Glasgow Coma Scale

Eye opening (4)		<1 year	>1 year
	4	Spontaneous	Spontaneous
	3	To shout	To command
	2	To pain	To pain
	1	None	None

Motor (6)		<1 year	>1 year
	6	Spontaneous	Obeys command
	5	Localizes pain	Localizes pain
	4	Withdraws pain	Withdraws pain
	3	Abnormal flexion	Abnormal flexion
	2	Abnormal extension	Abnormal extension
	1	None	None

Voice (5)

0-2 years

5	Babbles or coos appropriately
4	Cries, but is consolable
3	Persistent crying or screaming
2	Grunts or moans to pain
1	None

2-5 years

5	Appropriate words and phrases
4	Inappropriate words
3	Persistent crying or screaming to pain
2	Grunts or moans to pain
1	None

>5 years

5	Oriented and converses
4	Confused conversation
3	Inappropriate words
2	Incomprehensible sounds
1	None

Chapter 6

Environmental Emergencies
Drowning, Drugs, Bugs, Bites, and Radical Rashes

*The smallest children are nearest to God,
as the smallest planets are nearest to the sun.*
-Jean Paul Richter

Pertinent Pediatric Ponderings (NOTES)

CHAPTER 6
Sample Test Answer Sheet

1. _____	31. _____	61. _____	91. _____
2. _____	32. _____	62. _____	92. _____
3. _____	33. _____	63. _____	93. _____
4. _____	34. _____	64. _____	94. _____
5. _____	35. _____	65. _____	95. _____
6. _____	36. _____	66. _____	96. _____
7. _____	37. _____	67. _____	97. _____
8. _____	38. _____	68. _____	98. _____
9. _____	39. _____	69. _____	99. _____
10. _____	40. _____	70. _____	100. _____
11. _____	41. _____	71. _____	101. _____
12. _____	42. _____	72. _____	102. _____
13. _____	43. _____	73. _____	103. _____
14. _____	44. _____	74. _____	104. _____
15. _____	45. _____	75. _____	105. _____
16. _____	46. _____	76. _____	106. _____
17. _____	47. _____	77. _____	107. _____
18. _____	48. _____	78. _____	108. _____
19. _____	49. _____	79. _____	109. _____
20. _____	50. _____	80. _____	110. _____
21. _____	51. _____	81. _____	111. _____
22. _____	52. _____	82. _____	112. _____
23. _____	53. _____	83. _____	113. _____
24. _____	54. _____	84. _____	114. _____
25. _____	55. _____	85. _____	115. _____
26. _____	56. _____	86. _____	116. _____
27. _____	57. _____	87. _____	117. _____
28. _____	58. _____	88. _____	118. _____
29. _____	59. _____	89. _____	119. _____
30. _____	60. _____	90. _____	120. _____
			121. _____

Pertinent Pediatric Ponderings (NOTES)

Certified Pediatric Emergency Nurse (CPEN) Review IV

1) Rabies in the United States is most commonly associated with bites from:

A) Bats

B) Bears

C) Bulldogs

D) Bedbugs

A – Most cases of rabies in the United States are caused by bat bites. For the most part, bats stay away from humans. After all, we are much bigger than they are and they are happy flying around eating mosquitoes. However, when they get rabies, bats can do stupid things like fly out of the sky and bite people. Any exposure to bat bites, bat scratches, pretty much bat anything, unless the bat can be caught, tested, and proven not to be rabid, results in rabies prophylaxis. If rabies does develop, it is pretty darn close to a 100% death sentence. Raccoons, and of course non-vaccinated dogs, can also be carriers of rabies.

2) In addition to a shot of rabies vaccine (not in the same syringe or area as the RIG), the patient gets to come back on days 3, 7, and 14 for the rest of the rabies vaccination series:

A) Only once

B) With the same frequency as for an adult

C) On a frequency dependent on the child's weight

D) With a dose that is based on the weight of the animal

B – Rabies treatment frequency is the same for children as it is for adults. Rabies kills little children just as easily as it kills bigger adults and if treatment is indicated, it is anything but pleasant. Rabies immune globulin (RIG) is injected directly into the bite area itself and depending on the child's weight, into other body areas as well. But that's not all… In addition to a shot of rabies vaccine (not in the same syringe or area as the RIG), the patient gets to come back on days 3, 7, and 14, and for the rest of the rabies vaccination series. It's a whole lot of painful shots and very expensive (this is why many public health departments, and not ED's give the shots), but is certainly a better choice than a death sentence. Remember, rabies is easily prevented, but just about never cured.

3) The increased risk of tissue damage and infection from human bites compared to bites from animals is:

A) Two-fold

B) Unsubstantiated

C) Age dependent

D) Based on the weight of the child

B – Contrary to what many of us were taught in nursing school, the generally accepted view that human bites are worse than animal bites cannot be substantiated by the existing data. All mouths are dirty and getting bit by a 2-year-old child, dog, or cat is never a good thing. Hands are the most common site for bite injuries and the most common site of serious infection following both human and animal bites.

Environmental

Certified Pediatric Emergency Nurse (CPEN) Review IV

4) If it has been less than one hour since the substance was taken, activated charcoal may be indicated for ingestions of:

A) Iron

B) Bleach

C) Tylenol (acetaminophen, Panadol)

D) Kerosene

C – Activated charcoal is most likely to be effective if administered within one hour of a Tylenol (acetaminophen) ingestion. Activated charcoal can bind the drug and prevent further absorption. Charcoal is <u>not</u> contraindicated for Tylenol ingestions. It does not interfere with the action of N-acetylcysteine (NAC, Mucomyst) and is important, especially if the patient presents soon after the ingestion, to help minimize the absorption of the Tylenol. For many common pediatric ingestions, charcoal is appropriate, but it "PHAILS" with: "P"esticides, "H"ydrocarbons, "A"lcohols/acids/alkali, "I"ron, "L"ithium, and "S"olvents. Like most medications in healthcare, whether charcoal is "in vogue" continues to change, so it's always a good idea to call poison control first!

5) Romazicon (flumazenil, Anexate) is the reversal agent for which category of medications?

A) Opiates

B) Benzodiazepines

C) Anticoagulants

D) Antibiotics

B – Romazicon is the reversal agent for the benzodiazepines (commonly used as sedatives and anxiolytics.) Narcan (naloxone) is the drug that is used to reverse opiates (really good pain killers.) Little known medical trivia: What was Romazicon called when it first was introduced on the market? Reversed! However, the company didn't want health professionals to think it could only be used for Versed (midazolam), so they changed it from something incredibly easy to remember (Reversed), to Romazicon (go figure.)

6) Syrup of ipecac is indicated for which of the following ingestions?

A) Opiates and benzodiazepines

B) Acids and alkalines

C) Aspirin, acetaminophen, and ibuprofen

D) None of the above

Environmental

D – According to the American Academy of Pediatrics (and if you talk to "tox docs,") you should never routinely use syrup of ipecac. Many want ipecac gone from the drug stores, ambulances, kitchen cabinets, and EDs. In addition to there being no evidence that vomiting helps children who have ingested something, there is also the very real problem that vomiting can continue for upwards of several hours after being given the syrup of ipecac. Depending upon what the child ingested, they may be awake now, but unconscious 10 minutes later. If the now unconscious child keeps vomiting, we have a big problem! Also, if your patient is actively vomiting, he can't get charcoal, Mucomyst (NAC), etc. No more syrup of ipecac – Hallelujah!

7) Gastric lavage is **not** routinely indicated for which of the following ingestions?

A) Opiates and benzodiazepines

B) Acids and alkalis

C) Aspirin, acetaminophen, and ibuprofen

D) All of the above

D – The American Academy of Clinical Toxicology (the "tox docs") has a position statement indicating that gastric lavage is not routinely, if ever, indicated for the management of poisoned patients. Unless the child is unstable, intubated, and it is known that less than one hour has passed since the ingestion, the risks can far outweigh the benefits. The "golden hour of overdoses" means that after an hour, most drugs have gone past the pyloric sphincter. If the drug has gone "below" (the pyloric sphincter,) we shouldn't bother trying to get it out from "above." Adults present on average 3-4 hours post-ingestion and kids tend to show up 1-2 hours post-ingestion. For drugs that slow peristalsis such as opiates, lavage can be considered because the drug stays "above" for longer. The other possible indication for gastric lavage can be medications that "form concrete" such as aspirin or iron. Getting those two medications, if possible, out from "above" before they "go below" is preferred, but again, primarily if it has been less than an hour.

8) The use of activated charcoal with sorbitol for children is:

A) Recommended because the sorbitol sweetens the taste and makes the medication more tolerable

B) Not recommended for children under 1 year of age or for repeated doses

C) Recommended if the ingestion has taken place within 1 hour per year of age

D) Not recommended for diabetic children because of the artificial sweetener

B – Activated charcoal with sorbitol is not recommended for children under 1 year of age and should not be given beyond the first dose at any age. While sorbitol is given with charcoal to enhance the taste, more importantly, sorbitol helps the charcoal move on through the system by drawing more water into the stools. There have been reported deaths from intractable diarrhea/dehydration and subsequent hypovolemia/electrolyte imbalances in children who have received multiple doses of charcoal with sorbitol.

9) A babysitter brings in a 2-year-old child who was found next to a spilled bottle of "white liquid" in the garage. The babysitter states the child "can't stop drooling." Vitals show HR 138, RR 44, BP 93/60, and the oxygen saturations are 88% on room air. The child's skin is warm and moist and her pupils are small, equal and reactive. Auscultation of her lungs reveals bilateral diffuse wheezes. This child was most likely exposed to:

A) An organophosphate

B) A hydrocarbon

C) Antifreeze

D) Paint

A – This child, presenting with non-stop drooling and exposure to the "white liquid" in the garage is most likely suffering from organophosphate poisoning. Hydrocarbons include kerosene and gasoline and are pretty easily identifiable by sight and smell. Antifreeze is alcohol based and is rarely, if ever, white. Paint, even outside of its original container, is also easily recognized by sight and smell. The SLUDGE/BBB mnemonic is used to help remember the signs associated with organophosphate or nerve gas exposures:

(S)alivation - drooling

(L)acrimation - tearing

(U)rination - peeing

(D)efecation - pooping

(G)I symptoms – lots of them

(E)mesis - barfing

(B)ronchorrhea – lots of airway secretions

(B)ronchospasm - wheezing

(B)radycardia – self explanatory

10) You are advised by poison control to administer IV atropine to this patient. The ED nurse should:

A) Question the order, as atropine is indicated for symptomatic bradycardias and this patient is certainly not bradycardic

B) Administer the atropine as directed, as atropine is being ordered in this situation to increase the patient's blood pressure

C) Question the order, as atropine is contraindicated if tachycardia is present

D) Administer the atropine as directed, as atropine is being given to help decrease the production of the airway secretions

D – One of the main problems with organophosphate poisoning (organophosphates are used in fertilizers and weed killers) is the incredible amount of oral and airway secretions that result. IV Atropine, more IV atropine, and then even more IV atropine is given to help dry the secretions, decrease the bronchospasm, and treat the bradycardias. 0.1mg/kg of atropine is given IV every fifteen minutes as needed with a minimum dose of 0.1mg. Noting the tachycardia is appropriate, but if the secretions block the airway, the tachycardia will resolve itself, because the child will be dead. This case demonstrates why a call to Poison Control is so important. They can certainly be of help with "routine" cases such as Tylenol (acetaminophen) or toothpaste ingestions; however, for the type of cases that we don't encounter every day, they are truly invaluable.

11) A 13-year-old girl is brought to the ED by her mother who states that her daughter reportedly took (50) 500mg tablets of Tylenol (acetaminophen, Panadol) last night. The ED nurse knows that if traditional treatment is unsuccessful for this patient, the following complication is likely to occur:

A) Cerebral edema

B) Liver failure

C) GI bleed

D) Cardiotoxicity

B - When a toxic dose of acetaminophen is acutely ingested, liver failure, vomiting, jaundice, and eventually renal, then total body failure can quickly result. GI bleed is a more likely complication from a Motrin (ibuprofen, Brufen) overdose, while cerebral edema and cardiotoxicity are not commonly associated with acetaminophen overdose. In most cases, signs of liver failure don't appear until 24-72 hours following the ingestion. This is important to remember, as even with a toxic ingestion, the initial liver function tests may be normal in the ED.

12) Which laboratory studies are commonly elevated early in acute Tylenol (acetaminophen, Panadol) toxicity?

A) BUN

B) Liver function panel

C) Creatinine

D) BNP

B – Remembering that the liver is the primary organ affected with acetaminophen overdoses, look for lab studies specific to the liver to help clue you in as to the correct answer for this question. BUN and creatinine are tests related to renal function and BNP is helpful in ruling out heart failure.

13) The ED nurse is aware that the antidote for acetaminophen overdose is:

A) Activated charcoal

B) GoLYTELY (polyethylene glycol)

C) Mucomyst (NAC)

D) Narcan (naloxone)

C – It only takes caring for one Tylenol overdose for any ER nurse to get the correct answer on this one. Once you've played with oral Mucomyst, you will never forget the smell and the memory will be burned into your brain forever. IV NAC (Acetadote) is now available in the U.S. after having been used in other countries for over 20 years. No more nasty smell and taste!

14) A frantic mother arrives at the ED with her 2-year-old son who she thinks has swallowed 5 or 6 iron tablets Feosol (ferrous sulfate) sometime last night. The child is now vomiting and complaining of severe "tummy" pain. In this case, the nurse would expect the physician to order:

A) Syrup of ipecac

B) Gastric lavage

C) Abdominal x-rays

D) Stat serum iron level

D – Obtaining an iron level is essential to guide management. Mild toxicity is expected at doses above 20mg/kg of elemental iron. Severe toxicity is above 60mg/kg. Because it's not always stated on the label, you may need to calculate the amount of elemental iron in a given form (Don't worry, you won't have to figure this out on the test.) Feosol tablets have 65mg of elemental iron per tablet, so this child may have taken 30-40mg/kg. Children's chewable vitamins usually have no more than 20mg/tablet. As with Tylenol, children's vitamins have limits on the amount of iron they can contain as a protective measure. Since the implication is clear that the ingestion time took place more than one hour ago, syrup of ipecac and gastric lavage are not likely to be effective. With individual pills of undigested iron, abdominal X-rays can help to find a "ball of iron." Chewable vitamins may not show up on X-rays, even if they weren't chewed and swallowed.

15) Which assessment finding may indicate iron toxicity in the previous child?

A) Respiratory alkalosis

B) Severe abdominal pain and hemorrhagic gastroenteritis

C) Hypothermia

D) Renal failure

B – Severe abdominal pain is a truly scary sign in a child who has taken unknown amount of iron. Shock and the patient literally bleeding to death from hemorrhagic gastroenteritis can quickly follow.

16) A 2-year-old arrives at the ED after possibly ingesting automatic dishwasher detergent (alkali.) Vital signs are HR 110, RR 24, and oxygen saturation is 100% on room air. The child is found to be drinking a bottle of milk without drooling. As there are no visible oral burns, the astute ED nurse realizes that:

A) There is no need for a further workup

B) There may be extensive internal damage that is not externally visible

C) The patient is medically cleared, but should be considered a suicide risk

D) 2-year olds aren't able to get under a sink, so suspect child abuse

A – Unless there are clinical signs of aspiration or ingestion (respiratory compromise or oral burns), no further workup is needed. Though what you see around the mouth (external) is not necessarily indicative of what's happening on the inside (esophagus), if the patient is tolerating oral fluids, not drooling, and breathing fine, these are very reassuring signs. Dishwasher detergent is not pleasant tasting by any means and just a small amount in the mouth is enough to stop just about all 2-year-olds. Alkaline burns tend to be worse than acid burns, but in reality, neither of them is very pleasant, and they get worse with extremes of pH and longer duration of contact. Lastly, suicide is not an issue for 2-year-olds who are certainly able to get under and into a sink and seemingly everywhere else.

Environmental

17) Which specific symptom should the nurse assess for in the previous patient?

A) Renal failure

B) Liver failure

C) Drooling

D) Sepsis

C – Drooling should be a huge red flag for the nurse. Acid and alkali ingestions can cause chemical irritation and burns wherever they touch, and this includes the lips, tongue, mouth, and esophagus. Sepsis and liver/renal failure are not associated with ingestions of this type.

18) In 3 minutes, EMS will be arriving at the ED with a 2-year-old in severe respiratory distress. He was found in the basement next to a bottle of kerosene. RR 60, HR 158, BP 110/80, O_2 sat on 10 liters of oxygen by mask is only 88%. He is continuously coughing and lung sounds are coarse throughout. The ED nurse anticipates the initial management for this patient to include all of the following **except**:

A) Rapid sequence intubation (RSI)

B) Gastric lavage

C) Chest X-ray to rule out pneumonitis

D) Consultation with poison control

B – Gastric lavage is not the immediate concern for this child. In a slight variation of our ABCs, we should focus on the airway (possible RSI), breathing (evaluate for pneumonitis), and consult (call poison control.) This child is exhibiting classic signs of a hydrocarbon ingestion and aspiration. Most children don't voluntarily drink more than the smallest of sips of these chemicals as they taste very, very bad. But with hydrocarbons and children, they don't have to drink it. Just inhaling the fumes can quickly kill them. This child needs to get intubated much sooner rather than later and by someone very skilled in intubation as they may desaturate and crash very quickly. He can get a nasty pneumonitis (chemical, not bacterial) and respiratory failure. Ipecac, lavage, or charcoal are not indicated as the risk of further aspiration is incredibly high.

19) The ED nurse would anticipate the management of a teen with a history of depression who presents with a tricyclic antidepressant (TCA) overdose and cardiac arrhythmias to include the administration of:

A) Sodium bicarbonate or 3% saline

B) Magnesium sulfate

C) Haldol (haldoperidol)

D) Dilantin (phenytoin)

A – In cases of TCA overdoses, if nasty ventricular arrhythmias start popping up, sodium bicarbonate or 3% saline, not necessarily amiodarone or lidocaine, are the medications most commonly used (with poison control's guidance.) These patients can seize if you look at them funny and also are notorious for making you go through every algorithm in the PALS book. Overdoses involving TCAs such as Elavil (amitriptyline), Tofranil (imipramine), and Pamelor (nortriptyline) can be some of the nastiest that we take care of. Fortunately, we don't see them as often as we used to since prescribing practices seem to have moved toward different categories of medications for depression; but TCAs are still out there.

20) Which nursing action holds the **highest** priority during the initial management of a patient with a TCA overdose?

A) Obtaining a 12-lead ECG

B) Completing the suicidal risk checklist

C) Anticipating and initiating measures to prevent aspiration

D) Placing a peripheral IV with 0.9NS

Environmental

C – If you see aspiration, think airway, and anything involving airway is almost always the answer. Though A, B, and D should be quickly done, these patients, like hydrocarbon ingestions, can crash and code very quickly.

21) All of the following conditions commonly mimic the symptoms of acute alcohol intoxication **except**:

A) Hypoglycemia

B) Head injury

C) Drug intoxications

D) Hyperglycemia

D – Remember the 3 "polys" of hyperglycemia: Polyphagia (frequent hunger), polyuria (frequent urination), and polydipsia (frequent thirst.) These are not symptoms that resemble acute alcohol intoxication. On the other hand, who might act like a "rookie" on New Year's Eve? A diabetic or any sick kid with low glucose can certainly look like someone who is acutely intoxicated with alcohol. Head injuries and overdoses can also result in someone acting goofy. The wise ED nurse also rules out the serious medical and trauma possibilities (including checking a pulse ox and finger stick glucose) before considering a patient just "Drunk on Arrival" (a different DOA.)

22) Public swimming pools at which chlorine can be smelled:

A) May pose a risk for asthmatics

B) Pose no risk of infectious diseases

C) Assure swimmers of a proper pH level

D) Have reduced likelihood of eye and skin irritation because excess chlorine is evaporating

A – Swimming pools at which chlorine can be smelled can produce enough chemical byproducts (nitrogen trichloride, etc.) to aggravate or even induce symptoms of asthma. Chlorine will kill many organisms which cause infections, but if you have kids who have ever been to a public swimming pool, you know that infections can and still will happen. Chlorine is a known eye and skin irritant, so more chlorine means more likelihood of irritation, not less.

Environmental

23) The process of experiencing respiratory impairment from submersion/immersion in liquid is called:

A) Drowning

B) Near-drowning

C) Secondary drowning

D) Apnea

A - Drowning outcomes are classified as death, morbidity and no morbidity. Agreed upon terminology is essential to describe the problem and to allow effective comparisons of drowning trends. Thus, this definition of drowning as adopted by the 2002 World Congress on Drowning, should be widely used.

24) Cases of young children surviving submersion in cold water are thought to be related to the mammalian or diving reflex. This reflex includes all of the following as a result of being submerged in icy cold water **except**:

A) Peripheral vasodilatation

B) Decreased heart rate

C) Decreased cardiac output

D) Decreased cerebral oxygen demand

A – Massive peripheral vasoconstriction, not vasodilatation, kicks in to keep what oxygen is present where it really needs to be, i.e. the brain. The mammalian or diving reflex is summarized as your body quickly throwing itself into a hibernation-like state and everything slowing way down. Hypothermia appears to also be a crucial factor in survival. Remember, people drowning in water not cold enough to be icy are just cold and dead. Researchers are still trying to determine exactly how it is that we know of miraculous cases of children under the icy cold water for way too long who survive, and neurologically intact as well.

25) Which statement is **true** concerning submersion injuries?

A) Death is always from hypoxia as a result of water or vomitus filling the lungs

B) 10% of drowning victims are described as "dry drownings"

C) True drownings only occur in water deeper than the victim's height

D) Because of their recent emersion from a fluid-filled environment, newborns do not suffer submersion injuries

B – "Dry drowning" accounts for 10% of drowning incidents and is characterized by laryngospasm, rather than water in the lungs. Laryngospasm also can contribute to death because of inadequate exchange of oxygen in the lungs. Dry drownings can occur up to 24 hours after a submersion incident, and do not require the filling of the lungs. Water depth and age (while risk factors for drowning), are not factors in the definition of drowning.

26) Your neighbor brings her 13-month-old child to you. The child is wet, but appears alert with normal respirations. The mother states that she found the child face down in the bathtub and pulled the child from the water. The mother states that the child was blue, but after "shaking her," the child began crying. When the medics arrived on scene, the child is alert with normal vital signs. What should you advise the mother?

A) Not to worry since children learn quickly from an incident like this

B) Mom should watch the baby for signs of Shaken Baby Syndrome

C) The child should be taken to the Emergency Department for evaluation

D) Homeowners insurance, not medical insurance, will cover any expenses

C – This child definitely needs to be evaluated in the ED for several reasons. The child was submerged long enough to "turn blue" and we know that submersion injuries are not always immediately obvious. Respiratory and neurologic complications can arise hours after the incident. In addition, there are situational concerns. What was a 13-month-old doing alone in a bathtub? What exactly did the comment about "shaking" the baby mean? Though this could easily be a situation where the mom was giving the child a bath, and then ran to answer the phone, it also raises enough red flags for possible abuse. The child should definitely be evaluated and watched for a few hours.

27) An immediate intervention for children just pulled from a swimming pool:

A) Perform the Heimlich maneuver followed by aggressive CPR

B) Assess the airway

C) Provide rewarming techniques

D) Administer epinephrine

B – If airway is an option, it's probably the right answer. It is interesting to note that up until several years ago, it was thought that after a submersion incident, children would be in danger of dying due to an airway obstruction, as water was blocking the trachea. The thinking was that you can't get the air in, until you get the water out! However, current research reveals that it is not usually a matter of having an airway obstruction, but rather that these patients are horribly sick because they were under the water and not breathing for way too long. The Heimlich maneuver is still highly recommended for cases of choking, but not near-drowning. Rewarming is nice, but not immediately needed, and drowning victims need an open airway before epinephrine.

28) The leading cause of death in children found in a house fire is:

A) Burns and thermal injuries

B) Asphyxia from smoke and inhalation of toxic fumes

C) Child abuse

D) Blunt trauma

B – Statistically, 2/3 of people die in building fires without being burned before they suffocate. Carbon monoxide, cyanide and other noxious gases kill them before the flames ever would.

29) What is the **most** common cause of death with pediatric burns?

A) >50% body surface area (BSA) burns

B) Infection

C) Delayed fluid resuscitation

D) Inhalation injury

D – When in doubt… pick something that involves airway and chances are you will have the correct answer. A 2007 study of why pediatric burn patients died found that the most common cause of death was unpreventable lung damage due to the initial insult. Though ½ of your body being burned is an unbelievably bad injury, over the years, burn care has evolved to the point that more and more children survive truly horrible burns.

30) In conjunction with airway management and aggressive pain control, fluid resuscitation is vital for the burned child's survival. Though not universally accepted, the Parkland formula is commonly used to determine the amount of fluids to be administered. Which of the following is the **correct** amount of fluid to give a 50kg child who sustained 50% BSA burns?

A) 50ml/hr of LR or 0.9NS

B) Wide open 0.9NS or LR until the child arrives at a burn center

C) 10,000ml LR or 0.9NS over 24 hours, 5,000ml LR or 0.9NS over 12 hours, followed by 5,000 LR or 0.9NS over the next 12 hours

D) 10,000ml LR or 0.9NS over 24 hours, 5,000ml LR or 0.9NS over 8 hours, then 5,000ml LR or 0.9NS over the next 16 hours

D – To correctly answer this question, it's easy to rule out A and B as they don't involve any calculations. So that leaves C and D as possible answers. D is the correct answer as the Parkland formula divides the amount of fluid to be given in 24 hours into the first 8 hours and the next 16 hours. The actual formula is 2-4ml x kg x % BSA (body surface area) burned. It is important to remember that the timer starts at the time of the burn, not from when the patient arrives in the ED. Once you have figured out the total amount (C and D both started with the same amount), then ½ is given over the next 8 hours. The remaining amount is then given over the next 16 hours. The way that I've always remembered the 2-4ml x kg x BSA burn formula is:

4ml

Look at your arms and legs and count them? How many are there? Four. They hopefully aren't burned so you are doing better than the patient is.

Kg – "Big kid vs. little kid"

How much do they weigh? Big kids get more fluids than little kids.

BSA burn – "Bad burn vs. not bad burn"

How much are they burned? Bad burns (more BSA) get more fluids than not bad burns.

Multiply all three numbers together and that's how much fluid they get in the first 24 hours, but ½ in the first 8 hours, because that's when they do the most fluid shifting and subsequent swelling.

31) The Parkland formula shows that the child in the previous scenario should receive 5,000ml over 8 hours (625ml/hour) for the first 8 hours post-burn. However, if the child arrives in your ED two hours post-burn, what is the appropriate fluid rate?

A) 625ml/hour of LR or 0.9NS

B) 833ml/hour of LR or 0.9NS

C) 1,000ml/hour of LR or 0.9NS

D) 1,250ml/hour of LR or 0.9NS

B – 625ml/hour was appropriate when the child arrived at the ED shortly after the burn. However, when the patient doesn't arrive until much later or if access cannot be obtained until much later, then you have to play "catch up." In this case, the child still should receive 5,000ml of LR or 0.9NS, but now over 6, not 8, hours. The clock starts when they got burned, not when they arrived at the ED. Sometimes we just have to do the math!

Certified Pediatric Emergency Nurse (CPEN) Review IV

32) What is the minimum ml per hour urinary output goal in a 20kg burn child?

A) 20ml

B) 40ml

C) 60ml

D) 80ml

A – 1-2ml/kg/hour is the minimum amount of urine output that is desired, so the minimum goal in this case is 20ml per hour. With burns and associated shock states, urine output is important to watch as it is one of the first things to go. If urine output drops below 1-2ml/kg/hour, give more fluid. If that doesn't work, give more fluid. If it seems like you are giving way too much fluid, get over it, and give more fluid. The burn unit can recommend bicarb or mannitol or whatever they are into that particular week, but in the ED with few exceptions, you have to flush the pee-pee out!

33) EMS arrives with an 2-year-old who suffered full-thickness flame burns to his entire head and the front of his chest and abdomen. What percentage of body surface was burned?

A) 18%

B) 27%

C) 32%

D) 36%

D – The Rule of 9's teaches that there are two kinds of body parts: Little parts (worth 9%) and big parts (worth twice that amount – 18%.) In adults, "little parts" include the arms and head and get 9%. "Big parts" include the entire front of the chest and abdomen or the legs and they get 18%. However, remember that children have "big head, little body syndrome." So how much do they get for their heads? 18%. The front of the chest and abdomen still comprise a big part, so we add another 18%. Therefore 36% is a good approximation of the percentage of the body burned. Burn centers teach that children also have "short little leg syndrome" and they only get 14% for their legs. However, for us in the ED where most of us don't take care of critically ill burn patients every day, simply remembering "big parts and little parts" is much easier. When the patient gets to the burn center, they can more accurately assess the burn percentage using the Lund-Brower chart or other methods.

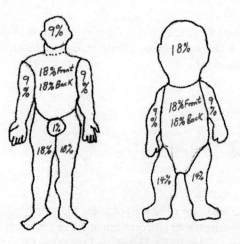

Adult and Pediatric Rule of 9's

Illustration by Nina DeBoer, then age 9 (my aspiring artist daughter, now aspiring baker daughter)

34) Which initial nursing action(s) would **not** be appropriate for the previous patient?

A) Removing all of the patient's jewelry

B) Removing the patient's wet clothing and covering him with sterile towels

C) Flushing the burned areas with cool water

D) All of the above

C – When the patient in still "on scene," briefly rinsing with cool water to stop the burning process is an appropriate intervention. However, this patient is in the ED and the time for stopping the burning process has passed (except with tar burns – much hotter and still cooking the skin.) Flushing the skin with cool water in the ED for thermal burns can quickly result in devastating hypothermia, so "clean and dry" or WaterJel (gel soaked dressing that eases pain and doesn't induce hypothermia – www.waterjel.com) and removing jewelry are appropriate actions.

35) Based on the Parkland fluid replacement formula, approximately how much isotonic fluid should this 40kg patient receive over the first 24 hours?

A) 96ml of LR or 0.9NS

B) 960ml of LR or 0.9NS

C) 5,760ml of LR or 0.9NS

D) 7,560ml of LR or 0.9NS

C – 2-**4**ml x kg x BSA burn. 4ml x 40kg x 36% BSA burn = 5,760ml over 24 hours, and ½ of that whole amount should be given in the first 8 hours post-burn. Sometimes we have to do the harder math.

36) Which statement **best** describes the reason for keeping a burn patient NPO while in the ED?

A) Esophageal edema can occur because of the burn injury

B) Keeping the patient NPO will help prevent aspiration from vomiting

C) Burn patients are prone to developing paralytic ileus

D) Keeping the patient NPO will help prevent sepsis from gut translocation of bacteria

C – Patients with "bad burns" are prone to developing a paralytic ileus as the body is focusing all of its efforts on surviving the burn, and not on digesting food. The burn unit can place feeding tubes for enteral nutrition; however, in the ED, as with any major trauma patient, NPO status is desired.

37) The human body's temperature regulation center is found in the:

A) Pituitary

B) Hypothalamus

C) Hyperthalamus

D) Cerebellum

B – The hypothalamus is the prime regulatory center in the body. One way to remember this is to associate hypothalamus with hypothermia. They both start with "hypo." There is no body organ known as the hyperthalamus, so hypothalamus is the closest sounding answer.

38) Adolescent athletes are:

A) Not at risk for heat stroke because they are in better shape than most of us

B) At risk for heat stroke especially with temperature extremes

C) Not at risk of heat stroke because of hormonal changes that take place during puberty

D) At risk for heat stroke because of hormonal changes that take place during puberty

B – Though adolescent athletes are in better shape than many of us, they are still at risk for heat stroke, especially at the beginning of sports season when they have not yet "acclimated" to the workouts and temperature extremes. While heat stroke is seen more often with the very young and the very old, teens are not immune from this illness. While puberty may do many wonderful and weird things to adolescents, it probably doesn't affect their inherent risk for heat stroke except for: a) The fact that they think it will never happen to them and b) Peer pressure may spur them to go beyond the point where they start feeling bad.

39) Which of the following statements is **true** regarding heat exhaustion?

A) Heat exhaustion can be distinguished from heat stroke as patients with heat exhaustion have altered mental status and a rectal temperature above 104F (40C)

B) Heat exhaustion patients in the ED should be categorized as Triage I (resuscitation) due to their potential for acute deterioration

C) Heat exhaustion is treated by removing the patient to a cool area and providing rest along with either oral or IV rehydration

D) Treatment for heat exhaustion include removing the child's clothing and applying ice-water soaked sheets

C – Heat cramps can occur in a patient who has been in the heat, has been sweating, and now due to a sodium imbalance and dehydration, they start experiencing cramping. Imagine that. In most cases, this is easily treated with rest, a cooler environment, and oral rehydration (Pedialyte, Gatorade, etc.) This is similar to heat exhaustion, but there is one significant differentiating factor. With heat exhaustion, the patient frequently has nausea and vomiting which tends to preclude oral rehydration attempts. But as with heat cramps, if they are in a nice cool environment (i.e. the ED), and are rehydrated, they do fine. So that's heat cramps and heat exhaustion. Two out of three isn't bad. The third heat condition, heat stroke, aka "heat prostration," is the one that we really worry about, as this can quickly kill a patient. Heat stroke is characterized by the body being so hot that it stops trying to cool itself (no more sweating) and is accompanied by mental status changes. Remember that if your rectal temperature is 106F (41C), your "inside organs" such as the liver can be even higher. With that in mind, quickly and safely cooling these patients is imperative in order to prevent permanent brain and other organ damage.

Environmental

40) All of the following nursing interventions are appropriate in caring for a patient with heat stroke **except**:

A) Applying ice packs to the axillae and groin

B) Instituting measures to prevent shivering

C) Continuing all cooling measures until the patient's body temperature reaches 98.6F (37.1C)

D) Administering room temperature IV fluids

C – Whichever cooling methods are chosen, the key is to cool them down, but only until the core temperature is 102F (38.9C.) Though 102F (38.9C) is still high, remember that after you stop active efforts to cool the patient, they still cool down a bit further. If you don't stop until they are 98.6F (37.1C), then they can keep cooling down until they are 93F (34C) and treatment for ER-induced hypothermia in the summer really looks bad. There are many methods for cooling patients. Simple measures like fans and "spray bottle misting" can be very effective. IV fluids will help cool the patient from the inside. Even room temperature fluids are much cooler than the patient. Placing cool packs where large blood vessels come closest to the skin (back of the neck, axillae, and groin) is another effective intervention. If you are thinking about something more dramatic, like an ice water bath, please think again. Immersion in ice water baths is not only not practical in the ED, but also not recommended because of the possible initiation of bradycardia and cardiac arrest due to stimulation of the mammalian dive reflex. ER induced cardiac arrests look really bad!

41) Which of the following would the nurse expect to see in the teen patient with heatstroke?

A) Elevated serum glucose

B) Low serum BUN

C) Respiratory acidosis

D) Elevated hematocrit

D – As dehydration is common with the body's pre-heatstroke attempts to cool down, an elevated hematocrit is to be expected. The glucose can be low due to vomiting and increased metabolic demands, the BUN would be high due to dehydration, and respiratory alkalosis occurs with increased respiratory rates (Picture kids with fevers or dogs panting and trying to cool down.)

42) Febrile seizures are **most** common in children of what age group?

A) 3 months to 6 years of age

B) 6 months to 5 years of age

C) 1-8 years of age

D) 10-14 years of age

B – Little ones from 6 months to 5 years are those we most commonly associate with febrile seizures. How fast, not how high is the key. It's not necessarily that they have a temperature of 104F (40C) and therefore they will seize, but how fast did they go from normal 98.6F (37.1C) to 104F (40C.) Either way, with febrile seizures, their temperature is high, lab studies are normal, but it's important for parents to know that recurrence is actually quite common. Febrile seizures do not cause brain damage and giving antipyretics "by the truckload" does not prevent febrile seizures. If they are going to happen, they are going to happen. Long term anticonvulsants are not generally recommended until the child has had 8-10 febrile seizures.

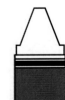

Environmental

43) Tylenol (acetaminophen, Panadol) should be administered every:

A) Hour

B) 2-3 hours

C) 4-6 hours

D) 6 hours

C – Tylenol can be administered orally or rectally every 4-6 hours as needed for fever or pain relief. This is important for parents, and staff, to remember, as Motrin (ibuprofen, Brufen) can be administered for similar reasons, but only every 6 hours.

44) Infants and young children are at an increased risk for infectious diseases for each of the following reasons **except**?

A) Their immune systems are immature

B) Many spend considerable amounts of time in areas like daycare and pre-school where infectious diseases thrive

C) They lack the ability to care for themselves in terms of hand washing and other methods to avoid exposure to infectious diseases

D) The hypothalamus is insufficiently developed for adequate thermal regulation

D – This answer sounds fancy, but clearly isn't true! As children, and their immune systems develop, they are exposed to more and more things (good and bad), and the chance of them "catching something" increases exponentially. Little ones who are in daycare and pre-school increase their exposure to kids and the things kids carry (bacteria, viruses, fungi, and Ebola.) Hand washing, blowing noses, covering mouths and noses when sneezing or coughing, and using tissues (not fingers and sleeves) are all great lessons to be learned, but often not regularly practiced until beyond the infant/young child state.

45) The mother of a 3-week old child arrives at triage stating "My baby's got a fever." The pediatric ED nurse knows that this child's ED workup will **most** likely involve:

A) Blood and urine cultures

B) Lumbar puncture

C) Chest X-ray

D) All of the above

D – Remember that a 3-year-old, or even a 3-month-old, with a fever is very different than a 3-week-old with a fever. During the first month of life if the child is "anything but healthy" (i.e. they have a fever), it's probably because they are septic. And if they are not septic, it's because they are about to be septic. And if they are not about to be septic, it's because they are thinking about becoming septic. During the first month of life, every baby with a fever or who looks bad is septic until proven otherwise. So expect cultures (of everything), pictures (chest X-ray if there are respiratory symptoms or positive lung findings), and punctures (LP and IV.) In addition, these kids will get admitted, with IV antibiotics for two days until the cultures are proven to be negative.

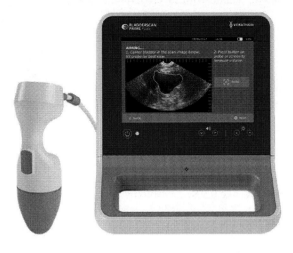

BladderScan Prime Plus to Ensure Urine is Present in the Bladder Prior to Catheterization

Photo Courtesy of Verathon

www.Verathon.com

46) When caring for a hypothermic child, the ED nurse should remember that the major area(s) of heat loss from the body is/are the:

A) Hands and feet

B) Head

C) Chest

D) Abdomen

B – "Big head, little body syndrome" strikes again. When little ones lose heat, most is lost through their "big heads." So covering their heads with hypothermia, or to maintain normothermia, is crucial.

47) Which statement regarding extreme hypothermia is **false**?

A) The myocardium is irritable

B) Profound vasodilatation is present

C) Hepatic function is decreased

D) Renal function is decreased

B – Vasoconstriction, not vasodilation, occurs to keep the warmest blood near the vital organs and away from the cold outside world. In profound hypothermia, everything slows way down, including the functioning of the liver (drugs don't get metabolized), kidneys (they let everything go through and out, aka cold diuresis), and the heart. Not only is the heart rate much slower, but more importantly, the myocardium or heart muscle, is very irritable. That's important because all these patients need is a funny look and they go into V-fib. Emergency interventions such as intubation, spinal immobilization, etc. are often still required, but please, just do them as gently as possible.

Certified Pediatric Emergency Nurse (CPEN) Review IV

48) The IV fluid of choice for a child with severe hypothermia is:

A) LR

B) D5.2NS or D5.45NS

C) D5W

D) 0.9NS

D – Though D5.2NS or D4.45NS are generally the "fluids of choice" for young children, in hypothermic patients, 0.9NS is where it's at. Just about everything you want to give is compatible with it, if the patient's pressure is low, you can bolus them with it, and it primarily stays "in the tank" (blood vessels) where you want emergency fluids to be. LR, like 0.9NS, is isotonic so it stays in the blood vessels, but remember that the "L" in LR stands for lactated. And where is that lactate broken down? In the liver. And what is that liver doing when you're are horribly hypothermic? Nothing. So, 0.9NS is the correct answer.

49) A 6-year-old boy is suffering from hypothermia post-submersion in an icy pond. He is unresponsive with a respiratory a rate of only 4-6 breaths per minute. A femoral pulse of 40 beats per minute is barely palpable and his rectal temperature is 84F (29C.) Management of this child's airway should:

A) Be limited to bag-valve-mask ventilation because insertion of a tracheal tube is likely to induce ventricular fibrillation

B) Be limited to supplemental oxygen via non-rebreather mask since the child is now breathing spontaneously

C) Include intubation, preferably by someone experienced in pediatric intubation

D) Include a BiPAP mask for pressure support

C - Having a person experienced in pediatric intubation place an endotracheal tube in this patient is not only recommended, but needed to prevent aspiration and maximize ventilatory support of the soon to be present ARDS. In the past, it was taught that interventions such as intubation would induce ventricular fibrillation. However, current research has disproven this thinking. In addition, think about it from a reality perspective. Could you bag-mask ventilate a child for hours while they warm up? Possibly. But would you want to? No. 4-6 breaths per minute may be present and spontaneous initially, but that isn't going to last long and BiPAP still relies on the patient's own spontaneous respirations.

50) Which rewarming method is **least** effective for a severely hypothermic pediatric patient?

A) Applying warming blankets

B) Administering warmed fluids via a nasogastric tube

C) Administering warmed IV fluids

D) Administering warmed and humidified oxygen

A – Warming blankets are an option for rewarming hypothermic patients, and are a quick and easy start in the ED, but they warm the patient from the "outside in." The other three answers (O_2/NG/IV) are methods that warm from the "inside out." This is important because hypothermia leads to vasoconstriction and blood being shunted away from the "outside" to the "inside." Therefore, warm the patient where the blood is.

Environmental

Certified Pediatric Emergency Nurse (CPEN) Review IV

51) In relation to hypothermia, "afterdrop" refers to the:

A) Continued drop of core temperature during rewarming

B) Inability to hold onto small objects until rewarming is complete

C) Peripheral flaccidity after near-drowning and before rewarming is started

D) Rebound bradycardia after a run of V-fib caused by intubation

A - The "afterdrop" or "afterfall" phenomenon refers to the continued drop of core temperature during rewarming. As with many things in medicine, it is controversial as to its actual occurrence or implications. The idea is that the patient has cold blood trapped in their periphery, and as the core temperature slowly increases through warming efforts and blood now starts to re-enter the periphery, the cold blood from the periphery now returns to the core and the temperature drops. Because of this theory, most practitioners advocate for rewarming patients with severe hypothermia from both the inside out and the outside in.

52) A 15-year-old patient is brought to the ED complaining of tingling and pain in the fingers of both hands after an afternoon of reluctantly shoveling snow to earn some spending money. The nurse notes that the fingers are soft, but the soft tissues fail to "pink up" after blanching. The ED nurse should suspect that this patient has:

A) Deep frostbite

B) Superficial frostbite

C) Peripheral neuropathy

D) Hyperventilation Syndrome (HVS) from overexertion

B – Both superficial and deep frostbite have frostbite in the diagnosis, which means it can't be good. The findings that lead the ED nurse to suspect that this is superficial frostbite is the fact that the fingers are still soft (not frozen solid) and he still has sensation (he complains of pain.) Peripheral neuropathy is generally caused by trauma or systemic illness, not shoveling snow, and Hyperventilation Syndrome is usually behavioral or psychogenic in nature, not due to exertion.

53) A 17-year-old intoxicated teen spent the night in a snow bank and now stumbles into the pediatric ER. He is awake and wants someone to "check his fingers and feet out." The triage nurse finds the digits to be cold and solid to the touch and his tympanic temperature is 91F (33C.) Which nursing intervention would be **most** appropriate to rewarm frostbitten digits?

A) Giving the patient alcohol to promote vasodilatation

B) Vigorously rubbing the affected areas to promote circulation

C) Allowing the digits to thaw at room temperature, spontaneously and gradually

D) Rewarming the digits rapidly in a water bath at 100F to 105F (38-40.5C)

D - Frostbite is a condition caused by ice crystals forming and then expanding in the intracellular space. If you've ever put a can or bottle of pop in the freezer, and later found it expanded out of shape or exploded, you can visualize what happens to your cells with frostbite. With this in mind, rapidly rewarming the digits (and the patient) is essential to prevent further damage. This can be done by warm water baths in conjunction with the administration of boatloads of IV narcotics. The affected areas don't hurt when they are frozen, but when they start to warm up, that's a very different story. Expect that those areas will really, really hurt. Room temperature doesn't warm them up fast enough, vigorous rubbing is likely to produce additional tissue damage, and the patient already has more than enough alcohol on board.

54) A 14-year-old presents in anaphylactic shock from a bee sting. Which of the following is the **most** important initial intervention?

A) Ensuring an open airway

B) Assistance with breathing

C) IV access for fluid resuscitation

D) Administration of epinephrine and antihistamines

A – Once again, airway wins! Though B, C, and D will certainly need to be done, airway trumps everything. When caring for patients in anaphylactic shock, burns, or other conditions in which airway edema is very real possibility, the immediate focus must be on maintaining a patent airway. This is especially true with pediatric patients as they don't have that much room to swell, so a little edema goes a long (and understandably bad) way!

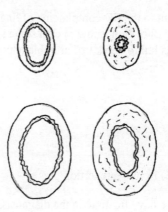

Pediatric vs. Adult Airway Edema

Illustration by Nina DeBoer, then age 9 (my aspiring artist daughter, now aspiring baker daughter)

55) The ED nurse knows that anaphylaxis in children is commonly precipitated by:

A) Insect venom

B) Food ingestion

C) Antibiotic use

D) All of the above

D - Bee and wasp stings are among the most common causes of anaphylaxis. Common food allergies which can lead to anaphylactic reactions include eggs, strawberries, milk, and seafood, and of course, peanuts. Common medications (and medically related items) which are among the "usual suspects" for allergic reactions include antibiotics, especially penicillin, but also aspirin, latex, and IV contrast media.

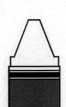

56) A patient can develop symptoms of anaphylaxis up until how long after exposure to an allergen?

A) 2-minutes

B) 20-minutes

C) 2-hours

D) 2-days

D – Though delayed onset reactions are rare, they can occur hours to even days after the initial exposure. Most children will have a reaction relatively quickly after exposure, and in general, the quicker the onset, the more severe the reaction.

57) Management of patients with anaphylaxis includes:

A) IV fluid administration

B) H_1 and H_2 blockers

C) IM or IV epinephrine

D) All of the above

D – Love, like the treatment of anaphylaxis, is a many splendored thing. The physical issues in anaphylaxis revolve around the release of boatloads of histamine. This release results in airway edema, bronchospasm, vasodilatation, and of course, itching. Airway edema is the #1 reason people die from anaphylaxis, so if a child says "it feels like my throat is swelling up," it's appropriate to be very concerned. A close runner up in the "why do they die" category is bronchospasm. If a child says "I can't breathe" and they have audible wheezing, or even worse, no air movement (silent chest), it's again appropriate to be very concerned, as bronchospasm is the #2 reason they die from anaphylaxis. Vasodilatation and shock complete the triad of death from anaphylaxis. Treatment for anaphylaxis involves fixing the symptoms and the problems. IV fluids help to "fill up the tank" and ward off shock. IM or IV epinephrine (earlier rather than later) and albuterol nebs help with the airway edema and/or bronchospasm. Histamine blockers for both types of histamine are also part of the management plan. Benadryl (diphenhydramine) blocks the stronger form of histamine (H_1) and is often given in conjunction with medications such as Pepcid (famotidine), Zantac (ranitidine), or Tagament (cimetidine), not for ulcer prophylaxis, but to block the other form of histamine, H_2.

58) A 15-year-old presents to the ED with a mosquito bite on his leg that occurred two hours ago. He is alert, vital signs are stable, and his chief complaint is itching at the site. Which nursing intervention is appropriate when treating this patient?

A) Carefully place a tourniquet proximal to wound

B) Tell the patient to go home because no interventions are necessary

C) Ensure that antivenom is available

D) Ensure that emergency airway equipment is available

D – We keep coming back to the airway and for good reason. Airway considerations (hence airway answers) are almost always our prime target. Happily, tourniquets and antivenom are not used for mosquito bites. Although, to be honest, you are probably thinking, "You have a mosquito bite... go home and scratch it" would be the correct response. However, EMTALA specifies that all patients must have a Medical Screening Examination, so telling them to go home from triage is not a correct option. This is a test question review book after all, so read all the answers before picking one, just to make sure that airway isn't an option.

59) The ED discharge instructions for a patient who suffered a bee-sting induced anaphylactic reaction should include all of the following **except**:

A) The importance of wearing a medical alert bracelet or necklace

B) The importance of carrying an epinephrine auto injector and knowing its proper use

C) Avoiding the use of perfumes, sprays, and brightly colored clothing because these can attract bees

D) The possibility of serum sickness

D – Serum sickness is associated with antivenin for snake bites, not with the treatment of insect or bug bites. Medical alert jewelry or identification cards can provide important information in an emergency, and being prepared with an epinephrine auto injector ("bee sting kit") is a great idea. Taking preventative steps, as identified in answer "C" may help avoid future problems. Especially if they "got sick" after a bee sting, prevention and notification as above, coupled with self-or family initiated emergency management are all important components of discharge teachings.

60) A 12-year-old Boy Scout is brought to the ED after having suffered a snake bite to his left ankle 30 minutes prior to arrival. The **most** appropriate initial nursing intervention is to:

A) Accurately identify the snake type

B) Immobilize and elevate the affected leg

C) Immobilize the affected extremity below heart level

D) Apply ice to the skin over the snake bite wound

C – Keeping the limb immobilized and below the level of the heart can help to minimize the distribution of venin (the toxic substances found in the venom of animals.) Elevating the leg will increase venous return (not desired) and placing ice is also not recommended by poison control centers. Also not recommended are attempts to suck out the poison, applying electric shock or tourniquets. Accurate identification of the type of snake would be helpful, but not a priority intervention for the nurse. If the patient is exhibiting severe local or systemic signs of envenomation such respiratory distress, hypotension, bleeding, or compartment syndrome, IV antivenin such as Cro-Fab should be administered with poison control guidance. If compartment syndrome is suspected, measured compartment pressures should be obtained to confirm the diagnosis before extremity fasciotomies are considered.

61) A 2-year-old child arrives at the ED with his parents after being bitten by a spider with a red hour glass on its belly. The child was **most** likely bitten by:

A) Days of our Lives spider

B) Black widow spider

C) Microsoft spider

D) Wicked Witch of the West spider

B – This is one of the "easy to answer" spider bite questions. Though famous hourglasses are also found on the opening of the soap opera (daytime drama) "Days of Our Lives" (Like sand through an hour glass…), in Microsoft Windows, and with the Wicked Witch of the West (both involve "just waiting"), when it comes to spider bite questions, an hour glass means a black widow spider. Management involves IV antivenin, analgesics, sedatives, and muscle relaxants if seizures or paralysis are present.

Certified Pediatric Emergency Nurse (CPEN) Review IV

62) A 14-year-old Girl Scout presents to triage after being bitten on the hand by a spider while on a camping trip last night. She now has 10/10 pain radiating up into the arm, abdominal pain, and vomiting. The ED nurse should suspect:

A) A brown recluse spider bite

B) A reaction to poison ivy

C) A bad case of homesickness

D) An infected mosquito bite

A – Nothing tricky here. When it comes to spider bites and emergency exams, there are usually only two types: black widow and brown recluse. The venom from these spiders contains a powerful necrotoxin (necro = death and toxin = poison) which hurts a little when you are bit, but then quickly progress to severe pain with redness, blistering, and scar formation. Management involves cool compresses, antibiotics, steroids, IV analgesics, and later skin grafting.

63) On physical exam, the ED nurse finds a teen patient with a "bull's eye" rash, fever, and joint pain. The nurse should suspect:

A) Lyme disease

B) Juvenile rheumatoid arthritis (JRA)

C) Influenza

D) Neisseria meningitis

A – When you see "bull's eye rash," think Lyme disease. Lyme disease is a tick borne disease which if untreated, can lead to conditions such as blindness, meningitis, cardiac arrhythmias, and even death. Diagnosis is made by history (living in the Northeast during the summer months), physical exam findings including flu symptoms and that bull's eye rash (though not all Lyme patients have the rash), and positive titers in the blood or CSF. Management involves carefully removing the tick if it is still present and oral or IV antibiotics depending on the severity of symptoms. Joint pain by itself might direct you to JRA, fever alone to influenza, and for Neisseria meningitis, you'd expect to see something about stiff neck or a bulging fontanel. The combination, and especially the bull's eye rash, point to Lyme disease.

64) Pain associated with stingray and jellyfish stings can be initially managed with any of the following **except**:

A) Meat tenderizer (MSG)

B) Immersion in fresh water or urine

C) Immersion in sea water or normal saline

D) Isopropyl alcohol or vinegar

B – Fresh water won't help with the pain from stingrays or jellyfish, and another medical urban legend bites the dust… peeing on the sting will make the other ED nurses certainly look at you funny, but it won't do anything to diminish the pain. Stings from rays or jellyfish can result in intense pain which can be decreased by sprinkling with meat tenderizer, immersion in sea water, normal saline, isopropyl alcohol, or even better, vinegar. Frequently, oral or IV analgesics are also required for adequate analgesia prior to carefully removing any remaining tentacles and certainly for continued pain relief.

Environmental

65) Impetigo is caused by:

A) E. Coli

B) Candida albicans

C) Staph. aureus

D) Helicobater pylori

C - Impetigo, a relatively easy to identify, nasty looking skin infection, is caused by Staph. aureus, or more recently, MRSA. With topical and/or oral antibiotics, as long as kids and/or parents don't play with it or try to "pop" it, impetigo will typically heal without scarring. However, remember impetigo is very contagious and is yet another scourge/product of day care. E. Coli infections often result in severe bloody diarrhea and abdominal cramps, while Candida albicans is responsible for candiasis (thrush.) H. Pylori is a gastric bacteria associated with stomach ulcers.

66) Staphylococcal scalded skin syndrome (SSSS) is associated with what sign?

A) Nikolsky's sign

B) SSSS sign

C) Nina's sign

D) Nicole's sign

A – Nikolsky's sign is defined as the slipping of the superficial layer of the epithelium with gentle pressure. The skin of SSSS patients looks very similar to the skin of burn victims, but these patients have no history of a thermal injury. Their sandpaper like skin can "slip off" with dressing changes and this is a both a defining and very worrisome sign of SSSS.

67) Which of the following treatments are recommended for Pediculosis Capitis (head lice)?

A) Petroleum jelly, oil, vinegar, butter, alcohol or mayonnaise shampoos

B) Shaving of the child's head

C) Spraying the area with insecticide

D) Nix (permethrin) or RID (pyrinate) cream rinse

D – Nix or RID, coupled with daily removal of nits with a nit or flea comb is the currently recommended treatment for head lice. Home remedies as described above, or even worse, shaving the child's head, not only don't work, but can be psychologically and physically traumatic to the child. Head lice can quickly spread though a class room or other "community" where children congregate. Prevention and management includes careful cleaning of clothing, bedding, or other personal items, and avoiding the sharing of hats, scarves, combs, brushes, and anything else that would make contact with the head and hair

Environmental

68) The **most** common complaint associated with scabies is:

A) Intense itching

B) Malodorous scabs

C) Blue/green discoloration of the skin

D) Nausea and vomiting

A – Pregnant female scabies mites (Sarcoptes scabiei) burrow under a layer of the epidermis to lay their eggs and feces. How gross is that??? Inflammation and itching may not kick in for 30-60 days after the initial contact (though much sooner if there is a return visit from more mites.) This is important as everyone the person has been in close contact with for the previous 60 days (except for those that are pregnant or breast feeding) should be treated with one application of a scabicide lotion or cream such as Elimite (permethrin) cream, from top to bottom and everywhere between (except the eyes, ears, mouth.) Not just the itchy parts – everywhere!

69) The nurse has just been notified that EMS is about to arrive with three pediatric victims from a dirty bomb attack. Which nursing intervention should be done after the patients' airways have been stabilized?

A) Remove all of the patient's clothing and jewelry, dispose of them in a lead lined container, and then scrub the patient with soap and water

B) Assess the amount of radiation with a Geiger counter

C) Administer activated charcoal

D) Debride open wounds or radiation burns

A – Keep in mind that the most immediate danger with a dirty bomb is blast injury, not radiation. Once the immediate threats to life (airway management and it's quite a challenge to intubate in haz mat suits), have been addressed, then decontamination can begin while other interventions are undertaken. Good old fashioned soap and water still work very well, not only for lacerations, but also for radiation exposure. 95% of radiation can be removed with soap, water, and removal of the patient's clothing. If, after adequate external cleaning, the Geiger counter still reveals radiation, then internal contamination should be considered. The START method of triage is utilized with mass casualty situations for adult triage, while JumpSTART should be utilized with pediatric patients.

70) Acute radiation syndrome (ARS) is composed of which of the following sub-syndromes?

A) Hematopoietic and gastrointestinal

B) Cardiovascular

C) Neurologic

D) All of the above

D – ARS is responsible for the majority of deaths within the first 60 days after exposure. As you can imagine, the higher the radiation exposure, the quicker the symptoms and subsequent death occur. High level lethal exposures can kill within minutes to hours, while victims with lower level exposures may survive for days to weeks. If the patient amazingly survives, full recovery can take months to years. Children are especially vulnerable to ARS because radiation affects actively growing cells, and who has got more growing cells than kids?

Environmental

Certified Pediatric Emergency Nurse (CPEN) Review IV

71) A young child presents to your ED with flu-like symptoms, including a nasty, productive cough, fever and extreme lethargy. You begin gathering your history and ask if the child has done anything out of the ordinary. The child's mother recalls that a couple of days ago the child was stabbing at a dead rat with a stick while they were camping in New Mexico. This new information combined with this history leads you to suspect:

A) Anthrax

B) Influenza

C) Pneumonic plague

D) Tularemia

C - The appropriate answer is pneumonic plague, which is the most dangerous form to the patient and their caregivers. By feasting on blood clots in dead animals, the ticks which cause plague can live for up to 3 months until they find a new host. In this case, the child presented a fresh blood supply and has become the new host. Every year, several cases are diagnosed in the U.S. Southwest. If there had been no rat, no camping trip, and the child lived in Maine, the suspicion would be for something else. Anthrax; the usual "other" in the differential diagnosis, presents with similar symptoms, minus the history of playing with dead rats. A big difference is that the cough associated with anthrax is not generally productive, and the chest X-ray can show a widened mediastinum rather than the "pneumonia/ARDS" look of plague. Treatment will be aimed at personal protective equipment (PPE) for staff, quarantine measures (droplet), and oral antibiotics for anyone who had contact with the child – including you!

72) A 12-year-old previously healthy girl presents to your ED this morning with severe respiratory difficulty. Her parents state she was fine last night when she went to a football game, but complained of tightness in her chest early in the morning. Since then, the symptoms have gotten worse. Your assessment reveals she is hypotensive, diaphoretic, and lung sounds are wet. If bioterrorism was a possibility, you would suspect which toxin or "bad bug"?

A) Ricin

B) Smallpox

C) Anthrax

D) Pneumonic plague

A – Ricin exposure matches these symptoms. Ricin is a naturally occurring "leftover" from castor bean processing. Making someone sick with Ricin would probably have to be intentional. Even though Ricin is not contagious, ED personnel need to be careful to avoid spreading it to the ED staff through contact with material such as clothing that has been contaminated. Keep in mind that only 24 micrograms of Ricin can kill a person weighing 80kg (176lbs) and Ricin is 20-50 times more toxic than the nerve agent Sarin! Smallpox characteristically presents with lesions on the head and extremities and progresses over time. Anthrax, as well as plague, presents with flu-like symptoms over several days (doesn't everything seemingly present with flu-like symptoms)?

Environmental

308

Certified Pediatric Emergency Nurse (CPEN) Review IV

73) The ED just received word from Health Department officials regarding alleged intentional contamination of food at a local family restaurant with botulinum toxin (aka. botulism.) The report states the alleged incident happened approximately 24 hours ago. Which of the following is **not** anticipated in the management of botulism in children?

A) Sufficient negative pressure airflow rooms for patient isolation

B) Administration of botulinum antitoxin

C) Intensive medical and nursing treatment

D) Ventilator support

A – According to the Centers for Disease Control (CDC), patients suspected of having botulism do not need to be isolated. Botulism/botulinum intoxication does not spread person to person. It's an intoxication, not an infection. Early administration of the antitoxin is effective in reducing the severity of the symptoms. As far as intensive nursing/medical treatment and ventilator support go, remember that Botox is BOtulinum TOXin. Think about why people get Botox injections. It's to paralyze the facial muscles and eliminate wrinkles. So if a little Botox works to paralyze the facial wrinkles, a whole lot of botulism paralyzes everything else including the respiratory muscles. As opposed to Guillain Barre, the botulism paralysis starts with cranial neuropathies (the head) and descends through the rest of the body. So watch for drooling, droopy eyelids, difficulty swallowing or speaking before it descends to the respiratory muscles. If those muscles get affected, just remember the American Lung Association motto: If you can't breathe… Nothing else matters!

74) A child in severe respiratory distress presents via EMS to the ED. Per the family, the patient complained of blurry vision and a severe headache prior to the onset of respiratory distress. The pupils are bilaterally pinpoint and reactive. He has lacrimation, salivation, and is profusely diaphoretic. In addition, at triage, he has uncontrolled vomiting, diarrhea and muscle twitching. The history and physical examination findings would lead you to suspect:

A) Sarin Exposure

B) Soman (GD)

C) VX

D) All the above nerve agents

D – These symptoms scream "something really bad" is going on, especially if there is more than one patient with similar symptoms. When you hear nerve gas, think about "everything opening up and the "**ing**." Tear**ing** (of the eyes), drool**ing**, sweat**ing**, vomit**ing**, twitch**ing**, and poop**ing**. These symptoms could be associated with any one of these nerve agents or many others not listed. SLUDGE/BBB and the "ings" are truly scary and unpleasant symptoms before you die!

(S)alivation - drooling

(L)acrimation - tearing

(U)rination - peeing

(D)efecation - pooping

(G)I symptoms – lots of them

(E)mesis - barfing

(B)ronchorrhea – lots of airway secretions

(B)ronchospasm - wheezing

(B)radycardia – self explanatory

Environmental

309

Certified Pediatric Emergency Nurse (CPEN) Review IV

75) An event at the local mall has sent dozens of patients to your ER complaining that "someone set off a smoke bomb" and they exhibiting classic SLUDGE/BBB symptoms of exposure to nerve gas. You know that the primary two medications in your auto injector (Mark 1) kit are:

A) Atropine and epinephrine

B) 2-PAM and atropine

C) Sodium bicarbonate and Valium (diazepam)

D) Versed (midazolam) and dopamine

B - Atropine and 2-PAM auto injectors are the primary medications in the nerve gas kit. Nerve impulses in the body are sent by the messenger acetylcholine (Ach.) But you need the impulses to "stop" at some point and that is where acetylcholinesterase (AchE) comes in. It is the "stop." Nerve gases, such as Sarin, VX, and Tabun, affect the body by blocking the work of the AchE, effectively removing the "stop" of impulses. Now think about the implications on electrical impulses in the heart or receptors in the brain. 2-PAM and atropine break the hold of the nerve gas on the AchE, and allow the body to return to its resting state. If SLUDGE/BBB sounds familiar, it should - this is essentially the same mechanism and symptoms as organophosphate poisoning.

Pediatric Use of the Mark 1 Kit (Courtesy of Lou Romig MD)

< 3 years (under 13kg)	May use one Mark I kit if life-threatening condition and no other dosage forms are available
3-7 years (approx 13-25kg)	May use one Mark I kit as maximum dose
8-14 years (approx 26-50kg)	May use a total of two kits
>14 years (approx >51kg)	May use a total of three kits

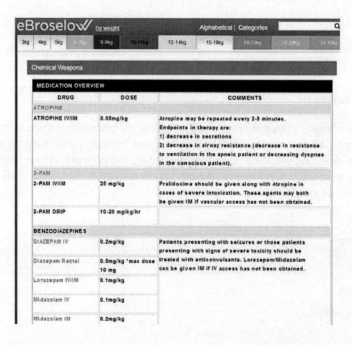

Color coded chemical warfare antidotes

Courtesy of James Broselow MD & Robert Luten MD - www.eBroselow.com

Certified Pediatric Emergency Nurse (CPEN) Review IV

76) A 16-year-old teen arrives via EMS from a local rave party. The medics report she experienced several generalized seizures which ceased after administration of IV Ativan (lorazepam.) A friend with the patient states that they both took ecstasy (MDMA) at the party. Which laboratory finding would be expected in this case?

A) Hyperglycemia

B) Hyponatremia

C) Hypernatremia

D) Hypocalcemia

B – Since the mid-1980s, Ecstasy (MDMA) has been increasingly popular as a recreational drug, especially at dance or rave parties. As the drug suppresses the need to eat, drink, and sleep, users can "party" for hours to days without a break. However, this can result in hyperthermia (heat cramps to heat stroke), profound dehydration and renal failure. Hyperthermia is managed with traditional cooling measures as detailed in previous questions. On the internet, to avoid the complications associated with dehydration, Ecstasy users are now promoting the idea of "drinking water like a fish." This practice may be especially harmful coupled with the fact that MDMA causes inappropriate secretion of ADH (SIADH), a unique toxicity associated with its use. This can result in symptomatic hyponatremia and resultant seizures which may require airway support and potentially the need for 3% hypertonic saline.

77) The following are always primary factors related to the injury potential of exposure to a chemical substance/chemical weapon **except**:

A) Proximity to the agent

B) The relative respiratory rate of the person exposed

C) Time before decontamination

D) How the agent is introduced into the body

B – Respiratory rate will only be a primary exposure factor in the event that the chemical was in a gaseous state or was in small enough particles to be inhaled. It is certainly true that a very effective way to spread a chemical agent is as a gas (or an inhaled substance) and it would typically produce more victims with significant exposure than other, non-inhaled chemical exposure. And in those cases, while respiratory rate could play a part in determining the amount of exposure, it is not an "always" consideration. When determining the danger from chemical exposure, remember that the toxic effects of chemicals (weapons or otherwise) are directly related to the amount of exposure the patient has to the chemical agent. The closer the patient was to the agent, the more exposure they would receive. The longer the patient is exposed (the time from initial exposure to decontamination), the worse the effects will be. Lastly, many chemical agents will cling to skin and clothing, and the patient will continue to receive toxic exposure. That is why decontamination, including removal of all clothing and jewelry, is vital to both the patient's care and the safety of the ED staff. The physical state (gas, liquid, solid) of the chemical contaminant/weapon is a direct factor in all of the above considerations relative to the amount of exposure.

Environmental

78) Several children from a local grade school are brought to your ED for triage. They were on a field trip to the local water park when they suddenly began complaining of difficulty breathing and "burning" eyes. Your patient is a first grader who is coughing uncontrollably, has shortness of breath with wheezing and rales, and is starting to go into respiratory failure. As you begin supporting the airway, you notice a strong chlorine odor and your throat begins to get scratchy. Your **first** and immediate intervention is to:

A) Begin positive pressure ventilation

B) Decontaminate the patient

C) Place an intraosseous line and give 2-PAM

D) Contact federal law enforcement to report a chemical weapon terrorist attack

B – It is obvious that this child is sick, and based on the history and presentation, there is a good chance this child is the victim of a "choking agent" such as chlorine. But what is more worrisome is that he has not been decontaminated (remember the strong chlorine smell) and now you are being affected as well. The number one intervention is rapid decontamination to reduce his exposure and protect you. Since the contaminant is most likely chlorine, which can be rinsed into the wastewater system safely, the fastest way to proceed may be to "decon" the patient and yourself quickly in a nearby shower. Once decontamination has taken place, you will not need any special protection. This will be followed by aggressive respiratory support and careful observation for hypovolemic shock (think of all the fluid he is losing into his lungs.) Choking agents cause mucous membrane irritation (eyes and upper respiratory tract,) but, in more significant exposures, they can cause a "dry land drowning." This occurs when the agent causes damage to the cell walls in the lower airways, allowing fluid to leak into those airways and results in a non-cardiac pulmonary edema. While chlorine and other choking agents can be used as chemical weapons, most cases in the ED are accidental exposures. Since there is no reason to believe that this incident is anything more than accidental, there is no reason to consider this as being a terrorist attack. Lastly, 2-PAM is indicated in cases of neurotoxin exposure, such as saran or VX gas.

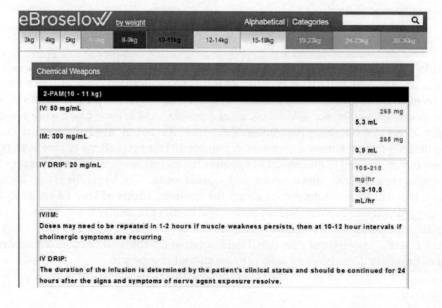

Color coded 2-PAM administration for chemical weapon exposure

Courtesy of James Broselow MD & Robert Luten MD - www.eBroselow.com

Certified Pediatric Emergency Nurse (CPEN) Review IV

79) A pick-up truck with horn blaring and tires screeching has pulled up to your emergency entrance. A man and woman jump out of the truck, and the woman is holding a small child who appears to be covered with a grey powder and is choking and coughing. There is a look of fear in the child's eyes and the lips appear cyanotic. The adults are also coughing and appear short of breath. They are screaming for you to do something to help their child. Your initial course of action should be:

A) Bring them directly to a room in the main ED (bypassing triage in accordance with the "immediate bedding" best practice policy) and begin your assessment

B) Stop them at the door and do an assessment and quick registration there

C) Keep them outside the entrance with the door locked and activate the facility hazmat response

D) Send additional staff out to undress, decontaminate, and then assess and register the family

C – Since you have no idea what is on this child or the adults, or what is causing their symptoms, the golden rule of the unknown is YOUR SAFETY FIRST. Although the first instinct for many of us is to rush in and help, in order to protect staff and patients already in the ED, you should lock the door and activate the hazmat system for your facility. Delaying the activation of the hazmat response team will most likely result in additional patients and increased levels of exposure. If you let these folks in, you run the very real risk of needing to shut down your entire facility for several hours of wide spread decontamination. In addition, not only will you need decontamination, but so will other staff members and probably the other ED patients as well. Even bringing other staff members outside may result in additional exposures and potentially additional patients (the staff) with fewer people available to provide care to the patients. Hazmat teams are trained to perform decontamination to the level that will provide a safe environment for you to take the patients into your hospital and complete their care.

80) Parents (and many medical care providers) have lots of misconceptions about childhood fever. Which of the following common parental beliefs about fever is **true**?

A) A fever of 100.4 (F) 38.0 (C) can cause brain damage.

B) Fever can cause seizures.

C) A high fever always means a worse infection.

D) Fever must always be treated, even if it means giving both acetaminophen and ibuprofen.

B – Fever can indeed cause febrile seizures in a select age group of children (6 months to 4-5 years) but these are usually benign and rarely have long-term complications. Fever is not a disease, but a symptom, and should be treated as such. In reality, other symptoms such as vomiting, diarrhea and bronchospasm are much more potentially dangerous than fever. Studies suggest that body temperature must be about 107°F (41.7°C) or higher to cause irreversible cell damage in susceptible organs such as the brain and liver. BUT children with normal brain function and thermoregulation don't get temperatures that high due to infection. Most cases of body temperature-related morbidity and mortality occur due to environmental hyperthermia. With very few exceptions, the degree of fever means very little prognostically. Defining fever as "low grade," "medium" or "high" is largely meaningless. The reason to treat fever in the great majority of children is to make them more comfortable. When the kids feel better, they'll be less cranky, have a better appetite and be more active. This also makes the caregivers more comfortable, which is half the battle in pediatrics! Many pediatricians and other medical professionals continue to recommend alternating acetaminophen and ibuprofen to improve fever control. Studies suggest that there's no consistent improvement in fever control when using both drugs and the process of alternating the drugs increases the chance that a child will receive an overdose of one or both medications. The same qualifications apply to using ibuprofen and acetaminophen at the same time – there's no proven benefit and more chance of medication errors.

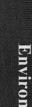

81) Which statement below best demonstrates a parent's correct understanding regarding fevers in a two-month old infant?

A) "Fever's dangerous, so I have to do whatever's necessary to bring the temperature down."

B) "Even though I hate doing it, I really should check my baby's temperature rectally if she feels warm."

C) "The best way to manage fever is to alternate acetaminophen and ibuprofen."

D) "Giving acetaminophen and ibuprofen together is perfectly safe."

B – The only correct statement above is B.

Additional Pediatric ED Attending Physician Insights: In children less than about three months of age, differences of tenths of a degree of body temperature may determine whether the infant needs no diagnostic tests, one or more tests, or a full sepsis work-up and admission to the hospital. The only commonly available method to measure fever with that degree of accuracy is rectal thermometry. Above 3-months of age, such accuracy isn't routinely required and it's usually OK to switch to taking axillary temps, when determining whether or not fever is present. (Note that you CANNOT just add one degree to an axillary temp to get a rectal equivalent; that old rule of thumb has been proven not to be true.) Tympanic thermometers are not accurate in infants because of their small and angled ear canals and accuracy is technique-dependent even with older children. Oral and temporal artery thermometers may also be used, especially for older infants and children. Surprisingly, with few exceptions, the height of the fever means very little about the infection itself, especially after the first year of life. The first matter of importance is an accurate assessment of whether or not a fever exists before any discussion of "control" takes place.

Fever is not dangerous unless a child has poor cardiac or pulmonary reserves that would be challenged by the increased metabolic state caused by elevated body temperature. These children may not tolerate the tachypnea, tachycardia and/or increased oxygen and glucose demands generated by fever. Some children with seizures (epilepsy) may have more seizures when febrile because the fever lowers the seizure threshold. Otherwise, fever in a reasonably healthy child does NOT pose the same risks as environmental hyperthermia, which may cause irreversible damage to the brain and other organs once the body temperature exceeds about 107.0°F (41.7°C) Fever (hyperthermia from infection) rarely exceeds 106.0°F (41.1°C) in children (without chronic problems with thermoregulation) and does NOT cause irreversible damage of any kind. Complications traditionally attributed to fever actually occur due to infection rather than to the fever itself. The exception is febrile seizures (a complication of the fever, not the infection) in the six month to five year age range; although often quite scary, simple febrile seizures rarely cause any lasting complications. The most important reason to treat fever is NOT to prevent complications, but simply to make the children (and the family!) feel better.

In the United States, acetaminophen and ibuprofen are commonly used to control fever. As with all medications, they should not be used indiscriminately or in excess. "Fever phobia" often leads to frantic efforts to control fever by giving either or both drugs too often and/or in inappropriate doses. Because the risks of fever itself are commonly overrated, inappropriate use of antipyretics is rampant and may represent more of a risk to children than the infections themselves. Simultaneous administration of acetaminophen and ibuprofen is not only unnecessary in efforts to reduce risk from fever, but also doubles the chance of dosing errors because two medications are being given instead of one. Alternating the two medications carries the same risk and provides only an inconsistent and minimal improvement in temperature control. Neither antipyretic alone has been conclusively proven to consistently provide better fever control.

In short, the younger the infant, the more important it is to accurately record the degree of fever. Rectal temps should be used for infant's less than about 3-months of age, but are commonly and correctly used up to a year of age. Fever is not a disease, but a symptom, and is usually no more dangerous than a runny nose. Fever is simply a signal that infection is present. The main reason to treat fever in usually healthy kids is to make them feel better. Just like a runny nose, sometimes you can effectively treat fever and sometimes you can't. Make sure the treatment isn't more risky than the symptom itself--it's safest to use a single antipyretic at the recommended doses and treatment intervals. Don't perpetuate fever-phobia!

Environmental

82) Which of these patients would be most likely to require a post-exposure rabies vaccination series? The bats involved in the exposures could not be captured or identified:

A) A three-year old child who was playing in guano (bat feces) from a nest removed by animal control

B) An 18-month old who was sleeping when parents saw a bat flying around in his room

C) A seven-year old who was looking at bats in a cave when one of them urinated on his head

D) A 12-year old who saw a bat flying around his house and chased it away using a tennis racquet

B – The U.S. Centers for Disease Control (CDC) recommends a dose of human rabies immune globulin and a four-dose rabies vaccine series (days 0 (day of the bite), 3, 7, & 14) for people bitten or who may have been bitten if the bat cannot be captured and tested. Bats have very small teeth, and their bites may not awaken a sleeping bite victim. The teeth marks may be difficult or impossible to find. The CDC recommends these precautions for people who awaken in a room with a bat, for unattended children, and for mentally impaired or intoxicated persons found in a room with a bat. The children in answers "A" and "C" are at low risk as rabies is not spread by urine or guano. The child in answer "D", though at risk for exposure, was awake during the encounter and did not report a bite. Approximately 6% of bats captured for rabies screening have tested positive. Rabies occurs in wildlife in the 49 continental United States, with Hawaii remaining consistently rabies-free. Moral of the story, if you are going to get bitten by a bat, do it in paradise! Mahalo!

83) A mother carries her 2-year old son into triage after finding him crying and lying next to a plugged in extension cord. Your exam reveals a painful, red area with a black center at the corner of the child's lower lip. You identify this wound as a probable:

A) Fever blister

B) Decubitus ulcer

C) Allergic reaction

D) Burn wound as a result of biting the extension cord

D – Children, especially under the age of three, often explore their environment with all of their senses, including taste. This means that anything that can be in the hand can also be in the mouth. Biting an electric cord can easily result in a burn on the lip. In this case, the affected area has a red or dark, charred appearance, common with burn injuries. Allergic reactions would involve swelling of the lips and as you can imagine, decubitus ulcers of the lips are rare to say the least. Though fever blisters certainly can be red and painful, the fact that the question specifically mentioned an electrical cord should be a clue that the answer involves an electrical injury.

84) The priority intervention for the previously described patient with oral burns is:

A) Airway assessment and control

B) Educating the mother about electrical safety in the home

C) Intravenous access

D) Arterial blood gas (ABG)

A – Remember the ABCs. If you don't have A, you don't have to worry about B and C because you will not have them very long. It is important to recognize the potential for edema in the mouth and on the lips that can affect the airway. Electrical cord injuries are low voltage burns, but when the electricity comes in

Environmental

contact with the moist oral mucosa, the heat generated by the electrical source can cause tissue destruction. Be sure to evaluate the inside of the child's mouth for burns as well. Most children with this type of injury can be observed for a short time in the ED and managed on an outpatient basis as long as their airway is unaffected, their initial ECG is normal and the urinalysis shows no evidence of myoglobinuria or "Pepsi™ Pee" (urine that resembles the color of a cola beverage.) Cardiac abnormalities are rare, but it is recommended that children have continuous cardiac monitoring for up to four hours, as well as an initial 12-lead ECG. It is important to confirm that the child has the ability to take in adequate oral fluids despite the burn to the mouth area. Perioral burns at the corner of the lips also have the potential to develop a labial artery hemorrhage from about 8-12 days post-burn. In those occurrences, the necrotic tissue separates from the healthy living tissue and the labial artery can become exposed with resultant bleeding. This is managed with direct pressure and evaluation in the ED, and is a crucial piece of information to be included in discharge teaching (along with home safety teaching.) IV access and ABGs would only be necessary if the patient's condition deteriorates.

85) EMS is transporting a 9-year old suspected lightning strike victim. Bystanders report the victim being struck by lightning, with immediate loss of consciousness. Bystanders also reported that the child gradually returned to his normal level of consciousness. The emergency nurse recognizes that this period of unconsciousness was possibly caused by which one of the following:

A) Metabolic acidosis

B) Asystole or ventricular fibrillation (V-fib)

C) Multi-system trauma

D) Subarachnoid bleed

B – While lightning strikes cause serious injuries, death from a lightning strike only occurs in about 10-20% of cases. The primary cause of death following a lightning strike is an asystolic or V-fib cardiac arrest. The massive DC (direct current) shock (like a defibrillator on steroids) causes the myocardium to depolarize. This can lead to the initial asystole or V-fib arrest. Additionally, respiratory arrest can occur from lightning damage to the neurological respiratory centers or by paralyzing the chest muscles themselves. Sometimes, even if the heart is able to restart itself after the initial "shock" of the lightning strike, respiratory arrest may lead to a secondary hypoxic cardiac arrest. But remember, unlike "big people" who often have a significant cardiac history (whether known or unknown), these children have good, strong hearts before they were unlucky enough to be struck by lightning.

86) Immediate priorities for the above lightning strike patient include all of the following **except**:

A) Cardiac monitoring

B) Airway control

C) Respiratory assessment

D) Neurology consultation

D – ABCs are always your immediate priority. Once the patient is stabilized, and based on the history, physical exam and diagnostic tests, consultations may include referrals to a neurologist, cardiologist or (if significant burns are involved) even a burn surgeon. Later consultations may include referral to a neuropsychologist, physical and occupational therapists, rehab and pain specialists and/or psychiatrist.

Environmental

Certified Pediatric Emergency Nurse (CPEN) Review IV

87) What is the minimum age for administration of Crotalidae Polyvalent Immune Fab (CroFab®?)

A) 1 year

B) 5 years

C) 8 years

D) There is no minimum age

D – There is no minimum age for CroFab®. Snakes don't care whether they bite an infant or an adult; they just bite. Because CroFab® contains mercury, there may be some risk for the developing fetus or if given to a young child; there is also a risk for neurological and renal toxicity, but first and foremost, they must survive the bite! So in the ED, antivenin, CroFab®, can be administered across the lifespan.

88) When administering Crotalidae Polyvalent Immune Fab (CroFab®) to a pediatric patient, the dose:

A) Is the same as an adult dose

B) Is less than an adult dose

C) Is greater than an adult dose

D) I'm doing a travel nurse assignment in Antarctica and we don't have snakes or children here

A – Remember: Snakes don't care who they bite; they just bite and usually only when stepped on by humans or provoked (famous last words… "Watch this!") A snake injects the same amount of venom regardless if the victim is a child or an adult, so the CroFab® dose is the same regardless of age. The initial dosing for CroFab® is 4-6 vials for all ages, but many more may be required (and they are incredibly expensive!) The pediatric patient may actually end up needing twice the adult dosage for a pit viper bite! Each vial is reconstituted with 10-25ml of sterile water and gently swirled (reconstitution is faster with 25ml than 10ml). The CroFab® is then diluted in a 250cc bag of normal saline and an infusion is started at a slow rate, evaluating for any reaction. If no reaction is noted, the infusion can be increased to run over one hour. CroFab® should always be administered with an IV infusion pump.

89) What is the relatively common side effect of Crotalidae Polyvalent Immune Fab (CroFab®)?

A) Urticaria

B) Coagulopathies

C) Petechiae at site of envenomation

D) GI upset

A – While urticaria (itchy rash) is the most commonly reported side effect of CroFab®, it is not nearly as common as with the earlier types of antivenin. Patients receiving CroFab® must be closely monitored for anaphylactic reactions, especially for those with a known allergy to papaya, due to the use of papain (a papaya extract) in the production of CroFab®.

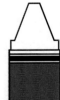

90) Crotalinae Polyvalent Immune Fab (CroFab®) is indicated for what type of envenomations?

A) Pit vipers

B) Arachnids

C) Gila monster

D) Cookie monster

A - CroFab® is indicated for the new world genera of the Crotalidae subfamily of vipers. The need for antivenins to treat arachnid (spider) bites in the US is rather low, and consequently arachnid antivenin is frequently unavailable in many parts of the U.S. No antivenin exists for Gila monsters (or Cookie monsters for that matter, but you knew that.) Gila monster bites are treated symptomatically with antihistamines, and antibiotics. (Cookie monster bites are treated with… you guessed it, cookies!) Of note, due to their extremely strong jaws, it is not unheard of for patients to present to the ED with the offending Gila Monster still firmly attached. (Admit it… That's a picture/video going straight from triage to YouTube!)

91) All the following are considered risks for envenomations (bites/stings in which venom is injected) **except**:

A) Brown recluse spider bite

B) Black widow spider bite

C) Centipede bite

D) Millipede bite

D - Millipedes are herbivores (they eat plants, not little kids), have tiny mouths, and even in the largest species, do not pose a venom risk to humans. Handling of some larger and more exotic species of millipedes can result in dermatological reactions. Millipedes do excrete a caustic liquid as a defense mechanism. Centipedes (particularly exotic species), black widow and brown recluse spiders and scorpions, certainly do pose a venomous risk to humans, especially to the very young, elderly or immunocompromised.

92) A 30kg (Broselow-Luten "Green") 8-year old boy presents to your ED with a suspected rattlesnake bite to his lower leg. He is crying and stating his "tummy hurts." His pulse rate is 138, respiratory rate is 24, blood pressure is 90/52, oral temperature 98.1°F (36.7°C,) and his oxygen saturation is 98% on room air. The ED nurse would anticipate the administration of CroFab® to include:

A) Two vials of CroFab® reconstituted with 10-25ml sterile water and shaken well

B) Two vials of CroFab® reconstituted with 10-25ml normal saline and gently swirled

C) Four vials of CroFab® reconstituted with 10-25ml sterile water and gently swirled

D) Four vials of CroFab® reconstituted with 10-25ml sterile water and shaken well

C - The standard initial dosing for CroFab® is four to six vials. CroFab® should be stored at near freezing temperatures and each vial is reconstituted with 10-25ml of sterile water. Unlike a James Bond martini, these vials must be swirled, not shaken. (Shaking the vial causes excessive foaming of the solution.) Vials must be gently swirled for up to 45 minutes in order to allow for adequate dissolving, so assign the job to someone as soon as you get the CroFab® in hand! After reconstitution, the solution should be further diluted in 250cc normal saline for administration over one hour with an infusion pump. CroFab® is indicated in this patient because he is demonstrating gastrointestinal involvement and possible early signs of shock (tachycardia.)

Certified Pediatric Emergency Nurse (CPEN) Review IV

93) A 12kg (Broselow-Luten "Yellow") 2-year old female patient arrives via EMS for a possible black widow spider bite. Your primary assessment reveals that this child's only response is to grimace and withdraw from painful stimuli. Her HR is 70 with good distal perfusion and she has a SpO2 of 88% on room air. EMS states that the patient was alert and crying during transport. Your **initial** intervention should be:

A) Preparation of antivenin

B) Airway positioning and bag-mask ventilation with 100% oxygen

C) Inspection of bite location for petechiae or bruising indicating coagulopathy

D) Initiating chest compressions

B - Airway ALWAYS takes precedence. Remember, it seems everything bad that happens in children is "something respiratory" and bradycardia in children is most frequently a result of hypoxia. In this child, the hypoxia is due to respiratory depression from the neurological effects of envenomation. A good rule of thumb is that if airway is offered as an answer, it probably is the correct answer, unless the question makes it very clear that the airway is patent.

94) A 36kg (Broselow-Luten Green) 10-year old girl presents to your ED after being stung by a yellow jacket on her left forearm. The triage nurse provided an icepack and the patient cries in pain whenever the ice pack is removed. Inspection of the site reveals a raised wheal around a puncture wound with no apparent retained foreign body. The patient indicates that the area is "itchy." Her parents state she had this same type of reaction last summer when stung by a bee. You would expect all the following interventions except:

A) Benadryl® (diphenhydramine)

B) Ice pack to injury site

C) Constricting band (tourniquet) 5-10cm proximal of site

D) Motrin® (ibuprofen, Brufen®)

C - Hymenoptera envenomations (stinging, flying insects such as bees, wasps, ants) result in significant local reactions in 17-56% of patients. Treatment includes antihistamines (Benadryl®) localized wound care and oral analgesics/anti-inflammatory medications such as Motrin®. Constricting bands are contraindicated in arachnid and insect bites. An estimated 5-10% of patients who have experienced large local reactions will progress to systemic reactions with subsequent stings. Therefore, monitoring this girl for early signs of anaphylaxis (airway edema, bronchospasm, hypotension) is also a very prudent intervention.

95) Which of the following is TRUE about envenomations in pediatric patients?

A) Due to their smaller size, children are at higher risk for systemic reactions to venom

B) Unless they have been stung before they will not have a systemic reaction

C) Girls are more likely to be stung by jellyfish

D) Residents of major metropolitan areas are at lower risk for envenomation

A – Most children have a higher baseline heart rate, smaller surface area and less body mass than their adult counterparts, so even first-time envenomations can result in systemic reactions. Because of a child's size, the effect of a single well-placed bite or sting can progress quite rapidly and dramatically. Due to encroachment on wilderness areas and the popularity of exotic pets, living in a major city is no protection against envenomations. Avoidance and prevention of bites remains the best way to remain healthy. And despite the "fact" that little girls are made of sugar and spice, there is no evidence that jelly fish are unusually attracted to the sweet and savory!

96) A 30kg (Broselow-Luten Green) 8-year old male is brought to your emergency room after stepping on a sea urchin while climbing on rocks at a local seaside park. He is able to tell you through snuffled crying that it hurts "really bad" and that it still feels "pokey." Inspection of the plantar surface of his left foot reveals two puncture wounds. You anticipate that his treatment will include all of the following **except**:

A) Soaking the foot in the warmest water tolerable

B) X-ray of the foot

C) Assurance of tetanus prophylaxis

D) Antivenin administration

D - There is no antivenin for Echinoidea (sea urchin) envenomation. Treatment consists of soaking the affected part in non-scalding hot water to inactivate heat sensitive toxins, as well as oral ibuprofen and oral antibiotics. Soft tissue radiographs should be obtained to rule out a retained foreign body (broken sea urchin spine), and tetanus prophylaxis should be administered as needed. In addition, surgical debridement is frequently required. If spines are present in the patient, carefully remove spines with forceps and protect your own hand with gloves. Vinegar and urine do not remove spines or reduce pain.

97) A 6-month old male presents to the pediatric emergency department with two days of vomiting and a history of cold symptoms for two weeks. The child initially had a fever and was treated by the pediatrician with antibiotics for a week for an ear infection. Although the fever resolved over a week ago, the mother tells you she's been giving the child both an over-the-counter (OTC) combination cold medicine "for the cold" as well as liquid Tylenol® (acetaminophen, Panadol®) "for the ear pain" for the entire two weeks. While in the emergency department, the nurse should consider what possible condition?

A) Tylenol® overdose

B) Child abuse

C) Esophageal foreign body

D) Asthma

A – The correct answer is Tylenol® overdose. Vomiting is a common early sign of acetaminophen toxicity. When reading the question, you should notice that the patient has been treated with OTC cold medicine and liquid Tylenol®. Many OTC cold medicines also have acetaminophen in them and toxicity can easily occur in patients who are "double dipping" (cold medicine with acetaminophen and additional Tylenol®.) In addition, it's very possible this child has been receiving acetaminophen infant drops, which has the confusing concentration and packaging of 80mg in a 0.8ml dropper. If it's sometimes hard for us to figure correct dosage, imagine what it's like for a parent with a sick child! The emergency room nurse should alert the physician, and obtain the names of the medications and doses the child has been receiving. It would even be helpful to have the parent explain or demonstrate what they have been drawing up for the child. And of course, call Poison Control if your suspicion is correct.

98) You are called to assist in the triage room for a 4-year old girl who is actively seizing. The father was in the process of giving the triage nurse a history, which included his daughter helping him in the garden that morning. She began to "look sick" and he brought her to the ED. She has no history of seizures, and is covered in dirt and powdered material. On initial assessment you also notice her pupils are 1 mm (miosis) and she is drooling. What do you suspect is the main cause of this child's condition?

A) Organophosphate poisoning

B) Anaphylaxis

C) Epilepsy

D) Brain damage from child abuse

A – Organophosphates are one of the most common causes of poisoning worldwide and include insecticides, herbicides and nerve gas. They are potent nerve agents that functions by inhibiting the action of AChE (Acetycholinesterase) in nerve cells. Basically, ACh (Acetycholine) is responsible for transmitting impulses along the nerves; AChE stops the impulse once it has completed the message. When organophosphates interfere with the AChE, it removes all the "stops," causing uncontrolled stimulation. Our impulses (nerve impulses, of course) go crazy! Imagine the secretions, sensory input, muscle spasms and electrical impulses in the heart all happening without order. One acronym used frequently to describe the signs and symptoms of organophosphate poisoning is SLUDGEM (salivation, lacrimation, urination, defecation/diarrhea, gastric upset, emesis, miosis). What is your very first intervention? Sorry, it's not airway in this case – it's rapid decontamination! Minimum protection is Level C (over-garments, respirator/gas mask) for staff. Removal of clothing and showering the patient is absolutely necessary or you may soon have additional patients, including you!

Additional Pediatric ED Attending Physician Insights: Actually, the dad should be decontaminated as well. It's a virtual certainty that he's been contaminated through contact with the patient. The triage area and all staff in contact with the patient and father prior to recognition of the threat are also going to have to be decontaminated. (By the way, did a security guard help this dad get the child out of the car? Don't forget ancillary staff that also may be contaminated!) This incident may shut down the ED for a while.)

99) While removing a tick from a child, the actual goal is to:

A) Prevent tick regurgitation

B) Get the whole tick out

C) Prevent patient regurgitation

D) Prevent an anaphylactic reaction

A – Gross as it sounds, we want to prevent regurgitation of infectious tick stomach contents. For this reason, NEVER squeeze the tick's body or irritate it by heating it or using topical anesthetics. While there are conflicting recommendations regarding smothering the tick (it might seem that this would only prolong the exposure time), the current ENA core curriculum DOES recommend the smothering technique. For safe removal, use fine tip forceps and wear gloves (you don't want to be exposed). Grasp the tick as close to the skin surface as possible, near the mouth parts, and pull gently in an upward motion. If the mouth parts do happen to stay, remember they aren't infectious, but can continue to cause local irritation. Afterwards, wash the bite area and your hands. Although getting the whole tick is certainly "nice to have," it is not a "need to have!" The take-home message: "Don't make the bug barf, or for the Aussie's, don't make the critter chuck!"

Certified Pediatric Emergency Nurse (CPEN) Review IV

100) You are receiving an obtunded 8-year old child found down after running a gasoline-powered generator in his "clubhouse" (Daddy's freestanding equipment shed/workshop). After the ABCs, management of this child will likely include:

A) Atropine sulfate

B) Hyperbaric oxygen therapy

C) Methylene blue

D) Sodium bicarbonate

B – This is the classic history for carbon monoxide poisoning. Whenever someone says "generator," think carbon monoxide (CO)! (After all, it is a gasoline powered engine.) After intubation, 100% oxygen and possibly hyperbaric therapy are the ONLY things that will improve this child's tissue oxygenation. Carbon monoxide competes with oxygen in binding to the hemoglobin molecule--and usually wins. CO has a 250 times greater affinity for hemoglobin than oxygen. Even a small amount of CO exposure can have really bad effects. Although there is no consensus regarding hyperbaric therapy, administering oxygen under pressure (a hyperbaric chamber) will raise the oxygen levels in the body's tissues. Atropine is for anticholinergics (exposure to nerve gas or fertilizers); methylene blue is for cyanide poisoning and methemoglobinemia; sodium bicarbonate is for tricyclic antidepressant overdoses and some other poisons.

101) You are caring for an obtunded and intubated 3-year old patient who was found unconscious on the garage floor next to a spilled jug of antifreeze. Initial labs show a serum pH of 7.09. While awaiting a peds ICU bed and emergent dialysis, you anticipate administering all of the following **except**:

A) Sodium bicarbonate

B) Warmed IV fluids to counteract the hypothermic effects of the suspected antifreeze ingestion

C) IV or nasogastric ethanol (alcohol) or IV Antizol® (fomepizole) if available

D) Appropriate hydration with IV fluids

B – You probably spotted this one right away. We are not aware of any documented cases of antifreeze induced hypothermia. The primary goals in the initial care for this patient are to correct the profound metabolic acidosis and to prevent renal damage and eventual kidney failure. Antifreeze (ethylene glycol) metabolizes in the body to oxalic acid, which then reacts with serum ionized calcium to precipitate into kidney-clogging (and kidney-killing crystals--calcium oxalate). Sometimes "antifreeze" is methanol, as in windshield washer antifreeze. Methanol is metabolized to formic acid, which is also highly toxic (beware of any end result containing the word "acid"!). Fomepizole can be used in either ethylene glycol or methanol poisoning to prevent the formation of these toxic metabolites; however, it is not always available. In children, as in adults, if fomepizole is not available, ethanol can be used to tie up the enzyme (alcohol dehydrogenase) that metabolizes the toxic alcohol or glycol. By competing for the enzyme and blocking it, fomepizole and ethanol can prevent the formation of the toxic chemicals, but fomepizole is more effective. Do not use fomepizole and ethanol together, as fomepizole is more effective and will prevent proper metabolism of the ethanol, leading to toxicity from the therapeutic alcohol itself.

Additional Pediatric ED and Toxicology Attending Physician Insights: "I would not give ethanol via the GI tract in this setting unless my back was against the wall. We really don't like to use ethanol in kids, as they are very sensitive to hypoglycemia."

Environmental

102) A 16-year old combative and obviously pregnant patient with multiple past visits to the ED for assaults and substance abuse is brought in with dilated pupils, tachycardia, tachypnea, hypertension, and chest pain. It is likely that she took any/all of the following **except**:

A) Methamphetamine (crystal meth)

B) Heroin (smack)

C) Crack cocaine (crack)

D) Phencyclidine (PCP, angel dust)

B – Based on the presentation, it is unlikely that this patient took heroin. Abusers of opiates, such as heroin, classically present with decreased levels of consciousness, pinpoint pupils and respiratory depression because things (respirations, levels of consciousness) slow way down. Meth, crack, and PCP all "speed things up."

103) The previously described patient with substance abuse is at risk for all of the following **except**:

A) Intracranial hemorrhage

B) Spontaneous abortion

C) Respiratory depression

D) Myocardial ischemia

C – We would not anticipate respiratory depression with this patient. Patients with meth, crack or PCP use are at risk for each of the other sequelae listed above, secondary to vasospasm and profound hypertension.

104) EMS is enroute to the ED with a 2-year old from a house fire with a one minute ETA. They report the child is saturating 100% on a non-rebreather mask, but has a hoarse voice, 30% full-thickness burns, and they are unable to obtain IV access. The **most** concerning portion of the above scenario is:

A) Hoarse voice

B) One minute ETA

C) 30% full-thickness burns

D) Lack of IV access

A – Though all of the above are certainly concerning with a pediatric burn patient, airway trumps everything. Remember that the airway of a child is essentially funnel-shaped and narrower than that of an adult; therefore, a little bit of edema goes a long way. Though the saturation of 100% is reassuring, the fact that the child has audible voice changes means that some serious airway edema is probably kicking in and this child may need to be intubated as soon as it's possible to do so safely--regardless of what his oxygen saturation may be. Airway edema is an equal opportunity killer! This patient will be best served by a controlled rapid sequence intubation, which means vascular access is critical. Consider rapidly securing an intraosseous line, which can be done through burned tissue if absolutely necessary.

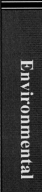

105) You are working a travel assignment at an ED in the southwestern United States. EMS reports they are bringing in a 3-year old male with confirmed multiple Centruroides (Bark Scorpion) stings to his hand approximately 30 minutes ago. You expect the child's symptoms to be mainly which system in nature:

A) Cardiac

B) Gastrointestinal

C) Neurological

D) Respiratory

C – You would expect to see primarily neurological symptoms. Centruroides sculpturatus, or Bark Scorpion, is the most prevalent poisonous scorpion in the southwestern United States. Although the venom includes multiple toxins and a variety of signs and symptoms may be elicited, the primary toxin associated symptoms associated with Bark Scorpion stings are neurological. In addition to relatively rare central nervous system effects (i.e. ataxia, global paresthesias, altered level of consciousness), bark scorpion neurotoxin has profound effects on the peripheral nervous system. These effects can include both the sympathetic and parasympathetic nervous systems. It is the release of epinephrine and acetylcholine that is responsible for the majority and severity of the neurologic symptoms. Remember sympathetic = "Fight or Flight" and parasympathetic = "Rest and Digest." Sympathetic symptoms will classically include tachypnea, tachycardia, agitation and hypertension while the typical parasympathetic symptoms can be remembered by the mnemonic SLUDGE - Salivation, Lacrimation, Urination, Diarrhea (Defecation) and Emesis. It is important to remember that acetylcholine also acts through the parasympathetic peripheral nervous system to cause contraction of airway smooth muscle (bronchoconstriction), which is of particular concern in pediatric patients. Fortunately, death is rare with bark scorpion stings, although children are more at risk of dying than adults.

106) You are caring for a 16-year old, 65 kg male with a confirmed intentional Elavil® (amitriptyline) overdose approximately 5 hours ago. He is displaying a consistently prolonged QRS and occasional runs of wide complex tachycardia, which seem to be occurring more frequently. The patient has two large bore IVs and 0.9NS is infusing. When the teen goes into sustained V-Tach, the intern (it's July 1st by the way) asks what he should order **first**:

A) Activated charcoal

B) Stat 12 lead ECG

C) Sodium bicarbonate

D) Lidocaine 20 mg IV push

C – Sodium bicarbonate is the appropriate choice in this case because we know an important factor from the history. Sodium bicarbonate is preferred over lidocaine (a very tempting choice) in tricyclic antidepressant (TCA) overdose because it works double time. The bicarbonate ion can act to reverse the metabolic acidosis that usually goes hand in hand with TCA overdose, while the high sodium load counteracts the conduction delay occurring through cardiac sodium channels. Bicarbonate should be administered as an initial bolus of 1-2 mEq/kg, followed by an infusion titrated to a QRS width of 100 milliseconds. Your pH goal is 7.45-7.55. It is too late for activated charcoal, which is recommended in the first one to two hours post ingestion. The stat 12 lead ECG, while nice to have, is not needed at this moment, as there are potentially lethal arrhythmias obvious on 3-5 leads. There is also a great risk of seizures in these patients, especially within the first 6-8 hours, so be ready with benzodiazepines such as Ativan® (lorazepam). Dilantin® (phenytoin) is NOT recommended, because it acts on sodium channels, which are the issue with TCA overdoses.

Additional Pediatric ED and Toxicology Attending Physician Insights: Correction of acidosis should be guided by arterial blood gases, electrolytes and clinical judgment. Attention should be directed to

Environmental

volume status and correction of poor perfusion in mild cases. Sodium bicarbonate may be used to correct the acidosis in severe cases with an initial push of 1 to 2mEq/kg IV (not to exceed adult doses). Infusion of sodium bicarbonate in an appropriate fluid for the patient's size and age may be guided by the base deficit on blood gases. Usually this requires 1 to 2 ampules of sodium bicarbonate per liter of IV fluids administered at a rate appropriate for the patient's weight. Additional added sodium bicarbonate or slow boluses may be required. A hypertonic solution with respect to sodium content should not be made. Sodium content should generally not exceed that of normal saline.

Finally, remember that in all cases like this, your friendly neighborhood Poison Control Center is your best friend

107) Despite initiating a bolus of sodium bicarbonate, the runs of wide complex tachycardia continue and the patient with a TCA overdose is now borderline hypotensive. Your next anticipated medication is:

A) Amiodarone

B) Magnesium

C) Bretylium

D) Procainamide

B – Magnesium is next because all of the rest of the medication choices are contraindicated in TCA overdose. Amiodarone and Bretylium both prolong QT interval, while Procainamide (avoid the "ides") will worsen the preexisting conduction delay by further blocking sodium channels.

108) Ringing in the ears (tinnitus) is a common finding in which overdose?

A) Selective serotonin receptor inhibitors (SSRIs)

B) Tylenol® (acetaminophen, Panadol®)

C) Tricyclic antidepressants (TCAs)

D) Aspirin (ASA)

D – Tinnitus is a hallmark of aspirin overdose and typically occurs at serum levels of 30mg/dL or higher. While tinnitus may theoretically (and rarely) occur with several of the above medications, if you see a question with ringing in the ears or tinnitus on the exam, chances are the answer is aspirin overdose. Aspirin is also known as Acetylsalicylic Acid (ASA.)

109) Patients with Reye's syndrome typically present afebrile, with an acute altered mental status, protracted vomiting and elevated liver function tests. It is commonly associated with which of the following:

A) Aspirin (ASA)

B) Monoamine Oxidase Inhibitors (MAO inhibitors)

C) Selective serotonin receptor inhibitors (SSRIs)

D) Tricyclic antidepressants (TCA's)

A – Although aspirin has NOT been identified as a definite cause of Reye's syndrome, research has identified aspirin as a major preventable risk for developing Reye's syndrome. Since the use of aspirin in children was actively discouraged, Reye's syndrome has virtually disappeared. Aspirin is NOT recommended for use in children under the age of 19 without expert consultation. Remember that aspirin is an ingredient in many over-the-counter medications used to treat viral symptoms, so be meticulous in taking history from parents. In the past, Reye 's syndrome occurred in children during recovery from a viral infection. Reye's syndrome is characterized by encephalopathy and fatty liver disease (also called hepatic lipidosis or hepatic steatosis). If you see Reye's syndrome in a test question, chances are the answer is something involving aspirin.

110) Which of the following correctly lists typical symptoms of Tylenol® (acetaminophen, Panadol®) overdose within the first 6 hours?

A) Nausea, vomiting, diarrhea, headache

B) Nothing, nonspecific, asymptomatic

C) Altered mental status, prolonged PR, QRS and QT intervals

D) Abnormal liver function tests, bradycardia, hypotension

B – Early acetaminophen overdose may be hard to identify because patients often exhibit "Nothing, Nonspecific, and/or Asymptomatic" symptomology. This is why obtaining an accurate patient history, empiric treatment, drawing initial/repeat labs and contacting Poison Control are so important in a suspected acetaminophen overdose. Patients may be asymptomatic for 24 or more hours, but the liver damage has begun before that point.

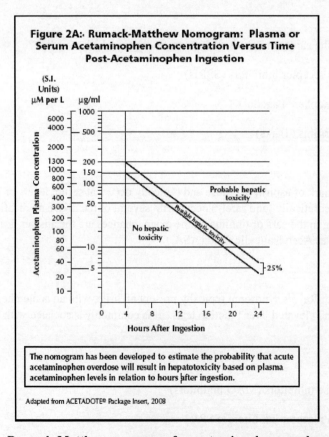

Rumack-Matthew nomogram for acetaminophen overdose

Courtesy of Cumberland Pharmaceuticals - www.cumberlandpharma.com

Certified Pediatric Emergency Nurse (CPEN) Review IV

111) Which of the following is an effective intervention for a non-pregnant, 16-year old teen with Type I diabetes who took, "I don't know…I just emptied the bottle…three handfuls, maybe 20 capsules…." of Tylenol® (acetaminophen, Panadol®) six hours ago?

A) Syrup of Ipecac

B) Gastric lavage

C) N-acetylcysteine (NAC)

D) Activated charcoal

C – N-acetylcysteine or NAC (Mucomyst® PO form, Acetadote® IV form) is the appropriate intervention in this scenario. Aside from the "guestimated" amount ingested, all of the other variables given are irrelevant distracters. Follow your local protocols and Poison Control guidance for N-acetylcysteine dosing guidelines. If possible, serum acetaminophen concentration will be determined and used, along with the estimated time and amount of ingestion, to guide treatment. Note that the toxicity nomogram starts at four hours. Serum acetaminophen levels drawn prior to four hours post-ingestion are of little use except to determine whether any of the medication was ingested. Aside from smelling like rotten eggs, Mucomyst® has few adverse side effects and may be given with little risk until the laboratory results are known. With few exceptions (i.e. Poison Control recommendation), syrup of ipecac and gastric lavage are no longer recommended, and even activated charcoal is falling out of favor unless the ingestion was within an hour of presentation to the ED.

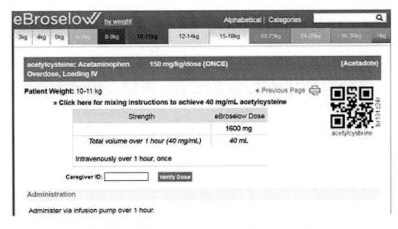

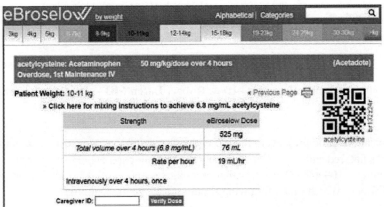

Color coded intravenous Acetadote® administration

Courtesy of James Broselow MD & Robert Luten MD – www.eBroselow.com

112) Which of the following acronyms is useful as a mnemonic for remembering the signs and symptoms of organophosphate poisoning?

A) CADET

B) MUDPILES

C) SLUDGE

D) HANG IV

C – The mnemonic SLUDGE is used to remember the symptoms of organophosphate poisoning, which classically occurs with a pesticide or nerve agents. The symptoms are: Salivation, Lacrimation, Urination, Diarrhea (Defecation) and Emesis. Organophosphates disrupt nerve conduction by blocking the enzyme acetylcholinesterase, which is used to control nerve impulses. Think of what happens if the messages to secrete/excrete all the various body substances are no longer controlled--you have all of the symptoms of SLUDGE! And these are mild when you consider what you would see in uncontrolled brain or cardiac impulses. In this case, atropine, atropine and more atropine is the treatment of choice to prevent these patients from drowning in their own secretions. Outside of the exam, in which the answer to questions involving exposure to fertilizer or nerve gas is SLUDGE and atropine, in real life, call Poison Control first - they love stuff like this! Oh yes, don't forget to contain and decontaminate the patient as your REAL first action; otherwise, you might be in no shape to call Poison Control!

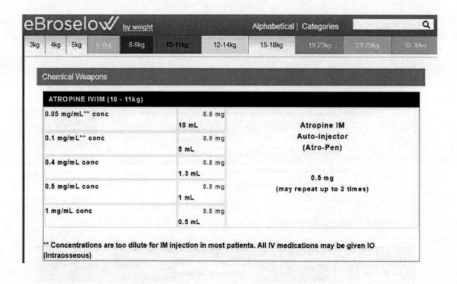

Color coded atropine administration for chemical weapon exposure

Courtesy of James Broselow MD & Robert Luten MD – www.eBroselow.com

113) An 8-year old child presents to the ED with a fever, itchy, reddened eyes, a runny nose, and a diffuse rash that is flat, red and covered in small bumps (maculopapular). His vital signs are: HR 92, RR 24, oral temperature of 100.4°F (38.0°C), with a room air saturation of 98%. He is alert, appropriate and in no respiratory distress. Which of the following should the triage nurse do **first**?

A) Place a surgical mask on the patient

B) Inquire if the patient has recently traveled outside of the United States

C) Inquire if the parents have recently changed laundry detergents

D) Inquire if the patient has recently traveled inside of the United States

A – Safety first… for the patient, but also for the others in the waiting room and registration and for your fellow staff members. Fever + rash = something icky and infectious (not just dermatitis or an allergic reaction) until proven otherwise. Even though we don't see measles nearly as often as in past years, it's still out there. Occasional outbreaks occur, especially among children who are under- or non-immunized. Measles is transmitted via respiratory droplets, so placement of a mask at triage, followed by placement in a private ED room is the goal. Safety first!

114) Scabies is the diagnosis for two children in the ED. Discharge instructions to the parents should include all of the following **except**:

A) Place any clothing that needs to be sent out for dry cleaning in a sealed plastic bag for 2 weeks before taking it to the dry cleaner

B) Your children will be contagious for 30-days after treatment

C) Your children's itching should subside within two-weeks after treatment

D) Clothing and linens that can be washed, should be double washed with hot water

B – As knowledge is power, parents and caregivers need to know not only how to treat the condition but also that 1) their child is only contagious for 24-hours post-treatment, 2) the symptoms may persist even though the condition is treated, and 3) the bugs are dead after following the treatment instructions. Scabies should be treated with 5% permethrin (Elimite®) lotion exactly as directed. It is crucial to ensure that parents understand the proper use of anti-scabies lotions, especially in regard to the frequency of application. Unfortunately, many parents or caregivers seem to think that if "now" and in a week is good, then "now" and every day for a week must be better. This is a huge problem because it was not uncommon for children to show up seizing from lindane (Kwell®) toxicity. One last common misconception: Clothing does not need to be thrown away or even worse, burned. If it can be washed and dried, then washed again with hot water and dried with hot air, and then the clothes should be okay. If the clothes must be dry cleaned, "bagging" the clothes for 2-weeks will kill the mites and dry cleaning can be done without potentially contaminating the dry cleaner's shop!

Additional Pediatric ED Attending Physician Insights: Anyone who buys "dry clean only" clothes for their kids should be asked to donate to the hospital, since it's obvious they have plenty of money!

115) A 2-year old presents to the ED after accidentally dousing his left arm with hydrofluoric acid. The Pediatric ED nurse knows that in addition to IV analgesics, the drug of choice for management of this exposure is:

A) Sodium bicarbonate

B) Fluoride

C) Calcium

D) Atropine

C – If given as an option, the most appropriate answer would be to address decontamination and the ABCs along with IV analgesics. However, given the choices offered in this question, the treatment for hydrofluoric acid exposure is calcium, calcium and more calcium. Let's neutralize that acid! Calcium gel applied liberally, IV calcium and, occasionally, even intra-arterial calcium (calcium gluconate only) is used. Calcium chloride should only be given intravenously, preferably through a central line or diluted with 1 part calcium chloride to 2 parts sterile water. Calcium gluconate can be used intravenously in a Bier block (given IV and kept in the venous system of the affected limb with a blood pressure cuff tourniquet device), but only by those experienced in the technique. Intra-arterial calcium gluconate can be administered via a radial artery catheter for serious hand or digit burns and also should be employed only by those experienced

Environmental

in this procedure.

Hydrofluoric acid (HF) is commonly found in rust removers (outdoor metal furniture cleaners) as well as cleaning fluids for bricks, air conditioners, aluminum, automobile wheels, and (less commonly) industrial-strength carpet, wall and tub cleaners. Skin exposure results in excruciating pain, either immediately (with higher concentrations) or hours later (with lower concentrations). As with necrotizing fasciitis and high-voltage electric burns, what you see on the outside does not even begin to tell you what damage is present on the inside. HF penetrates tissue easily, resulting in white burn marks, erythema, blistering and pus, among other symptoms. In the event of a hydrofluoric acid exposure, you should always contact the regional poison center in your area by calling 1-800-222-1222 (nationwide).

The relief of pain is a useful clinical indicator of successful treatment. Therefore, some advocate limited use of narcotic analgesics or nerve blocks, as they directly affect the reporting of pain without regard to the source. Nevertheless, the pain may be severe, especially with more concentrated forms of hydrofluoric acid, and intravenous narcotic pain relief may be warranted.

Do not underestimate the potential systemic effects of hydrofluoric acid burns, even those that are "only" 3% to 5% BSA burns. Patients have died from 5% BSA burns with concentrated HF (i.e. 60% to 70% HF). Skin burns can result in life-threatening hypocalcemia or hypomagnesemia because the highly-reactive negatively-charged fluoride ions search for positive ions like calcium and magnesium to combine with in our tissues. In addition, hyperkalemia may be present from release of potassium ions from lysed RBCs. This combination of electrolyte disturbances is a set-up that can lead to ventricular arrhythmias, especially ventricular fibrillation.

Ingestion of hydrofluoric acid, such as seen in suicide attempts, is almost always fatal. Animal studies have failed to show that oral antacids (calcium or magnesium based) are helpful. HF is cleared from the body through the kidneys, so hemodialysis may be used to help clear the poison if kidney damage has occurred. Meticulous supportive care has resulted in some case reports of survival after HF ingestion.

116) Evidence of chemicals used in "huffing" will show up on a:

A) Routine urine toxicology screen

B) Special blood or urine test

C) Routine blood test

D) "Breathalizer" type test

B – While metabolites from inhaled agents may occasionally be present in a urine tox screen, the abused chemicals themselves are generally absent. To confirm the presence of these metabolites, most hospitals will order special blood and urine tests. These may, along with other assays, include an "inhalant panel" or an "inhalant and metabolites panel." These specialized blood and urine tests are only available at selected commercial laboratories in the United States.

117) The most common factors leading to acute fatalities among "huffers" include all of the following **except**:

A) Hypoxia

B) Chemically induced pneumonitis

C) Arrhythmias

D) Aspiration of vomitus

B – Chemically induced pneumonitis is certainly a potential complication, but it is not an acute one. It can result either from aspiration or direct irritation by the inhaled agent. Emergency management of these patients ("huffers") is initially focused on airway and breathing, after which the management is largely supportive. Acute effects of "huffing" include direct CNS/respiratory depression and hypoxia. These often lead to death due to hypoxia and/or aspiration of vomitus. Hypoxia results from the fact that many inhaled agents are heavier than air and will displace oxygen in the lungs. Huffers usually pass out from hypoxia before all of the oxygen is displaced from their lungs. At that point, the bag, rag or bottle they were inhaling from typically will fall away from their face and the chemical exposure stops. However, if the person was huffing from a plastic bag, there is the very real potential for the plastic bag to remain over the mouth and nose after the huffer passes out, thereby causing further suffocation, vomiting, aspiration and death. Another likely and deadly complication of huffing is a sudden arrhythmia due to the inhalation of halogenated hydrocarbons. Halogenated hydrocarbons are sometimes used in computer keyboard cleaners which contain fluorinated hydrocarbons and sensitize the myocardium to electrical stimulation.

118) You are the nurse of a 12-year old with unknown drug ingestion. The patient complains of ringing in his ears. The emergency department staff should particularly evaluate the patient for what kind of overdose?

A) Benzodiazepines

B) Aspirin (acetylsalicylic acid)

C) Antibiotics

D) Iron

B – One of the textbook side effects of a large aspirin overdose is ringing in the ears or tinnitus. Acute aspirin overdose may lead to nausea, vomiting (sometimes with blood) and stomach pain. Another classic sign of aspirin overdose is hyperventilation, as the body attempts to compensate for the developing respiratory alkalosis (caused by for the ingested acetylsalicylic acid) by blowing off CO_2. Other signs and symptoms of aspirin overdose include: temporary deafness, dizziness, drowsiness, hyperactivity, seizures and even coma. One mnemonic used to remember how to treat overdoses or ingestions is SIREN: S-Stabilize the child's condition, I-Identify the poison, R-Reverse its effect and Reduce absorption, E-Eliminate the toxin, N-Need for consultation with poison control, ongoing physical care, and psychiatric consultation (was the incident a suicide attempt?)

119) A young child presents to the emergency department triage area with burns to the soles of both feet from stepping barefooted into an unknown liquid on the floor of a neighbor's garage. The patient is actively crying. What should be the FIRST intervention made by the ED nurse?

A) Initiate the decontamination process

B) Contact Child Protective Services about possible abuse

C) Assess the depth and percent of burns

D) Place an IV line for pain management

A – The first step with any possible chemical burn is to stop the burning process and to decontaminate the patient (without contaminating the staff or the emergency department). When reading the question, try not to read too much into it. The patient is crying, which should tell you they have a patent airway. After decontamination is complete, further assessment can be completed. Test tip: Note that the question was asking specifically for an intervention, not an assessment.

Environmental

Certified Pediatric Emergency Nurse (CPEN) Review IV

120) A child is brought to the ED 45 minutes after ingesting an unknown number of mom's prenatal vitamins with iron. He is awake, alert and vital signs are normal. You anticipate the approach to this patient will include:

A) Give 1 gm of activated charcoal per kilogram because it is more effective within one hour of ingestion

B) Give a weight-based dose of syrup of ipecac because the ingestion was so recent

C) Initiate lab work, including iron levels, complete blood count, liver function tests, glucose, type and screen. Obtain an abdominal X-ray

D) Discharge the patient after a brief observation period if his vital signs remain stable

C – Our biggest concern is with the iron, and the severity of iron poisoning is directly related to the amount of iron ingested. Prediction of the toxicity can be determined if the serum iron concentration is known and if the abdominal x-ray shows the presence and number of iron tablets in the GI tract. The antidote for iron is deferoxamine, not charcoal. Charcoal does not bind metals and cannot prevent their absorption from the GI tract. Deferoxamine is a chelating agent that binds free iron once it's absorbed into the bloodstream. Symptoms of iron toxicity can occur as early as 30 minutes after ingestion. Because of the risk of severe complications and death, a patient needs more than brief monitoring and observation if significant iron ingestion is suspected. And when in doubt, it is far better to assume that there was more ingested than less. With very few exceptions, toxicologists no longer recommend the administration of ipecac. Though charcoal and overdoses seemingly go hand in hand, remember iron is one of several cases where charcoal "PHAILS." Other items include:

- P-Pesticides
- H-Hydrocarbons
- A-Alcohols, acids, alkali
- I-Iron
- L-Lithium
- S-Solvents

121) Which of the following serum electrolyte abnormalities is a pediatric severe burn victim **most** likely to suffer initially?

A) Hyperchloremia

B) Hyperphosphatemia

C) Hypernatremia

D) Hyperkalemia

D – Hyperkalemia is likely to occur first. In burns, hyperkalemia initially results from damaged cells releasing K+ into the serum. Think about crush injuries and myoglobinuria. The "squished cells" are very unhappy they are squished and send lots of bad things "downstream" to the kidneys to get filtered out. The same idea applies with bad burns, in that the burned cells initially push potassium out of the cell into the bloodstream, causing hyperkalemia. The other electrolytes listed are typically depressed or "hypo" secondary to third spacing, swelling and associated fluid losses.

Environmental

Lundblom's Lessons

The grandmother came running in, holding her 3 year-old grandson and yelling, "I think he drank some poison!" The child was alert, anxious, drooling, and taken to a resuscitation bed for evaluation. History revealed that grandma and the child were in the garage when the patient found "something that was poured into a bottle." The grandmother was not sure what it was and said that the patient "took a big swallow and then began coughing and choking." The child's vital signs revealed tachycardia (anxiety/stress/scared vs. airway issues?), respiratory rate 28/min, oxygen saturation 96%, normal blood pressure and no fever.

Discussion started immediately with our attending physician about treatment plans for this child. I expressed my opinion that we needed to intubate him to protect his airway. Initially, she did not agree but as the next several minutes went by and his drooling worsened, it became apparent we had no choice. The intubation was very difficult due to significant airway edema. Ultimately, it was discovered that the patient had ingested caustic drain cleaner. He was chemically sedated/paralyzed and eventually successfully intubated. He was transferred to the Pediatric ICU, where he remained intubated for over 2 weeks, had multiple failed extubations and required placement of a gastrostomy tube for feedings due to very poor swallowing post-extubation. This child had a very lengthy recovery, requiring numerous GI procedures and ongoing care to repair the damage done to his esophagus by this caustic ingestion, but he did eventually recover.

Teaching points: You could spend hours discussing the endless substances these little ones get into. Why do children swallow/inhale/ingest and generally put everything into their mouth? Because they can! Children are full sensory beings--if they see it, they must touch it, they must taste it, etc. Nothing is safe in the little fingers of a toddler.

It's important to think ahead, especially with some specific kinds of pediatric chemical or drug ingestions. This presentation pointed to a rapidly-evolving toxic (likely caustic) ingestion involving the upper airway and GI tract. Although the child wasn't in distress initially, it was reasonable to think he was going to get worse before he got better. Knowing that the airway was likely to become more difficult to secure with time, early aggressive action was indicated.

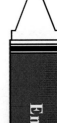

Certified Pediatric Emergency Nurse (CPEN) Review IV

Appendix 6-A

Radical Rashes and Bad Bugs

Type	Caused by:	Signs and Symptoms (systemic)	Signs and Symptoms (rash)	Management	Contagious Period	Route of Transmission
Chicken Pox	Virus	Flu	Chicken Pox rash	Benadryl (diphenhydramine) PO or lotion, Calamine lotion, time – Varicella-zoster immunoglobulin (VZIG) in high-risk kids	1 day before visible lesions until ALL lesions are crusted over	Primarily respiratory, but also direct contact with open lesions - Scabs are not infectious
Mumps	Virus	Fever/malaise x 24 hours, followed by "earache" that is aggravated by chewing – Then parotid gland swelling	None	Tylenol or Motrin Fluids	Most communicable immediately before and after swelling begins	Respiratory and saliva
Roseola	Virus	3-4 days of high fever in a cute kid – Fever goes away with rash	Discreet rose-pink rash – First on trunk, then to face and extremities – not itchy	Tylenol or Motrin	During the actively febrile period	Respiratory and saliva
Rubella (German measles)	Virus	None in most children	Pinkish red rash starts in the face and rapidly moves down – Disappears in same order it began and is usually gone by 3rd day	Tylenol or Motrin	7 days before rash to about 5 days after rash appears	Respiratory and saliva Isolate child from pregnant women (teratogenic)

Type	Caused by:	Signs and Symptoms (systemic)	Signs and Symptoms (rash)	Management	Contagious Period	Route of Transmission
Rubeola (measles)	Virus	Fever, malaise, and Koplik spots (red spot with a blue-white center found in the mouth)	Red rash – starts in face and becomes less red as it moves down the body	Rest, Tylenol or Motrin; antibiotics to prevent secondary infection in high-risk kids	4 days before rash until 5 days after rash appears	Respiratory and saliva
Fifth's Disease	Virus	"Flu" symptoms Usually afebrile	"Slapped face" appearance which disappears by 1-4 days, red, symmetrical, itchy rash moving proximal to distal	Tylenol or Motrin Antihistamines for itching	1-2 days before the rash starts until the rash appears	Respiratory and saliva
Scarlet Fever	Strep.	Malaise, high fever, and high pulse out of proportion to fever	Sandpaper-like red rash starting on the neck within 12 hours of fever	Penicillin or cephalosporins Tylenol or Motrin	First 10 days of symptoms	Respiratory and saliva

Appendix 6-B

Laboratory Detection of Drugs

Alcohol	12-24 hours
Amphetamines	2-4 days
Benzodiazepines	1-14 days
Rohypnol	36 hours
Cannabinoids	Occasional use: 1-7 days
Cannabinoids	Chronic use: 1-4 weeks
Cocaine	12-48 hours
GHB	4 hours (blood) - 12 hours (urine)
Opiates	1-3 days
PCP	Occasional use: 1-8 days
PCP	Chronic use: Up to 30 days

(Actual figures will vary due to metabolism, user laboratory, and excretion)

If someone asks how long a certain drug is detectable in their urine, what do you tell them???

Tell them whatever drug they asked about is detected in urine for 2 years!

Appendix 6-C

One Pill or One Swallow Killers

Agent or Class	Examples
Camphor	Camphor mothballs and camphor oil
Salicylates	Oil of wintergreen and methylsalicylate
Podophyllin	Podofilox (podophyllin)
	Also occasionally in herbal medications
Local anesthetics	Nupercainal (Dibucaine) ointment
Anti-arrhythmics	Quinaglute (quininide), Norpace (disopryamide), Enkaid (encainide), and Rhythmol (propafenone)
Anti-malarials	Quinine and chloroquine
Anti-hypertensives	Catapres (clonidine)
Tricyclic antidepressants	Elavil (amitriptyline), Tofranil (imipramine), and Pamelor (nortriptyline) - Depending on dose and size of child
Calcium channel blockers	Calan or Isoptin (verapamil), Cardizem (diltiazem), and Procardia (nifedipine)
Oral hypoglycemics (sulfonylureas)	Amaryl (glimepiride), Glucotrol (glypizide), and Glyburide (glibenclamide)
Opioids	Vicodin (hydrocodone with acetaminophen), Lomotil (diphenoxylate and atropine), and Duragesic (fentanyl) patch
Toxic alcohols	Windshield washer fluid (methanol) and antifreeze (ethylene glycol)
Theophylline	Theo-Dur, Theostat, and Theo-Dur Sprinkle

Thanks to James Rhee MD and Anthony Scalzo MD for their help with the creation of this chart

Appendix 6-D

Snakebite Tidbits from the Texas Poison Center Network - www.poisoncontrol.org

- The annual incidence of snake bite in the United States is 3-4 bites per 100,000 population; with only about 20 deaths reported each year. Rattlesnake bites are the most common envenomation, and the victim is often a young, intoxicated male who was teasing or trying to capture the snake.

- The potency of the venom and the amount of venom injected vary considerably. About 25% of all snake strikes are dry bites in which there is no envenomation.

- Fang marks from the Crotalidae (rattlesnake, copperhead, and the cottonmouth) may look like puncture wounds or lacerations.

- Coral snake envenomation is rare because of the snake's small mouth and fangs. The snake must hold on and chew for several seconds or more to work its rear fangs into the skin.

- **Red on yellow... Kill a fellow   Red on black... Venom lack**

- A child gets the same amount of antivenin as an adult.

- If platelets are low, give more antivenin... not more platelets.

- Do not pack the wound in ice or use a tourniquet.

- Never perform a fasciotomy unless compartment syndrome is documented with tissue compartment pressure monitoring.

- Electric shock treatment for snakebite is ineffective and is potentially dangerous!

Appendix 6-E

JumpSTART Pediatric Multicasualty Incident Triage

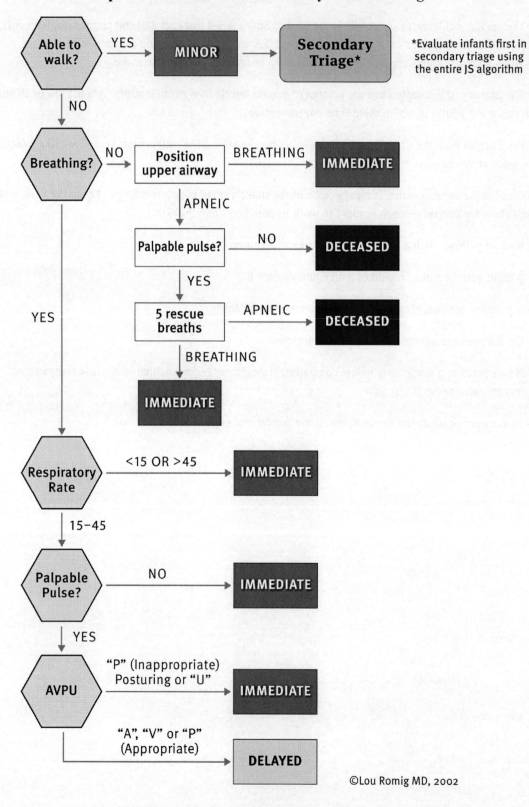

Photo Courtesy of Lou Romig MD, FAAP, FACEP

www.jumpstarttriage.com

Chapter 7

Abdominal and OB/Neonatal Emergencies
Bellies, Births, and Babies

Madam, there's no such thing as a tough child.
If you parboil them first for seven hours, they always come out tender.
-W.C. Fields

Pertinent Pediatric Ponderings (NOTES)

CHAPTER 7
Sample Test Answer Sheet

1. _____
2. _____
3. _____
4. _____
5. _____
6. _____
7. _____
8. _____
9. _____
10. _____
11. _____
12. _____
13. _____
14. _____
15. _____
16. _____
17. _____
18. _____
19. _____
20. _____
21. _____
22. _____
23. _____
24. _____
25. _____
26. _____
27. _____
28. _____
29. _____
30. _____
31. _____
32. _____
33. _____
34. _____
35. _____
36. _____
37. _____
38. _____
39. _____
40. _____
41. _____
42. _____
43. _____
44. _____
45. _____
46. _____
47. _____
48. _____
49. _____
50. _____
51. _____
52. _____
53. _____
54. _____
55. _____
56. _____
57. _____
58. _____
59. _____
60. _____
61. _____
62. _____
63. _____
64. _____
65. _____
66. _____
67. _____
68. _____
69. _____
70. _____
71. _____
72. _____
73. _____
74. _____
75. _____
76. _____
77. _____
78. _____
79. _____
80. _____
81. _____
82. _____
83. _____
84. _____
85. _____
86. _____
87. _____
88. _____
89. _____
90. _____
91. _____
92. _____
93. _____
94. _____
95. _____
96. _____
97. _____
98. _____
99. _____
100. _____
101. _____

[Remove page and cover rationale until after you answer questions.]

Pertinent Pediatric Ponderings (NOTES)

Certified Pediatric Emergency Nurse (CPEN) Review IV

1) A 15-year-old male involved in a fight arrives at the ED with a large knife protruding from his abdomen. **First** nursing actions should include:

A) Removing the object and applying a pressure dressing on the wound

B) Leaving the knife in place until the patient is taken to the operating room

C) Placing 2 large-bore IV lines, then carefully remove the object

D) Administering supplemental oxygen, ordering an abdominal CT scan, then carefully remove the object

B – The key here is to leave the "impaled" object in place, and even support it if necessary. We don't want that knife to do more damage by moving (or removing) it. While all of the other answers include later appropriate actions, they also include removing the knife. Removing the object outside of the operating room is not recommended (unless by a surgeon.)

2) A 14-year-old male arrives at the ED with a gunshot wound (GSW) to the sixth intercostal space. Anticipated workup for this patient would involve evaluation of the:

A) Chest

B) Abdomen

C) Pelvis

D) A and B

D – The unwritten motto of most trauma surgeons is simply, "Any penetrating injury below the level of the nipples is chest and belly until proven otherwise." Remember, you don't know at what point of inspiration or expiration they were in at the time they were lucky enough to get shot or stabbed.

3) The above patient arrives at the ED with a GSW to the sixth intercostal space. His abdomen is distended, tender, and gross hematuria is present. Which diagnostic test would the nurse expect the physician to order before surgery?

A) Diagnostic peritoneal lavage (DPL)

B) Abdominal x-ray

C) Intravenous pyelogram (IVP)

D) Abdominal CT scan

D – With a GSW to the abdomen, chances are the patient is going to surgery. An abdominal CT may be ordered as non-operative management of trauma is now extending from blunt to penetrating trauma. An IVP can quickly provide information about the status of the kidneys, however, helical CT scans will tell what's going on with the kidneys, and rest of the belly as well. The "new generation" of much faster CT scans, coupled with the high rates of non-operative intervention for liver and splenic lacerations in children, has resulted in DPL's or "belly taps" and IVP's not being done nearly as often as we used to.

4) When working with patients with a gunshot wound to the right upper abdominal quadrant, special consideration should be made for possible injury to the:

A) Liver

B) Transverse colon

C) Spleen

D) Kidney

A – Anatomically speaking, think about "what's where?" The liver is predominately in the right side and spleen is on the left. That being said, since in the majority of GSWs, we don't know where the bullet went, evaluation of other organs such as the stomach or colon is certainly appropriate. However, on a test, when a question is asked about right upper quadrant, think liver.

5) In children, like adults, esophageal varices are:

A) Primarily caused by abnormal circulation within the splenic artery

B) Primarily caused by alcohol, tobacco, or spicy foods

C) Primarily caused by hepatic carcinomas

D) Primarily caused by portal hypertension

D – Esophageal varices, or "varicose veins" of the esophagus, are primarily caused by portal hypertension of some etiology. Whatever the cause, pressure builds up in the portal hepatic system (liver, not spleen) and blood backs up causing dilation and possible rupture of the esophageal vasculature. If you see splenic, think spleen and hepatic refers to the liver. Alcohol, tobacco, and spicy foods are often the culprits in gastritis, so if only by process of elimination, the right answer is portal hypertension.

6) Chance fractures are commonly associated with which mechanism of injury?

A) Ejection from the vehicle

B) Low speed, vehicle vs. pedestrian incidents

C) Lap belt usage without other restraints

D) Air bag deployment

C – The most common etiology for a Chance fracture (flexion-extension fractures of the lumbar spine) is a motor vehicle crash with the passenger only restrained by a lap seatbelt. Here's an easy way to remember this: "You are taking a Chance if your child only wears a lap belt!"

Certified Pediatric Emergency Nurse (CPEN) Review IV

7) A 4-year-old girl presents to the ED with low-grade fever, vomiting, and abdominal pain for 12 hours. Pain in which quadrant is **most** commonly associated with acute appendicitis?

A) Right upper quadrant

B) Right lower quadrant

C) Left upper quadrant

D) Left lower quadrant

B – Though children with appendicitis can have abdominal pain "everywhere" in their abdomen, rebound tenderness at McBurney's point (in the right lower quadrant) is a classic finding with appendicitis. Interestingly, in the pediatric surgical journals, they have found that IV Morphine (or fentanyl) does not diminish the ability to diagnose appendicitis, but in fact, helps with confirming the diagnosis. So much for withholding pain meds until the surgeon completes her assessment. Think about it. If good drugs can get the child mellow and only screaming because the mean doctor is pushing on something that really hurts (not because the nurse is dressed in white and they know they are going to get a shot), aren't we the better for it?

8) Which type of fluid would the nurse expect to initially administer to a hypovolemic child with a liver laceration?

A) Hypertonic saline

B) Hypotonic (D5.2NS)

C) Isotonic (0.9NS) or lactated ringers (LR)

D) Whole blood

C – The "tank" (blood vessels) is empty, so you should fill it up. Isotonic fluids such as 0.9NS or LR are designed to "stay in the tank" and are commonly administered before blood products. The research on the use of blood products vs. whole blood continues to evolve, however for the purpose of the test, initial fluid resuscitation is still done with 0.9NS or LR.

9) Which of the following statements regarding splenic trauma is **false**?

A) The normal spleen is palpable below the lower right costal margin

B) The spleen and liver are injured more frequently than other abdominal organs

C) The significance of splenic injuries is directly related to the organ's high vascularity

D) Splenic bleeding can be associated with a positive Kehr's sign

A – The spleen is on the left and the liver is on the right. In addition, the spleen is sheltered by the ribs and normally is not palpable (Two chances to get this one right!) Solid organs, like the spleen and liver, are more susceptible to injury than hollow organs. When you hear left-sided abdominal trauma, think spleen and lots of bleeding due to the spleen's high vascularity. Kehr's sign or referred left shoulder pain without shoulder trauma is commonly associated with splenic trauma. Hint: Spleen begins with "S" and so does "Shoulder."

10) A child is involved in a high-speed motor vehicle collision. The ED nurse would suspect a splenic injury in the patient with trauma to the:

A) Bladder

B) Sternum

C) Right lower ribs

D) Left lower ribs

D – Again, with left sided trauma, think spleen and lots of bleeding. 10-20% of children with lower right rib fractures also have trauma to the liver, and similarly 10-20% of lower left rib fractures have associated splenic trauma.

11) A 10-year-old child with a history of several past abdominal surgeries is brought to the hospital complaining of severe abdominal cramping and abdominal pain. His mother states he has had "the flu" for the past few days with symptoms including vomiting and constipation. Within the last 12 hours, his pain has increased in intensity, and he has vomited small amounts of dark greenish liquid several times. He is diagnosed with a possible bowel obstruction. Classic signs and symptoms include:

A) Abdominal pain and distention, vomiting, and lack of stooling

B) No abdominal pain, but pronounced nausea, vomiting, and lack of stooling

C) Loss of bowel sounds, abdominal distention, constipation, and lack of stooling

D) Hyperactive bowel sounds, diarrhea, vomiting, and cramping

A – Abdominal pain and distention, vomiting, and constipation (not diarrhea) are the hallmark signs of a bowel obstruction. Think about what's going on. Things are obstructed. Fluids that cannot move down, then move up = vomiting) and little to nothing passes by the obstruction (constipation.) Abdominal distention and pain will progressively increase, and bowel sounds will become hyperactive, especially in the pre-obstruction portions of the bowel, as the body tries to keep moving things through.

12) In the emergency department, which is the correct sequence for assessing a child's abdomen?

A) Auscultation, percussion, inspection, and palpation

B) Auscultation, inspection, percussion, and palpation

C) Inspection, auscultation, percussion, and palpation

D) Inspection, auscultation, palpation, and percussion

C – Look at the abdomen first to see how it looks before you mess with it. Then listen to the abdomen before you mess with it and possibly create "false bowel sounds." Percuss next, before messing with the abdomen and altering the findings, and finally, do the painful palpation part of the exam.

Certified Pediatric Emergency Nurse (CPEN) Review IV

13) A 16-year-old teen is admitted to the ED after a high-speed motor vehicle crash (MVC.) He is conscious and alert. Skin is cool and dry. The EMTs report severe damage to the car with 20 minutes of extrication required. Which assessment finding is one of the **earliest** indications of impending shock?

A) Tachycardia

B) Hypotension

C) Narrowing pulse pressure

D) Cool and clammy skin

A – If you want to catch shock in its earliest stages, tachycardia (and subtle mental status changes) is where you start. Hypotension, narrowing pulse pressure (systolic/diastolic coming closer together) and skin changes will occur as shock progresses. The "tank" (blood vessels) is empty and the child's heart beats faster to make what little blood is still there circulate around and around.

14) False negative results of a diagnostic peritoneal lavage (DPL, "belly tap") may be found in a pediatric patient with a:

A) Hepatic hemorrhage

B) Diaphragmatic rupture

C) Bladder rupture

D) Retroperitoneal hemorrhage

D – Remember your abdomen is divided into two parts; the front (peritoneum) and the back (retroperitoneum.) DPL's can identify injuries in the front reasonably well (hence the peritoneal part of the name.) However, they can easily miss injuries in the back of the belly. This is important as the patient can have a perfectly normal DPL, but a severe and life threatening retroperitoneal hemorrhage.

15) Cullen's sign is characterized by:

A) Bruising over the flanks

B) Bruising around the umbilicus

C) Bruising around the perineum

D) Bruising around the xiphoid process

B – Cullen's sign is characterized by bruising around the umbilicus and can be a late sign of intra-abdominal or retroperitoneal hemorrhage (12-24 hours post-injury.) One way to remember it is that the first two letters in Cullen's sign are "CU." If you "C" bruising around the "U"mbilicus, that is Cullen's sign. More important than remembering the name of the sign is remembering that if you see it in a child, bad things are happening in their abdomen.

16) Grey-Turner's sign is characterized by:

A) Bruising over the flanks

B) Bruising around the umbilicus

C) Bruising around the perineum

D) Bruising around the xiphoid process

A – Grey-Turner's sign is characterized by bruising on the flank and can also be a sign of intra-abdominal or retroperitoneal hemorrhage. You might think about "Turn(er's) over on your flank" (Turners = Flank) as a way to remember this one. Again, more important than remembering the name of the sign is remembering that if you see this in a child, bad things are happening in their abdomen.

17) Which of the following signs are **most** important to assess when determining the resuscitation needs of a newborn?

A) Heart rate, muscle tone, and APGAR score

B) Presence of meconium, muscle tone, and color

C) Respiratory effort, heart rate, and color

D) Respiratory effort, presence of meconium, and muscle tone

C – Before handing the newborn baby to mom, the things you should check are: Is the baby working hard at breathing, yes or no? How's the heart rate, good or bad? Are they pink or purple? If they are breathing fine, the heart rate is good, and they are pink, give the baby to mom. However, if one of those three assessment components is not normal, interventions should immediately be undertaken.

18) Preferred methods for determining the heart rate in a full-term newborn who was delivered in the ED include each of the following **except**:

A) Palpating the femoral or brachial pulse

B) Palpating the umbilical pulse

C) Auscultating the apical pulse

D) Palpating the popliteal pulse

D – Assessing the popliteal pulse in adults in hard enough, but even more challenging in newborns. The simple answer is to find something that is pulsating and determine the heart rate. Brachial, femoral, or umbilical arteries (most babies have not one, but two, umbilical arteries screaming "feel me") are all appropriate places to check the heart rate. Palpating the baby's carotid pulse is not recommended as most babies have "no neck." Auscultation of the apical pulse is an option; however in a noisy environment such as most emergency departments, palpation is probably a better option.

Certified Pediatric Emergency Nurse (CPEN) Review IV

19) When palpating or auscultating the heart rate in a newborn, suggested methods include:

A) Listening/feeling for 60 seconds and multiplying x 1

B) Listening/feeling for 30 seconds and multiplying x 2

C) Listening/feeling for 10 seconds and multiplying x 6

D) Listening/feeling for 6 seconds and multiplying x 10

D – Listen/feel for 6-seconds and multiply by 10 (put a zero at the end.) Besides, it's poor form to listen/feel for up to 2-minutes to determine that the baby's heart rate is really bad. So, if the six second heart rate is 15, what's the actual heart rate? 150. Good – Celebrate! But if the six second heart rate is only 4, what the actual heart rate? 40. Bad - Do something!

20) When delivering positive-pressure ventilation (i.e. "bagging") a full-term baby, the respiratory rate should be approximately how many breaths per minute?

A) 10-20

B) 20-30

C) 30-40

D) 40-60

D – The American Academy of Pediatrics Neonatal Resuscitation Program (NRP) recommends 40-60 ventilations per minute. How fast should you "gently" squeeze the bag? Once again, NRP recommends a phrase to remember to help control the speed of breathing for babies: Squeeze while saying "one," quickly release, and then say slowly "two, three" before giving another breath. Remember, before you assist the baby's breathing, you should take a slow, deep breath or two to calm down and avoid potential barotrauma.

21) Assessment of a newly born infant reveals central and peripheral cyanosis. The heart rate is 140 beats per minute. He has spontaneous respirations at a rate of 40 per minute. Your **best** course of action would be to:

A) Perform immediate tracheal intubation

B) Reassess in 5 minutes

C) Begin chest compressions

D) Administer blow-by oxygen

D – The child is purple, but his heart rate and respiratory rates are normal. Think for a minute about adult "COPDers." Do you intubate them every time their lips get blue? No, or every one of them would be intubated every time they came to the ED. The same idea applies for babies. He is breathing and his heart rate is good, so giving a little extra oxygen via blow-by is an appropriate intervention to try first.

Abdominal / Perinatal

22) A 14-year-old girl with a history of heroin abuse delivers a baby in the ED. The baby has no spontaneous respirations, so after assisted ventilations are given, the ED nurse should anticipate all of the following **except**:

A) Providing assisted ventilations

B) The immediate administration of IV Narcan (naloxone)

C) Assessing the baby's pulse

D) Obtaining the APGAR scores

B – The call for the immediate administration of Narcan in these situations, like many things in emergency healthcare, is changing. Think about it. If mom is addicted (heroin, chronic pain issues, methadone maintenance), who else is addicted? The baby. And if you give Narcan to an opiate addicted baby, what does the baby do? Withdraw and very possibly seize. Remember, it's a lot easier to "bag" a baby than it is to make them stop seizing!

23) In the emergency department where a sick newborn has just delivered, Apgar scores should be:

A) Determined immediately after delivery

B) Determined at 1 and 5 minutes after delivery

C) Determined after initial resuscitation efforts are complete

D) Not assessed until the child is in the nursery

C – Ideally, Apgar scores should be assessed and determined at 1 and 5 minutes of life. However, life is not always ideal, so take care of the baby first and figure out Apgar scores later. There is no baby that ever came back to life because you could figure out an Apgar score while caring for the baby. Assess, and if needed, resuscitate the baby first; figure out numbers for the chart later.

24) A newborn infant in the emergency department is exhibiting signs of hypovolemic shock. An appropriate fluid bolus of 0.9NS would be:

A) 10ml/kg

B) 20ml/kg

C) 40ml/kg

D) 50ml/kg

A – While PALS (Pediatric Advanced Life Support) and ENPC (Emergency Nursing Pediatric Course) programs teach 20ml/kg for children, newborns are a different matter. Neonatology programs remind us that a little fluid goes a long way, so 10ml/kg is the suggested amount for newborns.

Certified Pediatric Emergency Nurse (CPEN) Review IV

25) A newborn infant has central cyanosis, with an unlabored respiratory rate of 40 and a heart rate of 130. When delivering blow-by oxygen, the oxygen flow rate should be approximately how many liters per minute?

A) 2

B) 5

C) 10

D) 15

B – Blow-by oxygen should be given at approximately 5 liters per minute to avoid possible hypothermia and vagal responses caused by flowing unheated oxygen near the face. Blow-by oxygen can be administered by taking some oxygen tubing and placing it near the face, placing a mask on or near the child's face, or by using an "anesthesia" bag. The technique of using a traditional "Ambu," or self-inflating bag, for blow-by oxygen is no longer recommended due to unreliable amounts of oxygen being delivered with this method.

26) Neonates often demonstrate what rhythm changes in response to hypoxia?

A) Bradycardia

B) Tachycardia

C) Ventricular fibrillation

D) AV blocks

A – If babies become hypoxic, one of the earliest signs is bradycardia. In the neonatal ICU, they describe babies as having "A's and B's" or apnea and bradycardias. Long before administering epinephrine or starting CPR, try supplemental oxygen first, because almost everything bad that happens to kids starts off with something respiratory.

27) In the emergency department, acceptable methods of stimulating respirations in a newborn include:

A) Squeezing the rib cage or dilating the anal sphincter

B) Firmly rolling the baby from front to back, applying chest thrusts and back blows, or shaking the baby and shouting, "Baby, Baby, Are you OK?"

C) Rubbing the back or flicking the soles of the feet

D) All of the above

C – Squeezing anything, dilating anything, and shaking anything are just wrong when trying to get a baby to breathe. It's as simple as that. In reality, if you do a really good job of drying the baby off and they are still not breathing, chances are they are not going to be breathing on their own, so you really should be "bagging".

28) Splenectomy is indicated for the management of:

A) All injuries to the spleen

B) Some injuries to the spleen

C) All injuries to the liver

D) Some injuries to the liver

B – Non-operative management of spleen (and liver) injuries is more and more common. It's a technique nicely described as "sit on your scalpel." This means the surgery residents want to operate so bad they can't stand it, but if you give the kid fluids, blood products, and bed rest, an amazing percentage do not need to go to the operating room. Splenectomy refers to the spleen and not the liver, but you knew that, right?

29) Management of gastroenteritis (sometimes referred to as "P and P" or pukin' and poopin') commonly requires:

A) IV antibiotics and antifungals

B) Intubation and cardiac monitoring

C) Rehydration, time, and patience

D) Benadryl (diphenhydramine) and H_2 blockers

C – Thankfully, most cases of gastroenteritis can be managed with PO/NG/SQ/IV rehydration, time, and patience. In the United States, most cases are viral in origin and as such, antibiotics or antifungals are not appropriate. Gastroenteritis is rarely serious enough to require intubation or cardiac monitoring, while Benadryl (diphenhydramine) and H_2 blockers are indicated for allergic reactions, not anaphylaxis.

30) Currant jelly stool is a finding classically associated with which condition in children?

A) Intussusception

B) Pyloric stenosis

C) Volvulus

D) Constipation

A – Though it is only rarely to occasionally seen in real life practice, currant jelly stool is the answer of choice if the test question involves intussusception.

31) Intussusception is **best** described to parents as:

A) A twisting of the bowel

B) A rupture of the bowel

C) A "telescoping" of the bowel

D) A cancer of the bowel

C – The analogy of a telescope is commonly used to describe intussusception. Most children with intussusception are stable, and barium or air enemas not only confirm the diagnosis, but also can help push the bowel back to where it needs to be. Avoiding surgery in many cases is accomplished by simply confirming the diagnosis. A twisting bowel is typically referred to as a volvulus. If the child has signs of hypovolemic shock or peritonitis which are signs of their belly already being perforated or "perfed," they are unstable and probably should go directly to the operating room (without passing GO or collecting $200.) Cancers generally have "oma" in the name, i.e. hepatoblastoma.

32) A child with pyloric stenosis usually presents with:

A) Non-bilious, projectile vomiting

B) Constipation

C) Tarry stool

D) Rebound tenderness in the right lower quadrant

A – Projectile vomiting is the "textbook answer" for pyloric stenosis, just as "currant jelly stool" is the "textbook answer" for intussusception. However, it is important to take a good history from the parents to determine what they consider to be projectile vomiting. Unless it's Linda Blair remaking her memorable scene from "The Exorcist," it's just vomiting.

33) A newborn infant in the ED is being bag-mask ventilated, but you don't see adequate chest rise. Your next action should be to:

A) Increase the oxygen flow to 15 liters/minute

B) Listen for equal breath sounds

C) Check the seal between the infants face and the mask

D) Squeeze the bag harder

C – Remember, "bagging" with a face mask is not as easy as it looks. The preferred technique of "bagging" is to have one person place the mask on the child's face to find the "sweet spot," while the other person squeezes the bag. If the seal on the face is not the problem, then assessing for pneumothoraces or the need for increased inspiratory pressures may be warranted, but try the easy stuff first.

34) When administering chest compressions to a newborn, the depth of compressions should be:

A) 1/3 the anterior-posterior diameter of the chest

B) 1.5-2 inches

C) 2/3 the anterior-posterior diameter of the chest

D) The diameter of the infant's little finger (Make 'em "pinky" depth)

A – Though chest compressions are rarely required in neonatal resuscitation since "bagging" (positive pressure ventilation + oxygen) fixes just about everything. If compressions are required, the depth should be 1/3 the anterior-posterior diameter of the chest or more importantly, deep enough to produce a palpable pulse! The "Make 'em pinky" answer sounds cute, but relates more to determining the ETT size, than chest compressions.

35) When placing a mask on an infant for bag-mask ventilation, the mask should cover all of the following **except**:

A) Chin

B) Mouth

C) Nose

D) Eyes

D – This should be an easy one. Masks should be sized to cover the chin, mouth, and nose. They should not cover the eyes to avoid damage to the eyes and possible vagal responses. The rule is: "Bridge of the nose to the tip of the chin."

36) Thirty seconds after birth, a newborn's heart rate is 80 beats per minute. The suggested next step is:

A) SQ epinephrine unless an IV is available

B) Administer positive pressure ventilation

C) Chest compressions

D) External pacing

B – Remember that if just about everything bad that happens in babies is respiratory, then it follows that "bagging" fixes just about everything bad. Most infants become bradycardic due to "something respiratory" (like hypoxia,) and therefore positive pressure ventilation or "bagging," should be the first intervention. Recheck the heart rate after 30 seconds of "bagging" to see if further interventions are required.

37) The Apgar score is:

A) Useful for determining which resuscitation efforts to initiate

B) Useful for documenting impressions of the newborn and can help predict future medical issues

C) Useful for trauma documentation when the child is too young to appropriately use the Glasgow Coma Scale or the Trauma Severity Index

D) Comprised of Appearance, Work of Breathing, and Circulation

B – Apgar scores are nice for helping to predict future medical (especially neuro) issues, but should not supersede providing care for the newborn. Remember, resuscitate first; figure out numbers and scores later. DO NOT use the Apgar score to determine what needs to be immediately done in the ED. Appearance, Work of Breathing, and Circulation are elements of the Pediatric Assessment Triangle (PAT.)

38) All of the following are effective methods to help minimize heat loss in a term newborn **except**:

A) Prompt drying of the newborn, removing wet linens, and placing a hat on the baby

B) Placing the newborn under a preheated warmer or heat lamps

C) "Mist" the newborn infant with sterile saline heated to body temperature to simulate the prenatal environment

D) Wrapping the newborn in clear (not colored) plastic "Saran" wrap or placing the newborn feet first in a "Zip-Lock" bag

C – Nice idea, but remember that when babies are wet, they are cold. And babies can do all sorts of bad things when they get cold, especially stop breathing! Drying the baby off, wrapping the baby in dry blankets, and placing a hat of some sort (an actual baby hat or even a piece of stockinette will do) are the first priorities. Don't forget to get rid of the wet blankets. People are often so excited the baby popped out that they do a great job of drying the baby off, but then they keep the baby wrapped in the same wet linen. If an overhead warmer, isolette, or BabyPod with wrapped warm packs is available, great, use them. But if none are available, what about using the warmer for the first nine months of life, i.e. mom? If the baby is sick (or the mom is sick) and unable to remain on mom's chest or abdomen, many transport teams and nurseries now wrap the baby in clear plastic wrap or place the baby (feet first please!) in a Zip-Lock bag and zip the bag up at the armpits. It looks really odd, but it works and does a great job of keeping the heat and the moisture in!

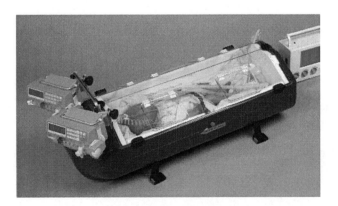

BabyPod II Infant Warmer

Photo courtesy of BabyPod

www.babypod.com

39) One of the **most** common causes of infant endotracheal tube migration is movement of the neck:

A) True

B) False

A – True – Baby's tracheas are much smaller and shorter than those of big kids, and therefore keeping the tube in the right spot is even more of a challenge. Moving their head and neck up or down can easily dislodge or "mainstem" an initially properly placed endotracheal tube. Remember, the tip of the tube follows the nose. Flexion of child's neck causes the tube to move down, while neck extension causes the tube to move up (and potentially out.)

Abdominal / Perinatal

40) Pain at McBurney's point is a sign of:

A) Meckel's diverticulum

B) Appendicitis

C) Hirshsprung's disease

D) Necrotizing enterocolitis

B – Right lower quadrant pain, specifically at McBurney's point, is one of the hallmark signs of appendicitis.

41) A 2-year-old with colicky abdominal pain, vomiting, and currant jelly stool may have which of the following?

A) Ingested foreign body

B) Pyloric stenosis

C) Intussusception

D) Constipation

C – The combo of 2-year-old with the infamous "currant jelly stool" is intussusception until proven otherwise. Again, it's one of those key words to make correctly answering the question easier.

42) Medications such as Imodium (loperamide) or Lomotil (diphenoxylate and atropine) are indicated in the emergency department treatment of:

A) Pediatric gastroenteritis

B) Endocarditis

C) Pyloric stenosis

D) None of the above

D – None of the above. Time and fluids are where it's at for gastroenteritis in kids. Anti-diarrheals, such as Imodium AD or Lomotil, are not recommended for children due to numerous side effects. As most cases are viral, the diarrhea will get better with time. The key is to keep them hydrated until it "passes." With this in mind, especially if oral dissolving Zofran (ondansetron) is given in the ED, the majority of children can tolerate oral rehydration therapy (50-100ml/kg over 4 hours) and do not require IV fluids or hospital admission. Antibiotics are appropriate for endocarditis and surgery is the treatment for pyloric stenosis.

43) Appendicitis may be diagnosed by all of the following methods **except**:

A) Abdominal ultrasound

B) Abdominal CT scan

C) 3-view abdominal series

D) Physical exam

Certified Pediatric Emergency Nurse (CPEN) Review IV

C – Plain radiographs can help to demonstrate problems such as free air or bowel obstructions, but are not commonly used to diagnose appendicitis. How appendicitis is diagnosed will depend on which medical center you work at and the surgeons/radiologists you work with. Many children's centers are now diagnosing appendicitis via ultrasound and/or CT scanning, however, the tried and true method of physical examination is still considered to be a valid method of diagnosis. Remember that when dealing with kids, referred abdominal pain from other causes (such as strep throat or pneumonia) can cause "it sounds like an appey" pain.

44) A potential sign of gastroesophageal reflux disease (GERD) is apnea:

A) True

B) False

A - True - GERD, or reflux of the stomach contents into the esophagus, can present with various signs including vomiting, choking, abdominal pain, irritability, and yes, even apnea. That is why the initial workup for an apparent life-threatening event (ALTE) or brief resolved unexpected event (BRUE) includes evaluation for GERD.

45) Which of the following statements is **not** true concerning pediatric gastroenteritis?

A) It is one of the leading causes of dehydration

B) Water should be encouraged to rehydrate the child

C) It is most commonly viral in nature, so antibiotics are not generally part of the treatment. In fact, antibiotics may be part of the cause.

D) It is still a significant cause of death in children worldwide

B – Oral Rehydration Solutions (ORS) such as Pedialyte, Infalyte, and Naturalyte, not water, are the "beverages of choice" when treating pediatric gastroenteritis.

46) Rehydration in a child with severe dehydration due to gastroenteritis might include:

A) One or more IV boluses (20ml/kg) of normal saline or LR

B) One or more IV boluses (20ml/kg) of D5/.45NS

C) Normal saline, wide open, until normal urine output returns

D) One of more IV boluses (40ml/kg) of normal saline or LR

A– In cases of severe dehydration where IV fluids are ordered, the only appropriate fluid choices are normal saline or LR and they are given in boluses of 20ml/kg. Remember with children, fluid boluses are always "something per kilo" and the magic number is 20. Save the sugar for maintenance fluids. In cases where dehydration is not severe, we know that there are other ways to give fluids without placing an IV. Sips of liquids, especially Oral Rehydration Solutions (ORS) at the start of every TV commercial, Pedialyte popsicles, nasogastric, or subcutaneous fluids (www.hylenex.com) can be very effective. If the child is exhibiting signs of severe dehydration, certainly IV rehydration is appropriate. However, especially if anti-emetics such as Zofran (ondansetron) are given, many children may not require IV placement for rehydration.

47) Failure to thrive (FTT) is thought to result from:

A) Infant organic disease

B) Dysfunctional parenting behaviors and/or disturbed parent-child interactions

C) Subtle neurological or behavioral problems

D) All of the above

D – Traditionally, FTT was thought to primarily result from disturbances in the parent-child interactions; however, there are several other physical causes as well. The causes of FTT are now categorized as: 1) Inadequate caloric intake, 2) Inadequate absorption, 3) Increased metabolism, or 4) Defective utilization. In most cases, the etiology of FTT is multifactorial and a multidisciplinary approach is required for proper diagnosis and management.

48) A 12-year-old hysterical, uncircumcised male presents to the ED with his penis stuck in his pants zipper. The **most** appropriate nursing action would be:

A) Carefully unzip the zipper after a local anesthetic has been administered

B) Carefully unzip the zipper as no anesthesia is required

C) Carefully cut the zipper around the injury which allows the tracks to separate

D) Prepare the patient for emergency circumcision

C – In most cases, if the zipper is cut below the foreskin, the tracks will separate and anesthesia/surgery is not required. Attempting to unzip the zipper first will likely cause more damage and pain. Circumcisions are certainly not required for this injury.

49) Which statement regarding urethral trauma is **true**?

A) Urethral trauma is difficult to diagnose because it is commonly painless

B) An indwelling urinary catheter (Foley catheter) should be inserted as soon as possible to maintain urethral patency

C) A suprapubic catheter may be required to divert urine away from the traumatized tissues

D) The patient typically suffers urinary incontinence as a result of sphincter damage

C – Think about where the urethra is. It's between the bladder and the urinary meatus (opening on the outside.) If there is an injury to the urethra, such as with a bicycle riding injury, suprapubic catheter placement may be required to allow for the drainage of urine and healing/surgical repair of the traumatized tissues. Urethral trauma hurts, and it hurts really, really bad. Please remember that blindly inserting a Foley catheter can turn a partial-tear into a completely transected urethra, so when urethral trauma is suspected, leave the Foley on the cart until the patient has been evaluated by urology.

Certified Pediatric Emergency Nurse (CPEN) Review IV

50) Anuria is a common symptom of all of the following **except**:

A) Urethral injury

B) Bladder injury

C) Acute renal failure (ARF)

D) Hyperglycemia

D – A symptom of hyperglycemia is polyuria, or the opposite of anuria. The medical prefix "A" means "none", and "uria" means "pee coming out". So, anuria means no pee coming out. Each of the remaining answers above can result in "no pee coming out" as the problem can be with not making urine (ARF), holding the urine (bladder), or allowing the urine to come out (urethral injury.)

51) In the pediatric ED, signs and symptoms of epididymitis may be easily confused with those of:

A) Priapism

B) Urinary tract infection (UTI)

C) Testicular torsion

D) Pyelonephritis

C – Epididymitis, or an inflammation of the testicles, can commonly present with symptoms similar to those of testicular torsion, so at the initial assessment, it can easily be confusing. Classically, if elevation of the testes provides relief from pain, epididymitis is more likely. However, if elevation of the testes causes increased pain, torsion is more likely. Either way, ultrasound imaging is commonly emergently performed to determine the true cause of the pain.

52) A 15-year-old male is brought to the ED after being involved in a fight involving baseball bats (he lost) with subsequent blunt trauma to the right flank. Chief complaint is right flank tenderness and bruising is noted to the flank and lower back. Urine dip reveals microscopic hematuria, however, other laboratory studies and vital signs are amazingly normal. Workup for this patient will most likely involve a high suspicion of:

A) Pulled muscles

B) Fractured pelvis

C) Retroperitoneal bleeding

D) Liver laceration

C – Remember there are two parts of the abdomen; the front (peritoneum) and the back (retroperitoneum.) Renal trauma can certainly cause hematuria, but more importantly, bruising around the flank (Grey-Turner's sign) and the mechanism of injury leads one to suspect a possible retroperitoneal bleed.

Certified Pediatric Emergency Nurse (CPEN) Review IV

53) An afebrile, 13-year-old male comes to the ED complaining of sudden onset of 20/10 pain to the testicular area, after a water skiing accident earlier that afternoon. The pain increases with elevation of the scrotum, radiates to the flank, and is accompanied by vomiting. The patient **most** likely has what condition?

A) Sexually transmitted disease

B) Pregnancy

C) Acute epididymitis

D) Testicular torsion

D – Though evaluation by nuclear medicine or ultrasound studies is quickly going to be undertaken, the fact that the patient is afebrile and the pain increases with scrotal elevation sounds much more like torsion, than epididymitis. STD's can happen, even in 13-year-olds, but the history points us elsewhere. Pregnancy in 13-year-old males remains remarkably rare.

54) Anticipated therapies for the child with a testicular torsion would include all the following **except**:

A) IV anti-emetics

B) Immediate orchiectomy

C) Cold packs to the scrotum

D) IV analgesics

B – Children with this condition are commonly in so much pain, that they are actively vomiting, "praying for death," or even suggesting that you just "cut them off!" The later would not be an appropriate intervention in the ED. Aggressive management of the vomiting and pain is appropriate. Cold packs can be used to decrease pain and edema. The goal is to make the diagnosis and intervene quickly to avoid the need for orchiectomy, or surgical removal of the testicle.

55) A 12-year-old with history of chronic renal failure and continuous ambulatory peritoneal dialysis (CAPD) presents with complaints of abdominal pain. While in the ED, the dialysate solution is difficult to drain from the abdomen. Appropriate nursing interventions to facilitate drainage include:

A) Repositioning the patient frequently from side to side

B) Syringe aspiration of fluid from the catheter

C) Flush the catheter with a heparinized syringe

D) Instilling a liter of warmed dialysate fluid

A – Repositioning the patient from side to side can sometimes allow the catheter to slightly reposition as well and results in increased dialysate drainage. Remember, when working with CAPD catheters, just like central lines, the less "breaks in the system," the better. Infusing additional fluid into a patient who is having trouble draining what's in there already doesn't make a lot of sense, nor does heparin for abdominal dialysate drainage.

Certified Pediatric Emergency Nurse (CPEN) Review IV

56) The previous patient with abdominal pain and CAPD use should also be evaluated for:

A) Periodontitis

B) Peritonitis

C) Perianal cystitis

D) Pericarditis

B – Yes, it starts with "peri" and ends with "it is," but don't be confused. Children on peritoneal dialysis with abdominal pain have peritonitis. And if they don't have peritonitis, they are getting peritonitis. And if they aren't getting peritonitis, it's because they are thinking about getting peritonitis. Certainly, evaluation for other causes of abdominal pain is appropriate, but an incredibly high percentage of these kids with CAPD and abdominal complaints have peritonitis.

57) A 14-year-old previously healthy female presents to the ED with dysuria, fever, and urinary frequency. She has lower abdominal/suprapubic tenderness upon palpation, but has no flank pain or costovertebral angle (CVA) tenderness. A tentative diagnosis of UTI is made. Which assessment finding is **not** a common characteristic of UTIs?

A) Dysuria

B) Non-menstrual vaginal bleeding

C) Hyperglycemia

D) Many bacteria and WBCs, positive nitrites, small blood, and no ketones in the urinalysis

B – Except for vaginal bleeding, for which a pelvic exam and pregnancy test should be done, all of the above in a healthy young female are the classic signs/symptoms of an uncomplicated UTI. However, if the patient were to look sick, have flank/costovertebral angle tenderness, or vomiting; that would lead one to consider pyelonephritis (infected kidneys) rather than just a simple UTI.

58) A 16-year-old with a 14-year history of poorly controlled, insulin dependent diabetes presents to the ED with acute shortness of breath. Physical exam reveals hypertension, generalized edema, and mid/lower lobe rales bilaterally. ECG shows sinus tachycardia with peaked T waves. Renal labs reveal BUN 70 mg/dl, creatinine 6.8 mg/dl, and potassium of 6.5 mEq/l. A diagnosis of acute renal failure is made. The tall, peaked T waves on the patient's ECG are indicative of:

A) Hypernatremia

B) Hyponatremia

C) Hypokalemia

D) Hyperkalemia

D – Hyperkalemia is too much potassium in the blood. The cascade from diabetes to renal failure takes patients to the place where they have problems with "pee." "Pee" begins with the letter "P." Potassium also begins with "P". So when you think of renal failure and the bad things that can potentially kill the child, you should think potassium. With the classic ECG finding of "P"eaked T waves. It's all about the "P"!

59) Anticipated therapies for the above patient with a serum potassium level of 6.8 mEq/l would include:

A) Boluses of IV dextrose and insulin

B) Boluses of IV calcium chloride or calcium gluconate

C) PO/NG Kayexalate (sodium polystyrene sulfonate) and albuterol nebulizers

D) All of the above

D – In the emergency setting, the goals of emergently treating hyperkalemia are two-fold. First, quickly bring the potassium level down. Then second, keep the potassium level down. Insulin helps to bring dextrose into the cells and potassium "piggybacks" with both of them into the cell. Calcium can be given, especially if the patient is hemodynamically unstable, to help protect and maintain cardiac function. Kayexalate is given to make the patient poop, and that's a good thing because it pulls potassium into the poop. How do you remember this? Kayexalate begins with "K" and the chemical symbol for potassium is "K." (You probably also remember that hyper or hypokalemia is also about the potassium.) In pediatric emergency medicine, albuterol has many applications. It not only helps wheezers, but can lower potassium levels as well.

60) EMS arrives at the ED with a 3-year-old with altered mental status, jaundice, and increased abdominal girth. He has a history of biliary atresia requiring a living-related donor liver transplant. The physician diagnoses probable hepatic encephalopathy. To reduce the ammonia level, the nurse would anticipate the administration of rectal:

A) Kayexalate

B) Lactulose

C) Albuterol

D) Tylenol

B – Lactulose. It's nice when the letters give you a hint. Lactulose begins with "L" and so does "L"iver. Hepatic refers to liver, so follow the "L."

61) A 16-year-old male who was involved in a high speed motor vehicle collision is brought to the ED. The patient is alert and complains of severe abdominal pain. The nurse notes blood oozing from his urethra. He is diagnosed with genitourinary trauma and urology is consulted. Which component(s) of the history lead the nurse to suspect a pelvic fracture?

A) Blood at the urethral meatus

B) Mechanism of injury

C) Pain upon light palpation to the pelvis

D) All of the above

D – Each of the above findings is commonly associated with pelvic fractures, especially pain with palpation of the pelvis. If it doesn't hurt, did they break it? Probably not. In an unconscious patient who can't tell you "it hurts," evaluating mechanism of injury and likely potential injuries is crucial. Blood at the urethral meatus or a "high riding" prostate are the other classic signs of a pelvic fracture.

Certified Pediatric Emergency Nurse (CPEN) Review IV

62) A 17-year-old girl presents to the ED after losing consciousness at home. She is now alert and oriented, hypotensive with a BP of 84/48 and complains of body aches and fever 104F (40C.) History reveals she finished her last menstrual period two days prior and uses super-absorbent tampons each month. The nurse would suspect the **most** likely diagnosis is:

A) Ectopic pregnancy

B) STD

C) Toxic shock syndrome (TSS)

D) Endometriosis

C – Toxic shock syndrome. Again, it's one of the key word association questions. If you see "super-absorbent tampons" in the question, think toxic shock syndrome as the answer. Could it be something else? Sure. But for the most likely answer, pick TSS.

63) What are the 3 classic symptoms associated with toxic shock syndrome?

A) Hypotension, fever, and diffuse rash

B) Hypertension, fever, and rash

C) Menses, hypotension, and LOC changes

D) Swollen spleen, swollen liver, and swollen tongue

A – The American Academy of Pediatrics defines toxic shock syndrome as when four of the following five criteria are met:

1) Sudden onset of fever of 102F (39C) or higher

2) Diffuse red rash

3) Desquamation (peeling) of skin, especially palms and soles, 1-2 weeks post-onset of illness

4) Hypotension

5) Multisystem organ issues

In addition, cultures of blood/CSF must be negative for anything except for Staph. Aureus.

Approximately 40% of the cases of TSS involve menstruating women. However, it has also been associated with sinusitis, pneumonia, catheter site infections, skin infections, post-op wound infections, and nasal packing in both women and men across the lifespan.

64) A 14-year-old girl presents to the ED with a complaint of vaginal discharge and painful urination for two days. She admits to being sexually active and her urine pregnancy test in the ED is negative. A diagnosis of STD is made. The nurse knows that anyone presumed to be infected with gonorrhea also should be tested for:

A) Chlamydia

B) Human immunodeficiency virus (HIV)

C) Syphilis

D) Herpes

A – Gonorrhea (GC) and chlamydia go hand in hand in emergency medicine. If you are going to test for one, you should test for the other as well. Depending upon physical examination and history findings, testing and treatment for HIV, syphilis, and herpes can also be performed. Whatever treatment is undertaken, in those who claim to be sexually active or not sexually active, urine pregnancy testing should be performed as pregnancy can definitely alter the treatment options.

65) A 13-year-old female is brought by EMS to the ED and states "I was raped." Her clothes are torn and she is visibly trembling and tearful. The patient is escorted by a nurse to a private room and the on-call sexual assault nurse examiner (SANE) is paged. The ED nurse knows that the most important message to convey to any assault victim includes:

A) The patient is now in a safe environment

B) All medical tests will be kept confidential

C) The examinations will be done as quickly/painlessly as possible

D) Medications are available to prevent possible STDs

A – Safety is probably the patient's first concern, so that is the message that should be conveyed first and foremost. Though all of the answers are appropriate and should be addressed, initially the most important message to the patient is that she is now safe. The availability of SANE nurses in pediatric and adult emergency care has truly been an asset for the staff, patients, and law enforcement.

66) When obtaining the initial history, it is important to determine if the patient has done any of the following **except**:

A) Urinated or defecated

B) Changed clothes

C) Dated the alleged attacker

D) Rinsed her mouth

C – Asking about prior contacts is inappropriate at this point. All of the other information is important in terms of evidence collection. If possible, it is preferred that the victim not urinate, defecate, change clothes, wash, shower, or even rinse her mouth prior to the collection of evidence. In addition to caring for the patient's medical and psychological needs, the goal in the ED is also to assist with the collection of forensic evidence. Regardless of what the patient may have done or not done, the forensic exam and evidence collection (commonly called a "rape kit") should be performed.

67) Which actions should be done when collecting this young patient's clothing?

A) Have the victim place all of her clothing together in one plastic bag

B) Have the victim fold each piece of clothing inside out and place each piece of clothing in a separate paper bag

C) Have the victim place all pieces of clothing together in one paper bag

D) Discard any clothing that may have been removed during the assault

Certified Pediatric Emergency Nurse (CPEN) Review IV

B – You may have a choice (paper or plastic?) at the grocery store checkout line, but when it comes to forensics in the ED, paper is the correct answer. Furthermore, the preferred method is to have the victim, not the nurse (we try to minimize extra fingerprints and trace evidence,) place each piece of clothing into a separate paper bag. Plastic bags can trap moisture which can potentially degrade the evidence. All clothing, not just those items with confirmed physical contact with the assailant, should be collected.

68) EMS calls with a 3-minute ETA for a 15-year-old, pregnant female involved in a high-speed, non-restrained motor vehicle collision. What would make the nurse **most** suspect possible abruptio placentae?

A) Painless vaginal bleeding

B) Mechanism of injury

C) Severe abdominal pain

D) B and C

D – Abruptio placentae occurs when the placenta has been torn <u>abruptly</u> from the uterus. Anytime something is torn, expect <u>pain</u>. And what can cause that abrupt tearing? Trauma, cocaine use, maternal hypertension, cigarette smoking, and alcohol consumption are among the more common causes. In this case, we have significant trauma in the form of an unrestrained person in a motor vehicle collision. The mechanism of injury in this trauma, along with the pain, point to the suspected diagnosis.

69) A 13-year-old female has just delivered a healthy newborn in the pediatric ED. She continues to have active vaginal bleeding beyond what is expected. Initial nursing intervention of choice would be:

A) Massage the fundus

B) Start a peripheral IV and infuse D5.2NS

C) Monitor the fetal heart rate

D) Position the patient on her left side

A – Post-partum hemorrhage, which is what this patient is experiencing, is commonly caused by a "boggy" uterus. Fundal massage or massaging the uterus is the initial intervention of choice to allow the uterus to "clamp down" and hopefully the bleeding will slow down or stop. If uterine massage is ineffective, medications such as Pitocin (oxytocin) may be added to the IV fluids to help with uterine contraction. Though D5.2NS is usually the maintenance fluid of choice for infants and toddlers, in this case, hemorrhage, not maintenance fluids, is the issue. Boluses of LR or 0.9NS would be administered if needed. Monitoring the fetal heart rate is not an issue as the baby is out of mom, and left side positioning is great before delivery, but not so important afterwards.

70) Signs of pre-eclampsia include all of the following **except**:

A) Proteinuria

B) Hypertension

C) Generalized edema

D) Increased urine output

D – Decreased or no urine output is a sign of pre-eclampsia. The pregnancy triad of hypertension (>140/90 mm Hg), proteinuria, and generalized edema are classic signs associated with pre-eclampsia. Many women experience dependent edema, especially in the ankles and feet, and this should not be confused with the "all over" edema which is present in pre-eclampsia.

71) The differentiating factor between pre-eclampsia and eclampsia is when:

A) The mother has a seizure

B) The edema resolves with rest and elevation

C) The mother's face becomes edematous

D) Diastolic pressure exceeds 100 mmHg

A – Quite simply, a seizure after pre-eclampsia defines eclampsia. So the goal in managing pre-eclampsia is to prevent the patient from becoming eclamptic, or having a seizure. Though there certainly are maternal risks with having a seizure, the bigger issue is the very real danger that they baby will become very sick or even die as a result of the mother's seizure. Pre-eclampsia is managed with decreased stimulation (turning lights down and closing doors for light and noise control), but also magnesium sulfate IV (bolus over 20 minutes, then continuous IV infusion.) Remember that magnesium sulfate may not stop mom actively having a seizure, but hopefully it keeps her from having a seizure. If she is actively seizing, benzodiazepines such as Valium (diazepam), Versed (midazolam), or Ativan (lorazepam) should be used to stop the seizure.

72) The pre-eclamptic patient receiving IV magnesium sulfate should be closely monitored for:

A) Hypotension

B) Polyuria

C) Respiratory depression

D) Pre-term labor

C – Magnesium sulfate is being given to "chill out" the central nervous system (CNS) and the muscles so she doesn't have a seizure. However, if the CNS or muscles (especially the diaphragm) gets too mellow (from too much magnesium), the main complication we worry about is that her body will forget to breathe. It's useful to remember that before she stops breathing, her deep tendon reflexes will progressively decrease. This is why you see OB nurses carrying reflex hammers in their scrub pockets. If the patient is getting too much "mag," you want to catch this when their reflexes are changing, not when she stops breathing. If respiratory depression or arrest does occur, like with any other patient, "bag" them with supplemental oxygen. While you are "bagging," IV calcium chloride or calcium gluconate can be administered to reverse the effects of hypermagnesemia. These patients get Foley urinary catheters to monitor urinary output, because we need to make sure the magnesium that is going in, is also going out. But as usual, airway and breathing are the first priorities.

73) An obviously pregnant 15-year-old presents to the peds ED with a chief complaint of painless vaginal bleeding for 2 hours. Physical examination finds a soft, non-tender abdomen, and a fetal heart rate of 140. The nurse suspects the patient **most** likely has:

A) Placenta previa

B) Hemophilia

C) Spontaneous miscarriage

D) Abruptio placentae

A – Placenta previa is characterized by painless vaginal bleeding, as opposed to abruptio placentae, which typically is painful, as any tearing usually is. Miscarriages or spontaneous abortions commonly are associated with abdominal cramping. Care of this patient is also care of the baby, so we need to be particularly mindful of how the baby is doing. It is also important to remember that nothing, not even fingers to determine dilation, should be "blindly" inserted into the vagina. Doing so can induce further bleeding. If vaginal examinations outside of Labor and Delivery must be done, use of a sterile speculum or ultrasound is recommended.

74) A 14-year-old female complains of severe lower abdominal pain that began this morning. Last menstrual period (LMP) was 2-months ago and current vital signs are BP 80/40, HR 120, RR 24, and Temperature 98.9F (37.2C.) Fluid resuscitation is begun, a Foley catheter is placed, and routine laboratory studies, including a Type and Screen are sent. To no surprise, the urine HGC is positive. Therefore which diagnosis does the nurse suspect while awaiting ultrasound confirmation?

A) Acute appendicitis

B) Acute bowel obstruction

C) Incomplete spontaneous abortion

D) Ectopic pregnancy

D – This patient is exhibiting the textbook signs of an ectopic pregnancy. She has severe lower abdominal pain and a positive urine HCG. Aggressive fluid resuscitation should be initiated, and this should be treated as a surgical emergency because even with early diagnosis and treatment, the maternal mortality rate can be quite high.

75) In pediatric blunt abdominal trauma, which internal organs are typically injured?

A) Liver and spleen

B) Liver and stomach

C) Stomach and kidneys

D) Bowel and bladder

A – In pediatric trauma, the liver and spleen are the two most commonly injured organs after the head. Though bowel, bladder, and other organs certainly can be affected, if the trauma is to the abdomen, bet on the liver and spleen.

76) A 6-month-old child is referred to the ED from the pediatrician's office with a diagnosis of rule-out volvulus. The ED nurse knows that this patient should be:

A) Given an oral fluid challenge

B) Triaged as a very high priority

C) Referred to a pediatric neurologist

D) Kept in strict isolation

B – Volvulus, most commonly caused from malrotation, is a life-threatening condition and must be triaged that way. It is caused by the intestine partially or completely twisting around itself, and can quickly result in intestinal necrosis, peritonitis, perforation, and death! The diagnosis is made through a history of bilious vomiting, acute and constant abdominal pain, signs of peritoneal irritation (if perforated), and upper GI series.

Certified Pediatric Emergency Nurse (CPEN) Review IV

77) Dustyn, a 15-year old female, presents to the Pediatric ED after striking her abdomen on the edge of the trampoline. What test might you expect to be repeated multiple times either in the ED or upon admission?

A) Urinalysis

B) Hemoglobin and hematocrit

C) Abdominal x-ray

D) Amylase

B – Repeated hemoglobin and hematocrit would be expected since the initial findings in a patient with acute blood loss can be normal until the patient's volume has equalized (with a subsequent drop in hemoglobin and hematocrit.) Urinalysis is often performed as a screening test for abdominal or genitourinary trauma, and if gross hematuria is noted, the test would not need to be repeated. There is ongoing controversy regarding the importance of microscopic hematuria in patients with blunt abdominal trauma and no other symptoms or signs of urinary tract injury. Placement of a urinary catheter alone may cause microscopic hematuria of no consequence. Plain radiographs may occasionally demonstrate signs of intra-abdominal injury (i.e. elevated hemidiaphragm, displaced gastric bubble or free abdominal gas); however, they are neither sensitive nor specific for these injuries. Elevated serum amylase may indicate intra-abdominal injury, but is not trauma specific and is much more likely to be due to a medical condition.

78) A 5-year old girl arrives to the emergency department via ambulance. She complains of pain in her abdomen and chest that goes towards her neck. She is afebrile, slightly short of breath and has difficulty swallowing. After speaking with her mother, you find out that the babysitter tried to force the child to eat lunch by pushing the food into her mouth and forcing it down her throat. What injury might you suspect?

A) Cardiac tamponade

B) Cardiac contusion

C) Esophageal perforation

D) Pneumonia

C – Inflicted esophageal perforation can result from foreign body ingestions, caustic ingestions, blunt external trauma and penetrating external trauma. Cardiac contusion (blunt cardiac injury) and cardiac tamponade are injuries commonly resulting from blunt chest trauma. Common causes of blunt chest trauma include rapid deceleration injuries such as motor vehicle crashes which result in the impact of the chest against the interior of a vehicle or vehicle ejection and fall injuries. There is no evidence in the question to suggest a chest injury or pneumonia. In this question, there is a specific history of food being forced down the patient's throat which, when coupled with abdominal and chest pain (the esophagus is in your chest after all) should clue you in as to the correct answer.

79) A 14-year old female presents to the ED with her parents. Her chief complaint is heavy vaginal bleeding. She denies any significant medical/surgical history, current illicit drug use, being sexually active or current abdominal pain. Upon exam, the clinician notes moderate, thick, dark vaginal bleeding, a swollen perineum and a large mass about the size of a grapefruit in the abdomen around the umbilicus. The **most** likely diagnosis for this patient is:

A) Uterine carcinoma

B) A first trimester spontaneous abortion

C) Bleeding uterine fibroid

D) A normal post-partum assessment

D – These findings are normal after a normal spontaneous vaginal delivery; notably a moderate amount of dark thick vaginal bleeding (lochia rubra), a swollen perineum (from the delivery of the baby) and grapefruit sized mass in the abdomen (post-partum uterus as it clamps down on itself.) The fact that the patient denies being sexually active means NOTHING, especially with her parents present with her at the bedside. Uterine cancer is uncommon in teens, and while vaginal bleeding may be present, the perineum will not be swollen. Spontaneous first trimester abortions may have vaginal bleeding, but will not present with a swollen perineum or a uterine mass. Uterine fibroids certainly may have vaginal bleeding, but are usually accompanied by abdominal pain and there would be no reason for the perineum to be swollen with uterine fibroids. * CRUCIAL NOTE: Immediately contact the ED charge nurse, house supervisor and/or social services. There is an immediate need to locate the infant!

80) A 14-year old patient is 34-weeks pregnant and presents to the ED complaining of "feeling wet down there." She has yellow/green vaginal discharge with a strong odor, a fever of 102.2°F (39.0°C), and diffuse uterine tenderness to palpation. Though she will go probably go straight to L&D, the Pediatric ED nurse knows the **most** likely cause for this presentation is:

A) Spontaneous rupture of membranes with chorioamnionitis

B) Pelvic inflammatory disease (PID)

C) Sexually transmitted disease (STD)

D) Infected ovarian cysts

A – Spontaneous rupture of membranes with chorioamnionitis ("chorio") is the most likely cause for the presentation. When the two layers of the amniotic bag (the amnion and chorion) become infected, they produce a vaginal discharge that has a very strong and unpleasant odor. Further evidence leading to this conclusion is the uterine tenderness on palpation. There may even be contractions present as the maternal host attempts to protect itself from the infected pregnancy. Pelvic inflammatory disease is possible, but very uncommon during pregnancy. The ascending infections from the vagina that might normally travel up through the uterus into the fallopian tubes are mechanically blocked by the presence of the mucus plug in the cervix. STDs certainly may present with foul smelling vaginal discharge, but are rarely associated with fever. Infected ovarian cysts are very uncommon.

81) An obese 16-year old female presents to the ED with chief complaints of shoulder pain, a terrible stomach ache and vaginal spotting. Which bedside lab is **most** important to run FIRST?

A) Fingerstick glucose

B) Blood or urine HCG (human chorionic gonadotropin)

C) Hemoglobin and hematocrit (H&H)

D) Urinalysis (UA)

B – HCG is the correct answer because the "common wisdom" is that all women between the ages of 12 and 50 who present to the ED are considered pregnant until proven otherwise. Determining pregnancy may very well impact many other treatment decisions. In addition, this patient's presenting symptoms are classic for a ruptured ectopic pregnancy. Her obesity makes it more likely that her menses are irregular, reducing the reliability of the date of her last period as a predictor of pregnancy. The patient's obesity may also hide external signs of uterine enlargement. The shoulder pain is most likely Kehr's sign (referred shoulder pain caused by peritoneal irritation from blood) caused by the ruptured ectopic. The presence of a "stomach ache" is a vague complaint, and may be abdominal pain also caused by the condition. Ruptured

Certified Pediatric Emergency Nurse (CPEN) Review IV

ectopic pregnancies are true surgical emergencies and must be aggressively managed. Adolescents in diabetic ketoacidosis (DKA) often present with abdominal pain of unknown etiology, but DKA is not associated with vaginal spotting and shoulder pain. Hemoglobin and hematocrit are important, but other earlier signs of impending shock such as skin parameters, capillary refill time, and tachycardia can clue you in to possible blood loss quickly and easily. Urinalysis is also helpful, as it can assess for signs of urinary tract infection or blood in the urine; however, there is nothing in a positive UA that can kill you. A missed ruptured ectopic can definitely kill you, so remember the first law of ED and pregnancy… Every female between 12 and 50 is pregnant until proven otherwise!

82) A 3-year old patient with a history of sickle cell disease presents with a distended and rigid abdomen, anemia, shock, and a palpable mass in the left upper quadrant. These clinical findings likely represent:

A) Aplastic crisis

B) Acute mesenteric infarction

C) Splenic sequestration crisis

D) Acute hepatic infarction

C – These findings strongly suggest splenic sequestration crisis. In splenic sequestration, the sickled red blood cells (RBCs) become trapped in the small vessels of the spleen (left upper quadrant), resulting in blood being trapped in the spleen. As this happens, the spleen enlarges with non-circulating blood, explaining the above symptoms. The liver (hopefully found in the right upper quadrant) should not be palpable in the left upper quadrant and mesenteric infarcts generally do not cause the formation of masses. While aplastic anemia can occur in the sickle cell patient, it does not present as described. It is important to note that not all splenic infarcts result in this sort of crisis. Children with sickle cell disease may actually become functionally asplenic by the age of 4 or 5 due to chronic/recurrent asymptomatic splenic infarcts. This sets them up for increased risk of infection by encapsulated bacteria such as Streptococcus pneumoniae and Hemophilus influenza.

83) You are caring for a lethargic 8-month old patient with a few hours of vomiting and dark red, mucous, jelly-like stools, as well as intermittent intense crying since early morning. You suspect:

A) Fecal impaction

B) Toxic mega colon

C) Intussusception

D) Appendicitis

C – This patient is presenting with classic signs and symptoms of intussusception: Vomiting, episodic severe abdominal pain and dark red "currant jelly" stools. Intussusception is the "telescoping" and incarceration of one segment of bowel into another. It occurs most commonly at the ileocecal junction (right lower quadrant), where the small bowel transitions into the colon. Needless to say, this is very irritating to the intestines! Similar to an incarcerated inguinal hernia, the edema caused by intussusception can cut off circulation to the affected segment of the gut. This causes necrosis of the gut and represents a surgical emergency, with a high mortality rate if left untreated. After all, we are talking about obstruction and the death of a segment of bowel. Texts will list one of the signs of intussusception as a sausage-shaped mass in the area of the obstruction; however, this may not be found that commonly. The "currant jelly" stool is a result of intestinal bleeding secondary to bowel ischemia. It's a relatively late sign, often absent at the time of diagnosis. Abdominal ultrasound is the diagnostic tool of choice. An air or barium enema will often reduce the intussusception and resolve the problem, but the chance of success lessens as time passes from the onset of symptoms. All intussusceptions not reducible by enema must be reduced surgically.

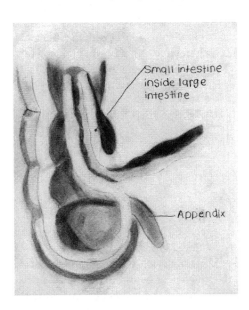

Intussusception

Courtesy of Nina DeBoer, my then 12-year old aspiring artist/baker daughter

www.ninasbeliciousbakery.com

84) Parents present to the emergency department with a lethargic, full-term, 18-day old infant with a history of two days of projectile vomiting. Upon physical exam, you note a sunken anterior fontanel, dry mucosa and poor skin turgor. You appropriately suspect:

A) Splenic engorgement

B) Pyloric stenosis

C) Intussusception

D) Necrotizing entercolitis (NEC)

B – These are classic signs and symptoms of pyloric stenosis. This is a condition where the pyloric sphincter is way too narrow or stenotic (hence the term pyloric stenosis) and hinders stomach contents from passing into the intestines. The stenosis occurs because the pyloric muscle becomes hypertrophied, bulging both inward and outward. With limited or no absorption taking place, this child is dehydrated and becoming shocky (lethargic). This case represents an extreme presentation of pyloric stenosis. Many infants are brought for evaluation before they become dehydrated simply because the projectile vomiting can be quite dramatic. In these cases it's the history that often leads to the performance of a pyloric ultrasound and the diagnosis. The presence of an olive-shaped mass in the epigastrium (the outwardly-bulging pyloric muscle) is a classic sign of pyloric stenosis; however, the diagnosis is now often made before the mass is big enough to be palpable. The big clue as to the correct answer is projectile vomiting. Pyloric stenosis beings with "P" and the vomiting is "P"rojectile. Splenic engorgement would not cause these symptoms. Intussusception is uncommon in children younger than 6-9 months. NEC can certainly cause vomiting and a very ill-appearing child, but it's quite uncommon, especially outside of the Neonatal ICU setting.

85) A 22-month old child presents to the Pediatric ED with the mother stating, "I think he might have swallowed a coin." The child is alert, interactive, lying down, pink and not drooling and exhibits no respiratory distress. A chest X-ray shows what appears to be a coin in his stomach. Based on the above information, the nurse should anticipate the next interventions to be:

A) Discharge home

B) Laryngoscopy

C) Bronchoscopy

D) Endoscopy

A – If the coin has made it past the esophagus into the stomach, the old adage that "this too will pass" will probably hold true. An ingested metallic foreign body is most often diagnosed via X-rays, but some emergency departments use hand-held metal detectors, similar to those used by airport security, to ascertain the position of the coin. If it is at the stomach or below, the child has no need for X-ray exposure. If the child was exhibiting respiratory distress, laryngoscopy and/or bronchoscopy should be anticipated. If a coin remains impacted in the esophagus (usually at the level of the second thoracic vertebra where the esophagus is narrowest), endoscopy may be needed to push coin into the stomach or remove it via the way it got in there (the mouth). In some facilities, surgeons or ED physicians pass a Foley catheter through the mouth, past the coin in the esophagus, using fluoroscopy. The balloon of the catheter is then inflated and the catheter is pulled out, hopefully bringing the coin with it. This can be a quick procedure, done without sedation or anesthesia, but it obviously has its own potential complications and should be done only by experienced staff with an abundance of caution. This question specifically addressed coin ingestions, but remember that little ones can and do put anything smaller than their head into their mouths. Some objects (such as bad things like button batteries) may have to be removed instead of just "passing in the poop."

86) Right upper quadrant pain post-trauma is **most** commonly associated with:

A) Splenic trauma

B) Bowel trauma

C) Liver trauma

D) Renal trauma

C – Basic Anatomy 101 strikes again. Right upper quadrant trauma is associated with liver injury. Trauma to the high left flank and left upper quadrant may involve the spleen. Bowels are throughout the belly and, if you think about boxers taking a kidney punch, you will remember the kidneys are in the flanks.

87) Feeding tubes are different from decompression tubes in that feeding tubes:

A) Have smaller lumens and fewer holes

B) Have smaller lumens and more holes

C) Have larger lumens and fewer holes

D) Have larger lumens and more holes

Certified Pediatric Emergency Nurse (CPEN) Review IV

A – Think about the nature, or reason for feeding tubes (Dobhoff™, G-tubes, J-tubes). They are made for short or long term feeding (putting food in, not sucking food out); therefore, they tend to be smaller, softer and have fewer holes than tubes made for decompression. Applying suction to a feeding tube generally just causes the softer, more compliant walls of the tube to collapse. In contrast to this are decompression tubes (NG/OG), which are made with the intended use of sucking things out. They tend to be bigger in diameter, more rigid and have more holes at the end to allow more stuff to get sucked out. Feeding tubes are made for feeding and should be used for feeding, not for suction.

88) Pediatric patients presenting with a positive "lap-belt sign" after motor vehicle crashes are likely to have injuries to the:

A) Bowel

B) Liver

C) Spleen

D) Kidneys

A – While motor vehicle crashes certainly can result in damage to the kidneys, liver, and spleen, patients with horizontal bruising over the lower abdomen (a "positive lap belt sign") are at increased suspicion for injury to the bowel and mesentery. These injuries occur when the vehicle suddenly stops, but the child and their internal organs keep moving forward, trapping the organs between the lap belt and the spine. Bowel rupture, hematomas, and peritonitis can be the result, and the patient may not show symptoms and signs for hours or even days after the collision. Therefore it is crucial to have a high index of suspicion for such injuries whenever you see a lap belt sign. Lap Belt = Bowel injuries. If a lap belt is used without a shoulder restraint belt, hyperflexion of the spine can also cause lumbar spinal cord injury in the event of a crash. Lap belt injuries can be largely avoided by assuring that lap and shoulder belts are always worn in combination.

89) You assume care of a one week old who was transported to the Pediatric ED from an outside hospital for "A's & B's" (episodes of apnea and bradycardia), abdominal distention and guaiac positive stool. Abdominal X-rays show pneumatosis. An orogastric (OG) tube was placed by the transport team, IV fluids started and antibiotics given. The patient was intubated and ventilated for prolonged apnea and is on a fentanyl drip for pain management and sedation. Based on the given information, you suspect:

A) Gastroschisis with necrotic bowel

B) Volvulus

C) Necrotizing enterocolitis (NEC)

D) Omphalocele

C – The presentation described above should lead you to suspect necrotizing enterocolitis (NEC) or bowel death. "Necro" means death, "entero" means gut" and "colitis" means inflamed/unhappy gut. All of the information presented is relevant and typical; pneumatosis intestinalis (gas inside the bowel wall) is a hallmark x-ray finding in NEC, especially when seen in combination with hepatic portal vein gas. Necrotizing enterocolitis is the most common neonatal GI emergency, with mortality rates as high as 50%, particularly if perforation of the bowel occurs. Gastroschisis occurs when the infant is born with a hole in the abdominal wall just to the right of the umbilical cord. This results in a situation that might be described as "bowel in the bed" or "intestines in the isolette." Omphalocele is another abdominal wall defect, and is the result of abdominal contents herniating into the base of the umbilical cord. Both of these conditions are immediately obvious at birth and would have been surgically corrected prior to discharge from the Neonatal ICU. Volvulus, is a twisting of the guts, and usually presents with rapid abdominal distension and bilious vomiting in a soon to be very ill-appearing neonate. Volvulus begins with "V" and is very, very bad!

Certified Pediatric Emergency Nurse (CPEN) Review IV

90) A 3-week old child presents with a recent 3-day history of vomiting. He appears very dehydrated. What should the Pediatric ED nurse do **first**?

A) Obtain abdominal radiographs

B) Detailed physical exam

C) Ensure airway patency

D) Check electrolytes

C – Though all of the above may indeed be done, the correct answer hopefully shouldn't be too hard to pick since the question asked for the first thing to do. Since safety doesn't appear to be a concern, "Airway trumps everything!"

91) The child with prolonged vomiting would be expected to:

A) Lose acid from above

B) Lose acid from below

C) Lose base from above

D) Lose base from below

A – Acid begins with "A" and children lose "acid from above." Additionally, hypokalemia commonly also occurs secondary to vomiting, so be sure to monitor and replace the potassium as well. Prolonged Puking and Potassium all begin with "P."

92) A 3-week old presents with a 2-day history of severe diarrhea. She is listless, tachypneic, with a sunken anterior fontanelle and poor skin turgor. You would expect the child to:

A) Lose acid from above

B) Lose acid from below

C) Lose base from above

D) Lose base from below

D – Remember you lose "acid from above" (vomiting) but "base from below." The loss of base (HCO3-) is from diarrhea and can lead to metabolic acidosis. Volume repletion with 0.9NS, in conjunction with maintenance dextrose administration, should be done until the diarrhea is "all better."

93) An 11-month old child awaiting a liver transplant presents to the ED with significant acute upper GI bleeding. Prior to endoscopy, the pediatric ED nurse should anticipate the administration of which medication:

A) Pitressin® (vasopressin)

B) Sandostatin® (octreotide)

C) Dopamine (dopamine)

D) Albuterol (all-better-ol)

Certified Pediatric Emergency Nurse (CPEN) Review IV

B – Patients of all ages with liver failure often have hepatic portal hypertension and esophageal varices that can cause life-threatening upper GI bleeding. In years past, Pitressin® (vasopressin) was commonly used to help vasoconstrict or clamp down bleeding GI vessels. The problem was, like dopamine, vasopressin not only clamped down the GI vessels, but many of the other peripheral (and cardiac) vessels as well. With this in mind, Sandostatin® is more commonly used in both the emergency and critical care environments, as it specifically decreases portal pressure (the pressure between the portal and hepatic veins) and has far fewer systemic hemodynamic effects than vasopressin. While in the emergency department, in addition to fluid resuscitation with 0.9NS and possibly blood products, other intravenous medications such as Zantac® (ranitidine) or Protonix® (pantoprazole) may be administered. Of special note to ED nurses: there is no evidence that gastric lavage has any therapeutic role in controlling GI hemorrhage and actually may make it worse by dislodging fibrin clots that are trying to form. Finally, endoscopy under general anesthesia (hopefully in the operating room or Pediatric ICU) can be performed to diagnose and hopefully treat the cause of the upper GI bleeding.

94) In pediatric patients, hemolytic-uremic syndrome (HUS) is considered to be a:

A) Food-borne illness

B) Blood-borne illness

C) Chilean-borne illness

D) Bourne Supremacy illness

A – Hemolytic-uremic syndrome (HUS) is a disease characterized by hemolytic anemia (hence the "hemolytic" part), acute (usually reversible) renal failure (hence the "uremia" part) and a low platelet count (this part doesn't fit into the title, but it's really important). Children between the ages of 6 months and 4 years are the most common victims of this syndrome. It is most certainly a medical emergency, as the child's kidneys, brain, and other end organs are at stake.

Classically, the child eats some sort of food contaminated with E. coli, and then quickly exhibits "flu" symptoms (everything bad begins with "flu" symptoms), bloody gasteroenteritis (bloody diarrhea-- a hallmark of HUS) or bloody emesis. The E. coli bacteria release an endotoxin which messes up the endovascular lining (inside of the blood vessels), especially in the kidneys. This can result in acute (and sometimes chronic) renal failure. Treatment is generally supportive in nature with dialysis as needed (9% of cases). In most children with post-diarrheal HUS, there is a good chance of spontaneous resolution; observation in hospital is often all that is necessary. With aggressive treatment, > 90% of children will survive the acute phase of HUS.

95) An obese teen is admitted to the ED for possible acute appendicitis. You quickly determine that she is actually in active labor and a short while later delivers a baby that appears to be about 25 weeks gestation. Your immediate interventions for the baby include all of the following **except**:

A) Wrapping the infant with food grade plastic wrap (e.g. Saran Wrap™), leaving only the face exposed

B) Attaching a pulse oximeter and maintaining 02 saturation between 85-95%

C) Airway support with bag-valve mask ventilation

D) Checking a blood glucose within five minutes

D - Fetal blood glucose is approximately 70% of maternal glucose levels. While it is very important to anticipate hypoglycemia in premature infants, if blood glucose is drawn immediately after delivery, it may be falsely and reassuringly high because much of mom's glucose is still in the baby. If the new mom appears ill, you'll want to make sure to check her blood glucose because hypoglycemia will affect both her and the baby. You'll get a more accurate reading of the baby's own blood glucose approximately 15-30 minutes after the delivery. All of the other actions would be appropriate for this newborn.

96) A one week old baby presents to the clinic with a rectal temperature of 96.4°F (35.8°C) and a history of only four wet diapers in the past 24 hours. The umbilical stump is still intact and dry; however, the skin surrounding it is reddened and warm. As omphalitis (infection of the umbilical cord stump) is a possible source of infection in newborns, you anticipate the emergency treatment will include all **except**:

A) Blood culture and complete blood count

B) Oral antibiotics and follow up with the primary pediatrician tomorrow

C) Checking a bedside blood glucose

D) Performing a lumbar puncture (LP)

B – This baby is sick and needs definitive treatment today, not tomorrow! Neonates with infections may present with hypothermia rather than fever, and only having four wet diapers in 24 hours may be indicative of poor feeding. This baby is clinically sick and only a week old, so a full sepsis workup, including an LP, should be seriously considered. Newborns are unable to localize infections well and, therefore, they should be admitted for continuous monitoring and treated with IV antibiotics until bacterial infection has been ruled out. Remember, during the first month of life, if a baby is "anything but cute" (and even worse if they have a fever or are hypothermic) it's because they are septic or thinking about becoming septic. In this case, the redness and warmth around the umbilical stump indicate that the baby may have an infected stump (omphalitis), which must be treated with IV antibiotics because it's always bacterial.

97) Two days ago, a baby was born via a difficult, vacuum-assisted vaginal delivery in a small community hospital. The mother brings the newborn back to the emergency department because the baby's head has a "funny shape." While the fontanels are soft and flat, the nurse immediately notices a significant "boggy" swelling in the infant's scalp. The baby is afebrile, but has a respiratory rate of 80, moderate retractions and a sustained tachycardia in the 190s. This baby appears to be **most** at risk for:

A) Hypovolemic shock and hyperbilirubinemia

B) Hydrocephalus

C) Bacterial meningitis

D) Hyperglycemia

A – The big clues here are the vacuum-assisted delivery and the "boggy" area of the scalp. Think about how badly scalp lacerations bleed. With this in mind, consider that vacuum delivery is the cause of 90% of subgaleal hemorrhages (bleeding between the skull and the scalp.) The subgaleal space can hold up to 50% of the TOTAL circulating blood volume of a 3 kg baby, making this child at significant risk for hypovolemic shock and associated hyperbilirubenemia which may occur when the body breaks down the accumulated scalp blood. Typically, both hydrocephalus and meningitis would exhibit signs of bulging fontanels. Nothing in the history or presentation suggests hyperglycemia, which is actually a very low risk for newborns. (Hypoglycemia is a much greater risk/concern when dealing with newborns!)

98) Intussusception is an acute abdominal emergency in the pediatric patient. The child may have the following symptoms **except**:

A) "Currant jelly" stools

B) Intermittent spasmodic pain in the abdomen

C) Projectile vomiting by a very young infant (<2 months) after feeding

D) Periods of screaming and crying followed by moments of calm and, sometimes, hypoactivity

C – Both pyloric stenosis and intussusception can cause either projectile or non-projectile vomiting; however, pyloric stenosis is diagnosed in infants from about 2 weeks to 2 months of age, while intussusception usually occurs in older infants (6-8 months) and toddlers. Projectile vomiting in a very young infant is a classic symptom associated with pyloric stenosis, not intussusception. Pyloric stenosis is caused by hypertrophy of the circular muscle of the pylorus (guarding the entrance from the stomach to the intestines). The hypertrophy causes constriction and obstruction of the gastric outlet. Intussusception occurs when two portions of the intestines telescope into each other and become stuck. The resulting swelling causes an intestinal obstruction. In addition, the circulation to the affected bowel may be cut off, causing strangulation and death of the segment of bowel. Left untreated, this can be a fatal problem.

99) You are caring for a 1-week old patient who presented with lethargy, abdominal tenderness, and bilious vomiting. You are not able to see or palpate any masses in the abdomen. You suspect:

A) Midgut volvulus

B) Intussusception

C) Gastroschisis

D) Pyloric stenosis

A – Forceful **bilious vomiting** in a neonate is one of the hallmarks of a volvulus (twisted gut) and should immediately increase your index of suspicion for this diagnosis. Radiographic studies are important in making the diagnosis. Differential diagnosis at this age: Bilious vomiting, diffuse large amounts of air in the proximal small intestine coupled with abdominal distension, and a really sick (i.e. potentially trying to die neonate) = volvulus. Non-bilious projectile vomiting, normal amounts of intestinal air and not usually horribly sick neonate = pyloric stenosis. Pyloric stenosis doesn't cause bilious vomiting or abdominal tenderness and the baby only tends to look sick if they have been vomiting for days and are dehydrated. Gastroschisis ("intestines in the isolette" or "bowel in the bed") is not even in the running as a correct answer. It's hard to miss this particular anomaly of intestinal contents outside of the body. Intussusception rarely occurs before 6-9 months of age and doesn't cause bilious emesis, but does sometimes have the infamous bloody "currant jelly" stools.

100) After ensuring airway patency, your initial care for the child with a volvulus will include all of the following **except**:

A) Isolation procedures

B) Gastric decompression

C) IV fluids and electrolyte replacement

D) Broad spectrum antibiotics

Certified Pediatric Emergency Nurse (CPEN) Review IV

A – Isolation is not necessary in this case. Gastric decompression along with IV fluids and electrolyte replacement should be obvious as the baby will be NPO and require IV fluids and an empty gut. Patients with volvulus are at high risk of sepsis and/or peritonitis due to strangulated, dying bowel, so broad spectrum intravenous antibiotic coverage is indicated. Then get the baby ready to go to (or transfer the kid for) immediate surgery--the definitive treatment for volvulus.

101) You are the triage nurse on a very busy night in a pediatric ED. There are four children who need an appropriate triage level determined. Which of the following children should be the **first** to be evaluated by the physician?

A) An 11-year old female with right lower abdominal pain. Onset was four hours ago. Nausea and vomiting two times since pain began. Mother states she has had a fever intermittently all day.

B) A 7-year old boy with sudden onset of left testicular pain and inability to walk. No known injury. He has pain radiating to his lower abdomen.

C) A 16-year old female with severe lower abdominal pain. No vaginal bleeding. Last menstrual period was two weeks ago. Denies being sexually active.

D) A 2-year old with lower abdominal pain and fever. History of frequent UTIs.

B – Twisting of the vessels of the spermatic cord can cause ischemia, swelling, and severe pain to the affected testicle. Patients may also have nausea, vomiting and abdominal pain. Patients with suspected testicular torsion should receive a higher triage priority because of the imminent danger to the testicle, which can be mitigated by rapid diagnosis and surgery. Testicular salvage is approximately 80-100% likely if the torsion can be resolved within six hours. Salvage is less than 20% with more than 12 hours of torsion and approaches zero percent after 24 hours.

Lundblom's Lessons

The rescue phone rang in the ED and dispatch told us that EMS is a few minutes out with a 4-day-old infant with a chief complaint of vomiting. The ED was told the infant "looks ok, vitals are fine."

When this baby arrived, the triage nurse had EMS bring the infant to the triage office. When I walked into the triage area to assist, I was stunned at the appearance of this pale, dehydrated and emaciated infant. The mother looked stressed and exhausted, stating, "She just keeps vomiting." I weighed the baby and found that she had lost almost 2 pounds from her birth weight. Mom stated that the infant has vomited every feeding, even before discharge from the hospital. "They said all babies spit up." Triage vital signs: rectal temp was 97.8°F (37.0°C), heart rate 230 at rest, blood pressure unable to be obtained. Respirations were 60/minute and oxygen saturation was normal. Skin was cool and dry, cap refill greater than 5 seconds, tenting was noted on the skin, and the anterior fontanel was sunken. The baby was taken to a resuscitation bed with an overhead warmer. IV access was obtained and labs were sent. The patient grimaced, but didn't cry when stuck. After several fluid boluses of 0.9 NS we were finally able to obtain a blood pressure and the infant's perfusion and mental status quickly improved.

Abdominal x-rays were done showing a "double-bubble" (a large proximal bubble is air in the stomach, and a distal smaller bubble is air in the dilated proximal duodenum). This finding is typically seen with congenital duodenal atresia. This condition occurs in 1:6,000 births and can usually be seen on prenatal ultrasound. About 30% of all patients with duodenal atresia are children with Down's syndrome (Trisomy 21). An orogastric tube was placed and NPO status was maintained until surgical repair was performed. The baby was discharged home weeks later after lengthy postoperative care.

Teaching points: What you hear from prehospital providers and what arrives may not always correlate! To us, this was a clearly a critically ill newborn, but her severe dehydration and hypotensive shock was not detected by the EMS providers. Prompt recognition and IV access/hydration were essential parts of care for this newborn, whose condition is usually diagnosed on the first day of life.

Our physicians called the newborn nursery that discharged this infant and described her presentation, history and diagnosis to ensure follow up in regards to this missed congenital defect. All of us in the medical field can be guilty of not listening to our patients' families; this infant could be the poster child for why listening is so important.

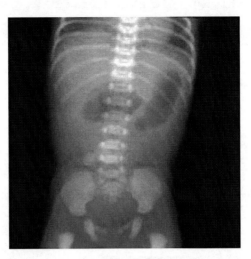

Double bubble & double trouble abdominal x-ray

Courtesy of Gerald A. Mandell MD - Phoenix Children's Hospital

Appendix 7-A

APGAR Scores

Element	0	1	2	Score
Appearance (skin color)	Body and extremities blue, pale	Body pink, extremities blue	Completely pink	
Pulse rate	Absent	Below 100/min	100/min or above	
Grimace (Irritability)	No response	Grimace	Cough, sneeze, cry	
Activity (Muscle tone)	Limp	Some flexion of extremities	Active motion	
Respiratory effort	Absent	Slow and irregular	Strong cry	
			TOTAL SCORE =	

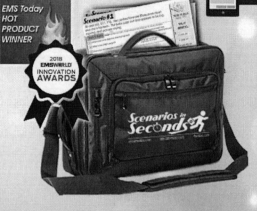

CHAPTER 8

Endocrine Emergencies
Hormones and Haagen-Dazs

*"The word **diabetes** is derived from the Greek word diabainein, which means to stand with legs apart (as in urinating) or to siphon. The most obvious sign of diabetes is excessive urination. Water passes through the body of a person with diabetes as if it were being siphoned from the mouth through the urinary system and out of the body."*

*"**Mellitus** comes from a Latin word that means sweet like honey. The urine of a person with diabetes contains extra sugar (glucose.) In 1679, the physician Thomas Willis, tasted the urine of a person with diabetes and described it as "wonderfully sweet" like honey."*

Pertinent Pediatric Ponderings (NOTES)

CHAPTER 8
Sample Test Answers & Rationales

1. _____
2. _____
3. _____
4. _____
5. _____
6. _____
7. _____
8. _____
9. _____
10. _____
11. _____
12. _____
13. _____
14. _____
15. _____
16. _____
17. _____
18. _____
19. _____
20. _____
21. _____
22. _____
23. _____
24. _____
25. _____
26. _____
27. _____
28. _____
29. _____
30. _____
31. _____
32. _____
33. _____
34. _____
35. _____
36. _____
37. _____
38. _____
39. _____

Pertinent Pediatric Ponderings (NOTES)

Certified Pediatric Emergency Nurse (CPEN) Review IV

1) Which of the following abdominal organs secretes insulin?

A) Pancreas

B) Liver

C) Spleen

D) Gallbladder

A - The pancreas is the sole organ responsible for the secretion of insulin.

2) A 10-year-old girl arrives at triage from school complaining of a headache, nausea, weakness, and being sweaty. She states that she has taken insulin for diabetes since the age of four. You suspect:

A) "The flu"

B) Hypoglycemia

C) Hyperglycemia

D) Food poisoning

B – As the question mentions diabetes, something related to sugar is probably the answer. Hypoglycemia, or low blood sugar, is most likely the case, especially with the clues of headache and weakness. Think about how you feel mid-way through most shifts. If you haven't had a chance to grab a meal or even a snack, you might have a headache and feel weak. Kids with low blood sugar feel the same way. Nausea and vomiting are common complaints with food poisoning, but this patient hasn't complained of vomiting. The complaints certainly could point towards "the flu," but the big clue here for the correct answer is the history of diabetes.

3) In some cases, it may be difficult to distinguish hypoglycemia from hyperglycemia. When in doubt, you should rely on:

A) The presence of "fruity" breath indicative of hyperglycemia

B) The patient's history of the last insulin dose

C) The knowledge that any diabetic patient with an altered level of consciousness has hyperglycemia

D) A finger stick glucose reading if available

D - With the new finger stick glucose meters allowing you to know the glucose level in less than two minutes, figuring out which is the hypo/hyperglycemia answer is easier than ever. But when in doubt, hypoglycemia is the answer. Hypoglycemia is easier and quicker to fix, and a little extra glucose will do a lot less damage to the hyperglycemic child than a little extra insulin would do the hypoglycemic child.

4) Which of the following statements is **correct**?

A) Hypoglycemia should be treated with PO (oral) glucagon

B) Hypoglycemia should be treated with PO or IV dextrose

C) Hypoglycemia should be treated with insulin therapy

D) Hyperglycemia should be treated with IM glucagon

B – Hypoglycemia is defined as a blood sugar less than 60 mg/dl and can be treated with PO or IV dextrose. Glucagon can be given IM to help stimulate the release of glycogen from the liver, but is not given PO. Glucagon given to a hyperglycemic patient would only make the sugar go higher. Treating hypoglycemia with insulin would simply kill the patient.

5) Which statement is **incorrect** concerning diabetic ketoacidosis (DKA)?

A) The onset of symptoms is gradual

B) The patient's symptoms are due to taking too much insulin

C) The patient's skin is usually dry

D) The patient complains of excessive thirst and frequent urination

B – DKA is caused by not enough, not too much insulin. This leads to hyperglycemia, not hypoglycemia. The symptoms associated with DKA generally develop gradually and can be remembered as being the "**3 Ps**:" **P**olyuria (pee all the time), **P**olydipsia (drink all the time), and **P**olyphagia (eat all the time.) The skin in DKA is dry due to dehydration from polyuria. Even though there is way too much sugar, the real problem is that, due to the lack of insulin, the sugar can't get into the cell. So the body tries to get more sugar by eating more (polyphagia.) Polyuria comes as the body tries to "pee out" the extra sugar and polydipsia is an attempt to replace the fluids lost through polyuria. Hypoglycemic patients commonly, but not always, have a fairly rapid onset of symptoms including diaphoresis and mental status changes.

6) Which of the following is an **early** indication of possible hypoglycemia in an infant?

A) Jitteriness

B) Lethargy

C) Increased urinary output

D) Increased feeding

A – As the brain uses glucose incredibly quickly, one of the earliest signs of hypoglycemia in infants is jitteriness. With infants, if something doesn't seem right, one of the first interventions should be to check a finger or heel stick sugar level. Hypoglycemic ED nurses get cranky… babies get jittery.

7) Initial treatment of an unconscious 6-month-old infant with hypoglycemia would include:

A) IV bolus of D5W

B) IV bolus of D10W

C) IV bolus of D25W

D) IV bolus of D50W

C – A 6-month-old child with hypoglycemia should get D25W. If D25W is not immediately available, simply dilute D50W 1:1 with sterile water if this is permissible in your facility. D50W boluses are most often reserved for teens and adults. In the neonatal ICU, D5W is commonly used with micro-preemies, while D10W is given for most of the other babies.

Certified Pediatric Emergency Nurse (CPEN) Review IV

8) Which of the following is **not** a common sign or symptom of hyperglycemia in patients with Type II (non-insulin dependent) diabetes?

A) Polydipsia

B) Polyphagia

C) Kussmaul's respirations

D) Glycosuria

C – The presence of Kussmaul's respirations, related to the body's attempt to "blow off" excess CO_2 in DKA, is not common with Type II, or non-insulin dependent diabetes. For these patients, the body produces some, but not nearly enough insulin. The insulin present is typically enough to prevent the extensive breakdown of fats for energy, which means that fatty acids are not produced. Consequently acidosis does not occur, and no compensatory Kussmaul's respirations are needed.

9) Kussmaul's respirations are described as:

A) Fast and deep

B) Fast and shallow

C) Slow and deep

D) Slow and shallow

A – Kussmaul's respirations are like "heavy breathers" on the phone, they are fast and deep. The body is acidotic due to the breakdown of fats and trying to compensate by "blowing off acid" or CO_2.

10) Which of the following statements is **correct** regarding the administration of potassium for patients in diabetic ketoacidosis?

A) IV potassium is contraindicated

B) IV potassium should only be given after the initial insulin bolus

C) IV potassium may need to be administered before or after insulin

D) IV potassium should be added to D5.2NS in the second and subsequent days of treatment

C – The potassium level of patients in DKA should be monitored regularly and IV potassium should be given based on serum levels. Early in hyperglycemia and acidosis, the patient may lose potassium through polyuria. However, once in DKA, the patient is pretty dry and potassium loss will slow down, often resulting in an increase in the serum potassium. The most common approach is to hold off on potassium until fluid volume has been restored and urine output returns. It is important to remember that insulin not only brings glucose into the cells, but it also brings potassium into the cells. The combination of increased urine output and increased potassium movement into the cells can cause a significant drop in serum potassium, so it is wise to be prepared for the very real potential for hypokalemia. In some cases, the patient will present with both a very high glucose and a very low potassium level. In those cases, potassium needs to be given before the insulin to prevent potentially deadly cardiac disturbances from the hypokalemia.

Endocrine

Certified Pediatric Emergency Nurse (CPEN) Review IV

11) A common initial indication that a child has developed type II diabetes is presentation to the pediatrician or ED with:

A) DKA

B) HHNC

C) ARDS

D) ABCD

B - Type II, or non-insulin dependent diabetics are much more likely to present with HHNC (Hyperglycemic Hyperosmolar Nonketotic Coma) than any of the other complaints. Although pediatric type II diabetes is on the rise, it is still uncommon to see children with HHNC. DKA is in many cases, the first presentation for newly diagnosed, Type I, or insulin-dependent diabetics. ARDS (Acute Respiratory Distress Syndrome) is not a likely occurrence with new-onset type II diabetes and ABCD are simply the first four letters of the alphabet.

12) An 11-year-old presents to the ED via ambulance with lethargy and tachypnea. Her skin is dry and flushed, and she has a fruity breath odor. The blood glucose level is 1,110 mg/dl and her UA reveals 4+ glucose and 4+ ketones. DKA is made as the diagnosis. Each of the following are commonly found in patients with DKA **except**:

A) Hyperkalemia

B) Hyperventilation

C) Jugular venous distention (JVD)

D) Delayed capillary refill

C – In the initial assessment of severe DKA, signs of dehydration, including lethargy, weakened peripheral pulses, and delayed capillary refill (>3 seconds) are commonly present in conjunction with Kussmaul's respirations. As the patient is dehydrated, JVD would not commonly be found.

13) When caring for the above patient in DKA, the ED nurse's **first** role would be to:

A) Administer IV fluids

B) Administer insulin IV

C) Administer IV fluids and prepare an IV insulin drip

D) Administer a bolus of IV insulin

C – Establishing IV access and administering IV 0.9NS and insulin will be required for this patient. However, most pediatric centers no longer give IV insulin boluses and only initiate a continuous insulin infusion.

14) Which type of IV solution would the nurse expect to use in the **initial** management of this patient with DKA?

A) Isotonic saline solution (0.9NS)

B) Hypotonic saline solution (0.45NS)

C) Hypertonic saline solution (3% NS)

D) Hypotonic dextrose solution (D5.45NS)

A – 0.9NS is the IV solution most commonly used for the initial management of patients with DKA.

15) During therapy for DKA, this child's serum potassium level is likely to be:

A) Initially elevated, then gradually decreasing

B) Initially decreased, then gradually increasing

C) Initially normal level, then gradually increasing

D) Initially decreased, then gradually decreasing

A – Hyperkalemia is commonly found in patients with metabolic acidosis (a part of the DKA process.) However, during treatment, the potassium level can and will decrease, frequently requiring potassium supplementation.

16) Which arrhythmia is **not** commonly found in young patients with DKA?

A) Sinus bradycardia

B) Sinus tachycardia

C) Tall T waves

D) Premature ventricular contractions (PVC's)

A – It would be very unusual to find sinus bradycardia in a patient with DKA. These patients are commonly dehydrated, and as such, we would expect to see sinus tachycardia. Tall or peaked T waves can be found with severe hyperkalemia as well. Since DKA patients can quickly go from hyperkalemia to hypokalemia, PVCs might also be expected. Sinus bradycardia in a really sick patient is never a good sign.

17) Which laboratory finding(s) would **not** support an initial diagnosis of DKA?

A) Decreased arterial or venous PCO_2

B) Elevated serum potassium level and decreased serum bicarbonate level

C) Elevated urine specific gravity

D) Decreased serum potassium level and decreased hematocrit

D – The patient in DKA is typically severely dehydrated, and as such, the hematocrit will be elevated, not decreased. It is also very likely the potassium level would be elevated, not decreased. Low CO_2 is a likely finding as the patient is trying to "blow off" excess CO_2 from the acidosis, and a decreased bicarbonate level is also expected as the patient is in metabolic acidosis.

Endocrine

Certified Pediatric Emergency Nurse (CPEN) Review IV

18) After initiating IV fluids and an insulin drip, the ED nurse should assess the patient for which potentially fatal treatment-related complication?

A) Hyperosmolar hyperglycemic nonketotic coma (HHNC) or syndrome (HHNS)

B) Acute renal failure

C) Cerebral edema

D) Respiratory acidosis

C - The most feared complication of DKA management is that of cerebral edema. <u>Very</u> rapid correction of DKA may lead to cerebral edema, a potentially fatal condition, which can be detected via changes in mental status (early) or CT scan (late.) The treatment for cerebral edema includes airway support, mannitol and/or hypertonic saline. The management of DKA has definitely changed over the years and current recommendations include cautious fluid resuscitation, <u>very</u> rare use of sodium bicarbonate (even with a pH of less than 7.0), and <u>very</u> rare use of insulin boluses (just start the drip.) Remember, the patient didn't develop DKA in a few hours, and therefore you shouldn't try to fix it in just a few hours. HHNC occurs primarily in type II, non-insulin diabetics, and is a very different condition than DKA.

19) Close monitoring of hourly lab results for the patient being treated for DKA is needed because which of the following complications can easily occur?

A) Hyperglycemia

B) Hyperkalemia

C) Hypercalcemia

D) Hypokalemia

D – Hypokalemia can easily occur even though the patient may initially present with hyperkalemia in addition to DKA. As the patient becomes euvolemic, urine output increases, and the insulin facilitates the movement of potassium into the cells, we should anticipate and prepare for the potential hypokalemia.

20) 18 hours after entering the ED, the DKA patient's serum glucose level decreases from an initial level of 710 mg/dl in the ED to 238 mg/dl. Which fluid therapy would the nurse expect to be administered next?

A) 0.45NS

B) 0.9NS

C) D5.45NS

D) Lactated Ringer's (LR)

C – Commonly, when the sugar level decreases to 250-300 mg/dl or so, dextrose containing solutions such as D5.45NS are initiated. As the sugar in the fluid (glucose in the serum) slowly decreases, plan on increasing the sugar in the fluid (from no sugar in the 0.9NS to D5.45NS.) The goal of DKA management is to drop the sugar slowly, but not too quickly (avoiding cerebral edema), and certainly not to a "way too low" level. This fluid choice helps prevents relative hypoglycemia from occurring while the insulin drip is continued until the acidosis is corrected.

Certified Pediatric Emergency Nurse (CPEN) Review IV

21) What type of insulin can be used intravenously to manage DKA?

A) Regular

B) NPH

C) Lantus

D) All of the above

A – Regular insulin is the only type of insulin given IV. Regular insulin, when given IV, has an onset of action within minutes and has a relatively short duration, making it very suitable for IV administration. Here's a helpful reminder for when you are preparing an IV insulin infusion: Once you have the tubing attached to the bag with the insulin solution, prime the tubing and flush through a small amount of the solution. Insulin can bind to the IV tubing and result in unreliable amounts reaching the patient initially. Priming the tubing first allows for some insulin to bind the tubing, and then the actual subsequent delivery of insulin through the tubing will be much more reliable.

22) An unconscious 12-year-old, obese child is brought to the ED via EMS. The child's mother reports that he has complained of weakness, frequent urination, and seemed to be drinking all the water he can get his hands on for the past week. The finger stick glucose at triage is "High." Soon after, the laboratory calls the ED with a panic value serum glucose reading of 1,104 mg/dl with a negative serum acetone. He is diagnosed with HHNC. When an arterial blood gas is done, the pH is 7.23. You realize from this:

A) With a glucose of over 1,000, this is probably an error and the test should be repeated

B) Though low, this is not an unexpected finding

C) The patient is experiencing respiratory alkalosis from hyperventilation

D) The patient is experiencing metabolic alkalosis due to frequent urination

B – By definition, Hyperglycemic Hyperosmolar Nonketotic Coma, does not involve severe acidosis (beyond dehydration acidosis,) so we would not expect a very low pH like we find in DKA. It is a complication of diabetes that involves very high blood sugars, without the breaking down of fat into ketones. Since signs of HHNC may include extreme dehydration and/or a high temperature, you might see a slightly lower pH. However, if the serum arterial pH is really 7.23, then something else, beyond HHNC, is probably going on. This patient is acidotic, not alkalotic, so C and D are not appropriate answers.

23) The nurse would expect the management of HHNC to differ from DKA because the patient with HHNC requires more:

A) Fluids

B) Insulin

C) Potassium

D) Bicarbonate

A – HHNC patients are very dehydrated and commonly require much more fluid resuscitation than those in DKA. The patients are typically type II diabetics, which mean that they produce some, just not enough insulin, and therefore we would not expect their insulin needs to be greater than those of a patient in DKA. Potassium levels may vary, but treatment should not be very different than with DKA. They are typically not severely acidotic and as such, would not require bicarbonate.

24) A child with severe hyperthyroidism is likely to be:

A) Bradycardic

B) Tachycardic

C) Hypotensive

D) Obese

B – A classic sign of hyperthyroidism is tachycardia. Though this disease is rare in children, other symptoms, like hypertension and weight loss are common enough to suggest an evaluation for hyperthyroidism. In contrast, think about how people with hypothyroidism look and act. They are tired and everything seemingly "slows way down." In extreme cases, this can lead to myxedema coma. Exactly the opposite occurs with hyperthyroidism in which seemingly everything is "hyper." Picture manic-depressive patients who are very much in the manic phase and you've got the picture of hyperthyroidism.

Endocrine

25) Chvostek's and Trousseau's signs are associated with which condition:

A) Hypocalcemia

B) Hypercalcemia

C) Hypokalemia

D) Hyperkalemia

A – Positive Chvostek's and Trousseau's signs are commonly found in patients with presumed hypocalcemia which lowers the excitation threshold of neurons. This lowered excitatory threshold results in spasms, which is the repeated response to a single stimulus. An easy way to remember these two signs is that Chvostek begins with "C" and tapping the "C"heek results in facial muscle spasm. The other hypocalcemia sign commonly asked on tests is Trousseau's sign. Trousseau's sign begins with "T" and is like what you do when you "T"ake a blood pressure for "T"oo long. If hand/wrist spasms result after a 3 minute inflation of the BP cuff (above systolic pressure) on the upper arm, this is considered a positive Trousseau's sign and is indicative of hypocalcemia.

26) All of the following are possible causes of diabetes insipidus (DI) **except**?

A) CNS infection

B) Brain injury

C) Pituitary tumor

D) Pancreatic disorders

D – Pancreatic disorders are associated with diabetes mellitus (DM), not diabetes insipidus. DI is very different than DM. The problem is not with glucose, but with antidiuretic hormone (ADH.) CNS infections, traumatic brain injury, or pituitary tumors (just remember bad brains) can result in little to no ADH being released. If you have little or no "antidiuretic" in your system, there is nothing to stop you from eliminating excessive water (a polite way to say you just pee and pee and pee.) And because the pee is mostly water, the urine specific gravity will be close to that of water.

27) Which laboratory finding would **most** likely be found in patients with acute diabetes insipidus (DI)?

A) Decreased serum sodium level

B) Decreased serum osmolarity

C) Increased urine osmolarity

D) Urine specific gravity of 1.001

D – Because of excess water elimination, the specific gravity of the urine of patients with DI is very low, perhaps as low as 1.001. When you hear DI, think about "peeing water" because of a lack of ADH (antidiuretic hormone.) These patients can become dehydrated quite quickly and as such, the serum sodium and serum osmolarity would increase, not decrease. Urine osmolarity will decrease along with the specific gravity.

28) A 14-year-old teen is brought to the ED by EMS from a pediatric long term care facility because he has been experiencing polydipsia and polyuria. His most recent medical history is significant for meningitis which resulted in severe neurological deficits. Laboratory studies reveal a serum sodium of 155 mEq/l and a urine osmolarity 248 mOsm/l. The patient is diagnosed with diabetes insipidus (DI.) The priority nursing intervention in this situation would be to:

A) Assess for hypovolemic shock

B) Institute seizure precautions

C) Repeat the laboratory studies in 60 minutes

D) Monitor the patient for arrhythmias

Endocrine

A – Excessive water elimination (too much pee, and it's mostly water) found with DI can lead to dehydration and hypovolemic shock, so this patient should be closely monitored for signs of shock. The other actions are appropriate, but the immediate priority is to assess for shock.

29) SIADH (syndrome of inappropriate antidiuretic hormone) and DI (diabetes insipidus) may be confusing because:

A) The clinical findings are so similar

B) They both involve ADH

C) They are both forms of diabetes

D) They are common in preschool children

B – While both SIADH and DI involve abnormalities in the release of ADH, they actually represent opposite extremes. DI results from little or no ADH and SIADH results from "inappropriately" excessive release of ADH. As you would expect, the clinical findings are opposite, and neither are forms of diabetes mellitus, nor are they common conditions at any age. They are similar in respect that both are associated "bad brains" such as trauma, CNS infections, or tumors.

Certified Pediatric Emergency Nurse (CPEN) Review IV

30) Which laboratory finding is commonly found in patients with SIADH?

A) Serum sodium of 120 mEq/l

B) Serum potassium of 6 mEq/l

C) Serum osmolarity of 348 mOsm/l

D) Urine specific gravity of 1.002

A – Hyponatremia, as evidenced by a serum sodium level of 120 mEq/l (normal range is approximately 135-145 mEq/l,) is a common finding in patients with SIADH. These patients do not release water (don't pee) enough, and as the body holds onto water, everything in the body gets diluted, especially the sodium. Excess water would also lower the serum potassium levels and decrease the serum osmolarity. Urine specific gravity would increase as very little water is leaving the body.

31) The nurse would expect the initial treatment of this patient in SIADH to include all of the following **except**:

A) Fluid restriction

B) 3% hypertonic saline:

C) Close monitoring of lab values and intake and output

D) Thiazide diuretics

D– If all the answers look intuitively appropriate, look for the tricky part of one that might be wrong. In this case, it's not the diuretic part that is wrong, although diuretics are rarely part of the treatment, but the thiazides that is wrong. Thiazides decrease free water excretion by the kidneys and can actually aggravate the already existing hyponatremia. These patients can't get rid of the water they take in, so limiting what does go in is a very good idea. In conjunction, as the sodium levels progressively drop, especially if neurological symptoms are present, hypertonic saline can be administered to help restore the sodium levels to normal levels. As with the glucose in DKA, rapidly correcting hyponatremia can result in severe CNS complications including cerebral edema and infarction.

32) Prevention of which complication is the primary goal for a patient with SIADH?

A) Tetany

B) Seizures

C) Hypotension

D) All of the above

B – Hyponatremic seizures are a serious complication of SIADH. We can also see hyponatremic seizures in babies who are given too much water, as might be the case with overly diluted baby formula, or merely substituting "Kool-Aid" like drinks for infant formula. There is way too much water in the system, so hypertension, not hypotension, is a more frequent finding. Tetany is associated with tetanus or hypocalcemia.

Certified Pediatric Emergency Nurse (CPEN) Review IV

33) Failure of which gland can result in Addison's disease?

A) Thyroid

B) Pancreas

C) Adrenal gland

D) Pituitary gland

C – Addison's disease is also called adrenal insufficiency, so there's your answer. Sometimes we get lucky and the letters match. The problems with Addison's disease are related to decreased levels of cortisol. When the adrenals secrete too much cortisol, the result is Cushing's syndrome. The adrenals are also responsible for the excretion of epinephrine and norepinephrine.

34) The clinical findings found with acute adrenal crisis or chronic Addison's disease are caused by decreased cortisol (steroid) levels:

A) True

B) False

A – True – Addison's begins with "A" and these patients "Aint" got enough steroids. Chronic steroid use triggers suppression of steroids by the adrenal glands. Whether acutely as with meningococcal sepsis, or abruptly stopping long-term steroids (i.e. teen asthmatics or kids on chronic steroids for autoimmune disorders), the lack of steroids is a true medical emergency, managed with IV, and later oral steroids.

35) The clinical findings found with Cushing's syndrome are caused by increased cortisol (steroid) levels and include all of the following **except**:

A) Weight gain

B) Facial puffiness (Moon face)

C) Hypotension

D) Hyperglycemia

C – Patient's with Cushing's syndrome often have hypertension, as opposed to hypotension. Other symptoms include weight gain, puffy faces, high blood sugars, easy bruising, and the classic "buffalo hump."

36) A common finding in teens with the onset of Addison's disease is:

A) Brown pigmentation of the skin

B) Weight gain

C) Hypertension

D) Edema

A – Though Addison's disease is most commonly found in middle-age adults, one of the early warning signs for teens is a "terrific tan" in February (without the benefit of visits to a sunny climate or a tanning parlor for that "fake-bake"). To pale teenagers, the brown pigmentation and often accompanying weight loss may seem like a great combination, but those symptoms are really the signs of a lifelong disease process. The other three possible answers are actually related to Cushing's syndrome patients who have way too much cortisol (steroids); they are swollen, hypertensive, and hold onto water. Those with Addison's, where they "ain't got nearly enough steroids" are the opposite of Cushing's in that they tend to have undesired weight loss and, when they're in adrenal crisis, are hypotensive (vascular collapse), not hypertensive. Addison's begins with "A" and it's all about the "Ain'ts." They ain't got enough steroids; they ain't got enough sodium; they ain't got enough water and, if they are really really sick, they ain't got a blood pressure!

37) Common causes of Cushing's syndrome involve each of the following **except**:

A) Pituitary tumor

B) Adrenal gland tumor

C) Chronic steroids

D) Suddenly stopping steroids

D – Cushing's begins with "C" and they have way too much of the steroid "C"ortisol. Stopping steroid usage would not cause Cushing's, but it could induce an adrenal crisis, as with Addison's disease. Although the increase in cortisol could be from pituitary or adrenal gland tumors, the most common cause is iatrogenic, meaning we caused it ourselves. This can occur from chronic steroid use, as may happen with patients with arthritis, lupus and other autoimmune disorders. Patients with Cushing's disease have way too much steroids, so the treatment involves slowly tapering the steroid medications and/or removing the brain or belly tumor.

38) With children in acute diabetic ketoacidosis (DKA), which of the following tests is generally sufficient in order to evaluate the acid-base status (pH and pCO2)?

A) Venous blood gas

B) Arterial blood hydrogenase

C) Partial pressure ketoacidotic blood saturation

D) Basic-acid chemical profile

A – A venous blood gas (VBG) can be utilized to provide information on the acid/base balance. An arterial blood gas (ABG) would also provide information on the acid/base balance, but since you are going to have to establish IV access for hydration and assessment of laboratory studies, just get a VBG while you're at it. Besides, ABGs hurt a lot, so why subject the child to unnecessary painful procedures? With most children in DKA, the problem is not with oxygenation, which the ABG would certainly show, but with the state of acidosis--shown well by a VBG.

Certified Pediatric Emergency Nurse (CPEN) Review IV

39) In a child being treated for DKA in the pediatric ED, when is it appropriate to add potassium to the maintenance fluid?

A) As soon as the initial maintenance fluid is hung

B) Once the bed side glucose is below 150

C) Once the bed side glucose is below 350

D) After the first documentation of urine output in the ED

D – In an acidotic state, potassium is pushed out of the cell and eventually out of the body. As insulin is administered and the pH slowly returns to normal, the potassium is then transported back into the cell causing a pseudo-hypokalemic state. But, if potassium is added to the maintenance fluid prior to knowing the renal status, this could be a bad thing. The reason is that generally there is a polyuric state as DKA develops, and depending on the amount of fluid loss and resulting dehydration during that polyuric state, the kidneys could have been damaged. (Remember, poly = lots of and uric = pee and the "p" in potassium follows the "p" in pee.) The decrease in renal function (which is very rare, but very serious) could result in the decreased ability to secrete potassium and a subsequent real (and dangerous) hyperkalemic state. Moral of the story: Once they pee (kidneys are present and accounted for,) potassium may be added.

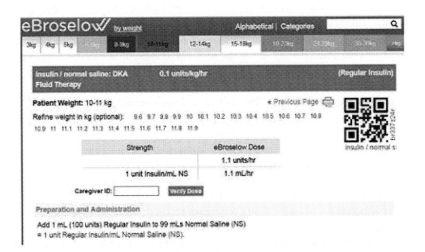

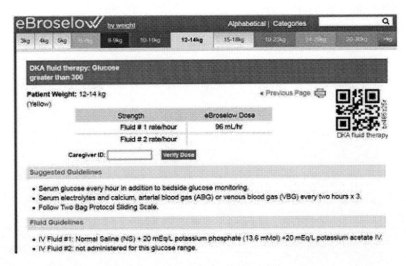

Color coded DKA intravenous insulin and fluid management

Courtesy of James Broselow MD & Robert Luten MD – www.eBroselow.com

Certified Pediatric Emergency Nurse (CPEN) Review IV

Lundblom's Lessons

EMS arrived with a 4 year-old male with a chief complaint of "not acting right" per the father. When asked what's going on, he stated the child was playing outside for a while then "came in and fell down." Upon arrival at the Peds ED, the patient had a generalized seizure, which was stopped with IV Ativan® (lorazepam). Watery diarrhea was noted post-seizure and the boy's abdomen was found to be distended. The patient remained responsive only to painful stimulus after the seizure. He began seizing again a short while later and did not respond to additional anticonvulsants. During the second seizure, the lab called to report critical sodium of 114 mEq/L. Treatment was initiated with 3% saline IV to correct the hyponatremia, which presumably, was causing the seizures. The child was intubated for airway protection. Chest and abdominal radiographs showed free air in the belly. Upon further physical exam, the patient's anus was found to have many abrasions and was continuously leaking watery stool. Pediatric surgery was consulted and emergently took patient to the operating room.

After lengthy discussion with another child (age 9) at the scene, police arrived at our facility and arrested the patient's father. The witness described how the father became angry with the child, "grabbed him and stuck the water hose in his bottom and turned it on." As a result, the child had absorbed a very large quantity of water, causing significant water intoxication. This caused the altered mental status, hyponatremia and seizures. The force of the water perforated the child's colon. Despite aggressive resuscitation efforts, the child died postoperatively, shortly after arrival in the PICU.

Teaching points: Again, what was called in and what actually arrived were very different. Not all parents/caregivers report the truth to medical personnel in the field or the hospital. Remember to think outside the box when the story just doesn't add up. Water intoxication is a relatively rare, but often-lethal condition in the pediatric patient. We used to see it a lot with young babies of disadvantaged families near the end of the month. Parents would intentionally dilute the formula to make it last until the next government check came, unaware of the potential detrimental effects to the infant. Broaden your suspicion to parents who may not be eligible for government aid, but are financially strapped and cutting costs by mixing/diluting formulas to make them last longer. This is also still seen occasionally with infants with GI illness who are given tap water instead of oral rehydration solutions such as Pedialyte®. Water intoxication with significant hyponatremia may result in cerebral edema, which carries a mortality rate of about 50%. (It is more prevalent in children than adults.) Increasing the sodium gradually with a 3% saline solution IV is indicated and should be continued until signs and symptoms of central nervous system compromise resolve.

Finally, we need to address the horrific NAT (non-accidental trauma) presented here. As opposed to this case, there are several documented cases of children being forced to drink copious amounts of water, but the outcomes are the same. Every ED nurse has a traumatic critical incident--a heartbreaking story--that keeps us awake at night. Make sure you keep your eyes open for NAT, as well as signs of critical incident stress in yourself and your colleagues.

Certified Pediatric Emergency Nurse (CPEN) Review IV

Appendix 8-A

Summary of Insulin Preparations

Insulin Chart

Each type of insulin has its own unique behavior. One difference among types of insulin is how long they take to start working at lowering blood-glucose levels. The "insulin peak" is the point at which the dose is working at its maximum, and the "duration" is how long the blood-glucose-lowering effect of the injection will last. The following is a list of insulin types available in the United States, along with how soon they start working, their peak, and how long they last. Talk to your healthcare provider about your insulin regimen.

Insulin Type	Onset of Action	Peak	Duration of Action
Lispro U-100 (Humalog)	Approx. 15 minutes	1-2 hours	3-6 hours
Lispro U-200 (Humalog 200)	Approx. 15 minutes	1-2 hours	3-6 hours
Aspart (Novolog)	Approx. 15 minutes	1-2 hours	3-6 hours
Glulisine (Apidra)	Approx. 20 minutes	1-2 hours	3-6 hours
Regular U-100 (Novolin R, Humulin R)	30-60 minutes	2-4 hours	6-10 hours
Humulin R Regular U-500	30-60 minutes	2-4 hours	Up to 24 hours
NPH (Novolin N, Humulin N, ReliOn)	2-4 hours	4-8 hours	10-18 hours
Glargine U-100 (Lantus)	1-2 hours	Minimal	Up to 24 hours
Glargine U-100 (Basaglar)	1-2 hours	Minimal	Up to 24 hours
Glargine U-300 (Toujeo)	6 hours	No significant peak	24-36 hours
Detemir (Levemir)	1-2 hours	Minimal**	Up to 24 hours**
Degludec U-100 & U-200 (Tresiba)	1-4 hours	No significant peak	About 42 hours
Afrezza	< 15 minutes	Approx. 50 minutes	2-3 hours

*Information derived from a combination of manufacturer's prescribing information, online professional literature sources and clinical studies. Individual response to insulin preparations may vary.

**Peak and length of action may depend on size of dose and length of time since initiation of therapy

***Premixed insulins are more variable in peak and duration of action. For instance, even though the literature states that the effects may last for up to 24 hours many people find that they will need to take a dose every 10-12 hours

Image courtesy of dLife.com

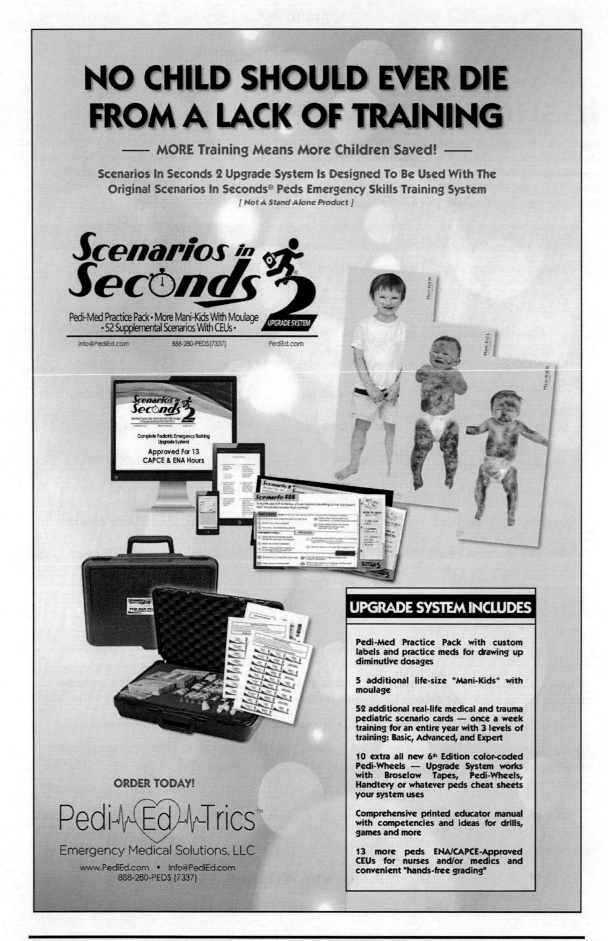

Chapter 9

Orthopedics and Pain Management

Bumps, Breaks, Morphine, and Monitoring

*Experts say you should never hit your child in anger.
When is a good time? When you are feeling festive?*
-Roseanne Barr

Pertinent Pediatric Ponderings (NOTES)

CHAPTER 9
Sample Test Answer Sheet

1. _____
2. _____
3. _____
4. _____
5. _____
6. _____
7. _____
8. _____
9. _____
10. _____
11. _____
12. _____
13. _____
14. _____
15. _____
16. _____
17. _____
18. _____
19. _____
20. _____

21. _____
22. _____
23. _____
24. _____
25. _____
26. _____
27. _____
28. _____
29. _____
30. _____
31. _____
32. _____
33. _____
34. _____
35. _____
36. _____
37. _____
38. _____
39. _____
40. _____

41. _____
42. _____
43. _____
44. _____
45. _____
46. _____
47. _____
48. _____
49. _____
50. _____
51. _____
52. _____

Pertinent Pediatric Ponderings (NOTES)

Certified Pediatric Emergency Nurse (CPEN) Review IV

1) A 14-year-old runs into the ED bleeding and screams, "My finger got cut off!" The **first** nursing intervention would be to:

A) Apply direct pressure to the bleeding vessels

B) Obtain pulse oximetry to assess oxygenation

C) Question the patient about how the amputation occurred

D) Evaluate the amputated part for possible reimplantation

A - Since he is screaming and able to run into the ED, chances are his airway and breathing are just fine. With the "A" and "B" of the ABC's assessed, "C"irculation is next. If the injury site is bleeding, we have good circulation (at least at the present moment), so the next thing to do is to stop the bleeding from the amputation. Most bleeding from complete extremity amputations will not kill the patient as the body doesn't want to die, and in its attempts not to die, the blood vessels will clot off, clamp down, and shrink up.

2) The ED nurse's next appropriate step would be to take the amputated part and:

A) Place it in a bottle of sterile normal saline solution

B) Wrap it in saline-dampened gauze and place it in a plastic bag

C) Place it directly on ice

D) Discard it because children's fingers are always contaminated

B - Amputated parts should be treated like a fine cocktail. You want them "chilled, not frozen." Current suggested management of the amputated part includes: 1) Rinse it off with some saline, but do not submerge it. If the part is floating in anything, it's not going back on. 2) After rinsing, wrap the part in gauze, then place the wrapped part into a bag. 3) Lastly, place the rinsed and wrapped (insulated) part in a bag on ice.

3) After falling on the playground, a 6-year-old presents to the ED with multiple facial lacerations. Prior to suturing, the emergency nurse should:

A) Irrigate the wounds with normal saline

B) Scrub the wounds vigorously

C) Apply Betadine (povidone-iodine) ointment

D) Provide a mirror for the patient to assess the injury

A - After the wound is anesthetized, it should be irrigated, not scrubbed, with normal saline. Don't even try to clean lacerations out before they are numb because the patient won't let you. Local anesthesia before cleaning the wound will not make the wound "dirtier," it's just humane. Betadine, like hydrogen peroxide and Hibiclens, is toxic to open tissues (like lacerations) and should not be used in this situation.

4) When suturing the lacerations, the physician orders lidocaine with epinephrine. However, when anesthetizing a nasal wound, lidocaine without epinephrine is commonly desired because:

A) Epinephrine is a vasodilator and will cause further bleeding

B) Epinephrine will cause profuse nasal discharge and contaminate the wound

C) Epinephrine is a vasoconstrictor and may cause tissue ischemia

D) Administering epinephrine in a child may cause ventricular arrhythmias

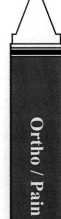

Ortho / Pain

405

C - Injectable lidocaine for local anesthesia in suturing lacerations comes in 2 strengths and is available with or without epinephrine. There are a couple important things for peds ED nurses to remember: 1) First, 2% lidocaine does not make you any "more numb" than 1%. It's just more concentrated. It has twice as much drug per volume. With very little patients, this may be a problem. Why have a little one lido toxic and seizing if they don't need to? 2) Where should you not use lido with epi? Fingers, ears, nose, toes, and hose (penis)! Epi is given with the lidocaine for its vasoconstrictive effects. It helps restrict or stop bleeding. However, for circulatory end points, most practitioners still recommend "plain" lidocaine for those areas to avoid potential distal ischemia.

5) Which statement is **true** about analgesics and sedatives?

A) Analgesics used to manage severe pain usually can cause sedation, but most sedatives do not provide analgesia

B) Sedatives used for patients in pain provide analgesia

C) Most sedatives eliminate the need for analgesia

D) Sedatives should not be used in conjunction with analgesics

A - This concept is crucial for pediatric ED nurses to remember. If you want to take away the patient's pain, give them an analgesic. If you want the patient to go to sleep, give them a sedative. However, if you want both effects, then with few exceptions (ketamine, nitrous, dexmedetomidine), that means you have to give them two separate drugs.

6) Which statement is **true** concerning pain and little children?

A) Very little kids don't feel pain because their pain receptors are immature and therefore they don't transmit the pain response to the brain

B) They won't remember it anyway, and it will hurt more to give them something for pain than the procedure itself

C) Both A and B

D) None of the above

D - None of the above. It's scary, but some medical professionals still think that way about pain and pediatric patients. Research has proven all of the previous statements to be false in infants, children, and adults! If you look at a child and say "that's gotta hurt," chances are it does.

7) All of the following are **true except:**

A) Respiratory arrest and hypoxia are common side effects associated with sedative use in the pediatric population

B) Unless specifically indicated otherwise, IV sedation should start with a small dose given slowly

C) SPO_2 and $ETCO_2$ measurements are both recommended for respiratory monitoring

D) There is considerable variability in sedatives, so you need to know what the drug does and doesn't do

A - Can hypoxia and respiratory arrest happen with sedative administration? Absolutely. Is it common? Happily, no. The keys to safe sedation are meds and monitoring. Meds - You have to know what the drug does (and doesn't do), and how long does it last. Remember, you can always give more. So especially with IV sedation, it's a good idea to "start small and slow." Monitoring - Does every sedated child need a pulse ox? Yes. It's as simple as that. When you think sedation and respiratory complications, pulse oximetry is the minimum standard of care. In addition, according to pediatric anesthesia professionals, end-tidal CO_2 ($ETCO_2$) monitoring, in conjunction with pulse oximetry, should be used for moderate and deep sedation.

8) Which of the following is **not** appropriate for a child in pain?

A) Distraction with toys

B) Allowing the child to cry himself to sleep

C) Massage therapy

D) Analgesic administration

B - Think about what you would want if your child was in pain. Toys, massage, and pain medication would probably all help. Infants and children do feel pain, and letting them cry themselves to sleep is not what you, as a parent, would want for your child.

9) Which statement is **true** regarding pediatric pain assessment?

A) It is not necessary since little kids don't feel or remember pain

B) If kids aren't crying, they aren't in pain

C) Methods for assessing pain in the pediatric patient will vary according to the age of the child

D) Published pain scales are inappropriate for use with very small children who can't verbalize pain

C - One pain assessment method does not fit all patients. There are several scales that have been validated to "work" for neonates, infants, and children. I highly recommend those taking the CPEN examination review the pain scales illustrated at the end of this chapter and in the ENPC textbook.

10) All of the following influence a child's response to pain **except**:

A) Previous experience with pain

B) Cultural background

C) Age

D) The specific pain scale being used

D - The scale used to record the response to pain doesn't cause the pain. Just as one scale doesn't fit all, the same procedure may hurt different children differently depending on previous experience, age, and even socio-cultural background. If they look like they are in pain, tell you they are in pain, or even if the procedure being done is expected to cause pain, chances are they are in pain and should be treated as such.

11) Medications used for moderate sedation/analgesia most often include:

A) Paralytics, barbiturates, and benzodiazepines

B) Benzodiazepines, opiates, and barbiturates

C) Paralytics, barbiturates, and opiates

D) Paralytics, opiates, and benzodiazepines

B - There is nothing "moderate" about paralytics (neuromuscular blockers.) Paralytics paralyze and that's all they do. Using paralytics means that the patient must be intubated for the procedure, and very significantly, they are unable to reliably tell or show you that they are in pain (or awake.) Benzodiazepines such as Ativan (lorazepam), Versed (midazolam), or Valium (diazepam), or barbiturates (pentobarbital) are great for sedation, but do nothing for pain. Opiates (morphine, fentanyl, or Dilaudid (hydromorphone) are great for pain, and may help with sedation as well, but their primary role is pain relief.

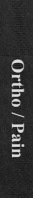

Ortho / Pain

12) A sleeping child:

A) Is not in pain

B) Is a sleeping child

C) Does not need pain medication

D) Has a pain level of 5 or less

B - All we really know is that the child is sleeping. Sedated or asleep does not mean they are not still in pain, it just means they are sedated or asleep.

13) All of the following would be appropriate initial non-pharmacological treatments for pain **except:**

A) Distraction

B) Parental comforting

C) Restraints

D) Massage and positioning

C - Just as with any other patient, medical and behavioral restraint use should follow policies according to the specific situation. Restraints are rarely, if ever, the first approach to pain control. In preparation for, during, and after painful procedures, a combination approach of non-pharmacologic (distraction, parental comforting, positioning, etc.) and pharmacologic interventions is appropriate.

14) Which of the following is the **best** resource to use in determining how much pain a child has?

A) Parent

B) Patient

C) Nurse

D) Doctor

B - It makes no difference whether they are verbal or not, the patient, not the parent or the healthcare professional, is the best authority regarding his or her pain.

15) Versed (midazolam) provides which of the following:

A) Sedation, amnesia, and analgesia

B) Sedation, amnesia, but not analgesia

C) Sedation, analgesia, but not amnesia

D) Sedation, but not analgesia or amnesia

B - For the vast majority of pediatric patients, Versed (midazolam) provides both sedation and amnesia, but it doesn't provide analgesia. It is truly a great drug for pediatric emergency care, in part because it can be given nasally, orally, IM, IV, or rectally, and once administered, if you can get the patient into a quiet area, chances are he or she will go to sleep in about 10 minutes. But it is crucial that ED nurses remember that Versed does NOTHING for pain! Even if the patient is asleep, and even if they may not actively remember being in pain, the body will still react to being in pain, and that is often unnecessary and avoidable. A small, but significant number of patients may experience a paradoxical effect of the medication. If that should happen, don't give more Versed to try to calm things down. It is likely to only make matters worse. Try to let the Versed wear off and consider a different sedative.

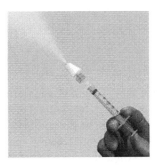
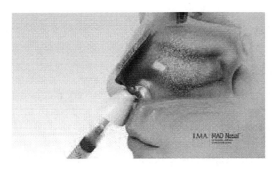

MAD Nasal Medication Delivery Device

Images courtesy of Teleflex

www.teleflex.com

16) Sublimaze (fentanyl) is primarily administered for which of the following?

A) Amnesia

B) Analgesia

C) Anxiolysis

D) Sedation

B - In the pediatric ED setting, fentanyl is primarily used for its potent analgesic effects (100X as powerful as morphine), short duration of action (30 minutes or so), and its excellent hemodynamic stability. If a 10-year-old with radius and ulnar fractures is screaming in pain, morphine may seem like a great choice, but fentanyl is probably a better one. Morphine lasts several hours, which is great if you need long term pain control with burn management. However, if you need short term pain control such as for a closed reduction procedure, or if you have a hypotensive patient, fentanyl is a fabulous drug!

17) Fentanyl, when pushed rapidly, can cause a life-threatening condition called:

A) Loose chest syndrome

B) Rigid chest syndrome

C) Paradoxical pain syndrome

D) Big head, little body syndrome

B - Rigid chest syndrome can occur when large doses of fentanyl are pushed rapidly. Though primarily seen in neonates, this can happen in older children as well and is a truly scary experience for all involved. The patient's chest "locks up" and you are unable to ventilate the patient. Though Narcan (naloxone) can be tried to reverse the situation, the only reliable cure is a neuromuscular blocker such as succinylcholine. Of course, after giving succinylcholine, we know that the patient won't be able to breathe on his own, so we'd better be prepared. Anesthesia professionals know that this syndrome can indeed occur, but they also teach that if fentanyl is pushed in dosages appropriate for analgesia, and most importantly, is pushed slowly (over a couple of minutes), rigid chest is very rare. So if you are pushing fentanyl, you have to keep this in mind. Push it slowly and always be prepared!

18) Ketalar (ketamine) provides which of the following?

A) Amnesia

B) Analgesia

C) Sedation

D) All of the above

D - Ketamine provides all three desired effects very nicely with one shot. Ketamine can (rarely) cause respiratory depression, so administer it carefully and watch the patient closely. In addition, there are a couple of additional considerations. 1) Ketamine can increase nasal/oral secretions, so if a child already has lots of "boogers pouring out of his nose," ketamine is not a good choice in meds. Until recently, many practitioners administered atropine or Robinul (glycopyrrolate) in the same syringe to reduce secretions, but several recent studies have shown that though it sounded like a good idea, atropine or Robinul didn't really make a difference in the secretions. 2) Ketamine can make people wake up "a little nutty." This is medically described as children having "emergence reactions." Recent ketamine research reveals that if the patient goes to sleep nicely, there is an excellent likelihood that he or she will wake up nicely.

19) Nitronox (nitrous oxide, Entonox) is primarily administered for which of the following?

A) Amnesia

B) Analgesia

C) Sedation

D) All of the above

D - Nitrous oxide is colorless, odorless, and tasteless and more importantly, does all 3 things (sedation, decreased pain, amnesia) without a shot. Many EDs use Nitronox which is 50% oxygen and 50% nitrous oxide. As long as a 50/50 mixture is used and no additional sedatives/analgesics (i.e. fentanyl or Versed (midazolam) are given, respiratory depression is very, very rare.

20) A 16-year-old with a crush injury to the leg and compartment syndrome asks why the pain is so horrible. The peds ED nurse tells him that the pain is most likely caused by all of the following **except**:

A) Pressure on the nerves in the leg

B) Lack of blood flow to the leg muscles

C) Pressure on deep tendons in the leg

D) Bleeding into the leg muscles

C - The pain from compartment syndrome does not usually come from deep tendon pressure; the pain comes from the other three answers. The large muscle groups (arms/legs/and even the abdomen) are "shrink wrapped" in a membrane. Compartment syndrome occurs when there is edema or bleeding into the muscle group and the nerves, veins and arteries "get squished." As the pressure continues to build, this can result in decreased blood flow (ischemia) to the muscle tissues and severe pain.

Ortho / Pain

Certified Pediatric Emergency Nurse (CPEN) Review IV

21) The ED nurse knows that the signs and symptoms of increased compartment pressure include paralysis, parasthesia, pallor, pain, increased pressures and:

A) Prolonged capillary refill

B) Purple extremity

C) Palpation

D) Pulselessness

D - Pulselessness is the missing "P" in what is classically described as the "6 P's" of compartment syndrome: Pain, Paralysis, Parasthesia (diminished sensation), Pallor, Pressures (increased in the compartment), and Pulselessness. But that can be way too much to remember, and so we might be happy if we can remember and understand two of the six. First remember pain that is disproportionate to the injury. It hurts, and it should hurt, because it's broken. However, if the patient is screaming "cut my leg off!" there is a really good chance that compartment syndrome is developing. The reason the first sign, disproportionate pain, is so important, is that if we don't catch things quickly, the second thing that must be remembered, pulselessness, will follow. If the distal pulse is lost, there is a good chance that the limb may be lost. If so much pressure has built up that the nerves, veins, and high pressure arteries are squished, the muscle ischemia is horrible and amputation is a likely outcome.

22) Which symptom is considered the classic sign of a developing compartment syndrome?

A) Tenseness of the extremity or abdominal compartment

B) Chest wall rigidity with dyspnea

C) Pain that is out of proportion to the injury

D) No pain with passive stretch of the affected muscles

C - When you see compartment syndrome as a test question, just remember pain and pulses. The classic initial sign is out of proportion pain, while the parasthesias, pallor, paralysis and pressures all progress until the limb is eventually pulseless.

23) The emergency nurse knows that if compartment syndrome develops, the expected treatment in the ED or operating room involves:

A) Elevation of the affected extremity

B) Application of ice packs

C) Application of warm packs

D) Fasciotomies

D - Fasciotomies may be required if compartment syndrome develops. If you understand what is going on inside the injured area, you know what needs to be done to the area outside the injured area. The extremity is swollen, but elevation won't help because the blood vessels are squished and elevation will only make it harder for blood to get to the tissues. So elevation is not an appropriate intervention. Neither heat nor cold will effectively relieve the cause of the increased pressure, so we would not expect to proceed with those treatments initially.

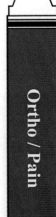

Ortho / Pain

24) If a patient is suspected to be a victim of child abuse, the ED nurse should anticipate orders for any of the following diagnostic tests **except:**

A) Radiographic skeletal survey

B) Nuclear medicine bone scan

C) PET scan

D) CT scan

C - A PET scan would not be expected for a child abuse victim. For most children with suspected child abuse, skeletal surveys (X-raying from top to bottom) are done in the ED to look for old and new fractures. In some cases, nuclear medicine bone scans are ordered to provide a more definitive identification of the status of fractures and other orthopedic injuries. In addition, if neurological trauma is suspected, a head CT scan is certainly warranted.

25) Which statement is **true** about Duchenne's muscular dystrophy (DMD)?

A) DMD is the most common and most severe type of childhood muscular dystrophy

B) DMD is the most common and least severe type of childhood muscular dystrophy

C) DMD is the least common and most severe type of childhood muscular dystrophy

D) DMD is the least common and least severe type of childhood muscular dystrophy

A - Duchenne's muscular dystrophy (DMD) is the most common and the most severe type of childhood muscular dystrophy. Between 3 and 5 years of age, male children typically start having difficulty in running, biking, or climbing stairs. Their gait becomes more unsteady until usually by the age of 12, they are unable to walk. Immobility leads to atrophy and contractures, but the facial, oral, and respiratory muscles are usually spared until the end stages. Respiratory infections or cardiac failure are often what eventually kills these patients. It is crucial to remember that the muscles of DMD kids are horribly affected, but their brains are intact. They are just kids trapped in a progressively deteriorating body. Children with DMD definitely get the attention of anesthesia providers when sedation is required, as these children have a higher chance of cardiac arrest, malignant hyperthermia, and aspiration associated with anesthesia. If these children require procedural sedation, a quick call to anesthesia for their input is highly warranted.

26) Cerebral palsy results in motor developmental delays:

A) Always

B) Frequently

C) Rarely

D) Never

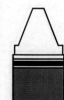

A - Cerebral palsy (CP) always affects muscle coordination and body movement. It is defined as a "non-specific term applied to neurologic disorders characterized by early onset and impaired movement and posture." Though it is commonly thought to be due to birth asphyxia, recent research is finding that over 80% of cases are from unknown prenatal factors. Either way, all children with CP have delayed gross motor development, but it is important to remember that 40-50% of CP kids have <u>normal</u> intelligence; just abnormal motor tone or performance. Test tip: Generally, you will want to avoid answers that use the words "always" or "never", unless, as is the case in this question, "always" is the defining characteristic of the situation.

Certified Pediatric Emergency Nurse (CPEN) Review IV

27) Which complication is most feared in a pediatric patient with a fractured pelvis?

A) Pneumothorax

B) Ruptured bladder

C) Intestinal perforation

D) Retroperitoneal hemorrhage

D - The problem with truly messed up pelvic fractures is not necessarily the broken bones, but the nearby blood vessels. Though rare in pediatrics, crushed pelvic bones can quickly result in hemorrhagic shock and death. In the past, and for many years, MAST (military anti-shock trousers) were used by EMS and ED professionals in an attempt to combat hypovolemic shock and stabilize pelvic fractures. However, their use has dramatically decreased over the years. Currently, pelvic stabilization devices such as the Pelvic Sling (www.sammedical.com), T-POD (www.tpod.com), or even a bed sheet can be used as temporary stabilization devices. If the patient is hemodynamically questionable, interventional radiology can attempt embolization to clot the bleeding vessels from the inside out. Once the patient is hemodynamically stable, definitive surgical stabilization of the fractures can be done.

28) A 10-year-old male was riding his bike when he fell and straddled the bicycle. While performing a secondary survey, the nurse notes blood at the urethral meatus. This finding suggests that:

A) Foley or urinary catheterization should be immediately performed

B) Foley or urinary catheterization should not be performed

C) There is a probable bladder rupture

D) The patient has a retroperitoneal hematoma

B - Blood at the urinary meatus suggests a possible urethral injury and is an absolute contraindication for urethral urinary catheterization, at least until the patient has been evaluated by urology. Moral of the story, if you see this in a trauma patient, do not attempt to place a Foley catheter as this could turn a partially transected urethra into a completely transected urethra.

29) A 16-year-old patient arrives at the ED after being the unrestrained driver in a high-speed MVC. The patient reports that his knees struck the dashboard and his "hip is killing him." During the secondary survey, the nurse notes the right leg is shortened and internally rotated. Based on these findings, the ED nurse suspects that this patient has:

A) An anterior hip dislocation

B) A posterior hip dislocation

C) A patellar fracture

D) A comminuted fibula fracture

B - A posterior hip dislocation will typically present with the affected leg shortened and internally rotated. But if you have trouble remembering the signs and symptoms, think about what happened, or what is referred to as the mechanism of injury. Picture the vehicle moving at a high rate of speed. Everything inside the vehicle is also moving at a high rate of speed. All of a sudden, the vehicle suddenly stops due to an impact. The vehicle and everything firmly attached to the vehicle, like the dashboard, stops. Our unrestrained driver, however, does not stop... at least not all of him and not all at the same time. First his knees hit the dashboard. The dashboard isn't moving, so his knees aren't moving any more either. And, the hips aren't moving any more either. But the rest of his body (pelvis, trunk, head, etc.) is still moving forward, and at that high rate of speed, until something else, such as the steering wheel, stops him. At that precise moment, his hip was stopped, but the pelvis was still moving. Enough speed and force combined to move the pelvis forward and away from the hip or femur. The pelvis moved forward and left the hip behind, or posteriorly dislocated. Other injuries such as fractures to the patella and/or fibula could certainly also have occurred.

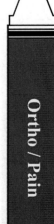

Reducing the dislocated hip back into place is a true emergency and should be done as soon as possible (with appropriate IV sedation/analgesics) to prevent possible neurovascular damage.

30) A 16-year-old rugby player arrives at the ED per EMS. He is holding his left arm by his side and appears very uncomfortable. He reports that he was injured during a game and developed sudden and severe shoulder pain. The patient resists all movement of the arm and has a loss of shoulder symmetry. Based on the above assessment, the ED nurse suspects that the patient has:

A) An anterior shoulder dislocation

B) A posterior shoulder dislocation

C) A fractured clavicle

D) An acute tear of the rotator cuff

A - Over 90% of shoulder dislocations in the ED are anterior in nature, and this teen has a classic anterior shoulder dislocation. Your clues are the history, the position of the arm (at the side versus against the front), the resistance to movement, and the fact that one side doesn't look like the other. An X-ray will quickly confirm the diagnosis and procedural sedation with IV analgesics (fentanyl) and sedatives (Versed (midazolam) will probably allow for the humane relocation of the shoulder.

31) An 8-year-old girl arrives at the ED after a sledding accident. She is alert and crying and has gross deformity of her right leg with exposed bone. Assessments of distal CMS (circulation, motor, and sensation) are grossly intact and bleeding is controlled. The ED nurse would expect orders for all of the following **except**:

A) IV antibiotic administration

B) Preparation for surgical repair

C) Long leg cast application

D) Posterior mold application

C - A long leg cast application is not appropriate in this situation, as it would completely enclose the still dirty wound and hinder further pre-operative assessments. With this exposed wound, antibiotics are absolutely to be expected. This child will be going to surgery to debride the wound and repair the fractures, so any of the other pre-op preparations above, including a posterior mold for stability are also appropriate.

32) A 2-year old, previously healthy child presents to triage with a refusal to move his left arm. The mother states that while walking and holding the child's hand, she tried to keep him from falling and he hasn't moved his arm since. There is no visible swelling or deformity and distal neurovascular function is intact. Based on the history and presentation, the ED nurse suspects this patient has likely suffered what type of injury:

A) Radial head fracture

B) Tennis elbow

C) Nursemaid's elbow

D) Supracondylar humerus fracture

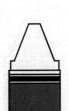

Ortho / Pain

C - Nursemaid's elbow occurs when a ligament in the arm slips over the head of the radius, into the joint space, and becomes entrapped. A common scenario for this type of injury would be when a child is falling and the individual holding the child's hand doesn't let go. Another common mechanism of injury is simply swinging a child by the hands. Reduction is easily performed in the emergency department, and providing there is immediate return of active movement, no orthopedic follow-up is necessary. Although there are no known sequelae, there is a relatively high incidence of recurrence. Parents should be informed of this fact and the mechanism of injury should be explained.

33) The preferred intramuscular (IM) injection site in infants and children under three years of age is the:

A) Vastus lateralis (anterior lateral thigh)

B) Ventrogluteal (lateral hip)

C) Dorsogluteal (upper outer buttock)

D) Deltoid (shoulder)

A - The vastus lateralis is the IM site of choice in children under the age of three as it's the largest muscle group in young children and is free of important nerves or blood vessels. The lateral hip is a close second for infants and adults, especially those requiring a large injection volume. The dorsogluteal area or "the butt" can tolerate larger injection volumes, but there is the danger of hitting the sciatic nerve and it's embarrassing to the child. The deltoid is fine for small volumes (0.5-1ml) and works great for many injections, especially in older children. The ENPC textbook is an excellent review source for this information and is highly recommended.

34) Which of the following medications can be given intranasally (IN) for pediatric pain management?

A) Versed® (midazolam)

B) Aspirin (aspirin)

C) Sublimaze® (fentanyl)

D) Tylenol® (acetaminophen, Panadol®)

C – Note that the question specified pain management. Atomized intranasal fentanyl is becoming very popular in pediatric and adult emergency care as an option for pain relief until intravenous access can be obtained. (Additional information is available at www.intranasal.net and www.wolfetory.com.) You may be more familiar with intranasal Versed®, and while Versed® certainly can be administered intranasally for seizures or sedation, and has sedative and amnestic effects, it does NOTHING for pain. Neither aspirin nor Tylenol® are administered intranasally. Per the ENA CPEN Exam outline (and common sense), pediatric patients receiving opiates and/or sedatives should be monitored for respiratory depression.

35) Which of the following medications can be given intranasally (IN) for pediatric sedation?

A) Versed® (midazolam)

B) Toradol® (ketorolac)

C) Sublimaze® (fentanyl)

D) Tylenol® (acetaminophen, Panadol®)

A – Once again, pay close attention to the wording in the question. Of the medications listed, only Versed® is considered for sedation. It can be administered orally, sublingually, rectally, IM, IV, and intranasally. The best way to administer Versed® intranasally is have it sprayed and atomized in, not dripped in. Dripping Versed® into the nose burns and it tends to get swallowed down or squirted out that way. Versed® is very versatile; pick an available route and appropriate dose and follow it with patient monitoring and 10-30 minutes in a quiet setting (for your patient, not necessarily for you). Your patient should go to sleep quite peacefully. All of the other medications listed are used for their analgesic and/or antipyretic effects, but not for any sedative effects. In addition, while Toradol® and fentanyl can be given intranasally, Tylenol® cannot.

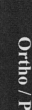

36) Intranasal medications can be used for all of the following emergencies **except**:

A) Seizures

B) Near-drowning incidents

C) Opiate overdose

D) Benzodiazepene overdose

B – While there are many medications that can be administered intranasally, none of them are specifically for near-drowning. Seizures can be managed with intranasal Versed® (midazolam) or Ativan® (lorazepam), opiate overdose with intranasal Narcan® (naloxone), and benzodiazepine overdose with intranasal Romazicon® (flumazenil, Anexate®). Helpful Hint: When reversing opiates with Narcan®, the desired endpoint of reversal therapy is to restore the spontaneous respiratory drive, not to fully wake up the patient.

37) You have no IV access and your uncooperative 3-year old patient who requires reduction of a dislocated fracture begins having a mild asthma attack. Which one of the following medications would be the ideal choice for intramuscular (IM) sedation?

A) Robinul® (glycopyrrolate)

B) Versed® (midazolam)

C) Ketalar® (ketamine)

D) Amidate® (etomidate)

C – Ketamine is a great choice in this child for multiple reasons. It can be given IM. It provides sedation, amnesia, and analgesia and bronchodilation. This sounds like just the thing for an asthmatic with no IV access and a painful extremity injury. None of the other drugs provide this combination of sleeping/forgetting/pain control/breathing. When preparing ketamine for administration, it is important to remember that ketamine is available as 10mg/ml, 50mg/ml, and 100mg/ml. (Those dose differences and decimal points really make a difference!) Although both Robinul® and Versed® can be given IM, Robinul® is an anticholinergic (decreasing secretions and drying up the goobers) and Versed (as well as other benzodiazepines such as Ativan® (lorazepam) or Valium® (diazepam) which do provide sedation, but do not provide analgesia. Etomidate is not given IM. Drawbacks of ketamine include: increased oral and respiratory secretions, the fact that it can't be reversed and possible hallucinations or agitation upon emergence. If necessary, secretions can be managed with intramuscular Robinul®. Hallucinations are unlikely to occur in a preadolescent child, especially if he is in as quiet an environment as possible. IM benzodiazepines may be given to help with emergence delirium but, in most cases, if they go to sleep nicely on ketamine, they wake up very nicely on ketamine. Minimizing stimuli pre- and post-ketamine administration is crucial. In the emergency department with kids that are "SAABing," ketamine has four beneficial effects: Sedation, Analgesia, Amnesia, and Bronchodilation!

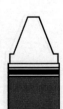

Ortho / Pain

38) Your 8-year old male patient with a history of Duchenne's muscular dystrophy (DMD) requires emergent intubation and ventilator support. After sedation, which neuromuscular blocker or "paralytic" is absolutely contraindicated?

A) Rocuronium ("Rock," Zemuron®)

B) Vecuronium ("Vec," Norcuron®)

C) Succinylcholine ("Sux," Anectine®)

D) Pancuronium ("Pav," Pavulon®)

C – Succinylcholine is contraindicated for multiple reasons in Duchenne's muscular dystrophy (DMD.) For patients with DMD, succinylcholine can cause severe spikes in serum potassium levels and lead to life-threatening cardiac arrhythmias. Succinylcholine is also a highly suspected trigger for malignant hyperthermia (where the patient's temperature goes to "a million" and they die in front of your eyes) in patients with DMD. In addition to seeing that "one of these things isn't like the others," it might be helpful to remember that muscular dystrophy "sucks" as a diagnosis, so NO SUX!

39) Your patient with DMD from the previous question is now intubated and on a ventilator. You are using end-tidal capnography. Over the course of 45-minutes, while waiting for a PICU bed, you notice your patient's heart rate, temperature and end-tidal CO2 steadily climbing. His limbs are stiff and hard to move. This patient is **most** likely experiencing:

A) Inadequate sedation

B) A normal response to intubation

C) Malignant hyperthermia (MH)

D) Inadequate pain control

C – This is certainly not a normal response to intubation, and while it is regrettable that inadequate sedation and pain control are still huge issues in pediatric emergency care and may seem tempting as correct answers, they do not explain the increasing temperature, rigidity, and end-tidal CO2. These are hallmarks of malignant hyperthermia and include muscle rigidity, rhabdomyolysis (rapid breakdown of skeletal muscle), and a hypermetabolic state which can quickly result in death. If you have a patient with Duchenne's muscular mystrophy (DMD) who's crashing with a fast and furious fever, think sepsis or possibly malignant hyperthermia.

40) Treatment for the previous patient with malignant hyperthermia includes:

A) Prostigmin® (neostigmine) and Robinul® (glycopyrrolate)

B) Rubbing alcohol bath

C) Cooling and Dantrium® (dantrolene sodium)

D) Romazicon® (flumazenil, Anexate®), Narcan® (naloxalone), and Amidate® (etomidate)

C – Dantrolene sodium is the only treatment currently available and approved for malignant hyperthermia. It is classified as a fast-acting skeletal muscle relaxant, and is given IV in these situations. The initial adult dose of 1 mg/kg is also the pediatric dose. In the very rare occasion that this happens in the ED, a call to anesthesia and pharmacy is highly, highly recommended as they are the experts in the management of this condition.

41) All of the following pieces of equipment should be readily available at the bedside during procedural sedation **except**:

A) Bag-valve mask with appropriate size mask attached to 100% O2

B) Suction device with a rigid tonsil tip (Yankauer®) device

Ortho / Pain

C) Bedside ultrasound or C-Arm radiography to ensure proper anatomical placement of minimally invasive catheters

D) Monitoring equipment including pulse oximetry and (ideally) capnography (EtCO2)

C – Don't be fooled by a long answer with lots of big words. Seriously, when a patient requires sedation for the completion of a procedure, it is referred to as "procedural sedation." Sedatives have the potential to slow the patient's respirations, so the use of capnography through an EtCO2 monitor provides early detection of hypoventilation (often even before the pulse ox.) Remember, if you suddenly stop breathing, it may take quite a while (longer than you would expect) for the pulse ox to drop below 90% and the alarms to start going off. Long before you see this pulse ox drop, you will see the CO2 rise as your patient's breathing slows. Anesthesia and emergency medicine research shows that the combination of pulse oximetry and EtCO2 monitoring (often done through a specialized nasal cannula device) will let you know if the child is running into trouble long before they desat, brady down, or even worse, arrest. Clinicians may intervene via stimulation, supplemental oxygen, assisting ventilation, or giving pharmacological agents such as Narcan® (naloxone – for opiates) or Romazicon® (flumazenil, Anexate® – for benzodiazepines). Having suction at the bedside is necessary for removing excess secretions or in the event the patient vomits. And that brings up an interesting question. Do children have to be NPO (nothing by mouth) for a specific period of time prior to procedural sedation? The literature is divided on this topic. While some recommend that the patient have only clear liquids for two hours prior, and no solid food for at least six hours prior to procedural sedation, other researchers have reported their positive experiences with "no wait, just sedate." NPO for 2-6 hours prior to a procedure may be the ideal, but not always a reality, so be prepared!

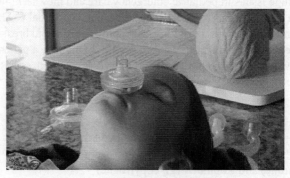

Mask that is "too small"

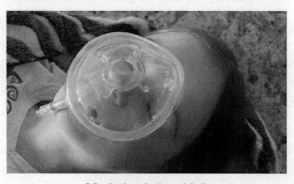

Mask that is "too big"

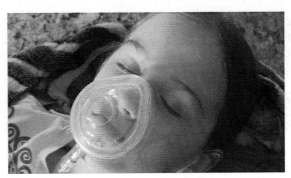

Mask that is "just right"

Photos courtesy of Joshua DeBoer, my then 14-year old aspiring computer genius son – Summit Studios Games

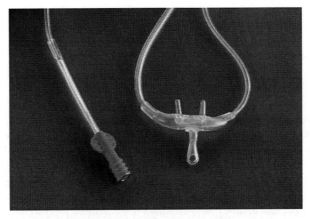

Pediatric nasal cannula capnography device
Note the ability to administer supplemental oxygen and monitor end-tidal CO_2 for both "nose & mouth breathers"

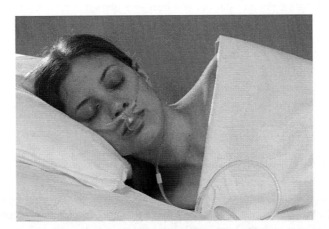

Nasal cannula capnography in use

![Normal ventilation capnograph with points A, B, C, D, E marked, CO2 axis up to 40]

Normal ventilation capnograph
Capnography images courtesy of Oridion Medical - www.oridion.com

42) What is the **correct** reversal agent for fentanyl?

A) Narcan® (naloxone)

B) Romazicon® (flumazenil, Anexate®)

C) Prostigmin® (neostigmine)

D) There is currently no reversal agent available for fentanyl

A – Fentanyl is an opiate, and Narcan® is the antidote for the opiates (the really good pain killers). It is commonly given for suspected opiate overdose. It may be administered IV, IM, nasally, SQ, or via the ET tube. Romazicon® is the reversal agent for benzodiazepines (the let's go to sleep no drugs). Like Narcan®, Romazicon® can be administered (cautiously) to patients with a history of addiction to avoid possible withdrawal seizures. While overdose or addiction is rarely cause for concern with the smaller children or in cases of procedural sedation, it certainly can be a concern with older kids, teens, and adults, and it's something you have to keep in mind. Neostigmine is an acetylcholinesterase inhibitor and is used in the operating room to reverse chemical paralysis from non-depolarizing muscular blockers following surgical procedures.

43) As you are passing the nursing station, you hear an ambulance crew calling in a radio report on a 7-year old patient. Another nurse acknowledges the call and says to you "sounds like Waddell's triad." Based on this comment, what kind of patient would you expect?

A) A little league baseball player hit in the chest with a fast pitch

B) A child struck by a car

C) A little league baseball player hit in the head with a baseball bat

D) A child with an upper respiratory infection

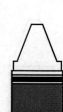

B - When young children waddle into the street and are hit by a car, the ensuing injuries are sometimes described as Waddell's triad. (Seriously, we didn't make this up!) Typically presentation of Waddell's triad is: 1) Femur fracture (contact with the bumper) 2) Intra-thoracic and/or intra-abdominal injuries (impact from the car grill and/or hood,) and 3) Head injuries (being thrown into the air by the car and the eventual impact of the head landing on the ground.) While it is true that not all children struck by a car will present with all of these injuries, or even with these specific injuries, it is important to remember that children involved in high-energy impact will rarely display isolated injuries. It is much more likely to see multiple traumas from multiple secondary impacts (car vs. body, body vs. street, etc.). Waddle's triad actually was initially used to describe adult, not pediatric, injuries associated with pedestrian vs. automobile collisions. Though a frequent test question, as kids and cars come in all different shapes and sizes, research has shown this triad not to be reliable in predicting pediatric injuries. An impact to the chest, as in answer A, may cause cardiac tamponade, which would present with Beck's triad (distended neck veins (JVD), distant heart sounds, hypotension) or commotio cordis. Head trauma patients with severely increased intracranial pressure would display Cushing's triad (hypertension with widening pulse pressure, bradycardia, agonal respirations.) A child with an upper respiratory infection might present with Dayquil's triad (cough, nasal congestion and a sore throat) and really shouldn't be in an ambulance anyway. (Okay, we made up the Dayquil® triad. Just checking to see if you were paying attention!)

44) You are treating a 13-year old obese child who is complaining of right hip pain. The patient tells you that she does not remember any incident that may have caused an injury, but that the pain worsens with activity. The pain has been present for 2 months. What is the **most** likely source of her hip pain?

A) Osteoporosis

B) Femoral vein thrombosis

C) Slipped capital femoral epiphysis (SCFE)

D) Fibromyalgia

C – Pediatric and adolescent patients who present with acute or ongoing hip pain with difficulty walking or a limp should be evaluated for a slipped capital femoral epiphysis (SCFE). This condition is triggered by instability of the femoral growth plate that causes the articular surface of the femur to literally slide off the rest of the head of the femur, similar to a scoop of ice cream sliding off the top of an ice cream cone. Patients with knee pain of similar nature should also be evaluated for SCFE since hip pain can be referred to the knee. Evaluation should include a clinical exam and radiographic imaging (plain films and occasionally MRI). Patients with "stable" SCFEs are those who are able to walk with or without crutches. "Unstable" SCFEs are those who are unable to ambulate at all. This is an important distinction as, not only can they not walk, but more importantly, they are at higher risk for avascular necrosis of the femoral head (no blood to the hip). Frequently, these patients will undergo an outpatient operative internal fixation. Twenty to 40 percent of teens with one slipped hip go on to develop bilateral slipped hips within 18 months. The key words that should lead you to pick SCFE as the correct answer are "obese" and "hip pain."

45) In order to ensure safety and provide adequate procedural sedation and analgesia for the profoundly developmentally delayed child, the emergency nurse must be especially alert to vital signs and other physical cues because:

A) Families of these patients are very likely to sue healthcare practitioners without cause

B) These patients often pose physical threats to caregivers

C) Families of these patients often have very limited knowledge about the conditions of the children

D) These patients may have altered communication, cognition, and sensation abilities.

D – These patients may not be able to verbally communicate discomfort. Increased heart or respiratory rates may be your primary clues. It cannot be overemphasized how important vigilant reassessment is in the developmentally delayed child. Prior to sedation, taking the time to speak with parents or caregivers to establish the child's developmental baseline is generally helpful because the parents/caregivers are typically well informed. Neither the patients, nor the parents pose unusual threats.

Certified Pediatric Emergency Nurse (CPEN) Review IV

46) The triage nurse is evaluating an 8-year old who fell from a tree. He has an obvious deformity of his right wrist, with what appears to be an open fracture. All of the following would be appropriate triage interventions **except**:

A) Cover the wound with a sterile dressing

B) Applying a traction splint to reduce pain, restore blood flow and minimize the risk for nerve and tissue damage

C) Splint the extremity to prevent further damage and assist with pain control

D) Assessing the circulation, motor and sensation (CMS) of the extremity

B – There is no traction splint for a wrist injury. (Femur fractures, yes, and used for the reasons mentioned above.) In addition to appropriate concerns regarding pain management, the issues concerning open fractures revolve around infection prevention and regular assessments of circulation, motor, and sensation. Covering a wound such as this with a sterile dressing is certainly appropriate and IV antibiotics before possible operative debridement are quite possibly in this child's near future. (Remember to keep the child NPO for possible surgery!) In addition to assessing CMS before and after splinting the joints above and below the injured area, regular reassessment of CMS should be undertaken to detect compromise to the extremity sooner rather than later.

47) A 9-year old with an isolated obvious mid-femur deformity arrives via ambulance with a traction splint in place. The EMS provider states the patient had good circulation, motor, sensation (CMS) prior to the traction splint application. Your initial assessment reveals a cool, pale, and pulseless foot. Pulselessness is confirmed via doppler. Your **first** intervention would be to:

A) Place injured extremity in dependent position

B) Call orthopedics to have compartment pressures measured to confirm compartment syndrome

C) Immediately reduce the splint traction to the point where circulation is restored

D) Ice and elevate the extremity and order a bilateral femur films (for comparison views)

C – If CMS was intact prior to splint application and absent following splint application, the current recommendation is to release traction. Although releasing the traction may be painful to the patient, the preservation of vascular integrity supersedes concerns about causing pain. Once circulation is restored, pain management should be addressed. The patient would definitely need intravenous access and the administration of narcotics for pain control. Putting the extremity in a dependent position will not restore circulation to the pulseless foot and is contradictory to the normal recommendation of ice and elevation. Compartment syndrome, although possible, is an unlikely cause of the pulseless extremity due to the acuteness of the situation. In addition, there is likely to be a time delay in obtaining the equipment and staff to get a compartment pressure, and the immediate need is to restore circulation. The femur is obviously deformed, so a film is not needed immediately to confirm the fracture. And the foot is already cool and pulseless, so ice and elevation won't solve the problem!

Ortho / Pain

Certified Pediatric Emergency Nurse (CPEN) Review IV

48) A 6-month old infant is suspected by the triage nurse to have multiple fractures. The parents state the baby rolled off the couch and also tell you he is being worked up for possible osteogenesis imperfecta (OI). Which of the following should you consider when treating this patient?

A) This is most likely a case of child abuse since the story (six-month old rolling off the couch) doesn't match the injuries

B) The parents are hiding something since OI is an adult onset disease

C) Children with OI will require special care to avoid additional injuries

D) You will be able to determine whether this patient has been a victim of abuse by a simple assessment of the injuries

C – OI is a congenital bone fragility caused by genetic mutations. The body of an OI child produces decreased or defective collagen, which results in fragile bones that are easily broken. Therefore, special care should be exercised with these patients. It is not uncommon for an individual to experience dozens of fractures over the course of his life. It is important to note that the fractures that occur with OI may be mistaken for child abuse because of their frequency of occurrence, the involvement of multiple bones and/or the seemingly minor mechanisms of injury. Parents of OI children often carry documentation to make ED personnel aware of their child's condition in order to avoid this diagnostic pitfall. X-rays of children with OI will usually show that even the bones that aren't acutely fractured, also are not normal. Neither the initial nurse's nor physician's exams may definitively determine whether or not the fractures of a child with OI are due to intentional injury. (Remember that OI children can be victims of abuse, too!) As with all cases of possible intentional injury, the suspicion is based on all the information gained via history, exam and diagnostic tests. This 6-month old should be able to roll over, so the alleged mechanism is developmentally appropriate. A funduscopic exam that shows retinal hemorrhages or evidence of other internal injuries on exam would suggest abuse, since these are not caused by OI alone. X-rays may reveal certain types of fractures that are typically seen in intentional injuries; however, some of those may also be seen in children with OI. The distinction is one that would likely not be made in the ED. Nonetheless, if there is any doubt, actions should be taken to initiate an investigation by appropriate authorities.

49) While in the ED, children with osteogenesis imperfecta should always have which of the following:

A) Supplemental oxygen

B) Suicide precautions as these children are understandably very depressed

C) A replacement trach "jump kit" at the bedside with at least a "1 size smaller" trach

D) Special padding to fill in gaps between the child and the mattress or wheelchair

D – Ideally these children will arrive or be provided with a special gel pad to protect their abnormally soft skulls, as well as wedges and blanket rolls to fill any gaps between the child and the mattress or wheelchair. These children often have bowed legs and spines, so it is important to pad well under and around these curvatures. Most importantly, we need to understand how to position and handle the child (slow, gentle movements that provide a maximum of support) in order to avoid causing fractures. We deliberately threw in the patient safety (suicide precautions), airway (extra trach), and breathing (supplemental oxygen) options to remind you not to read too much into the question.

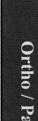

Ortho / Pain

Certified Pediatric Emergency Nurse (CPEN) Review IV

50) Which of the following is a special positioning consideration for children with osteogenesis imperfecta?

A) They should be provided with special neck braces and collars to support the abnormally large head

B) They should not be placed in a wheel chair

C) They should not be positioned on their stomachs for sleeping

D) They should be positioned in a lateral recumbent posture to promote drainage of secretions

C – Children with OI should NEVER be positioned prone because the child's body weight can compress the abnormally soft ribs causing fractures and potential suffocation. Children with OI do not have abnormally large heads, and wheel chairs with sufficient padding are just fine. These children do not normally have any problem clearing their own oral secretions.

51) After cutting his leg on a piece of metal several days ago in the backyard, an 11-year old presents to the ED with a complaint of "it looks infected." It is important for the ED nurse to verify his immunization status due to concerns about:

A) Tetanus (Clostridium tetani)

B) Pertussis (Bordetella pertussis)

C) Lyme disease (Borrelia burgdorferi)

D) Plague (Yersinia pestis)

A – The answer is Clostridium tetani (more commonly known as tetanus). Many of us learned about tetanus from our parents or grandparents and urban legends about the dreaded lockjaw. In children who are fully immunized, tetanus is not really a concern, although many believe it is. Wound care and infection are the real issues in this case. In the under- or non-immunized pediatric (or adult) patient, tetanus is certainly still a consideration that must be addressed with tetanus toxoid (booster shot) and possibly Hypertet® (tetanus immune globulin) for tetanus prone wounds. Pertussis (whooping cough) is making a huge comeback, so current recommendations are to give a combined tetanus/pertussis booster instead of just tetanus toxoid whenever possible. Lyme disease (Northern US) and plague (Southwestern US) are possible issues as well, although vaccines against these infections are either not available (Lyme disease) or not routinely available (plague). And neither Lyme disease, plague nor pertussis fit the story. For the test… if you read anything involving honey, chances are the answer is botulism. If you read anything involving aspirin, chances are the answer is Reye's syndrome (or Kawasaki's, but as a treatment, not a risk factor) and if the question involves punctures, lacerations or abrasions, chances are, the answer is tetanus.

52) The FACES pain rating scale is a helpful tool for evaluating pain in children. Which of the following is **true** regarding the FACES pain rating scale?

A) The nurse should be able to look at the patient's face and determine the appropriate number on the scale from 0 to 10

B) FACES is a self-reporting tool where the patient identifies which face represents how she or he is feeling

C) FACES is not useful in children over 3 years of age

D) FACES stands for: Fine, Angry, Crying, Emotional, Stoic

Ortho / Pain

B – The FACES scale is a self reporting tool for pain assessment that has been proven very effective for small children. Before asking a child to use it for the first time, you should explain it to the child. The child should look at the cartoon faces and understand that each face is for a person who feels happy because there is no pain or sad because there is some or a lot of hurt. The child should pick the face that best describes his or her pain. This scale can be used for children as young as 3 years of age.

Translations of Wong-Baker FACES Pain Rating Scale

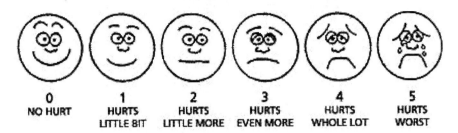

Original Instructions:
Explain to the person that each face is for a person who feels happy because he has no pain (hurt) or sad because he has some or a lot of pain. **Face 0** is very happy because he doesn't hurt at all. **Face 1** hurts just a little bit. **Face 2** hurts a little more. **Face 3** hurts even more. **Face 4** hurts a whole lot. **Face 5** hurts as much as you can imagine, although you don't have to be crying to feel this bad. Ask the person to choose the face that best describes how he is feeling.

Rating scale is recommended for persons age 3 years and older.

Brief word instructions: Point to each face using the words to describe the pain intensity. Ask the child to choose the face that best describes their own pain and record the appropriate number.

Wong-Baker FACES Pain Rating Scale, from Hockenberry, M. & Wilson, D. (2009)
Wong's essentials of pediatric nursing, 8th edition. Mosby: St Louis.
Used with permission. Copyright Mosby.

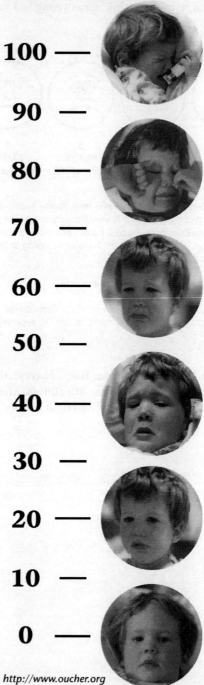

Caucasian boy OUCHER™ scale was developed and copyrighted in 1983 by
Judith E. Beyer, PhD, RN, University of Missouri-Kansas City School of Nursing, USA.

OUCHER!

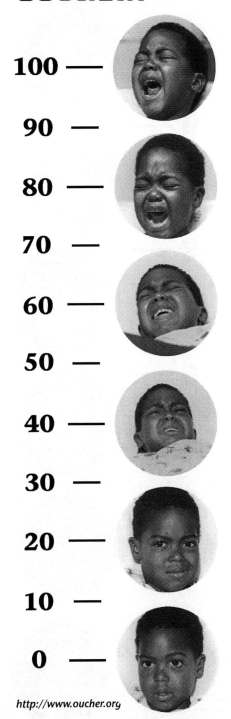

http://www.oucher.org

African-American boy OUCHER™ scale was developed and copyrighted in 1990 by Mary J. Denyes, PhD, RN (Wayne State University) and Antonia M. Villarruel PhD, RN (University of Michigan) USA. Cornelia P. Porter PhD, RN and Charlotta Marshall RN, MSN contributed to the development of this scale.

Ortho / Pain

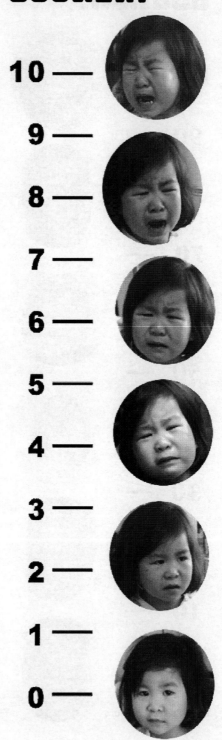

Asian girl OUCHER scale were developed and copyrighted in 2003 by C.H. Yeh and C.H. Wang (Chang Gung University), Taiwan.

Certified Pediatric Emergency Nurse (CPEN) Review IV

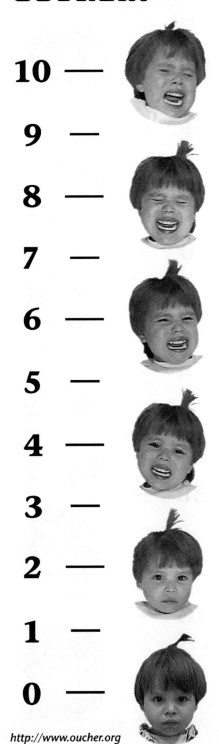

http://www.oucher.org

First nations girl OUCHER™ scale was developed and copyrighted by Carla Shapiro RN, MN, Canada, 1997.

OUCHER!

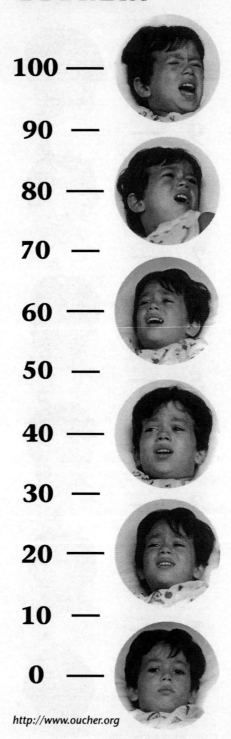

http://www.oucher.org

Hispanic boy OUCHER™ scale was developed and copyrighted in 1990 by Antonia M. Villarruel PhD, RN (University of Michigan) and Mary J. Denyes PhD, RN (Wayne State University), USA.

OUCHER™ scale images courtesy of Judith Beyer RN, PhD - www.OUCHER.org

Lundblom's Lessons

EMS arrived with a 4-year old who was hypothermic and in full cardiopulmonary arrest. They were called to the home by the grandmother who said she went in to wake him up from a nap and found him "not breathing." The patient's "down-time" was unknown. The child had no significant medical history, was on no medications and immunizations were up to date.

It was noted by the physician during intubation that the patient had a "sticky spot" on his forehead. The child was pronounced dead after all resuscitative measures failed. As a result of many discussions between ED staff, police and grandmother, both during resuscitation and after death, the grandmother finally admitted to having placed one of her Duragesic® (fentanyl) patches (she was being treated for cancer) on his forehead so he would "take a nap." Postmortem urine toxicology screen was positive for opiates, i.e. fentanyl.

Teaching points:

In dealing with pulseless electrical activity (PEA) and pediatric arrest patients, make sure to address the "H's and T's"
Stress possibility of hyperkalemia for any patients with known renal disease

Stress hypothermia for newborns/infants, because so many very competent ED staff members seem to forget that one.

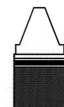

Ortho / Pain

Appendix 9-A

Common Pediatric Orthopedic Emergencies

Name	What is it?	Signs and Symptoms	Diagnostics	Management
Septic arthritis	Infection of the joint space – Bacteria spread from somewhere else, such as otitis, URI, cellulitis, etc.	Fever and/or chills Decreased ROM of joint Limping Palpable effusion	CBC, ESR, blood cultures, arthrocentesis (test of choice), vaginal, rectal, oral cultures to rule out N. gonorrhea infection, X-rays to rule out osteomyelitis	IV antibiotics Oral analgesics
Osteomyelitis	Bone infection – Bacteria spread from somewhere else, such as trauma, puncture wound, open fractures, etc.	Fever Focal bone pain Unwilling to bear weight or move limb	CBC, ESR, blood cultures, bone and chest X-rays (rule out TB), wound culture, bone scan	IV antibiotics IV analgesics Immobilize the extremity Possible surgery
Transient Synovitis	Inflammation of the membrane of the hip joint – Not sure why it occurs	Acute groin pain Non-traumatic knee/thigh pain Usually afebrile	CBC, ESR, X-rays, ultrasound, or MRI of hip	NSAIDS Bed rest with no weight bearing until pain free

Certified Pediatric Emergency Nurse (CPEN) Review IV

Name	What is it?	Signs and Symptoms	Diagnostics	Management
Slipped femoral capital epiphysis (SCFE)	Spontaneous displacement of the proximal femoral epiphysis which causes displacement of the femoral head relative to the femoral neck – Not sure why it occurs – Most common adolescent hip disorder	Severe hip pain (acute) External rotation with shortening (acute) Several months of pain, limping, and out-toed gait (chronic is most common type)	Pelvic X-rays	Oral analgesics No weight bearing Traction Surgical repair
Osgood-Schlatter Disease	Microfracture of the tibial tubercle – Running and jumping	Anterior knee pain Point tenderness at the tibial tubercle	Knee X-rays	NSAIDS Decreased activity x 2-3 weeks
Osteogenesis Imperfecta (OI)	"Brittle bone disease" - Most common osteoporosis syndrome in childhood – Genetic cause	Variable fractures, blue sclera, less fractures post-puberty (with most common type of OI)	Genetic testing (not in ED) X-rays and history Rule out abuse	Oral or IV analgesics Fracture care Gentle handling
Juvenile Rheumatoid Arthritis (JRA) – Now called Juvenile Idiopathic Arthritis (JIA)	Chronic inflammation of joints with eventual erosion, destruction, and fibrosis of the cartilage – Rarely "rheumatoid" type in children	Arthritis symptoms	ESR, rheumatoid factor (only + in 10% of cases), X-rays	NSAIDS Methotrexate Steroids
Childhood Accidental Spiral Tibial (CAST) fracture – aka Toddler's fracture	Spiral fracture of the lower 1/3 of the tibia caused by twisting/rotating the leg with the foot fixed in place (i.e. foot caught in something)	Limping or unwilling to bear weight No history of trauma (if unwitnessed) and no fever	Radiographs Bone scan Rule out abuse (most commonly midshaft or upper tibia)	Oral analgesics Long leg cast for several weeks

CBC - Complete blood count
ESR - Erythrocyte sedimentation rate
MRI - Magnetic resonance imaging
NSAIDS - Non-steroidal anti-inflammatory drugs
TB - Tuberculosis
URI - Upper respiratory infection

Appendix 9-B
Wong-Baker FACES Pain Rating Scale

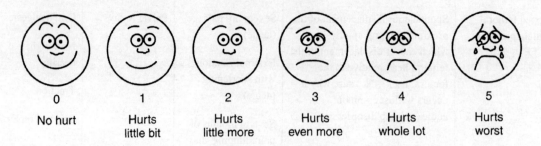

Brief word instructions: Point to each face using the words to describe the pain intensity. Ask the child to choose the face that best describes his/her own pain and record the appropriate number.

Original instructions: Explain to the person that each face is for a person who feels happy because he has no pain (hurt) or sad because he has some or a lot of pain. Face 0 is very happy because he doesn't hurt at all. Face 1 hurts just a little bit. Face 2 hurts a little more. Face 3 hurts even more. Face 4 hurts a whole lot. Face 5 hurts as much as you can imagine, although you don't have to be crying to feel this bad. Ask the person to choose the face that best describes how he is feeling.

Rating scale is recommended for person's age 3 years and older.

From: Hockenberry, M. and Wilson, D. (2009). <u>Wong's Essentials of Pediatric Nursing</u>, 8th Ed. Mosby: St. Louis. Used with permission: Copyright Mosby.

Appendix 9-C
International Use of FACES Scale

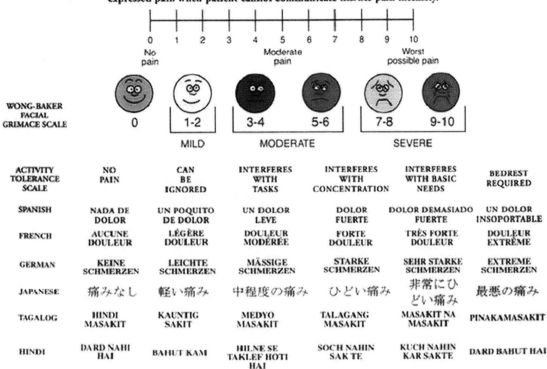

Appendix 9-D
FLACC SCALE

CATEGORIES	SCORING		
	0	1	2
FACE	No particular expression or smile	Occasional grimace or frown, withdrawn, disinterested.	Frequent to constant quivering chin, clenched jaw.
LEGS	Normal position or relaxed.	Uneasy, restless, tense.	Kicking, or legs drawn up.
ACTIVITY	Lying quietly, normal position moves easily.	Squirming, shifting back and forth, tense.	Arched, rigid or jerking.
CRY	No cry, (awake or asleep)	Moans or whimpers; occasional complaint	Crying steadily, screams or sobs, frequent complaints.
CONSOLABILITY	Content, relaxed.	Reassured by occasional touching hugging or being talked to, distractable.	Difficulty to console or comfort

Appendix 9-E
Neonatal/Infant Pain Scale (NIPS)

Pain Assessment Tools
Neonatal/Infant Pain Scale (NIPS)
(Recommended for children less than 1 year old) - A score greater than 3 indicates pain

Pain Assessment		Score
Facial Expression		
0 – Relaxed muscles	Restful face, neutral expression	
1 – Grimace	Tight facial muscles; furrowed brow, chin, jaw, (negative facial expression – nose, mouth and brow)	
Cry		
0 – No Cry	Quiet, not crying	
1 – Whimper	Mild moaning, intermittent	
2 – Vigorous Cry	Loud scream; rising, shrill, continuous (Note: Silent cry may be scored if baby is intubated as evidenced by obvious mouth and facial movement.	
Breathing Patterns		
0 – Relaxed	Usual pattern for this infant	
1 – Change in Breathing	Indrawing, irregular, faster than usual; gagging; breath holding	
Arms		
0 – Relaxed/Restrained	No muscular rigidity; occasional random movements of arms	
1 – Flexed/Extended	Tense, straight legs; rigid and/or rapid extension, flexion	
Legs		
0 – Relaxed/Restrained	No muscular rigidity; occasional random leg movement	
1 – Flexed/Extended	Tense, straight legs; rigid and/or rapid extension, flexion	
State of Arousal		
0 – Sleeping/Awake	Quiet, peaceful sleeping or alert random leg movement	
1 – Fussy	Alert, restless, and thrashing	

Certified Pediatric Emergency Nurse (CPEN) Review IV

Appendix 9-F

Probable Causes and Examples of Adverse Sedation Events

Probable Causes	Examples of Actual Reported Events
Drug-drug interaction - an event that was likely drug-related and for which a combination of drugs had been administered	"The six-week old infant received Demerol, Phenergan, and Thorazine for a circumcision and was found dead six hours later"
Drug overdose - at least 1 drug was administered in a dose > 1.25 times the maximum recommended dose	"The child received 6000 mg of chloral hydrate"
Inadequate monitoring - this could have occurred during or after the procedure	"The child was not on any monitors"
Inadequate resuscitation - the records indicated that the individuals involved did not have the basic life support or advanced life support skills or did not appropriately manage the emergency	"The heart rate decreased from 98 to 80, the nurse anesthetist gave oxygen and atropine, the pulse decreased further into the 60's, the nurse anesthetist gave epinephrine, 4 minutes later the nurse gave Narcan, 3 minutes later the nurse gave Antirilium, 12 minutes later the ambulance was summoned, 10 minutes later the patient was intubated, the ambulance drivers found the child on no monitors, EKG revealed electromechanical dissociation, the patient was transported from the dental office to a hospital"
Inadequate medical evaluation - lack of evaluation or appreciation of how underlying medical conditions would alter the patient's response to sedative drugs	"A child was transferred from Mexico and received 60mg/kg of chloral hydrate for a cardiology procedure; respiratory depression and bradycardia were followed by cardiac arrest. Autopsy revealed a ventricular septal defect, pulmonary hypertension, and elevated digoxin levels"
Premature discharge - the patient developed the problem after leaving a medical facility before meeting recommended discharge criteria	"The child became stridorous and cyanotic on the way back to his hometown"
Inadequate personnel - either the medication was administered at the direction of a physician who then left the facility, or there were inadequate numbers of individuals to monitor the patient and carry out the procedure at the same time	"The physician administered the medication and left the facility leaving the care to a technician"
Prescription/transcription error - if patient received incorrect dose either because of a transcription or prescription error (nursing or pharmacy)	"The patient received tablespoons instead of teaspoons"

Inadequate equipment - if an emergency arose and the equipment to handle it was not age - or size - appropriate or not available	"An oxygen outlet was available, but flow meter was not - only room air for the first 10 minutes"
Inadequate recovery procedures - this category included cases where there was not a proper recovery period, where no one was observing the patient after the procedure, or if an emergency occurred and the necessary equipment was not available	"If they made nurses stay after 5PM, they would all quit" (*my personal favorite - SLD*)
Inadequate understanding of a drug or its pharmacodynamics	"The patient was given 175mcg of Fentanyl by IV push; chest wall/glottic rigidity was followed by full cardiac arrest" - Narcan or muscle relaxant never administered
Prescription given by parent in an unsupervised medical environment	"The mother gave two prescriptions of chloral hydrate at home"
Local anesthetic overdose - if child received more than the recommended upper limits or if an intravascular injection occurred	"A 22.7kg child received 432 mg of mepivacaine for a dental procedure. Seizures were followed by respiratory and cardiac arrests"
Inadequate fasting for elective procedure	"The child received a bottle of milk prior to a CT scan"
Unsupervised administration of a drug by a technician	"The drug was administered by a technician; there was no physician or nurse in attendance"

Edited from Cote, C. et al. (2000). Adverse sedation events in pediatrics: A critical incident analysis of contributing factors. <u>Pediatrics</u>. 105(4). 805-814.

Appendix 9-G

Analgesia and Sedation Continuum

	Minimal Sedation (Anxiolysis)	Moderate Sedation/Analgesia "Conscious Sedation"	Deep Sedation/ Analgesia	General Anesthesia
Responsiveness	Normal response to verbal stimulation	Purposeful response to verbal or light tactile stimulation	Purposeful response following repeated or painful stimulation	Unarousable even with painful stimulation
Airway	Unaffected	No intervention required	Intervention may be required	Intervention often required
Spontaneous Ventilation	Unaffected	Adequate	May be inadequate	Frequently inadequate
Cardiovascular Function	Unaffected	Usually maintained	Usually maintained	May be impaired

Adapted from American Society of Anesthesiologists

www.asahq.org

Appendix 9-H

Sedatives and Analgesics Commonly Utilized in Pediatric Emergency Care

Drug	Route	Dose	Onset	Duration
TAC (tetracaine, adrenaline, and cocaine) NOTE: Never near mucous membranes	TD	-	15-30 minutes	45-60 minutes
LET (lidocaine, epinephrine, and tetracaine)	TD	-	15-30 minutes	45-60 minutes
EMLA (lidocaine and prilocaine)	TD	-	60 minutes	1-2 hours
L-M-X (lidocaine)	TD	-	30-60 minutes	2-4 hours
Synera (lidocaine and tetracaine)	TD	-	20-30 minutes	2 hours
Lidocaine (xylocaine, lignocaine)	SQ	5mg/kg max (plain) 7mg/kg max (with epinephrine)	1 minute	1-3 hours
Marcaine (bupivicaine)	SQ	2.5mg/kg max (plain) 3.0mg/kg max (with epinephrine)	1 minute	4-12 hours

Drug	Route	Dose	Onset	Duration
Tylenol (acetaminophen, Panadol)	PO, PR	10-15mg/kg PO or PR	30-60 minutes PO 60-180 minutes PR	4-6 hours PO or PR
Motrin (ibuprophen, Brufen)	PO	10mg/kg PO	30 minutes PO	6 hours PO
Toradol (ketoralac)	IM, IV	0.5mg/kg IM (max 60mg) 0.5mg/kg IV (max 30mg)	10-20 minutes IM 5-10 minutes IV	6-8 hours IM/IV
Narcan (naloxone)	IM, IN, IV	0.1mg/kg IM/IN/IV peds 0.4-2.0mg IM/IN/IV adults	5-10 minutes IM 3-10 minutes IN 1-4 minutes IV	60-90 minutes IM 20-40 minutes IN 20-40 minutes IV
Romazicon (flumazenil, Anexate)	IM, IN, IV	0.02mg/kg IM/IV peds 0.04mg/kg IN peds (0.2mg max single dose) 0.2mg IM/IN/IV adults (up to 1mg in 5 divided doses)	5-10 minutes IM 2-4 minutes IN 1-2 minutes IV	60-90 minutes IM 90-120 minutes IN 20-40 minutes IV

Certified Pediatric Emergency Nurse (CPEN) Review IV

Drug	Route	Dose	Onset	Duration
Zofran (ondansetron)	IV	0.1mg/kg IV (max 4mg)	10 minutes IV	3-4 hours IV
Morphine	IM, IV	0.1mg/kg IM/IV	10-15 minutes IM 5 minutes IV	3-4 hours IM/IV
Demerol (meperidine)	IM, IV	1-2mg/kg IM/IV	10 minutes IM 5 minutes IV	2-3 hours IM/IV
Sublimaze (**fentanyl**)	IN, IV, TM	2mcg/kg IN 1-5mcg/kg IV 5-15mcg/kg "lollipop"	5-10 minutes IN 2-3 minutes IV 20-30 minutes TM	45-60 minutes IN/IV 60 minutes TM
Succinylcholine ("**Sux**", Anectine, Quelicin) For reversal of fentanyl-induced "rigid chest"	IM, IV	4mg/kg IM 2mg/kg IV	1 minute IV and "Be ready to bag"!	10 minutes IV
Ketalar (**ketamine**) + with atropine or Robinul (glycopyrrolate) and Versed (midazolam) (adjunctive therapy)	IM, IN, IV, PO, PR	4mg/kg IM 10mg/kg IN 0.5-1.0mg/kg IV 5-10mg/kg PO 5-10mg/kg PR	2-10 minutes IM 10-20 minutes IN 1 minute IV 10-30 minutes PO 10-30 minutes PR	60-90 minutes IM 1-2 hours IN 5-10 minutes IV 1-2 hours PO 1-2 hours PR

Drug	Route	Dose	Onset	Duration
Nitronox (**Nitrous oxide**, Entonox)	INHL	50% N2O/50% O_2	3-5 minutes INHL	3-5 minutes INHL
Versed (midazolam)	IM, IN, IV, PO, PR	For seizures: 0.2-0.3mg/kg IN 0.1mg/kg IV 0.5mg/kg PR For sedation: 0.1mg/kg IM 0.4-0.5mg/kg IN 0.1mg/kg IV 0.5mg/kg PO 0.5mg/kg PR	10-20 minutes IM 5 minutes IN 2-3 minutes IV 10-30 minutes PO 10-30 minutes PR	1-2 hours IM 30-60 minutes IN/IV 60-90 minutes PO 60-90 minutes PR
Chloral hydrate (Nembutal)	PO/PR	50-100mg/kg PO/PR	15-60 min PO/PR	1-2+ hours PO/PR
Diprivan (**Propofol**)	IV	100mcg/kg bolus IV (loading dose) then 50-100mcg/kg/min (maintenance infusion)	<1 min IV	10-15 min IV

Certified Pediatric Emergency Nurse (CPEN) Review IV

Drug	Route	Dose	Onset	Duration
DPT Demerol, Phenergan, and Thorazine – meperidine, promethazine, and chlorpromazine)	IM	Just say no!	Just say no!	Up to 19+ hours (This is just one of the many reasons you that you should just say no)!
Seconal **(Pentobarbital)**	IM, IV, PR	5mg/kg IM 1-6mg/kg IV 3mg/kg PR	10-20 min IM 1 min IV 15-60 min PR	1-4 hours IM 15 min IV 1-4 hours PR
(Amidate) **Etomidate**	IV	0.2mg/kg IV	30 seconds IV	10 minutes IV
Precedex ("Dex", dexmedetomidine)	IN, IV	1-1.5mcg/kg IN 1mcg/kg/IV over 10 min (loading dose) 0.2-1.0mcg/kg/HOUR (maintenance infusion)	45 min IN 6-10 min IV	3 hours IN 2 hours IV

Legend

IM – intramuscular, IN – intranasal, INHL – inhalation, IV – intravenous, PO – oral, PR – rectal
SQ - subcutaneous, TD – transdermal, TM - transmucosal

(Thanks to Madelyn Kahana MD, Tim Wolfe MD, and Michelle Webb RN, MS, CRNA for their invaluable assistance with the creation of this chart)

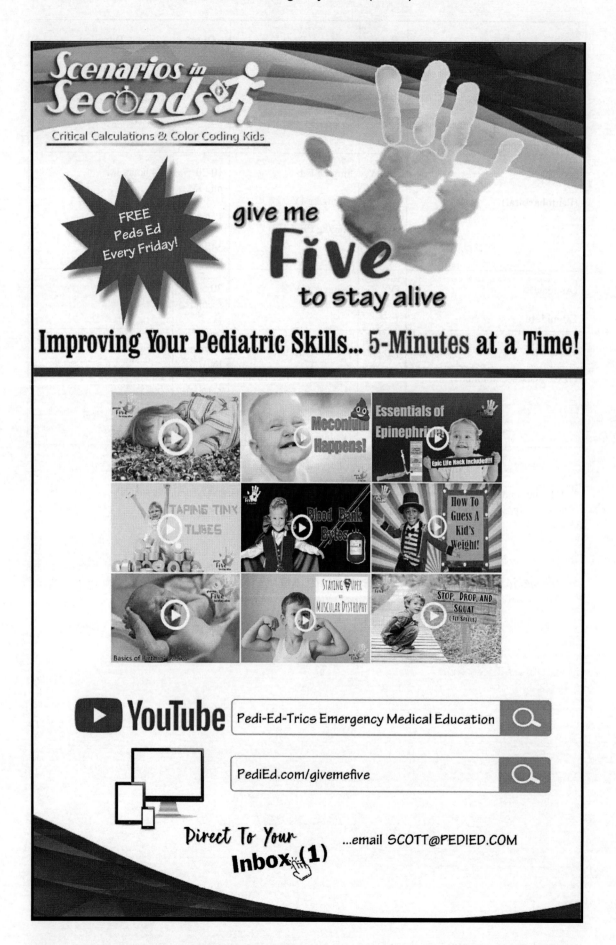

Chapter 10

Miscellaneous Medical Remaining Reminders

*There are only two things a child will share willingly –
Communicable diseases and his mother's age.*
    -Benjamin Spock

Pertinent Pediatric Ponderings (NOTES)

CHAPTER 10
Sample Test Answer Sheet

1. _____
2. _____
3. _____
4. _____
5. _____
6. _____
7. _____
8. _____
9. _____
10. _____
11. _____
12. _____
13. _____
14. _____
15. _____
16. _____
17. _____
18. _____
19. _____
20. _____
21. _____
22. _____
23. _____
24. _____
25. _____
26. _____
27. _____
28. _____
29. _____
30. _____
31. _____
32. _____
33. _____
34. _____
35. _____
36. _____
37. _____
38. _____
39. _____
40. _____
41. _____
42. _____
43. _____
44. _____
45. _____
46. _____
47. _____
48. _____
49. _____
50. _____
51. _____
52. _____
53. _____
54. _____
55. _____
56. _____
57. _____
58. _____
59. _____
60. _____
61. _____
62. _____
63. _____
64. _____
65. _____
66. _____
67. _____
68. _____
69. _____
70. _____
71. _____
72. _____
73. _____
74. _____
75. _____
76. _____
77. _____
78. _____
79. _____
80. _____
81. _____
82. _____
83. _____
84. _____
85. _____
86. _____
87. _____
88. _____
89. _____
90. _____
91. _____
92. _____
93. _____
94. _____
95. _____
96. _____
97. _____
98. _____
99. _____
100. _____

Pertinent Pediatric Ponderings (NOTES)

Certified Pediatric Emergency Nurse (CPEN) Review IV

1) An 8-year-old African-American child with a history of sickle-cell disease (SCD) arrives at the ED with complaints of severe abdominal and joint pain for the past 16-hours. He is **most** likely experiencing:

A) Aplastic crisis

B) Sequestration crisis

C) Painful crisis

D) Anemic crisis

C – Hopefully, this one is easy to answer. The chief complaint is pain, so chances are the answer involves pain. Painful events, formerly called vasoocclusive crisis, occur when the sickle shaped red blood cells (RBC) clog up to the point of causing ischemia to certain tissues. A concept that is important to remember is that while pain is certainly an issue, if the ischemic tissues are in the lungs or the brain, acute chest syndrome or even stroke can result. Aplastic or anemic crisis is usually triggered by a virus and results in greatly diminished RBC production and possibly CHF requiring packed RBC transfusion. Sequestration crisis occurs when large quantities of blood pool in the spleen and occasionally in the liver, resulting in shock.

2) ED management for most pediatric patients with sickle cell disease (SCD) involves all of the following **except**:

A) IV fluid rehydration

B) IV analgesics

C) IV exchange transfusions

D) Oral rehydration

C – Exchange transfusions are only done in cases of severe acute chest or stroke in the pediatric ICU. Remember, obtaining a "normal" hemoglobin (Hgb) level of 11.5-14.5 g/dl is contraindicated in these patients as it can lead to viscous blood and a high risk of stroke. When you think SCD; think pain and ways to decrease the pain, such as IV analgesics via intermittent IV push, PCA pump, or continuous infusion. Oral and IV fluids are given to promote hydration and decrease viscosity. In addition, supplemental oxygen should be administered in patients who are hypoxic or in respiratory distress. However, routine oxygen administration does not help patients in painful crisis, as it does not reverse sickled RBCs.

3) Which analgesic would the nurse **not** expect to administer to a patient in painful crisis?

A) Dilaudid (hydromorphone)

B) Morphine

C) Aspirin

D) Tylenol (acetaminophen) with codeine (Tylenol #3)

C – We should not expect to give aspirin in this case. Except in rare diseases such as Kawasaki's disease and some arthritis cases, we just don't give aspirin that much anymore. The fear of Reye's syndrome after aspirin administration has been drummed into our heads for so many years that we have a hard time even thinking aspirin and kids. Aspirin and myocardial infarctions are another situation altogether.

4) Outpatient management of sickle cell disease (SCD) in pre-school age children should include all of the following **except**:

A) Antibiotics

B) Antivirals

C) Analgesics

D) Fluids

B – Antivirals are not routinely part of outpatient SCD treatment. We already know about fluids and analgesics, but the tricky one here is antibiotics. Among children under five with SCD, infection is the most common cause of death and therefore prophylactic penicillin is recommended to "ward off" pneumococcal infections for children at home and when they are admitted to the hospital.

5) Demerol (meperidine) can cause all of the following complications in children **except**:

A) Anxiety

B) Tremors

C) Generalized seizures

D) Dry mouth

D – Several things cause dry mouth, but Demerol (meperidine) is not among them. Many facilities have formal protocols for the ED management of painful crisis and Demerol is less and less common as it has fallen out of favor with many practitioners due, at least in part, to the complications listed above. In addition to anxiety and tremors, a bigger problem is that normeperidine, a metabolite of Demerol, is a central nervous stimulant which can cause really nasty seizures.

6) A 10-year-old boy is brought to the ED after injuring his right knee in a bicycle accident. He is known to have hemophilia and presents with symptoms indicating hemarthrosis (bleeding into a joint) of the right knee. The ED nurse should be prepared for all of the following **except**:

A) IV administration of Factor VIII

B) Arthrocentesis

C) "RICE"

D) Comfort and reassurance

B – Arthrocentesis or "tapping a knee" is not recommended for patients with hemophilia. Putting a big needle into a joint to suck out blood in someone who can't clot very well in the first place and is likely to keep bleeding after the procedure is just not a great idea. These patients are treated with immediate IV administration of Factor VIII, as well as RICE (rest, ice, compression, and elevation.) Providing comfort and reassurance to children is always appropriate.

Certified Pediatric Emergency Nurse (CPEN) Review IV

7) When assessing a patient with hemophilia, all of the following can be common bleeding sources **except**:

A) Gums

B) Soft tissue

C) Inner ears

D) Joints (knees, elbows, and ankles)

C – Inner ear bleeding should not be common for anyone. It is important to remember that there are two types of bleeding associated with hemophilia; "not so bad" bleeds and "really really bad" bleeds. "Not so bad" bleeds are those we can treat quickly. These places include anywhere that minor trauma occurs. Gums can bleed from teeth brushing or flossing. Soft tissue and joint bleeding can result from even minor traumas, like falling off of a bicycle. Spontaneous hematuria can also happen. "Really really bad" bleeds include those in the head, airway, or GI tract as we can't quickly or easily treat those and the complications can be deadly.

8) All of the following are true about patients with Factor VIII deficiency **except**:

A) Factor VIII administration can be given prophylactically

B) Patients needing Factor VIII replacement must come to the hospital for administration and admission

C) Patients with this condition do not need to be kept in isolation while hospitalized

D) Home care and self-infusion programs have made patients more self-sufficient

B – Like many things in health care, we are now doing more and more things at home, to keep patients out of the hospital, and more importantly for us, out of the ED. Factor VIII is frequently administered prophylactically, and sometimes even acutely, at home by the patient or their care giver.

9) One of the **most** common causes of death in a patient with hemophilia is from bleeding into the:

A) GI tract

B) Heart

C) Cranium

D) Joints

C – Bleeding in general is never a good thing, especially for a patient with hemophilia. If you are asked about the worst places you could bleed, in and around the brain should be your top choice. Yes, we've come a long way since the days of barbers and bloodletting (which was still practiced as recently as the times of President Andrew Jackson.)

10) Aplastic anemia is characterized by an acute decrease in all of the following **except**:

A) Leukocytes

B) Osteocytes

C) Thrombocytes

D) Erythrocytes

B – Osteocytes relate to bones, not blood and the "nemia" in the name of the disease is your hint that we are talking about blood. In addition, any time you see a medical diagnosis beginning with "A," think "none" or not enough of something. Apnea means "no breathing." Asystole means "no systole." Aplastic comes from aplasia which means not enough blood cells are being made and anemia refers to low blood counts (in this case, all three types of blood cells; leukocytes (WBCs), Thrombocytes (platelets), and erythrocytes (RBCs.)

11) A 4-year-old boy with a history of acute lymphocytic leukemia is admitted to the ED with a fever. His mother states that he underwent chemotherapy 10 days ago. The nurse would expect treatment in the ED for this child to include all of the following **except**:

A) Oral Motrin (ibuprofen, Brufen)

B) Cultures of everything

C) Rectal Tylenol (acetaminophen, Panadol)

D) Isolation and IV antibiotics

C – In children with presumed neutropenia, most centers do not recommend rectal medications to avoid a possible break in the skin. A febrile child with a history of cancer, especially one who is actively undergoing chemotherapy or radiation therapy, is a true medical emergency. They are neutropenic (low WBC neutrophils) and should be considered septic and unable to fight off whatever infection may be present. You should immediately place this child in a private room, pan-culture (i.e. everything that can be easily cultured, will be cultured), and quickly follow with appropriate IV antibiotics. Oral Motrin should make the child feel more comfortable.

12) Which of the following is **not** an initial sign or symptom of leukemia?

A) Fever

B) Bruising

C) A lingering cold

D) Hair loss

D – Hair loss is associated with chemotherapy, not with the initial symptoms of leukemia. Most children with leukemia, or cancer of the blood forming tissues, exhibit remarkably few symptoms. A child may have a cold that "just doesn't go away" or unexplained weight loss, fatigue, fever, or bruising.

13) Leukemic patients are at higher risk for infections because they have:

A) Elevated WBCs

B) Decreased WBCs

C) Elevated RBCs

D) Normal level of WBCs

B – One of the initial defining findings in acute leukemia (and the reason for the high risk for infection) is a decreased total white blood cell count. Bone marrow aspirates may show an overproduction of immature white blood cells or "blasts," but the total WBC count is low. In addition, there may be a decrease in the red blood cell count and platelets. Remember the question asked about infection, so the answer needs to focus on WBCs. If the patient had asked about where the patient can get an infection, you would know that any break in the skin is a potential site for infection in these children.

14) A hepatoblastoma is a neoplastic disease of the:

A) Liver

B) Spleen

C) Brain

D) Kidneys

A – "Hepato" is the prefix for something involving the liver and "oma" (meaning a neoplastic disease) is never a good thing to have in a diagnosis. Lymphoma is a neoplastic disease involving the lymphatic system – "lymph" and "oma." Osteosarcoma is a neoplastic disease involving the bone. Nephroblastoma or Wilm's tumor is a neoplastic disease involving the kidney. Retinoblastoma is a neoplastic disease involving the eye. Astrocytoma and glioma are neoplastic diseases involving the brain (astrocytes or glial cells are found in and around the brain.) Any time you see "oma" in a question, think cancer of somewhere.

15) Which of the following are treatment options for Candidiasis?

A) Topical and/or oral antibiotics

B) Topical and/or oral antifungals

C) Oral antimalarials

D) Oral antivirals

B – Candidiasis is a common fungal infection in patients undergoing chemo or radiation therapy. As it is a fungal disease, antifungals such as Nystatin, Diflucan (fluconazole), or Amphotericin B are indicated. Antibiotics, antivirals, and antimalarials are not good options knowing the problem is fungal in nature

16) The **initial** sign associated with Hodgkin's disease is an enlarged lymph node in the:

A) Neck

B) Groin

C) Axillae

D) Toes

A – The "classic" first sign of Hodgkin's lymphoma is an enlarged, non-tender node in the neck; though nodes in the clavicle, axillae, or groin can be present. Hodgkin's disease primarily involves the lymph nodes and is very rare in children under the age of five. However, in teens between 15 and 19 years of age, it occurs almost as commonly as leukemia.

Certified Pediatric Emergency Nurse (CPEN) Review IV

17) Which of the following would be the priority ED nursing intervention for a pediatric patient experiencing thrombocytopenia?

A) Monitor for infection

B) Be ready to treat with granulocyte stimulating factor (GCSF)

C) Monitor for bleeding

D) Place the patient in isolation

C – The priority here is monitoring for bleeding because thrombocytopenia means not enough platelets which are crucial for clotting. Isolation and infection concerns would be appropriate for leukemia and GCSF is given to stimulate granulocytes (a type of WBCs.)

18) A 16-year-old with a history of non-Hodgkin's lymphoma presents to the ED in respiratory distress. Initial assessment finds an indwelling central line in the right upper chest, moderate respiratory distress, orthopnea, JVD, and facial edema. He is immediately placed on 100% oxygen by non-rebreather mask and a chest X-ray is obtained. The peds ER nurse suspects:

A) Pneumonia

B) Superior vena cava syndrome

C) ARDS

D) Asthma

B – This teen has classic symptoms of superior vena cava syndrome (SVCS.) This occurs when either an external (tumor) or internal (central line clot) mass occludes the superior vena cava. The result is a significant decrease in blood return to the heart. This patient has two huge risk factors for SVCS, non-Hodgkin's lymphoma and a central line. Remember that the "veins are the drains," so if the heart and head can't drain, everything backs up. Immediate treatment includes raising the head of the bed to help with breathing, supplemental oxygen and preparation for possible intubation. Additionally, emergent surgery, radiation, chemotherapy, or stent placement may be needed. Until the reason for the SVCS is determined, the central line should not be used as dislodging a big catheter clot is typically followed by even bigger problems.

19) In a "heme-onc" patient, acute renal failure is often associated with:

A) Superior vena cava syndrome

B) Leukemia

C) Lymphoma

D) Tumor lysis syndrome

D – Tumor lysis syndrome is caused by the rapid release of metabolites during the initial treatment of lymphomas and leukemias. This is a fancy way of saying the chemo killed lots of bad things which in turn released lots of other bad things. All of these bad things have to get filtered out somewhere and the kidneys are where that happens. Tumor lysis syndrome treatment includes efforts to avoid dialysis through the use of diuretics, alkalinization and hydration. Additionally, allopurinol may be given to reduce uric acid formation. If these are unsuccessful, then dialysis and/or exchange transfusions may be necessary to remove or reduce the bad things.

Certified Pediatric Emergency Nurse (CPEN) Review IV

20) A 14-year-old teen with a history of lymphoma arrives via ambulance with a complaint of difficulty walking and lower extremity weakness. With this history, the pediatric ED nurse immediately suspects:

A) Tumor lysis syndrome

B) Spinal cord trauma

C) Spinal cord compression

D) Cerebrovascular accident

C – In "heme-onc" patients, especially those with lymphoma or myeloma, one of the most feared complications is spinal cord compression (SCC.) This occurs when a tumor invades the spinal epidural space and compresses the spine (hence the diagnosis of spinal cord compression.) Diagnosis is made via history, physical, and MRI when possible. It is important for ED nurses to remember that more than 75% of the patients who present ambulatory will be discharged ambulatory. However, only 15-30% of patients who come in partially or fully paralyzed will be able to walk upon discharge. As you can imagine, ED treatment is focused on relieving the cord compression through the administration of IV Decadron (dexamethasone) before definitive chemotherapy, radiation therapy, or surgery can be undertaken. Either way, just as a "heme-onc" kid with a fever is a true emergency, a "heme-onc" kid with lower extremity weakness is a true emergency as well.

21) Infectious mononucleosis is treated with:

A) 14 days of oral penicillin

B) 7 days of oral penicillin

C) 3 days of oral penicillin

D) Rest and time

D - Mononucleosis or "mono" is viral in origin, so antibiotics are not indicated (unless a concurrent bacterial infection such as strep throat is present.) Though commonly referred to as the "kissing disease," transmission is via oropharyngeal secretions, so not sharing drinking glasses, tableware, etc. is vital. Treatment simply involves time, rest, and not kissing until the teens feel well enough to kiss again. Mono patients frequently have splenic enlargement associated with the disease and therefore are at higher risk for splenic rupture. Test hint: If one of the answers is clearly different from the others, there may be a very good reason!

22) A 4-year-old child arrives via EMS at the ED after falling from a 2-story window. He is hemodynamically stable and the patient's blood is typed and cross-matched for possible transfusion. His blood type is found to be AB positive. Which statement about type AB blood is **true**?

A) The plasma contains both A and B antibodies

B) The plasma contains both A and B antigens

C) The red cell contains both A and B antigens

D) The blood group possesses neither A or B antigens

Certified Pediatric Emergency Nurse (CPEN) Review IV

C – The red cells carry the antigens, and in this case, both A and B antigens, which mean that in an emergency, this patient could receive not only type O blood, but either type A or B as well. As he is not only type AB, but AB-positive, in an emergency, he is considered to be the "universal recipient," meaning he can receive any blood type until properly cross matched blood is available. Blood type O-negative is considered to be the "universal donor" as A and B antigens do not react to type O, and Rh negative blood works for both Rh positive and negative blood types. That's why in emergency situations such as major trauma, patients receive O-negative blood, until type specific or type and cross matched blood is available.

23) The nurse who administers packed RBCs to the above patient must be cognizant of standard transfusion practices. Which statement about blood transfusions is **true**?

A) LR is the only solution to be used when administering blood products

B) In the absence of a blood warmer, a microwave oven may be used

C) An 18g catheter or larger must be used during a blood transfusion

D) None of the above

D – None of the above answers are true. 0.9NS, not lactated ringers (LR) should be used with blood products and microwave ovens work fine for rewarming that dinner that you missed, but not for blood products. Lastly, many of us remember being told that if you try to give blood products, especially packed RBCs, through any IV catheter smaller than an 18g that that the blood would hemolyze. We are happy to report that, indeed, blood will flow safely through a much smaller catheter. Stories to the contrary, simply are not true. Think about an approximately one pound (500gm), 24-week preemie in the neonatal ICU. Blood is given through 24g IVs all the time without hemolysis. In an emergency… any vein is a good vein. Any size IV is a good size IV. And if they need blood… give them blood.

24) One hour after the transfusion was started, the patient is visibly shivering and complains of a headache. He remains neurologically intact and is hemodynamically stable, but his temperature has increased to 103.1F (39.5C.) Based on these findings, the ED nurse determines the patient is probably experiencing a:

A) Febrile, nonhemolytic transfusion reaction

B) Hemolytic transfusion reaction

C) Delayed hemolytic transfusion reaction

D) Allergic transfusion reaction

A – This child is most likely having a febrile, nonhemolytic transfusion reaction in which the body reacts to WBC, platelet, or plasma antibodies. Leukocyte-poor RBCs are less likely to cause this reaction. It is treated by stopping the transfusion and administering Tylenol (acetaminophen, Panadol.) Allergic transfusion reactions act like other allergic reactions and this doesn't look like your standard allergic reaction. The most feared transfusion reaction is the hemolytic type. These reactions occur from ABO incompatibility and are the most frequent cause of death from blood transfusions. The most common reason for a hemolytic reaction is human error (giving the wrong blood type or mislabeling the blood product.) The bad news is that since no one is perfect, accidents will happen. The good news is that because we know the cause, we can take safeguards and develop policies and systems to minimize the risk to our patients. Regardless of the type of reaction, the blood that was being given, along with blood and urine samples from the patient should be sent to the blood bank for their further testing.

Certified Pediatric Emergency Nurse (CPEN) Review IV

25) Children on long term anticoagulants such as Coumadin (warfarin) should have which blood level(s) regularly monitored?

A) PT (protime) or INR (International Normalized Ratio)

B) PTT (partial thromboplastin time)

C) PT and PTT

D) CBC

A – Patients on Coumadin need to regularly have their PT (and INR) checked regularly. Patients on Heparin need to have the PTT checked. This is important, especially with attempts to minimize healthcare expenses by only checking what really needs to be checked. Three suggested ways to remember the difference: 1) "Coumadin **P**revents **T**hrombus while **P**hysicians **T**reat **T**hrombus with Heparin" (Thank you, Kelly Begley CCEMTP), 2) "In physician handwriting, the TT in PTT is shaped like an H, so the PTT goes with Heparin." (Thank you, Dawn Plier RN) and 3) "You take Coumadin PO, so with the PO, check the PT." (Thank you, Clay Odell RN.)

26) A 16-year-old girl arrives at the ED after an abortion with complaints of heavy bleeding and severe lower abdominal pain. The physician suspects retained products of conception. While the patient is in the ED, her lab studies reveal an elevated PT/PTT as well as a hemoglobin of 7 g/dl. The physician diagnoses disseminated intravascular coagulation (DIC.) The nurse would expect to observe bleeding from which site(s) in a patient with DIC?

A) Mucous membranes

B) Venipuncture sites

C) GI tract

D) All of the above

D – The correct answer for DIC is to expect bleeding from anywhere and everywhere. Disseminated intravascular coagulation is a cascading condition which occurs when the body's clotting mechanism is abnormally triggered by conditions such as major trauma, shock, sepsis, or retained products of conception. Essentially what happens is that there is way too much clotting going on and this leaves way too few platelets being left over. The clotting then activates the body's fibrinolytic mechanisms (to break down clots) which in turn results in more bleeding. It's a vicious circle that can easily result in the patient bleeding out from everywhere and is managed with the administration of platelets and fresh frozen plasma (FFP, clotting factors.) We know that IV heparin is most commonly used to inhibit clotting and while it makes little sense to give it to a critically ill patient who is already bleeding too much, for patients with DIC who are not getting better despite platelets and FFP, IV heparin can be given to inhibit thrombin formation and break the clotting/bleeding cascade. Note: In obstetric patients who normally are hypercoaguable, heparin is not routinely used for DIC and they are managed with lots and lots of blood products.

27) In children under the age of thirteen, Human Immunodeficiency Virus (HIV) is **most** commonly acquired from:

A) Hemophilia and blood product transfusions

B) Casual contact with friends and family

C) Perinatal transmission from a HIV positive mother

D) Contact with contaminated eating utensils

C – 91% of pre-teen children with HIV acquired it perinatally from their mothers. Happily this rate is dropping as more and more pregnant moms are screened for HIV and the use of perinatal antivirals has increased. But it is still the number one way infants and pre-teen children get HIV. When children become teenagers however, sexual contact and IV drug use take the lead in terms of how the disease was acquired.

28) Which of the following is **not** commonly seen in children with HIV?

A) Pneumocystis carinii pneumonia (PCP)

B) Kaposi's sarcoma

C) Failure to thrive

D) Chronic diarrhea

B – Unlike adults in which the Kaposi's sarcoma, with its characteristic purplish skin lesion is a hallmark sign of HIV infection, less than 1% of children infected with HIV exhibit this sign. Much more common in children are recurrent bacterial infections, failure to thrive, chronic diarrhea, and Pneumocystis carinii pneumonia (PCP.) Management of HIV in children is very similar to adults in whom CD4 counts are regularly monitored and Bactrim (trimethoprin-sulfamethoxazole) is given for PCP prophylaxis. In addition, multiple antiviral medications (HAART - highly active antiretroviral therapy) are also part of the treatment.

29) All of the following are true of ITP (idiopathic thrombocytopenic purpura) **except:**

A) There is an increased risk for developing ITP following certain viral illnesses, such as chickenpox, measles, or mumps

B) The hallmark of the disorder is a low platelet count

C) Medications used in the treatment of ITP include prednisone, IVIG, Anti-D antibody, and Rh immune globulin.

D) Acute ITP is characterized by a greatly increased platelet count

D – ITP is characterized by decreased, not increased, platelet counts. Even if you've never taken care of a patient with ITP, that's OK, you can still get the correct answer on the test. The easiest way to ascertain the correct answer is to figure out what the name means. Idiopathic is a fancy way of saying, we really don't know why it happens. Although the actual cause of ITP is unknown, there is an increased risk about 3 weeks after certain viral illnesses, such as chickenpox, measles, or mumps. It is thought to be an autoimmune response to those viruses. Thrombocytopenic is a big word made up of 2 parts. "Thrombocyto" refers to Thrombocytes and is a fancy way of saying platelets. "Penia" is a fancy way of saying that there is a lack of whatever we identified before this part of the word (platelets in this case.) Purpura is a fancy way of saying bruising. Think about it. Not enough platelets = bruising. Makes sense, right? Acute ITP most commonly occurs in the 2-6 year old age group and the low platelet count occurs when the body "accidentally" makes antibodies that stick to platelets. The body then recognizes these platelets as foreign and destroys them. It is important to remember that with ITP, the only component of the blood word that is really way out of whack is the platelets. That information is crucial for differentiating ITP from leukemia which rarely presents only with a low platelet count. Symptomatic patients are treated with medications such as prednisone, IVIG, Rh immune globulin, or Anti-D antibody, however, these are not curative therapies. If the child is asymptomatic, many believe that no treatment is needed as the platelet count appears to recover at the same rate with or without therapy. The majority of children with acute ITP recover just fine on their own, but a small percentage go on to develop chronic ITP and require ongoing therapies.

30) A 5-year-old boy is diagnosed with acute ITP in the emergency department. The child's platelet count is 18,000. Which of the following statements made by the parents would indicate the need for additional discharge teaching?

A) We will not allow him to go ice skating until the doctor informs us that he has recovered

B) We will not give him aspirin or Motrin (ibuprofen, Brufen)

C) He will most likely need to have a splenectomy

D) The most serious complication we have to worry about is bleeding into his brain

C - Splenectomy is typically only considered for older children who have gone on to develop chronic ITP which is refractory to medical management. It would not be considered early in the course of acute ITP, as there are several medication options that may be very effective in treating this disorder. The most serious complication of ITP is intracranial hemorrhage, so it is very important that parents understand the importance of avoiding head injury and trying to ensure a safe environment. As aspirin and ibuprofen type medications mess with the platelets, they should be avoided in ITP. The platelets are already messed up enough.

31) The EMTALA legislation states that unstable patients can be transferred if:

A) The patient doesn't have insurance

B) The patient or their family requests transfer

C) The risks of transfer are less than the risks of not transferring

D) B and C

D – The Emergency Medical Treatment and Active Labor Act (EMTALA) was initially introduced to prevent hospitals from refusing to treat patients without insurance. Over the years, it has evolved to become the standard regarding the legalities of patient transfers as well. Stable patients cannot be transferred to another medical facility unless the following conditions are met: 1) The patient must be stabilized within the skill and capability of the referring hospital. Simply stated, you have to treat the patient the best you that you can before transfer. 2) The patient or a legally responsible person acting on the individual's behalf has requested the transfer. This prevents patients from being transferred without having told them or their family that they are going on a road trip. 3) The physician must sign a form stating that the medical benefits of transfer outweigh the risks of the transfer itself. In other words, the physician must affirm that not transferring the patient is more likely to be worse for the patient than keeping them where they are. 4) The accepting facility must have an accepting physician, space, and personnel to care for the patient. 5) Applicable medical records must accompany the patient. This means actual chart copies and actual copies of X-rays/CTs/etc., not just the reports, will go with the patient. 6) The transfer must utilize qualified personnel and equipment as determined by the referring physician. All six criteria must be met, not only for a safe patient transport, but to avoid an EMTALA violation as well.

32) When transferring a patient to another facility, who is responsible for determining the mode of transport?

A) The receiving (accepting) physician

B) The transferring (sending) physician

C) The transporting agency

D) The patient or family in accordance with the insurance company rules

Miscellaneous

B – The transferring physician is legally responsible for the patient until they arrive at the referring facility, and therefore, they, not the accepting physician, are responsible for determining how best to get the patient there, whether that be via BLS, ALS, or critical care team. While it is common and appropriate for a knowledgeable receiving physician to recommend a certain mode of transport or provider, the ultimate decision rests with the referring physician. The decision to accept a patient cannot be tied to the use of a particular mode of transport or provider. Remember, only the transferring staff determines how patients are transferred.

33) Appropriate methods of assisting parents who have experienced the death of a chronically ill child in the ED include all of the following **except**:

A) Telling the family that the death was for the best as the patient was sick for a long time and now is at peace

B) Calling the child by name

C) Allowing the family to spend time with their child

D) Allowing the family members to cry and tell you their feelings

A – Remember that just about anything that involves allowing patients or family members to safely express their feelings are the right things to do. This situation is no different. We don't want to tell the parents what they should feel or think, or what our opinions are (like it is good their child died.) That is up to them, not us, to decide. Their son or daughter, alive or dead, is still their child and calling them by name is the least we can do. Again, as the song says… "Feelings… nothing more than feelings…" Think airway, breathing, and feelings to get the correct answer.

34) A child with end-stage cancer in hospice care is brought to the ED by EMS with agonal respirations. Which action is appropriate when dealing with this situation?

A) Restricting family access to the patient in accordance with hospital and department visitor policy

B) Not withholding analgesics or comfort measures even though a co-worker states that the medications may hasten the onset of death

C) Completing all insurance and registration materials immediately in case the patient dies suddenly and the family gets distracted

D) Preparing the Code Cart in the likelihood that the patient will require intubation and resuscitation medications

B – Thank goodness for hospice and palliative care, as they are truly one of the greatest things to hit pediatric healthcare in decades. This child is going to die, but we can still provide care. Death is inevitable… suffering is optional!

35) In which circumstance may a nurse use physical force against a patient?

A) Under no circumstances as it could affect the patient's airway

B) To help a screaming teenager regain his senses

C) To assess an unconscious patient's level of reaction to physical stimuli

D) In self-defense, but only if the nurse has reasonable grounds to believe that he or she is being, or is about to be, attacked.

Certified Pediatric Emergency Nurse (CPEN) Review IV

D – Remember that airway trumps everything EXCEPT for safety. D is the correct answer not only because it has the most words, but also because it involves nurse safety. The "how didn't this get an Academy Award" movie classic, Airplane, has one of the greatest slapping back to senses scenes, but it is not appropriate for psychiatric patient care.

36) Which statement about verbal physician orders is **true**?

A) Verbal orders should be followed with written orders to comply with standards and policy and to ensure the nurse's legal protection

B) Verbal orders are illegal in most states

C) Verbal orders are only valid when witnessed by another person

D) Verbal orders should be carried out only when verified and countersigned by another physician

A – In the controlled chaos of the pediatric ED, verbal orders are still very frequently used. Joint Commission recommendations discourage verbal orders, but if verbal orders are used, they should be signed by the physician as soon as possible.

37) A 6-year-old is about to undergo procedural sedation for closed reduction of an extremity fracture. If the child's mother does not understand the information that was just given by the physician during an informed consent, the nurse should:

A) Answer the mother's questions

B) Notify the ED charge nurse

C) Notify the physician

D) Do nothing as the consent is already signed

C – Remember that describing the procedure and medical benefits/risks of the procedure for informed consent is the responsibility of the physician, physician's assistant (PA), or nurse practitioner (NP), not the ED nurse. Witnessing the signing of the consent form is only that; the nurse is witnessing that the person signed the paper. The nurse is not witnessing that the person who signed the consent understands anything or everything about the procedure. If your "gut" says that the patient or the parents don't understand, "take a time out" and have the physician/PA/NP talk with the patient and/or family prior to continuing with the procedure.

The act of signing the consent form is only one of the steps in "obtaining" of informed consent. It is the final step in the process where the parent acknowledges, by signing the form, that there has been an informed consent process. This process can range from discussion to providing reading materials to showing a video. The nurse is not responsible for this process unless s/he is the person performing the procedure (i.e. insertion of a PICC line.) The nurses' role is to obtain the parent's signature and to verify that the parent has the capacity to sign the form. Although there is no legal obligation, most agree that the nurse has a moral obligation to follow up if: (1) the parent has additional questions or doesn't understand; or (2) if the parent states that s/he has not previously had a discussion with the performing practitioner.

38) Administering a medication to a patient against her will is an example of:

A) Assault

B) Negligence

C) Battery

D) Invasion of privacy

C – Administering a medication to a patient without consent may be considered battery because it involves (directly or indirectly) touching the patient. This differs from assault which does not necessarily involve contact; it can be threatened as in a verbal assault. Negligence doesn't consider patient consent and the action of giving medications is not a matter of patient privacy.

39) Which of the following is necessary for negligence to have occurred?

A) The wrong therapy must have been given

B) Injury must have resulted

C) A change in the patient's condition must have been overlooked

D) An error in judgment must have been made

B – Negligence is when something happened that shouldn't have happened (commission) or when something that should have happened didn't (omission) and an injury or harm has occurred as a result of it. Both parts must be present; cause and effect. Giving 350mg of Tylenol instead of 325mg is a medical error, but is not likely to cause injury to the child. However, if after giving 3,325mg of Tylenol instead of 325mg the patient develops liver failure, well, that's a very different story.

40) Each of the following are responsibilities of the triage nurse **except**:

A) Preventing cross-contamination of suspected infectious patients

B) Performing a complete and comprehensive patient assessment

C) Initiating patient or family education

D) Fostering good public relations

B – Complete histories and physical examinations should be done after the initial sorting, or triage, has been done. Triage comes from the French word for sorting and is really more of a process than a place. Patients coming in simultaneously via ambulance can be triaged in a hall without going to a desk or room near the front entrance. The nurse responsible for triage, in most places, also has responsibility for the waiting room patients. As such s/he would need to help figure out which patient has got something nasty that can easily be given to other patients, and keep those who are probably contagious from sharing with others. Providing appropriate teaching to patients and families, as well as fostering good PR, are additional responsibilities of not only the triage nurse, but all nurses.

Certified Pediatric Emergency Nurse (CPEN) Review IV

41) Pediatric ED nurses should give telephone medical advice in which of the following situations?

A) When it is a medical, as opposed to a trauma question

B) If the call comes in after normal office or clinic hours since no one else is readily available

C) If the nurse has had personal experience with the situation in question

D) None of the above

D – None of the above. ED staff nurses giving phone advice is a troublesome and potentially legally messy situation. Many facilities have formal policies regarding this subject and specifically what, if any, advice should be given over the phone. In the absence of formally trained telephone triage nurses, even if it's for simple questions involving fever management or chicken pox, the safest advice to give is none. Both the American College of Emergency Physicians and the Emergency Nurses Association highly discourage telephone medical advice. If the parent or patient feels that they would like to be seen, tell them to come in, or call their regular physician. That is the safest answer for everyone.

42) The ED nurse knows that properly obtaining and securing evidence is known as:

A) Maintaining the chain of custody

B) Preventing custodial interference

C) Providing and protecting prima facia evidence

D) Preparing forensic anthropology

A – Maintaining the chain of custody (of potential evidence) to facilitate law enforcement investigations and possible later prosecutions is why many EDs have begun utilizing programs like SANE (Sexual Assault Nurse Examiners), SAFE (Sexual Assault Forensic Examiners), and SART (Sexual Assault Response Team.) These types of programs have nurses and other medical personnel who have been specially trained not only in the physical and psychological care of these specific patients, but also in evidence collection and preservation. Whether with cases involving battery, sexual assault, alcohol abuse, or non-accidental trauma, caring for the patient and the evidence is crucial.

43) The nurse knows that in a police investigation, law enforcement agents in the ED are entitled to:

A) The patient's name, address, and age

B) All patient information

C) A copy of the patient's medical record

D) No information without a court order or patient consent

A – In the post-HIPAA age in which we currently work, all we can legally tell law enforcement agents is "name, rank, and serial number." Everything else, including medical information, history, medical records, blood alcohol levels, etc. requires patient consent or a court order

44) The parent or legal guardian of a patient suspected of being a victim of child abuse or neglect can:

A) Withdraw consent for the child's treatment

B) Remove the patient from the facility against medical advice

C) Be prevented by law enforcement from taking the minor out of the hospital

D) All of the above

C – Safety first… for the nurses and for the patient. If abuse or neglect is suspected, then law enforcement can physically prevent parents or care givers from removing the child from the hospital environment. If abuse or neglect is seriously being considered, you should notify hospital and/or community law enforcement early in the process to help defuse any situations which might develop. This will help prevent the adults from running away with or without the child. We all must do what we can to keep the child in a safe place.

Some states have laws that allow the hospital to take a child into protective custody if it is believed that the child would be in imminent danger if returned to the care and custody of the parent or guardian. The test for taking protective custody is whether there is reasonable cause to believe that the circumstances or conditions are such that continuing in his or her place of residence or in the care and custody of the parent, guardian, custodian, or other person responsible for the child/adolescent's care presents an imminent danger.

45) The son of the city mayor is brought to the ED after an attempted suicide. The ED nurse receives a phone call from a newspaper reporter asking about the incident. Which nursing action is appropriate in this situation?

A) Give the reporter the information requested as stipulated by the Freedom of Information Act

B) Give the reporter the general patient information as dictated by hospital policy

C) Allow the reporter to interview the patient when his condition permits

D) Notify your Public Relations Department, the hospital administrator or nursing supervisor and providing no information to the reporter

D – Placing the caller on hold and allowing your Public Relations Department, the hospital administrator or nursing supervisor to handle the call is highly suggested.

46) A 15-year-old female arrives in the ED after being struck by a car while walking home from school. She has suffered moderate head, neck and chest injuries. The patient's father arrived in the ED with her and is pacing at the bedside. While he and the physician are discussing the potential need for a blood administration if the patient's condition worsens, the mother, who is divorced from the father, arrives at the ED nurses station and declares that the patient will not have a blood transfusion because it is against her religious beliefs. The **most** appropriate action by the nurse is:

A) Ignore the mother's demand and politely ask her to have a seat in the waiting room while waiting for social services

B) Quickly determine which parent has legal custody and only listen to that parent

C) Notify the physician of the issue and have the father confer with his ex-wife in the "Quiet Room" to resolve the blood transfusion consent issue

D) Have a risk manager or your hospital attorney confer with the physician and the family to untangle this complex situation

D - State laws vary widely in situations like this, especially when teenagers are involved. Some state courts have ordered blood transfusions for a child when the medical evidence demonstrates that there is no reasonable treatment alternative and where the risk of death is likely without transfusion. Such court decisions must balance the decision making authority of the parent(s) in the context of religious freedom against the interests and well being of the child. This analysis is more common for younger children when the objection to transfusion is based on the parent's (and not the child's) religious beliefs. Since teenagers may be of sufficient maturity to be able to make decisions about their own religious beliefs, a court may determine that the "mature minor" has the right to exercise her or his religious freedom. Knowing current case law in your state is the only way to ensure that you aren't ensnared in a legal endgame.

47) A 14-year-old female arrives via EMS to the emergency department after tripping on the bleachers at a high school pep rally. She is complaining of isolated pain in her left knee. While the knee appears to be obviously dislocated, distal pulses are strong and sensation and movement are intact distally. The history reveals that she is five and a half months pregnant. There are no other obvious injuries, her vital signs are stable, and there is no reason to suspect further injury. The school has contacted her parents and the patient's mother is enroute to the hospital to meet her daughter. Consent for treatment of the child's knee injury won't be a problem because:

A) At present, the nature of her injury does not pose a risk to either life or limb, and therefore can wait for further treatment until a parent can give appropriate consent

B) As a pregnant teenager, she is able to make her own decisions and authorize treatment

C) Because she is a minor, the doctrine of implied consent applies

D) She meets a universal exception for minors requiring immediate services for alleviation of all pain

A – Treatment can wait until appropriate consent is obtained. Generally speaking, pregnancy and motherhood among adolescents has created a number of seemingly inconsistent rules and many states deal with these situations differently. For example, in Florida, an unmarried pregnant minor may consent to medical and surgical care related to her pregnancy, but she cannot consent to medical treatment for herself that is not related to her pregnancy. What constitutes "related to pregnancy" is not defined by law. Once the minor girl gives birth, she can consent to treatment for her child, but not for herself. Likewise, in Maryland, a pregnant female over the age of 16 is considered "emancipated with respect to matters concerning the pregnancy." This means that she has the right to control her own decisions about her pregnancy. In Utah, parental consent is explicitly required for a minor to seek even general medical health services for themselves. In some states a pregnant minor can consent to any and all treatment regardless of whether the treatment is related to pregnancy. Emergency nurses should be aware of the laws and statutes in their own area as to when a child can provide consent, either for themselves, or their child.

48) A 3-year-old child is carried into the triage area of the emergency department. The sick child is accompanied by a neighbor. The parents are unavailable, but the neighbor pleads with the nurse to get the child treated. The child's condition appears to be serious, but you cannot tell how serious without doing further tests and beginning treatment. You should decide to:

A) Treat the child under the doctrine of informed consent

B) Withhold treatment until the parents can be contacted and consent obtained

C) Treat the child under the doctrine of implied consent

D) Withhold treatment because the parents could sue the hospital for unauthorized treatment of the child

C - The decision to treat the child or not to treat the child has to be made. This child is sick and needs

Certified Pediatric Emergency Nurse (CPEN) Review IV

treatment, and consent in this case is implied, not informed. If the hospital treats the child and the condition was in hindsight, an emergency, there is no legal difficulty. If the hospital does not treat the child, and the child recovers uneventfully, again there is also no legal difficulty (although it might be a PR disaster.)

The legal requirement for obtaining consent before rendering care has always been moderated by the privilege to render emergency medical care without the patient's consent. This privilege is based on the theory of implied consent. The law assumes that a patient who is unable to consent would in fact consent to emergency care if able. Remember, that implied consent can never overrule the explicit rejection of medical care. This is a very important consideration and can cause a great deal of confusion in an emergency room.

Problems arise if the child was treated in the absence of an emergency, or if no treatment was provided, and an emergency did exist. In the first case, assuming non-negligent treatment, the parents could sue the hospital for unauthorized treatment of the child, but not for malpractice. In the second situation, if care was denied because there was no one available to give a legally binding consent, and the child had a serious condition, that, left untreated, worsened, the parents could sue the hospital for failing to render care. The hospital would be in a position of needing to defend the lack of care, assuming that it would have saved the child's life, by proving that it was not negligent in assuming that there was no emergency. The jury would be presented with a devastated family, possibly the story of a dead child, a neighbor who will testify that he begged the hospital to treat the child, and a health care provider who tries to explain that the child was not treated because of a technicality in the consent law. Whose side would you want to be on?

49) A 16-year-old female presents to the emergency department after being involved in a multi-vehicle collision. She has significant lower extremity injuries that will most likely require surgical intervention. In the trauma bay, she asks that you call the local high school to advise her 18-year-old husband and ask him to come to the ED to be with her. Consent to treat her injuries is **best** obtained by:

A) Having her sign the consent because she is an emancipated minor.

B) Waiting for her husband to arrive, because since she is only 16 and still a minor, her husband must be present to give consent

C) Contact the parents, because even though she is married, she is a minor and still requires parental consent

D) Contact social services to report potential neglect and possible statutory rape

A – Generally speaking, marriage "emancipates" a minor, and that person (even if under 18) can give consent for treatment. In most states, the age of 18 is considered the age of majority, and children are said to be fully emancipated from parental control (Parents are also considered emancipated from the children at that point.) For certain children under 18, these adult-level responsibilities are already a reality. Emancipation is not available in every state in the United States, but in states that allow it, emancipation is a legal process by which minors can attain certain (not all) rights and privileges of adulthood before reaching the legal age to do so. Each state has different laws governing emancipation and some states simply have no law or legal process concerning emancipation.

50) Pain associated with hemophilia is best pharmacologically managed with which of the following:

A) Naprosyn® (sodium naproxen)

B) Aspirin (aspirin)

C) Tylenol® (acetaminophen, Panadol®)

D) Motrin® (ibuprofen, Brufen®)

C – Tylenol® has less negative effect on platelet formation or function than other non-steroidal anti-inflammatory drugs (NSAIDs) such as Naprosyn®, Motrin®, or aspirin. For those with hemophilia, acetaminophen is considered to be safe when used in normal doses. Opioid analgesics such as morphine or Dilaudid® (hydromorphone) offer another treatment modality that does not increase the risk of bleeding. Second only to bleeding out from massive total body trauma, head injuries with secondary intracranial hemorrhage represent the most serious complication of hemophilia and the highest probability of death or permanent impairment.

51) Steroids can be used to treat which of the following:

A) Hemophilia A and/or B

B) von Willebrand's disease

C) Disseminated intravascular coagulation (DIC)

D) Idiopathic thrombocytopenia purpura (ITP)

D – Steroids are used primarily for their anti-inflammatory and immunosuppressive effects and ITP is the only disease process listed above in which immunosuppression would help. Platelet transfusions are used in DIC and rarely with ITP, while the hemophilias use Factor infusions and von Willebrand's disease use DDAVP® (desmopressin.) In the case of scheduled surgeries, intravenous immunoglobulins (IVIG) may be used to temporarily help decrease the platelet destruction (and therefore increase platelet count and reduce bleeding risk.) However, this is a very expensive treatment with a very temporary effect. Most, but not all, cases of ITP in children resolve without treatment in a few months.

52) Potential triggers for sickle cell crisis include all of the following **except**:

A) Dehydration

B) Bed rest

C) Cold weather

D) Altitude

B – Dehydration, cold, and hypoxia (in this case secondary to elevation) are all well-known common triggers for sickle cell crisis. "Sicklers" should be kept oxygenated, warm, hydrated and pain-free as much as possible. Keep them "pink, warm, & sweet" (acting sweet as their pain is controlled) is the name of the game.

53) When reviewing the history for children with sickle cell disease, especially those under the age of five, you should routinely expect to find:

A) A daily penicillin regimen

B) A daily opiate regimen

C) A special diet

D) Strict restrictions in physical activity

A – Prescribed penicillin prophylaxis can be expected to be found in preschoolers with sickle cell disease. This regimen is designed specifically to protect against infection by Streptococcus pneumoniae (Pneumococcus, S. pneumo), the most common causes of bacterial pneumonia in children and a leading cause of bacterial sepsis among unvaccinated children. Any type of pneumonia can lead to acute chest syndrome, one of the most common causes of death in sickle cell patients. Lung infections lead to hypoxia, which precipitates sickling. This further occludes/infarcts the pulmonary vasculature. Additionally, sickle cell patients have impaired immune function due to splenic damage during childhood and are especially susceptible to infection by encapsulated bacteria such as Pneumococcus and Hemophilus influenza (H. flu). Routine pediatric vaccination against S. pneumo and H. flu have reduced the incidence of these infections in all children, but are not completely protective against all strains, so penicillin is still commonly prescribed for "sicklers" under five years of age. Pain medications, including opiates, are certainly appropriate, but only as needed. There is no special diet required in sickle cell anemia and all children, not just those with sickle cell disease, are encouraged to be as physically active as possible, with adequate hydration and opportunities for rest.

54) In patients with HIV/AIDS, the **most** significant indicator of infection may be:

A) Redness at the site of the infection

B) Fever

C) Swelling at the site of the infection

D) Warmth at the site of the infection

B – For patients with HIV/AIDS, fever may be the most significant indicator of infection. Redness, swelling and warmth at the site of the infection are classic symptoms of infection in the healthy individual and result from the body's phagocytic response. Unfortunately, this response is often impaired or non-existent in immune-compromised individuals such as those with active HIV/AIDS; therefore, infection may occur without signs of redness, warmth or swelling. Fever should always be taken seriously in these patients. Remember that serious infections may also occur without fever in these patients.

55) For AIDS patients with possible acute infections, after the ABCs, your priorities for patient care involve all of the following **except**:

A) Immediate antibiotic therapy

B) Identifying the source of infection

C) Protecting the patient against further infections

D) Social service consult

D – While a social service consult may be appropriate in certain circumstances, it is not an immediate priority for any patient with an acute infection. Patient safety (protecting against further infection) and identifying and treating the infection, which can be life-threatening, are all immediate priorities. Regardless of whether immune system depression is a result of cancer therapies or AIDS, the priorities are the same.

56) Systemic Lupus Erythematosus (SLE) is characterized by/as:

A) A predictable disease course

B) A single organ dysfunction

C) An infectious origin

D) A multisystem autoimmune disease

D – Systemic Lupus Erythematosus (SLE, lupus) is an autoimmune disease that simultaneously targets multiple organ systems in an unpredictable progression. It results in an overactive immune response that attacks otherwise healthy organs and tissues. It has no known underlying cause, is seen far more in females than males, and varies from mild to severe enough to cause death. The key to managing SLE is constant vigilance. Even your "frequent fliers" may not present the same way twice.

57) Although Systemic Lupus Erythematosus (SLE) has diverse presentations and progressions, it rarely manifests before age 8 and is often characterized by all of the following **except**:

A) Purple, non-blanching rash

B) Macular "butterfly" rash on the midface

C) Proteinuria

D) Pancytopenia

A – Remember, if you see a "purple, non-blanching rash," think meningococcemia. If you see a facial "butterfly" rash, chances are the correct answer is lupus. Often the patient's immune system will simultaneously attack alveolar (lung) and glomerular (kidney) membranes, resulting in pulmonary hemorrhage and nephritis/renal failure. In addition, children may present with neurologic symptoms, including psychosis, seizures, peripheral neuropathies, cognitive disorders, etc. Children who die from SLE typically die from some combination of the "Big Four:" Nervous system involvement (cerebral inflammation), infection, renal failure, and /or pulmonary hemorrhage.

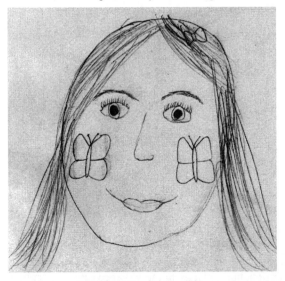

SLE "Butterfly Rash"

Courtesy of Nina DeBoer, my then 12-year old aspiring artist/baker daughter

www.ninasbeliciousbakery.com

58) Tumor Lysis syndrome (TLS) is **most** likely to occur with which of the following cancers?

A) Small, slow growing tumors

B) Small, rapidly growing tumors

C) Large, slowly growing tumors

D) Large, rapidly growing tumors

D – Tumor Lysis Syndrome (TLS) is typically seen with a large, rapidly growing/responding tumor burden, which is the typical presentation of the leukemias. You have to have a lot of "T"umor cells to "L"yse to get a "S"yndrome (TLS.) While this occasionally results from large, solid tumors such as meningiomas, it is most often seen in rapidly growing cancers such as acute lymphocytic leukemia (ALL), acute myeloid leukemia (AML) or lymphomas.

59) You have noticed a gradual, but increasingly significant change in behavior of a nursing colleague. This change includes erratic behavior, sudden outbursts of anger and agitation with fellow staff and patients. The pediatric emergency nurse identifies that these signs are consistent with behaviors exhibited by a person who may be abusing illicit substances. The nurse should:

A) Ignore the observations and hope the behavior improves

B) Discuss his/her concerns with a fellow staff member

C) Bring his/her concerns to their immediate supervisor immediately

D) Confront the colleague and tell them they need an intervention

C – Emergency nurses have a responsibility to recognize the signs and symptoms of impairment, especially if it should appear in colleagues or co-workers at any level. When impaired behavior patterns are recognized, a system that allows for confidential referral for the purpose of problem identification and evaluation should be utilized.

60) One of the **most** common triggers of violence in Emergency Departments is:

A) Inadequate or nonexistent English skills

B) Unexpected death of a family member

C) Prolonged waits to be treated

D) Request for co-payment

C – Prolonged waits for treatment is one of the most common causes of violence in the ED. With ED overcrowding continually on the rise, waiting times often become longer; the longer the waiting time, the more frustrated (and often angry) the patient and family members become. Patients and families may not understand why higher acuity patients, who arrived after them, are brought to the treatment area before them. They may also feel that the staff isn't working hard because they can't see what's going on behind closed doors. Communication problems, whether from a lack of explanations or language barriers certainly may lead to frustration, but typically not to violence (unless a really bad translation occurs.) While money may be a sore subject, discussions of payment arrangements rarely cause violence unless serious compounding conditions are present. Also, as a rule, people do not usually react with violence against health care professionals when a loved one dies, especially if the family has been included in the resuscitation efforts, and if possible, even the decision to terminate medical care.

61) A "red flag" that a patient or visitor in the waiting room may become violent is:

A) Crying

B) Speaking loudly

C) Sitting quietly

D) Laughing

B – One of the sure signs of increasing agitation is an increase in the tone and timber of the voice, especially when it becomes loud enough so that others around the area suddenly turn to see what's going on, or involves cursing and/or threats (making a scene). There can be many appropriate reasons for crying in the ED, and would not usually be considered a warning sign for violent behavior. Laughing, although certainly sometimes inappropriate, would also not necessarily indicate potential for violent behavior. Sitting quietly would typically not raise any concerns, even if it seems so unusually rare in most ED waiting rooms.

62) A child with a "hem-onc history" presents to your ED with complaints of abdominal spasms, painful urination, and pink-tinged urine. Your interview reveals recent administration of the chemotherapy medication Cytoxan® (cyclophosphamide.) This child is **most** likely experiencing:

A) Urinary tract infection (UTI) symptoms

B) Thrombocytopenia

C) Tumor lysis syndrome

D) Hemorrhagic cystitis

D – The recent administration of Cytoxan® puts this child at risk for hemorrhagic cystitis. Hemorrhagic cystitis (inflammation of the bladder leading to gross hematuria) may occur hours or even years after administration of chemotherapeutic agents. While the presenting symptoms may be indicative of a simple UTI, the medical and medication history points to likelihood of hemorrhagic cystitis. A child with thrombocytopenia may present with dark stools, bruising, and frank blood in the urine. The presentation of tumor lysis syndrome would be decreased urine output with "Pepsi™-Pee" rather than hematuria.

63) A 4-year old child with a history of sickle cell disease presents to the ED with a decreased level of consciousness. He appears drowsy, has a rapid, weak radial pulse of 180 and a BP of only 70/40. Based on these assessment findings, you suspect:

A) Aplastic crisis

B) Acute chest syndrome

C) Sequestration crisis

D) Bplastic crisis

C – This child is in shock as evidenced by changes in his level of consciousness and vital signs. Remember, the drop in BP is a late, bad sign. Of the choices given, sequestration crisis is the most correct answer; however, this child must also be assumed to be in septic shock. Sequestration crisis occurs when large quantities of blood pool in the spleen or liver and are trapped there, robbing the rest of the body of circulation (thus – shock!). It usually occurs in the younger SCD patients. Acute chest syndrome classically causes chest pain, signs of respiratory distress and hypoxia. Aplastic crisis is an acute, but fortunately transient, decrease in blood cell production (of all cell lines) in the bone marrow. Aplastic crisis may be seen post-Parvo virus exposure or in sickle cell disease. Lastly, there is no such thing as a Bplastic crisis.

64) You are assessing a 10-year old boy who fell off his bicycle about one hour prior to arrival. The child has a history of hemophilia A. Which assessment finding would be the **most** cause for concern?

A) Left knee ecchymosis

B) Decreased level of consciousness (LOC)

C) Epistaxis

D) Hematuria

B – Changes in LOC in any child, but especially in a child with hemophilia, is a huge big red flag! Although the other complaints are certainly important in any patient with hemophilia A, the symptoms of a possible intracranial bleed/injury take priority.

65) Appropriate discharge instructions for caregivers of a child with Idiopathic Thrombocytopenic Purpura (ITP) would include:

A) Treating fevers with aspirin or Motrin® (ibuprofen, Brufen®)

B) Return to the ED in 24 hours for follow-up

C) Use a toothpick after tooth brushing

D) Wear a helmet while bike riding

D – In children with ITP, it's all about preventing bleeding! Kids with ITP have way too few platelets (hence the term thrombocytopenia – thrombocytes are a fancy way of saying platelets and "penia" means you don't have nearly enough of them.) Treating a fever with aspirin or ibuprofen can increase the risk of bleeding rather than reduce the risk for bleeding. Remember, we don't use aspirin in children nearly as often as in the past due to the risk of Reye's syndrome. The relatively rare exceptions are for children with arthritis or Kawasaki's disease. As a side note, if you see "aspirin" in the question, chances are Reye's syndrome is the answer. Using a toothpick after tooth brushing increases the risk of additional bleeding. Although EDs are often used by many individuals for primary care, a pediatrician and/or hem-onc specialist would be the most appropriate follow-up providers for this child. Wearing a helmet when bike riding is always a good habit, and especially so for children with ITP. Kids with ITP have way too few platelets and therefore they have a decreased ability to stop bleeding in their brains if they fall!

66) A 7-year old child with a history of acute lymphocytic leukemia (ALL) is brought to the Pediatric ED by her parents, who state she has been bruising more than usual over the past 24 hours. They also report that she has had black, tarry stools today. The child appears drowsy and pale. Her radial pulse is 130 and weak, RR 28, Temp 100.2°F (37.9°C) and her BP is 80/50. Appropriate **initial** interventions for her coagulopathy would include:

A) Administering supplemental oxygen

B) Placement of a central line for intravenous access

C) Placement of a nasogastric (NG) tube

D) Applying a cooling blanket for a fever

A – Airway, Breathing and Circulation always take precedence, so administering supplemental oxygen is the most appropriate initial intervention. This child bleeds if you look at her funny, so she should have as few invasive procedures as possible. In other words, obtaining central IV access in the ED (especially since there was no mention of the inability to get a peripheral IV) would not be recommended, and neither would placement of an NG tube to check for upper GI bleeding. It is very likely that this child already has central venous access for her chemotherapy, so make use of that line whenever possible. Making the child hypothermic with a cooling blanket, which can exacerbate a coagulopathic state and make her bleed more, would definitely not be in this child's best interest.

67) The nurse in the ED is providing education regarding firearms to an adolescent. Which of the following pieces of information should be included in the conversation?

A) Adolescents are too young to carry a gun for hunting

B) Non-powered air-rifles or BB guns are harmless

C) Gun carrying is only a problem in the inner city

D) Adolescence is the peak age for being a victim or an offender

D – As more and more teens are carrying guns, there has been an increase in chances that adolescents will be either shooters or victims of a shooter or both. Teen gun possession is on the rise and is definitely not limited to the inner city. Many teens participate safely and responsibly in gun-associated hunting activities. In fact, there are many classes adolescents can and should take that teach gun and hunting safety. Anyone carrying a gun should be aware of laws restricting the presence of firearms in or near places such as schools. These restrictions hold true even for those with permits to carry firearms. And as far as air rifles and BB guns are concerned, they can cause injuries just like traditional firearms can. Just ask Ralphie from the Christmas movie classic, "A Christmas Story." He was told, "You'll shoot your eye out!"

68) Which of the following is **true** regarding obtaining consent from the parent or legal guardian of a thirteen-year old prior to testing the teenager for a sexually transmitted disease (STD)?

A) The nurse must obtain consent from the parent or legal guardian since the patient's life is not in imminent danger, parental consent is required.

B) Parental or guardian consent is required unless the teenager is considered an emancipated minor.

C) Since it is a routine test, regardless of the nature, the nurse does not need to get consent from a parent or legal guardian.

D) Consent is not required because all states allow minors over the age of 12 to have STD testing without parental consent.

D - All US states allow minors over the age of 12 to seek diagnosis and treatment of an STD without parental consent. (Don't let the "all" in the answer fool you!) In addition, most states allow minors to seek treatment for sexual abuse or assault without parental consent; however, many states require the minor's parents or guardian to be notified of the sexual abuse, unless the physician has reason to believe the parent or guardian was responsible for the sexual abuse.

Historically, parental consent was required for almost any type of medical treatment. Laws held that minors were not considered competent to make medical decisions. The past 50 years have witnessed a gradual expansion of the rights of minors, and health care has been no exception. Minors who previously had no medical rights are now in the position of making critical decisions about the most intimate medical procedures.

Some areas of the law surrounding the medical treatment of minors are still controversial, especially as it relates to certain procedures and conditions such as induced abortion and sexually transmitted diseases. There is a wide variation in the way that states allow minors to determine the course of their medical treatment.

Certified Pediatric Emergency Nurse (CPEN) Review IV

Informed Consent: In the case of children, can they offer informed consent or does that informed consent have to be provided by their parents? Beyond this simple question is an important set of underlying questions pertaining to, for example, the age at which a child may become capable of informed consent, and whether there are certain procedures in which informed consent is more important than others.

In general, for most medical procedures, the parent or legal guardian of the minor still has to grant consent in order for the procedure to be performed. While the state can challenge a parent's decision to refuse medically necessary treatment and can, in some cases, win the authority to make medical decisions on behalf of the child, the minor cannot make his or her own medical decisions.

This general rule nearly always applies regarding any sort of medical treatment before the minor enters their teenage years. No state or court has ever authorized minors younger than 12 years of age to make any sort of medical decision for themselves. But after the minor becomes a teenager, states begin to differ in terms of the responsibility the minor can take for medical decisions. Exceptions have been carved out for various medical procedures that allow teenage minors to have final say in their medical care.

Family Planning: Many states have laws that explicitly give minors the authority to consent to contraceptive services and specifically allow pregnant minors to obtain prenatal care and delivery services without parental consent or notification.

Emergency: All states allow parental consent for treatment of a minor to be waived in the event of a medical emergency if: The parent of the minor is incapacitated to the point of being unable to make an informed choice; The circumstances are life-threatening or serious enough that immediate treatment is required and no guardian is immediately available or it would be impossible or imprudent to try to get consent from an appropriate guardian. In these cases, consent of the parent is presumed, since otherwise the minor would suffer avoidable injury.

Sexually Transmitted Diseases: Every state currently allows minors over the age of 12 to receive testing for sexually transmitted diseases, including HIV, without parental consent. Most of these states also allow minors to receive treatment for all sexually transmitted diseases without parental consent; however, some states do not allow minors to receive treatment for HIV without parental consent. One state requires that parents be notified in the event of a positive HIV test. Many states allow doctors to notify the parents of the results of tests and treatment for sexually transmitted diseases, though they do not require consent for the test.

69) A 17-year old male is on leave at home after finishing basic training for the United States Army. He presents to the pediatric emergency department for an isolated fracture of his ulna after tripping and falling while visiting his old high school. Is parental consent required before treatment may begin?

A) Yes. Since the patient's life is not in imminent danger, parental consent is required

B) Yes. Parental consent is required in all situations, without exception.

C) No. The doctrine of implied consent exists

D) No. The patient is considered an emancipated minor

D – "Emancipated minor" is a term that is used far too often by people who really don't understand that it is a legal definition, and not a description of a child's living situation. Let's review what emancipated minor means. In the United States, there are three ways for a teenager to earn emancipated minor status. The first method is to demonstrate to a court that he or she is financially independent and the parents or legal guardians have no objections to his or her living arrangements. Another recognized way to earn emancipated minor status is to become legally married. This option does not supersede other laws governing the age of consent. A 12-year old girl seeking emancipated minor status cannot become legally married until she has reached her state's minimal age of consent. The third avenue for becoming an emancipated minor is to enlist in any of the armed forces of the United States. Once a minor is officially inducted into military service, he or she is automatically granted emancipated minor status for as long as he or she is an active member of the armed forces.

Certified Pediatric Emergency Nurse (CPEN) Review IV

70) A 16-year old teenager presents to the emergency department with flu-like symptoms. You know from his initial history that he lives under a highway overpass with other teen runaways, but that his parents still live in the local community. Is parental consent required before treatment may begin?

A) No. The patient is considered an emancipated minor since he says he doesn't live at home any longer.

B) No. The doctrine of implied consent exists (the parents would most certainly agree to treatment for their child) negating the otherwise necessary formality of obtaining consent.

C) Yes. Since the patient's life is not in imminent danger, parental consent is required.

D) Yes. Since the patient is a minor, parent consent is always required

C – Regarding this pediatric patient, unless the injury or illness is life threatening, he is a minor requiring parental consent for medical treatment until he reaches the age of 18. (The "always" in choice "D" should help with your choice of answers.) You might think that because the child is living on his own as a runaway, that he is an emancipated minor, but no…that is not correct! "Emancipated minor" is a legal designation that is the result of a court proceeding or other formal arrangement.

Once a child reaches the age of majority at 18-19 (depending on individual state laws), he or she is said to be fully emancipated from parental control. This means he or she can enjoy many of the privileges and responsibilities of adulthood such as voting, marriage and financial independence.

71) The Federal law designed to prevent hospitals from refusing to treat patients or transferring them to another hospital due to inability to pay is known as:

A) Health Insurance Portability and Accountability Act (HIPAA)

B) Emergency Medical Treatment and Labor Act (EMTALA)

C) United States National Health Care Act (USNHCA)

D) Health Care and Education Reconciliation Act (HCERA)

B) – The Emergency Medical Treatment and Active Labor Act (EMTALA) was created out of a concern that patients were being denied emergency medical treatment because of their inability to pay. The initial intent of EMTALA was to address the allegations that some hospitals were transferring, discharging, or refusing treatment to patients who did not have insurance (a practice sometimes referred to as "patient dumping"). The two basic requirements of the EMTALA law of 1986 are to: 1) Provide a medical screening examination (MSE) to anyone who seeks examination or treatment for a medical condition in order to determine if an emergency medical condition exists and 2) Stabilize the medical condition revealed by the MSE, using the staff and facilities available at the hospital, before transferring or discharging the patient.

72) A screech of tires and a slamming door are heard coming from the street just outside the ambulance entrance to the stand-alone children's hospital. Without going outside of the locked ED, the nurse can visualize an adult male lying on the sidewalk. He is not moving and blood appears to be soaking the front of his shirt. What action is required of the Pediatric ED nurse?

A) Call 9-1-1 because the patient is on the street, and not in the hospital

B) Immediate notification of the in-house supervisor in accordance with the "Safe Haven" policy

C) Respond, assess and begin stabilization of the emergency medical condition

D) No action is required because the patient is an adult and this is a pediatric facility

C – When considering the implications of EMTALA, pretend that your facility is surrounded by a 250-yard/meter "I am also responsible for this" zone. EMTALA rules apply to any person who presents on the hospital campus and requests or requires emergency medical services. The "250-yard/meter rule" obligates hospital staff to respond when a visitor, employee, or anyone on the hospital campus is in need of a medical screening examination. This area includes the sidewalks and parking lots adjacent to the building. Exceptions to this rule are any businesses that are not part of your hospital (such as a pharmacy or gas station) and contracted physician offices/ancillary services (an oncology clinic that is on your grounds). In those settings you would call 9-1-1 in accordance with your policy.

73) For EMTALA to apply, a patient must come to the emergency department. Which of the following conditions meets the criteria of coming to the emergency department?

A) A person is struck by a vehicle in the hospital's on-site parking garage.

B) A person collapses in a private physician office building next door to the main entrance of the hospital

C) A person is assaulted at the community/hospital partnership methadone clinic in the local library

D) A person choked on a piece of food in the McDonald's across the driveway from the ED

A – While the parking garage may not be attached to the hospital, it is still considered part of the facility and therefore within the 250 yard/meter rule. It is also important to remember that there are exceptions to the "250 yard/meter – I am responsible for this" zone. Examples of these would be non-medical businesses (eliminates D), private physician offices (eliminates B), as well as non-emergent clinical outpatient services (and that takes care of C).

74) EMTALA requires hospitals with specialized capabilities to accept transfers of patients with emergent conditions from a hospital with inadequate capabilities:

A) After reviewing the findings of the referring hospital's medical screening examination (MSE) to determine whether an emergency medical condition exists

B) When CMS coverage eligibility is confirmed that reimbursement for tertiary care is available

C) Before the patient is stabilized at the referring facility

D) When space and qualified personnel are available to treat the individual

D – An often forgotten requirement is that EMTALA only comes into play when the patient has an emergent condition and the sending hospital has inadequate capabilities to care for that patient. The receiving hospital is required to accept the transfer when they have space and personnel to take care of the patient. Can you imagine what would happen if this wasn't in place? Ambulances full of patients would simply show up at the tertiary center doors regardless of whether they had open beds or staff to take care of them! Referring hospitals are allowed to release the emergent patient for transfer when:

- The emergency medical condition has been stabilized; or

- The emergency medical condition has not been stabilized, but the treating physician certifies that the benefits of transfer outweighs the risk; or

- The patient or health care proxy requests transfer, regardless of whether the emergency medical condition has been stabilized; or

- The on-call physician at the referring hospital fails or refuses to appear within a reasonable period of time and, without the services of the on-call physician, the benefits of transfer outweighs the risk.

Interestingly enough, a patient in labor (having contractions) is not considered "stable" until the fetus and the placenta have been delivered.

Certified Pediatric Emergency Nurse (CPEN) Review IV

75) A 3-year old female presents to the emergency department via EMS with an unintentional gunshot wound to the left abdomen and chest. The child is rapidly taken to the operating room, where her chest and belly are opened. The surgeon cannot manage the extent of the trauma inflicted. He wants to arrange air transport to the pediatric trauma center, transferring the child in a hypotensive state with blood products infusing, and leaving the surgical site open, but packed. To avoid an EMTALA violation:

A) The surgery must be completed and closed and the hypotension resolved

B) An EMTALA violation cannot be avoided because the child has not been stabilized

C) The surgeon must acknowledge and document the poor decision to attempt to fix the damage in the OR/theatre

D) The treating physician must certify that the benefits of transfer outweigh the risks

D – For the purpose of EMTALA, a patient with acute symptoms of sufficient severity that, without immediate medical attention, could reasonably be expected to result in placing the health of the individual in serious jeopardy, serious impairment to bodily functions, or serious dysfunction of any bodily organ or part, is by definition, unstable.

Once a patient's condition has been stabilized, they can be transferred without violating any EMTALA guidelines. This patient, however, is obviously quite unstable. However, in the event that the referring physician certifies that the benefits of transferring an unstable patient outweigh the risks of the transfer itself, it is not an EMTALA violation. Many patients transported by air or ground teams would be considered "unstable," but the benefits tip the scales in favor of transfer.

Ideally, the decision to transfer an unstable patient should be made in concert with the responsible staff at the receiving hospital. All efforts should be made to assure that the patient will receive the best possible care during the transport and that the receiving hospital will be adequately prepared to immediately assume care upon the patient's arrival. Proper communication and documentation is required, even with the transfer of an unstable patient.

Depending on the individual's condition, there may be situations in which the presence of a physician or other qualified provider (nurse, paramedic, respiratory therapist, etc.) might be indicated during interfacility transfer.

76) A parent may be allowed access to their minor child's health care records:

A) When the minor is the one who consents to care and parental consent is not required

B) When a parent is the child's "personal representative" or when access is not inconsistent with state or other applicable law

C) When the minor obtains care at the direction of a court or a person appointed by a court

D) When a parent agrees that the child and the care provider have a confidential relationship

B – The federal privacy regulations issued under HIPAA provide important protection of confidentiality for minors. HIPAA includes rights for adolescents and grants legal significance to agreements that favor adolescents receiving confidential care. When a minor has the legal right to consent for care, HIPAA allows the minor to assume the right to control access to information and records of their care on the same basis as adults. The minor is treated as an "individual" who can exercise his/her rights under this rule. This applies when:

1)   The minor legally consents to health care, such as for treatment of STDs,

2)   The minor receives care without parental consent, but with court approval of care, or

3) When the parent consents to an agreement of confidentiality between the adolescent and the health care provider.

In these cases, the parent does not necessarily have the right to access the minor's protected health information (PHI). According to HIPAA, the parent's right to access PHI is determined by "state and other applicable law." However, the minor may request that the parent act as a personal representative and, if she does so, the parent may have access to information. State or other applicable laws may give the right to control access to the information to the minor or may grant discretion to a physician.

77) The legal duty to exercise the degree of knowledge, care and skill that is expected of a comparably trained practitioner in the same class in which he or she belongs, acting in the same or similar circumstances, is **best** defined as:

A) Standard of care

B) Direct liability

C) Negligence

D) Vicarious liability

A – What a reasonable, prudent and careful nurse in a same or similar circumstance would have done is the standard of care. Negligence is the failure to act, and liability reflects the degree or extent of responsibility for actions.

This book is not intended to act as a definitive text on medical-legal issues. If you are unfamiliar with the local/state/federal laws that are pertinent to your practice, please investigate further through your hospital or agency's legal resources.

78) Tumor lysis syndrome (TLS) is **most** likely to occur with which of the following cancers?

A) Small, slow growing tumors

B) Small, rapidly growing tumors

C) Large, slowly growing tumors

D) Leukemias

D – TLS is typically seen with a large, rapidly growing/rapidly responding tumor burden. You have to have a lot of tumor cells to Lyse to get a Syndrome. While this may occasionally occur with large solid tumors such as meningiomas, it is most often seen in rapidly growing cancers. Answers A, B, and C all specifically mention tumors, and it sure seems like one of them must be the correct answer. But remember that most tumors take time to grow into really big tumors. On the other hand, "emias," like acute lymphocytic leukemia (ALL) or acute myeloid leukemia (AML) and "omas," such as lymphomas grow a whole lot faster.

79) Which of the following signs and symptoms correspond to the emergently life threatening electrolyte abnormalities typically seen in Tumor Lysis Syndrome (TLS)?

A) Positive Brudzinski's sign, inverted or flattened T waves, shortened QT interval

B) Positive Chvostek's sign, peaked T waves, bradycardia

C) Positive Kernig's sign, U waves, shortened PR interval

D) Negative Chvostek's sign, peaked T waves, shortened RR interval

B – The emergently life threatening electrolyte abnormalities typically seen in TLS are HYPERkalemia and HYPOcalcemia secondary to HYPERphosphatemia. (Calcium goes down when the phosphate goes up – remember the see-saw that occurs with pH and potassium in DKA – same idea.) Think about the common sign of TLS, which is dark, icky, concentrated looking urine. Since the issues are all about the "P," and the fact that their kidneys are clogged up and therefore not peeing well, the answer is "P"otassium or "P"hosphate (they don't pee either away). This situation will result in muscle weakness (calcium needed for muscles to move), peaked T waves ("P"eaked T waves begin with "P"), and cardiac conduction delays in the "P"ump." Chvostek's sign is seen in hypocalcemia, while Kernig's and Brudzinski's signs are not found with electrolyte disturbances, but with meningeal irritation.

80) After assessment of airway, breathing and circulation (ABCs), the **most** important consideration when caring for a febrile patient with suspected or confirmed significant neutropenia is:

A) Initiation of reverse isolation precautions

B) Administration of oral antibiotics

C) Administration of intravenous antibiotics

D) Administration of Colony Stimulating Factors (CSFs)

C – Intravenous, not oral, antibiotics are indicated for these patients with a depressed immune system and the inability to fight off infections. While important to attempt, true reverse isolation in the ED is nearly impossible and doesn't help combat any infections the patient already may have. It simply helps protect the patient from acquiring a new infection. Colony Stimulating Factors (agents that increase white blood cell production) are used later on the inpatient side. In the ED, the most important consideration is preventing full-blown sepsis.

CLINICAL PEARL: Febrile neutropenia is clinically defined as:

Oral temperature > 38.0° Celsius / 100.4° Fahrenheit

Absolute Neutrophil Count (ANC) < 1000/mm3

ANC = Total White Blood Cell (WBC) count x (% Neutrophils + % Bands)

81) All of the following are contraindicated in febrile patients with neutropenia **except**:

A) Rectal temperatures

B) Foley catheters

C) Digital rectal examinations

D) Venipuncture

D – Venipuncture, although a potential source of infection (like the other options), is necessary for labs and IV antibiotics. This question is included to further hammer home a rule about neutropenia. ANYTHING that would disrupt the patient's protective epithelial/mucosal linings separating the blood stream from the "outside world" (and those dangerous and opportunistic pathogens) should be avoided. Anything, that is, except obtaining IV access.

Certified Pediatric Emergency Nurse (CPEN) Review IV

82) Disseminated Intravascular Coagulation (DIC) will commonly present with which of the following conditions and laboratory findings?

A) Thrombocytopenia, decreased fibrinogen, prolonged PTT, prolonged PT, elevated fibrin split products

B) Thrombocytopenia, increased fibrinogen, shortened PTT, shortened PT, decreased fibrin split products

C) Thrombocytopenia, increased fibrinogen, normal PTT, normal PT, elevated fibrin split products

D) Thrombocytopenia, decreased fibrinogen, prolonged PTT, prolonged PT, decreased fibrin split products

A – To get the correct answer on this question, one simply needs to think about the last time you took care of a patient in true DIC. What do you remember from the occasion? They bleed, bleed, and bleed! So, with that in mind, think back to what you learned in physiology class about what your body needs to stop bleeding--thrombocytes (platelets), fibrin, fibrinogen and other clotting factors. Each answer mentions thrombocytopenia (not nearly enough platelets), so that's not much help. Answers B and C mention increased fibrinogen which would help, not inhibit, clotting. That rules out B and C as correct answers, so you are now up to 50/50 odds of picking the correct answer. Answers A and D mention prolonged PT and PTT which makes sense considering the patient is actively bleeding. But the key is with the Fibrin. Fibrin is essential for clotting. When the clots are "split" and not sticking together (causing the patient to bleed all over the place), the fibrin is "split." So patients in DIC have elevated fibrin split products. This leaves only A as the correct answer. The primary treatment for DIC is to treat the underlying cause while also administering platelets, fresh frozen plasma (FFP,) cryoprecipitate ("cryo") and, in the case of microemboli, heparin.

CLINICAL PEARL: In patients with DIC, FFP must be given before heparin or the heparin will not have the Antithrombin III it needs for anticoagulation.

83) Disseminated intravascular coagulation (DIC) is treated by all of the following **except**:

A) Treating the underlying cause

B) Replacing red blood cells (RBCs), clotting factors and platelets

C) Heparin therapy

D) Tissue plasminogen activator (tPA®).

D – The primary treatment for DIC is to treat the underlying cause and stop the intravascular coagulation cascade. Replacing depleted platelets, clotting factors and RBCs is absolutely essential. In the case of thrombosis or microemboli, heparin may be used. The use of heparin is controversial, but (Hint!) it is listed in the ENA Core Curriculum. Although tPA® may seem tempting, as it's an anticoagulant too, we need to remember that tPA® breaks clots down, which is quite different from Heparin which prevents clots from forming in the first place.

84) All of the following are contraindicated in febrile patients with neutropenia **except**:

A) Rectal temperatures

B) Rectal suppositories

C) Digital rectal examinations

D) Reverse isolation precautions

D – Reverse isolation may be appropriate while all the other choices would be relatively contraindicated for febrile patients with neutropenia. This question is sort of a "gimmee," but it is included to further hammer home the fact that ANYTHING that would disrupt the epithelial/mucosal linings that protect against invasive pathogens (separating the blood stream from the "outside world") should be avoided. Although not stated in the question, scrupulous sterile technique must be observed when starting or accessing intravenous or intraosseous lines in these patients.

Pediatric Oncology Nurse Insight: We have never put our kids on neutropenic precautions because of the idea that we don't want to make them feel isolated. So even though their ANCs are less than 500 and we have many kids whose ANCs are at zero, we don't gown and mask, etc. We do urge them to avoid crowded places and especially anyone who is sick. If we get anyone in who has had a bone marrow transplant in the last 6 months, we usually mask and glove. We use masks and gowns and sterile gloves for accessing ports or central lines. We use sterile gloves and masks for certain types of central line lab draws and regular gloves when we do anything with the line, even changing the IV bag, hooking up more tubing to existing tubing, etc., and of course always using alcohol preps. I am forever getting report from EDs that they have put our kid on "neutropenic precautions" and I just say "OK" because that is probably a good thing to do in an ED environment anyway.

85) A well-known "frequent flyer" teen with sickle cell disease presents to the Pediatric ED in pain crisis. He has received several doses of IV Dilaudid® (hydromorphone) and Benadryl® (diphenhydramine) but still complains of 9/10 joint pain. His heart rate is 84, respiratory rate is 18, and room air saturation is 98%. At this point, the ED nurse should anticipate:

A) Discharge of the patient to home

B) Administration of additional IV analgesics

C) Administration of oral analgesics

D) A psychiatric consult for drug-seeking behavior

B – Pain is what the patient says it is, so forget the psychiatric consult. This is especially true for patients with poorly-controlled sickle cell disease, patients for whom pain is an everyday event. Many medical providers use vital signs to determine if the pain complaint is valid; however, normal vital signs do not always mean that the child or teen is not in pain. Think about it this way: The body cannot respond with tachycardia, tachypnea and hypertension every minute of every day in people with chronic pain issues. Therefore, unless there are compelling reasons not to believe the patient is in pain, treat the pain. In this patient, who has already received IV pain meds, it would not be appropriate to take pain management a step backwards and give oral analgesics unless they're used in conjunction with additional IV meds.

Certified Pediatric Emergency Nurse (CPEN) Review IV

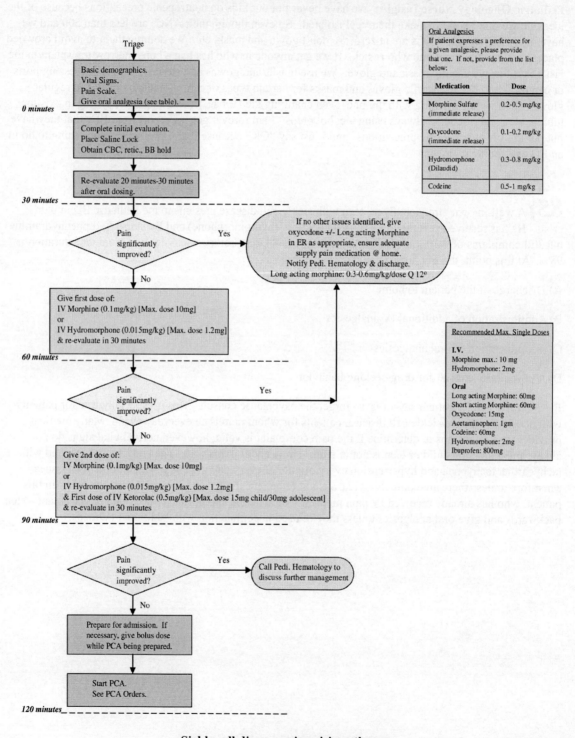

Sickle cell disease pain crisis pathway

Courtesy of William Zempsky MD & the New England Pediatric Sickle Cell Consortium

www.nepscc.org

Certified Pediatric Emergency Nurse (CPEN) Review IV

86) You are teaching new ED nurses how to properly collect evidence and maintain the chain of custody during physical exam in cases of known or suspected sexual assault. You stress that evidence items should be:

A) Collectively placed in a plastic bag

B) Individually placed in paper bags

C) Collectively placed in a paper bag

D) Does not matter what it is placed in so long as your initials and date are clearly marked

B – All items collected as evidence should be placed in individual paper bags. Individual bags prevent cross contamination between evidence items. In addition, paper is preferred over plastic because it "breathes" and does not promote bacterial growth the way that relatively impermeable plastic does. There are multiple dimensions of care, physical assessment and evidence collection that must be scrupulously attended to for these extremely vulnerable patients.

87) What is your **first** priority regarding a child who may have been sexually assaulted?

A) Evidence collection

B) Assuring the child's safety

C) Injury treatment

D) Comprehensive interview

B – If the question involves patient care and the word "safety" appears in one of the answers, then it's very probably the right answer! With this question, it should be a no-brainer. Making sure the child is safe includes reporting to the right agencies or individual, not leaving the child alone with alleged/suspected perpetrators and assuring the child that he or she is safe now. Treatment of injuries, unless they are life threatening, is ideally done after documentation of the injuries and evidence collection. Evidence collection is a vital part of our initial steps and includes the initial exam. Lastly, a comprehensive interview is not performed at this time, as the initial interview is narrowly focused for evidence collection purposes. It is crucial to remember that once evidence is collected, the Chain of Custody documentation must be scrupulously maintained from the initial examiner/collector on down. If this chain is broken, the evidence may be questioned or possibly even be inadmissible in court.

Additional Pediatric ED Attending Physician Insights: Limit the number of times the child is examined. These are not kids who need exams by the triage nurse, nursing student, assigned nurse, medical student, resident and attending physician! If a forensic exam is NOT to be performed at the facility during the initial exam, then the initial exam should be limited to identifying potentially life threatening injuries.

88) Severe complications from sickle cell disease can include all of the following **except**:

A) Heart failure

B) Ischemic stroke (CVA)

C) Acute chest syndrome

D) Diabetes mellitus

D – Diabetes mellitus is not a complication of sickle cell anemia. Congestive heart failure can result from chronic anemia and hypoxia, although this is uncommon in children. Ischemic stroke occurs at a 5-10%

rate in this patient population and has a high incidence (50-90%) of reoccurrence if they are not treated with transfusions and hydroxurea. CVAs and acute chest syndrome result from sickling cells obstructing capillary blood flow and causing downstream infarctions.

89) In pediatric patients, Idiopathic Thrombocytopenia Purpura (ITP) commonly follows all of the following **except**:

A) Recent viral illness

B) Recent bacterial illness

C) Primary immune deficiency syndrome (PIDS)

D) Acquired immune deficiency syndrome (AIDS)

B – In pediatric patients, ITP most commonly follows a viral infection (i.e. a cold or gastroenteritis), but it can also be seen in primary and acquired immune deficiency syndromes such as AIDS. Children with ITP make abnormal antibodies which bind to platelets, making them targets them for elimination by macrophages in the spleen. When the body cannot increase platelet production to compensate for this destruction, ITP results. As platelets given via transfusion are "chewed up as fast as you can give them," they are commonly only given prior to surgery or for an intracranial hemorrhage. For the exam, the answer for ED management of ITP is intravenous immunoglobulins (IVIG) or steroids, which may be used to temporarily help decrease the platelet destruction (and therefore increase platelet count and reduce bleeding risk). Most, but not all, cases of ITP in children are temporary and fortunately resolve without treatment in a few months.

Additional Pediatric ED Attending Physician Insights: Nobody knows why a recent viral infection is a risk factor for ITP or why only a tiny percentage of people get ITP after a viral infection. It would seem like the post-viral immune system might be hyped up (overactive), unlike with those patients with primary or acquired immune-deficiencies and baseline low immune activity.

90) In pediatric patients with HIV/AIDS, the **most** significant indicator of skin or joint infection may be:

A) Redness at the site of the infection

B) Fever

C) Swelling at the site of the infection

D) Warmth at the site of the infection

B – Fever is the most likely significant indicator of infection in pediatric HIV/AIDS patients. Redness, swelling and warmth are classic symptoms of infection in the healthy individual and result from the body's phagocytic response at the site of infection. Unfortunately, this response is impaired or non-existent in immune-compromised individuals, including those with active HIV/AIDS. In these patients, fever may be one of the only signs of skin or joint infection.

91) For febrile children with AIDS, after the ABCs, your priorities for patient care involve all of the following **except**:

A) Immediate antibiotic therapy

B) Identifying the source of infection

C) Safe sex counseling

D) Protecting the patient against further infections

C – Hopefully you identified counseling as not being a priority for treatment. Please see the discussions on febrile neutropenia. Regardless of whether immune system depression is a result of cancer therapies or AIDS, the priorities are the same.

92) Neutropenic patients are considered to be at very high risk for infections if they have an Absolute Neutrophil Count (ANC) of less than:

A) 500-1000/mm3

B) 1000-1500/ mm3

C) 1500-2000/ mm3

D) 2000/ mm3

A –The normal ANC is 1500-2000mm3, and patients with an ANC of less than 500-1000mm3 are considered to be at a really high risk for catching and being unable to fight off infections. While some people consider 500-1000 as indicative of moderate increased risk of infection, and < 500 is severe risk, most folks just consider anything <1000 to be risky.

The Absolute Neutrophil Count (ANC) indicates the number of neutrophils (specific types of white blood cells) in the blood. Neutrophils are the white blood cells that fight bacterial infections. The ANC is calculated by adding the percentages of the "segs" (mature neutrophils) and the "bands" (immature neutrophils) and multiplying that number by the total number of WBCs. If the total WBC count is 8,000 with segs of 20% and bands of 5% (segs + bands = 25%), the ANC = 25% of 8,000 = 2000. (Remember that the lab gives us the abbreviated count. What they report as "10" is really 10,000.)

Our big concern with patients who have low ANCs is the possibility catching bacterial infections, which tend to be more complicated than viral infections. The white blood cell count (WBC) is the total number of available resources available. The reason that the ANC is important because neutrophils specialize in fighting bacterial infections, while other white blood cells (lymphocytes and monocytes) respond more to viral infections. If infections are like enemy spies, our body (like our government), has two separate "spy fighting" groups. Just as there are domestic spies (fought by the FBI) and foreign spies (fought by the CIA), there are bacterial infections (our body fights bacterial infections with neutrophils) and viral infections (our body fights viral infections with lymphocytes and monocytes). That is why knowing the differentiated WBC is so important.

93) Hyperleukocytosis is defined as:

A) Extremely high levels of red blood cells

B) Extremely high levels of white blood cells

C) Extremely high levels of platelets

D) Extremely high levels of plasma

B – For questions such as this, if the word sounds way too big and complicated, simply break it down piece by piece. Chances are you can pick the correct answer. "Hyper" is defined as being "above and beyond." Leuko(cytes) are white blood cells. Cytosis means "more than the usual number of cells." So, hyperleukocytosis means that the body is pumping way too many white blood cells into the bloodstream (>100,000mm3), which can lead to clogged up organs. Most conditions of hyperleukocytosis are caused by malignancy affecting the bone marrow. If your patient has hyperleukocytosis, you can expect to flush, flush, flush in the ED followed by chemotherapy/exchange transfusion in the Pediatric ICU.

Certified Pediatric Emergency Nurse (CPEN) Review IV

94) The display board in the ED waiting room is used to educate patients and families on injury risks and prevention strategies. This month, the information is on teen driving risks and behavior. Which piece of the important information below is **false**?

A) Teens approach decision making and risks of driving differently than adults

B) The crash rate for newly licensed novice drivers is low due to restrictions on night driving

C) Listening to loud music, changing the music on the radio, or talking or texting on the phone while operating a motor vehicle is considered to be distracted driving

D) Teen drivers are often over-confident which can lead to dangerous driving behaviors

B – Teens differ greatly from adults in their approach to risk and decision-making. Each uneventful drive a teen makes results in their perception of risk decreasing and the perception of benefit (or being a skilled NASCAR driver!) increasing. As a result, the teen becomes overconfident of their driving skills and less vigilant about safety. Young drivers are at a significantly higher risk than older drivers, with crash rates decreasing dramatically from the first month to the seventh month (41%) then a gradual decrease through the twenty-fourth month (60% overall reduction) after receiving a restricted license. This is why delaying full licensure for teens is important for everyone's safety. Distracted driving is getting behind the wheel and allowing outside factors to pull your concentration away from the road. Texting, applying makeup, messing with an iPod™, talking on the phone, loud music, loud friends--all of these are examples of things that can decrease your ability to drive safely. Simply stated: Distracted Driving = dead drivers, dead passengers or dead innocent, non-distracted others.

95) EMS arrives with an unresponsive 13-year old boy found hanging by a belt from his bunk bed. Mom is understandably distraught, repeating "I don't understand. He is such a good, happy kid. He's popular and smart. Why would he do this?" Based on the reported presentation, you know this possibly fits the profile of:

A) Non-Accidental Trauma (Child Abuse)

B) Autoerotic Asphyxiation

C) The Choking Game

D) Suicidal Ideation

C – While there are pieces of this scenario that fit each answer, the most complete picture is "The Choking Game." This is a risky activity that is played primarily by the younger teenage population to get a "drugless high." It can be played in a group (bear hugs), in pairs (throttling) or alone (using belts or ligatures). Players are usually in the "tweens" and early teens. Eighty to 90 percent of the participants are males. In the Choking Game, the patient experiences a hypoxic state, followed by a "high feeling" as circulation (and the oxygen supply) to the brain is restored. Most often, these kids are well adjusted and have good grades and an adequate circle of friends. Of course, the greatest danger is if the child passes out prior to being able to release himself from the cord or belt. While the majority of deaths occur when children play the game by themselves, children can suffer from prolonged hypoxia even when playing the game with others, who may not realize that the child is in trouble. The Choking Game differs from Autoerotic Asphyxiation primarily (just looking at the name) because the latter commonly involves an older male restricting oxygenation for sexual arousal. Sexual arousal is not generally part of the Choking Game. The mechanism stated in the question is rarely seen as an indicator of intentional injury (child abuse). It's possible this was a suicide attempt, even though the mother is unaware of any indicators of depression in her son; however, the age, sex and known psychological profile of the patient make the Choking Game most likely.

Certified Pediatric Emergency Nurse (CPEN) Review IV

96) EMS is enroute with a 3-week old male whose mother said he "stopped breathing and turned blue during feeding." Upon presentation, the child is alert, well perfused and in no respiratory distress; however, he has a rectal temperature of 100.6°F (38.1°C) and has had 3 days of cough and cold symptoms. Anticipated workup for this child with an apparent life-threatening event (ALTE) or brief resolved unexpected event (BRUE) will most likely include all the following **except**:

A) Full sepsis workup and IV antibiotics

B) Tylenol® (acetaminophen, Panadol®) and discharge home if the fever doesn't elevate and he remains otherwise asymptomatic

C) Screening for respiratory illnesses such as RSV, influenza and pertussis

D) Admission

B - We need to find out why this child did what he did, so he isn't going home with a dose of Tylenol® and a pat on the head. This child's Brief Resolved Unexplained Event (BRUE) formerly was referred to as an Apparent Life-Threatening Event (ALTE), "near-miss sudden infant death syndrome (SIDS)" or "aborted crib death." Experts now recommend abandoning these terms, as they imply an incorrect close association between BRUEs, ALTEs and SIDS. BRUEs describes an event that: 1) Occurs in a child younger than 1 year of age, 2)Lasts less than 1 minute (typically 20-30 seconds), 3) Has one or more of the following: Central Cyanosis or Pallor - Absent, Decreased, or Irregular breathing - Marked change in tone -Altered level of responsiveness 4) Resolves and patient returns to baseline & 5) Has a reassuring history, physical exam, and vital signs during ED evaluation. BRUE is used only when another condition cannot be discerned as the etiology of the event. It is important to remember that BRUEs/ALTEs and SIDS are two different conditions. The most important concept for parents to come away with is that the vast majority of children who have an BRUE/ALTE do not go on to die of SIDS. Approximately 25-50% of BRUE/ALTE incidents have no identifiable cause. When a cause is found, the most common reasons are gastroesophageal reflux disease (GERD), upper and lower respiratory tract infections, pertussis, and seizures. This infant is only three-weeks old with an BRUE/ALTE and a mild fever, so he's septic, possibly septic, or thinking about becoming septic until proven otherwise. Therefore, he gets the full sepsis workup, including a lumbar puncture and admission for IV antibiotics until he is proven to be cute (non-septic) and the BRUE/ALTE evaluation has been completed.

97) A 12-year old who just finished a "round" of chemo four days ago presents to the ED with a fever and shortness of breath. He has a port in his right upper chest for venous access and asks the Pediatric ED nurse to please utilize the port for blood sampling and IV antibiotic therapy. A non-coring "Huber" needle is placed, but no blood can be aspirated. The next step should be to:

A) Ask the patient to cough or bear down

B) Place the patient in Trendelenburg position

C) Immediately remove the needle

D) Inject heparin solution

A – If you can't draw blood from an accessed port, appropriate steps would be to: A) Ask the patient to perform some sort of a Valsalva maneuver, such as bearing down or coughing, B) Raise the patient's arms over their head and/or turn them on either side or C) Both of the above. These interventions can sometimes help to reestablish blood flow through the port and are reasonably quick and easy to perform. Placing patients who are short of breath in Trendelenburg, (standing on their head) makes breathing much more difficult. Heparin should not be injected if the needle may not be in the correct position. Lastly, don't immediately remove the needle. Think "What's the first rule of impaled objects in the ED? Don't pull them out!" The same idea applies here. Take that one step further and think about putting a urinary catheter in female patients. If you miss the urethra the first time and go into the vagina instead, you never take out the Foley. You leave it in to show you where NOT to go with the next attempt. If the first attempt at accessing the port didn't work, leave the needle in as a guide to show you where NOT to go and then try again in a nearby area. If two attempts are unsuccessful, I suggest seeing if a heme-onc nurse can "please or pretty-please with sugar on top" come play and help out as they are simply amazing in their abilities to access ports.

98) An 8-year old child with a double-lumen peripherally inserted central catheter (PICC) presents to the Pediatric ED with signs of gastroenteritis. The ED nurse knows that which of the following statements are **correct** regarding PICC lines?

A)   A 10 ml or larger syringe should be used to flush the PICC line

B)   Only continuous, non-turbulent, flush techniques should be used

C)   Fluids must continuously be infusing in a PICC to prevent clotting

D)   Placing the patient's arms over their head may create an internal line obstruction

A – For flushing PICC lines, the idea for syringe sizes is simply "Go big or go home." Though it may seem like you should use smaller syringes (1-5 ml) for smaller patients, the smaller the syringe, the higher the psi and the higher the change of "popping" the PICC! Like peripheral IV lines, PICC lines certainly can be capped and patency maintained via intermittent flushes, preferably with the "push a little-stop-push a little" technique recommended to help remove build-ups in the catheter. Lastly, as with chest central lines or ports, if blood is not easily aspirated, then carefully changing the arm/patient position or having the patient perform a Valsalva maneuver can sometimes assist to remove, not create, internal catheter obstructions.

99) "…an unexpected occurrence involving death or serious physical or psychological injury, or the risk thereof. Serious injury specifically includes loss of limb or function" is part of the definition of a(an):

A) Occupational Safety and Health Administration (OSHA) regulation violation

B) Emergency Medical Treatment and Active Labor Act (EMTALA) violation

C) Sentinel event

D) Malpractice

C – The Joint Commission (formerly JCAHO), established the core definition of a Sentinel Event, and it is used throughout the healthcare industry. It is referred to as a Sentinel Event because it is a "signal" for an immediate response.

> Starting in 1998, the Joint Commission (JCAHO) began requiring the reporting of one specific type of medical error or serious adverse event termed a sentinel event. JCAHO updated their definition of a sentinel event in 2007 as follows:
>
> - A sentinel event is an unexpected occurrence involving death or serious physical or psychological injury, or the risk thereof. Serious injury specifically includes loss of limb or function. The phrase "or the risk thereof" includes any process variation for which a recurrence would carry a significant chance of a serious adverse outcome.
>
> - Such events are called "sentinel" because they signal the need for immediate investigation and response.
>
> - The terms "sentinel event" and "medical error" are not synonymous; not all sentinel events occur because of an error and not all errors result in sentinel events.
>
> http://www.premierinc.com/safety/topics/patient_safety/index_3.jsp#Sentinel%20events%20and%20alerts

Certified Pediatric Emergency Nurse (CPEN) Review IV

100) You are triaging a 16-year old stable patient brought in by police after he ran a red light and hit a parked car. During your assessment he states, "I don't know what the big deal is--I'm just a little buzzed." All of the following statements about being "buzzed" are true **except**:

A) Buzzed" is a slang expression comparable to "stoked" or "fired up" and reflects a heightened level of excitement or anticipation of an event

B) "Buzzed" is the same as "tipsy" which is the same as "impaired"

C) "Buzzed" is just another way of saying "I'm not as drunk as I would like to admit I am."

D) If you have been drinking enough to "feel buzzed," then you are probably already driving illegally.

A – "Buzzed" refers to a feeling one gets after drinking alcohol; not before an exciting event. Alcohol related driving incidents are still a significant cause of injury and/or death to young drivers, even though there has been good response to the "Friends Don't Let Friends Drive Drunk" campaign. In researching this question, the Ad Council, in partnership with the National Highway Traffic Safety Administration (NHTSA), found that many young people believed that "drunk" meant falling over your feet and drooling drunk, but didn't apply to them after only a few drinks. "Buzzed Driving is Drunk Driving" has been the message of these national agencies since 2005.

Lundblom's Lessons

A new mom called the local ED (thankfully, not ours) to ask advice regarding what to do with her 3-year old who had been experiencing vomiting and diarrhea for 2 days. The mother reported that she was told that it was just a virus that had to run its course. With that "advice," the mom left for work to do her usual night shift job. When she arrived back at home at 6:30 a.m. the following morning, she found her child "looking terribly sick." She elected not to call EMS, but instead drove to the ED with her child in her own vehicle. In triage, the child was observed to be very tachycardic and hypotensive, and was rushed to the resuscitation area. The child was determined to be in hypovolemic shock, and to no surprise, proved to be a very difficult IV stick. Vascular access was finally obtained after 60-minutes (this was before intraosseous access had really made a comeback) and labs could not be drawn during this time. After the child received multiple boluses of IV fluids, labs were drawn with ease and revealed BUN 58 mg/dl and Creatinine 2.8 mg/dl. The child was completely nonverbal during the initial assessment with no response to painful procedures. After the initial hydration, the child became awake, cried and asked for oral fluids. In short, she began and acting like a regular 3-year old again! Again, the patient was found to be rotavirus positive, and was discharged after 4 days.

Teaching points:

Stress the importance of NOT giving telephone advice

Some parents do a very poor job of accurately describing the child's current condition

With diarrhea, you may be unable to determine the last urine output due to the presence of watery stool. Incidentally, this is sometimes easier with young boys because they pee in the front of their diaper/underwear and poop toward the back (unless there's diarrhea everywhere!)

Hypovolemic shock due to GI fluid loss is the most common pediatric shock

In hypotensive shock, EMERGENT vascular access is needed, and early intraosseous access is indicated (maximum three quick PIV attempts)

In hypovolemic shock, for rapid infusion, consider using a pressure bag or even better, draw up the bolus in big syringes and use a stopcock to pull-push the bolus

Remember to reassess the patient frequently

In a patient with altered mental status, consider the possibility of hypoglycemia and draw a bedside glucose.

If glucose is indicated for a pediatric patient, give:

Newborns/Infants – 2ml/kg D10W

Children – provide either

5 – 10 ml/kg D10W

2 – 4ml/kg D25W

1 ml/kg D50W diluted 1:1 with NS or even D5W prior to administration to keep from losing the precious IV access! (yes, using D5W to dilute the D50 will obviously increase the glucose concentration, but only a bit)

Chapter 11

Medical Maladies & Trauma Trivia

We spend the first twelve months of our children's lives teaching them to walk and talk, and then the next twelve telling them to sit down and shut up.
                    -Phillis Diller

Pertinent Pediatric Ponderings (NOTES)

Certified Pediatric Emergency Nurse (CPEN) Review IV

CHAPTER 11
Sample Test Answer Sheet

1. _____
2. _____
3. _____
4. _____
5. _____
6. _____
7. _____
8. _____
9. _____
10. _____
11. _____
12. _____
13. _____
14. _____
15. _____
16. _____
17. _____
18. _____
19. _____
20. _____
21. _____
22. _____
23. _____
24. _____
25. _____
26. _____
27. _____
28. _____
29. _____
30. _____
31. _____
32. _____
33. _____
34. _____
35. _____
36. _____
37. _____
38. _____
39. _____
40. _____
41. _____
42. _____
43. _____
44. _____
45. _____
46. _____
47. _____
48. _____
49. _____
50. _____
51. _____
52. _____
53. _____
54. _____
55. _____
56. _____
57. _____
58. _____
59. _____
60. _____
61. _____
62. _____
63. _____
64. _____
65. _____
66. _____
67. _____
68. _____
69. _____
70. _____
71. _____
72. _____
73. _____
74. _____
75. _____
76. _____
77. _____
78. _____
79. _____
80. _____
81. _____
82. _____
83. _____
84. _____
85. _____
86. _____
87. _____
88. _____
89. _____
90. _____
91. _____
92. _____
93. _____
94. _____
95. _____
96. _____
97. _____
98. _____
99. _____
100. _____
101. _____
102. _____
103. _____
104. _____
105. _____
106. _____
107. _____
108. _____
109. _____
110. _____
111. _____
112. _____
113. _____
114. _____
115. _____
116. _____
117. _____
118. _____
119. _____
120. _____
121. _____
122. _____
123. _____
124. _____
125. _____
126. _____
127. _____
128. _____
129. _____
130. _____
131. _____
132. _____
133. _____
134. _____
135. _____
136. _____
137. _____
138. _____
139. _____
140. _____
141. _____
142. _____
143. _____

Pertinent Pediatric Ponderings (NOTES)

Certified Pediatric Emergency Nurse (CPEN) Review IV

1) Which of the following are the **most** common routes of absorption of methamphetamine by <u>very young</u> children?

A) Injection and smoking

B) Transdermal and ingestion

C) Smoking and transdermal

D) Ingestion and injection

B – Transdermal and ingestion are the most common routes of absorption of drugs of abuse by very young children. Little children do not commonly deliberately smoke or inject drugs of abuse. Those are learned behaviors. Thus, we can eliminate answer choices A, C, and D. The processing of methamphetamine often produces a fine powder or dust that is easily absorbed through the skin and mucous membranes. Young children are at particular risk for transdermal absorption since they frequently contact surfaces where the methamphetamine dust may settle, such as floors, countertops, beds, etc. Depending on the developmental age, children will be found crawling, playing on the floor, or being put down for naps. With regard to ingestion, one simply has to remember that young children often put their hands in their mouths. So if the child has been crawling on the floor of a methamphetamine lab, it would be natural to expect that what might be in contact with the hands, would soon be in contact with the mouth, and subsequent oral ingestion may result. Regardless of the actual agent, this "age associated" pattern of encounter and absorption/ ingestion is well worth remembering when asked about children and potential toxins that they are likely to encounter.

2) Which of the following signs and symptoms are typically observed with the use of synthetic cannabinoids ("K2", "Spice", or MAM-2201)?

A) Bradycardia, confusion, and seizures

B) Tachycardia, hypotension, and vomiting

C) Bradycardia, hypotension, and seizures

D) Tachycardia, hypertension, and seizures

D - Products containing synthetic cannabinoids can cause side effects such as hypertension, tachycardia or irregular heart rate, and seizures, in addition to vomiting, hallucinations, and agitation. It is worth noting that synthetic cannabinoids such as K2 or Spice do not actually contain Tetra-Hydro-Cannabinol (THC), which is the active cannabinoid ingredient in marijuana. Even though they are called "synthetic marijuana," the symptomology presents very differently than the name might lead one to believe. The symptoms might be exaggerated due to the fact that these drugs OVER-stimulate the cannabinoid receptors. Other symptoms might be related to the "mystery" chemicals involved in manufacturing. The exact symptoms differ related to the batch and source of the drug

3) Which of the following statements is **untrue** with regards to alcohol soaked tampons?

A) Alcohol absorbed either rectally or vaginally will irritate the epithelial mucosa

B) Alcohol absorbed either rectally or vaginally is undetectable by breathalyzer

C) Alcohol may be absorbed either rectally or vaginally, by either males or females

D) Alcohol absorption, either rectally or vaginally, is more rapid compared to oral ingestion

B - Alcohol is absorbed into the bloodstream through the epithelial mucosa, regardless of where the mucosa is located, and a breathalyzer has the ability to measure that alcohol. It does not matter if the mucosa in question is found in the rectum, the vagina, or the stomach; the alcohol will eventually find its way into the bloodstream.

Stomach acid delays absorption which is why option "D" is incorrect. At least for rectal absorption, there is no sex discrimination for the potential for this behavior; therefore "C" is also not a correct option. Last but not least, alcohol is VERY irritating to the epithelial mucosa making option "A" a true statement. Our readers may have observed this oral mucosal irritation for themselves, simply by retaining alcohol in their mouths (vs. swallowing.) Note: There is some debate as to the prevalence of the use of alcohol soaked tampons. We were unable to find any actual documented case studies; however, there were several instances of anecdotal reports.

Hypothetical difficulties include physical deformation of the tampon when soaked with alcohol, which in turn, complicates digital insertion. In addition, the previously mentioned intense mucosal membrane irritation and the difficulty in physically retaining the liquid within the desired cavity after insertion pose some potential tactical challenges. That being said, the urban legend that it provides a more rapid, intense, and most importantly, undetectable intoxication are provided as reasons for possible experimentation. In theory, since the body's natural defense mechanism against excess oral ingestion (the gag reflex) is taken out of the equation, it would be possible for someone to rapidly progress to toxicity and unconsciousness. However, given the small amount of liquid that even a "super-sized" tampon will hold (approximately 1 oz.), even with extremely potent alcohol, this seems unlikely.

Filed under the heading of "anything is possible, especially in the ER," our take home message is that given a patient presenting with decreased mental status and a strong odor of alcohol in their pelvic region, the provider may wish to consider a thorough physical exam, to include rectal and vaginal inspection in order to rule out this route of intoxication. Bystanders may prove to be valuable sources of information. And as always, document proper consent, chaperones, etc. NOTE: This is also applicable to "Butt Chugging" a colloquial expression for what is, in effect, an alcohol enema. Cases of severe ethanol toxicity resulting from "Butt Chugging" are well documented.

Medical Maladies & Trauma Trivia

4) When so-called "energy" drinks are mixed with alcohol, all of the following effects may be observed **except**:

A) Tachypnea from over-exposure to chemical stimulants

B) Exacerbation of underlying or previously undiagnosed cardiac dysrhythmias

C) Excessive alcohol consumption due to stimulants masking the effects of intoxication

D) Dizziness, tachycardia, and impaired judgment

A - Instead of tachypnea, overconsumption of caffeine and other stimulants commonly included in "energy drinks" can lead to over stimulation of the sympathetic nervous system, resulting in shortness of breath. Dizziness and tachycardia can also occur. Additionally, the effects of the stimulants may mask the effects of ethanol, resulting in the so-called "Wide Awake Drunk." This results in consumption past the point where the patient would start to feel drunk, and has resulted in several deaths from alcohol poisoning. At least one death, a patient with known QT prolongation has been linked to the consumption of alcohol and "energy" drinks. The FDA has issued warning letters addressing the dangers of premixed ethanol and energy drinks and several states and college campuses have banned them outright.

Certified Pediatric Emergency Nurse (CPEN) Review IV

5) The toxic effects of the "psychedelic N-Bomb" (25I-NBOMe) result from overstimulation of which receptors?

A) Dopaminergic

B) Serotonergic

C) Cholinergic

D) Adrenergic

B - Serotonergic. Drugs similar to the "psychedelic N-Bomb" (25I-NBOMe) are VERY powerful serotonin stimulants that produce hallucinogenic effects. It has been anecdotally reported that a single drop may be lethal. In pediatric patients, serotonin toxicity typically results from the accidental or intentional overdose of medications such as Zoloft®, Prozac®, or Paxil®. In N-Bombs (also referred to as "Solaris" or "Smiley"), the drug increases the amount of serotonin in circulation and may result in a life threatening characteristic triad of cognitive, autonomic, and somatic effects. Agitation, tachycardia, hypertension, hyperthermia, and tremors are typical. Additionally, increased risky behaviors may result in serious injury or even death. MDMA or Ecstasy is another example of a powerful serotonergic agonist. Although management may include serotonin ANTAGONISTS, due to the sudden onset and severity of the reactions, initial treatment is largely symptomatic and aimed at sedation with benzodiazepines, hydration to prevent rhabdomyolysis, and aggressive cooling.

6) Mephedrone, Methylenedioxypyrovalerone (MDPV), and other drugs known as "Bath Salts" are chemically **most** similar to:

A) Amphetamines

B) Barbiturates

C) Catecholamines

D) Dromotropics

A - Amphetamines. "Bath Salts" are synthetic cathinones, the active ingredient in the khat plant. In the Middle East, the leaves of khat are chewed for their stimulant effect. Mephedrone has been marketed in the United Kingdom as "Meow-Meow" (playing on the similarity to the words "cat" and "khat.") Bath salts mimic amphetamines and cocaine in that they cause rapid alterations in the serum levels of dopamine and/or serotonin. When hearing of bath salts in the emergency department context, think of "Excited Delirium" as opposed to relaxing in a nice warm bath! Sedation, cooling, and hydration are mainstays of treatment. In severe reported cases, general anesthesia may be required. Like cocaine overdoses, AVOID beta blockers for tachycardia and hypertension in bath salt overdose. The unopposed alpha adrenergic effects can result in lethal hypertension, coronary vasospasm, etc.

7) The **most** appropriate initial dose range for dopamine in pediatric carcinogenic shock is:

A) 2-20 mcg/kg/min

B) 2-5 mcg/kg/min

C) 5-10 mcg/kg/min

D) 10-20 mcg/kg/min

C - 5-10 mcg/kg/min is the most appropriate initial dose range for dopamine in pediatric cardiogenic shock. This question tests your knowledge of the dose dependent effects of dopamine on adrenergic receptors. At doses < 5 mcg/kg/min, dopamine has little effect on the beta-1, or CARDIAC adrenergic receptors. At doses > 10 mcg/kg/min, dopamine's primary effect is to increase afterload, which results in vasoconstriction and an increase in systemic vascular resistance (SVR.) The increased SVR leads to a greater workload demand on an already failing pump. THIS IS UNDESIRABLE IN CARDIOGENIC SHOCK. In theory, if you had to use dopamine (vs. milrinone or dobutamine) in pediatric cardiogenic shock, 5-10 mcg/kg/min would optimize cardiac rate and contractility, without increasing myocardial workload through increased vasoconstriction and afterload.

Ultimately, maximum dosage will be guided by evaluating the ongoing patient presentation and vital signs such as cardiac output (CO), systemic vascular resistance (SVR), and myocardial oxygen consumption (MVO2.) If a decreasing cardiac output, especially when combined with increasing SVR and/or MVO2, may be an indication to limit or reduce dopamine dosage.

8) Dopamine is <u>relatively</u> contraindicated in which of the following shock states?

A) Cardiogenic

B) Septic

C) Neurogenic

D) Obstructive

B – Though frequently still used in clinical practice, multiple studies have shown that in fluid refractory septic shock, dopamine is associated with higher morbidity and mortality than norepinephrine (Levophed®.)

Pediatric emergency medicine and critical care attending physician insights: Agreed, however in the ER you are most likely to grab dopamine 1st since it is pre-mixed.

9) A one-year-old presents to the ED in shock after "licking a blood pressure patch" of Catapress® (clonidine.) Anticipated initial management would most likely include fluids and which of the following:

A) Analeptics such as Dopram® (doxapram)

B) Intravenous pressors (dopamine and/or epinephrine)

C) Beta blockers such as Lopressor® (metoprolol)

D) Romazicon® (flumazenil)

B - Clonidine causes vasodilatory effects which reduces preload, so aggressive fluid resuscitation (to address the preload problem by "filling the tank"), and pressors (such dopamine and/or epinephrine) will form the mainstays of your front line treatment for clonidine overdose. Analeptics such as Dopram® (doxapram) are contraindicated in cases of clonidine overdose. Beta blockers would slow the heart rate and lower the blood pressure, which is clearly not the desired result. While some studies indicate that Narcan® (naloxone) has been shown to be helpful, Romazicon® (flumazenil) is specifically indicated for benzodiazepine overdose, and is not indicated for clonidine exposures. And one more thought: Since unintentional clonidine exposure or intentional overdose in children is not something most of us encounter, as with other toxic exposures, a phone consultation with the friendly and always available experts at poison control is highly suggested.

Pediatric emergency medicine and critical care attending physician insights: Understanding the mechanism of action of clonidine may help people understand why fluids and pressors are needed. Clonidine treats high blood pressure by stimulating alpha-2 (α2) receptors in the brain, decreasing cardiac output and peripheral vascular resistance and lowering blood pressure. It has specificity towards the presynaptic alpha-2 (α2) receptors in the vasomotor center in the brainstem. This binding decreases presynaptic calcium levels, and inhibits the release of norepinephrine (NE.) The net effect is a decrease in sympathetic tone.

10) Rohypnol® (flunitrazepam) has been reportedly used in Drug-Facilitated Sexual Assault (DFSA) or "Date Rape" cases. The exact incidence of Rohypnol® Facilitated Sexual Assault is difficult to determine because of which effect:

A) Anterograde amnesia

B) Retrograde amnesia

C) Sedation amnesia

D) Hypnotic amnesia

A – Rohypnol® causes anterograde amnesia. Although this is designed as a teaching question and meant to illustrate an important point in the epidemiology of date rape, a correct answer to this question is obtainable without knowing ANYTHING at all about Rohypnol®. Sedation amnesia and hypnotic amnesia are simply provided as distracters. The key to answering this question comes down to understanding the difference between anterograde and retrograde amnesia and applying that difference to the question at hand. Anterograde amnesia means not being able to recall events AFTER the incident in question. (It may help to remember that both "after" and "antero" begin with "A.") Retrograde amnesia refers to not being able to recall information BEFORE the precipitating event. Think about "retro" nights at the local bar. The music being played is the finest of all time, i.e. from the 80s. Which sort of amnesia would make it difficult to determine if sexual assault had occurred? Anterograde amnesia. The individual literally cannot remember if they were assaulted or not, which in turn, can make them reluctant to seek medical attention.

11) Because it preserves respiratory drive to a greater extent than many other agents, Precedex® (dexmedetomidine, "dex") is becoming increasingly utilized for procedural sedation. In addition to sedation, which of the following broad pharmacologic profiles **best** consistently fits dexmedetomidine?

A) Amnesia and analgesia

B) Occasional amnesia and analgesia

C) Occasional amnesia and occasional analgesia

D) Neither amnesia nor analgesia

B - In addition to its anti-hypertensive effects, dexmedetomine also consistently produces both sedation and analgesia. It shares a common pathway with opioids. It has been clinically demonstrated that pediatric patients on dexmedetomine often have reduced requirements for narcotics. Dexmedetomine also has been observed to have amnestic effects. However, these effects are inconsistently observed. Therefore, when reliable amnesia is clinically desired, additional agents ARE required.

12) When administering Precedex® (dexmedetomine) the prudent nurse would anticipate the possibility of all of the following side effects **except**:

A) Bradycardia

B) Hypotension

C) Hypertension

D) Tachycardia

D – Tachycardia has not been identified as a side effect of Precedex® (dexmedetomine). Bradycardia, hypotension and even transient hypertension have all been associated with Precedex® administration.

Pediatric emergency medicine and critical care attending physician insights: It is important to note that in procedural sedations with Precedex®, it is recommended to give a bolus of the Precedex® first, and then run a drip. It is very common to have HYPERtension with the bolus. However, during infusions you may see bradycardia and HYPOtension.

13) Paracelsus, the father of modern toxicology said: "All things are poison, and nothing is without poison; only the dose permits something not to be poisonous." Jimson weed (Datura stramonium) is a perfect example of this. It can be used in treating asthma or migraine headaches, but may easily be toxic when accidentally ingested by a child. With the guidance of poison control, ingestions of Jimson weed can be managed with which of the following:

A) Physostigmine

B) Dopamine

C) Lysergic acid diethylamide

D) Romazicon® (flumazenil)

A - Datura contains several anticholinergic compounds, the most notable of which is atropine, and physostigmine is the antidote for anticholinergic overdose. The toxidrome may be remembered as "red as a beet, dry as a bone, blind as a bat, mad as a hatter, and hot as a hare." Patients are flushed and dry, with grossly dilated pupils, confused, and febrile. Management of suspected datura ingestion is often symptomatic; sedation, particularly with benzodiazepines, often forms a mainstay of treatment. Romazicon® reverses the effects of benzodiazepines and therefore defeats the purpose of sedating these patients. Lysergic acid diethylamide, more commonly known as LSD, in a patient who is already hallucinating would not be your best choice of medications!

Pediatric emergency medicine and critical care attending physician insights: Physostigmine's mechanism of action: It is an inhibitor of acetylcholinesterase, the enzyme responsible for the breakdown of acetylcholine in the synaptic cleft of the neuromuscular junction. Therefore it increases acetylcholine and stimulates both nicotinic and muscarinic receptors.

14) All of the following statements regarding pain associated with intraosseous (IO) access are correct **except**:

A) Two percent (2%) preservative-free lidocaine without epinephrine (i.e. cardiac lidocaine) has been shown to be effective in minimizing (IO) *infusion* pain

B) The discomfort associated with intraosseous (IO) *insertion* is generally considered minimal to moderate

C) The discomfort associated with intraosseous (IO) *infusion* under pressure is generally minimal

D) Local administration of two percent (2%) preservative-free lidocaine without epinephrine (i.e. cardiac lidocaine) has been shown to alleviate intraosseous (IO) *insertion* pain

C – When the fluids start infusing through an IO device, there may be considerable discomfort from pressure sensors in the intraosseous space. Following intraosseous needle insertion, IO anesthetic (2% preservative-free lidocaine without epinephrine) may be considered for use to block these sensors. Due to the minimal discomfort involved, intraosseous *insertion* does not generally require local anesthesia, but it may be a nice touch to consider in <u>awake</u> patients. Of course, in the pediatric population, the local may be as frightening as the actual IO insertion. Always refer to your institution's policy regarding IO insertion and infusion practice.

Certified Pediatric Emergency Nurse (CPEN) Review IV

PURPOSE

This procedure describes a process for nursing and/or pharmacy personnel* to administer lidocaine through an intra-osseous catheter to decrease infusion related pain in a conscious patient. IO insertion may cause mild pain in conscious patients but IO infusions may cause severe discomfort. Lidocaine is meant to be used as an anesthetic and not as analgesia.

Broselow Color	Weight (KG)	0.5 mg/kg Lidocaine (mg)	20mg/ml Lidocaine (ml)	Normal Saline (ml)
Grey	3	1.5	0.08	0.92
Grey	4	2	0.1	0.9
Grey	5	2.5	0.13	0.87
Pink	6-7	3.4	0.17	0.83
Red	8-9	4.25	0.21	0.79
Purple	10-11	5.25	0.26	0.74
Yellow	12-14	6.5	0.33	0.67
White	15-18	8.25	0.41	0.59
Blue	19-22	10.37	0.52	0.48
Orange	24-28	13	0.65	0.35
Green	30-36	16.5	0.83	0.17

For **PEDIATRIC** patients who may or are able to perceive pain after the IO device is placed and position has been confirmed and secured. **CONTRAINDICATED** in pediatric patients with acute seizures or history of non-febrile seizures.

1. May give 0.5 mg/kg (Max 20mg) of 2% lidocaine (without preservatives or epinephrine) IO as a slow bolus
2. Diluted with Normal Saline to a total volume of 1 ml. (See table below)
3. Wait at least 30 seconds then flush with 5mls of normal saline.
4. If necessary, step 1 may be repeated as needed to maintain anesthetic effect.
(Do NOT exceed 3mg/kg/24hr)

This table represents approximate dosing based Broselow's weight breakpoints.

The volume of lidocaine recommended in pediatric patients is not enough to prime the tubing. A small amount of normal saline is used to ensure the volume is the correct amount to prime the tubing and complete the lidocaine flush. Because of the familiarity and ease-of-use of the Broselow system, we based our lidocaine chart (see chart below) on the weight-based tape recommendations.

ADULT patients- For patients who may or are able to perceive pain after the IO device is placed and position has been confirmed and secured.

1. May give 20-40 mg (1-2 mL) of 2% lidocaine (without preservatives or epinephrine) IO as a bolus over 1 minute.
2. Wait at least 30 seconds then flush with 10 ml of normal saline.
3. If necessary, step 1 may be repeated as needed to maintain anesthetic effect. (**Do NOT exceed 3 mg/kg/24 hr**)

*Medication must be ordered by physician or LIP.

Color-Coded Intraosseous Lidocaine

Chart courtesy of Stacie Hunsaker RN, MSN – Intermountain Healthcare, Provo, UT

15) Which statement below is **correct** regarding lidocaine administration in the conscious patient after intraosseous (IO) insertion?

A) Rapid infusion of the lidocaine dose will allow time for the anesthetic to take effect

B) After the initial administration, wait approximately one minute for the lidocaine to fully take effect

C) Use a syringe with normal saline to slowly flush the line in order to gently clear the medullary space for optimal flow

D) Once an initial dose of lidocaine is administered, no additional lidocaine may be given

B – The medullary (IO) space is filled with a thick, non-collapsible fibrin mesh. The increased pressure caused by the infusion of fluids through the IO catheter stimulates pressure sensors in the mesh, often resulting in pain during initial fluid flow. Lidocaine has proven to be the preferred analgesic, as it stops pain at the source. When using lidocaine for infusion pain, it must be administered slowly to avoid being sent into the central circulation. It is then crucial to wait 30 – 60 seconds for the full effect to be reached prior to beginning fluid infusion. Because the Lidocaine is meant to be used as an anesthetic and not an analgesic, it may be necessary to give additional doses.

16) It is possible to use blood drawn from the intraosseous site for laboratory results. Ideally, 2–3 ml of the sample should be discarded and the additional sample must be labeled "bone marrow specimen" prior to giving it to the lab. IO specimens for all of the following laboratory tests are typically found to be statistically similar to venous samples **except**:

A) Blood cultures

B) Electrolytes

C) Hemaglobin & hematocrit "H&H"

D) CBC

D - The intraosseous and peripheral lab values of WBC, RBC, and platelets do not correlate (will be elevated) because IO samples are being drawn directly from "the factory" (i.e. the bone marrow) where they are produced. If blood cultures are ordered, the first 2–3 ml of the specimen can be used. Since the intraosseous space is lined with a viscous fibrin material, if no cultures are ordered, it is important to discard the first 2 – 3 ml withdrawn. Transfer the blood to test tubes immediately, because blood obtained from the IO clots faster than venous blood. In several studies, IO blood proved to be reliable for the blood tests you "really need" versus those you "would like."

Intraosseous Clinical Nurse Educators Insight: What you "really need" in a sick kid, i.e. H&H, lytes (glucose, sodium, potassium,) lactate, type and cross, bicarbonate, and blood cultures can be done via IO just fine.

17) A 4-day old infant who was born at home comes into the ED with abdominal distention, vomiting, and "no bowel movements since birth." The pediatric nurse practitioner is ruling out Hirschsprung's disease. What is the **most** definitive diagnostic test to confirm Hirschsprung's disease?

A) Barium enema

B) Abdominal plain film

C) Rectal suction biopsy

D) Colonoscopy

C – Though radiographic techniques (plain films/barium enema) or colonoscopy can be used to help exclude other causes of "babies with big bellies & no poop," the definitive diagnosis is made by suction biopsy. (And it should go without saying that anything involving rectum and suction can't be good!) Hirschsprung's disease is a congenital disorder of the colon in which certain nerve cells, known as ganglion cells, are absent, thus causing a functional obstruction. Often this presents as constipation. Hirschsprung's is otherwise known as congenital aganglionic megacolon. To better understand it, break it down. Congenital = present at birth. Aganglionic = there are no ganglions. Megacolon = not just a big colon, it's a megacolon! This is a baby whose distal bowel (starting at the anus) is missing nerve endings and therefore poop gets stuck. It is suspected in a baby who has not passed meconium within 48 hours of delivery. Normally, 90% of babies pass their first meconium within 24 hours, and 99% within 48 hours. Other symptoms include green or brown vomit, swelling of the abdomen, lots of gas and bloody diarrhea. When you hear "newborn with constipation that hasn't passed any meconium yet," think Hirschsprung's.

18) A three week-old child presents to the emergency department with a rectal temperature of 104.0F (40.0C,) HR 188, RR 52, capillary refill > 4 seconds, BP 60/40, and saturations of 91% on room air. To no surprise, which of the following is the presumed diagnosis?

A) Sepsis

B) Sepsis

C) Sepsis

D) Sepsis

A – Sepsis (or B, C, D.) Remember that during the first month of life, every baby who has a fever and is anything but cute is septic, very nearly septic, possibly septic, or thinking about becoming septic. Fever is the most common presenting sign of children with SIRS (systemic inflammatory response syndrome.) Therefore, they get the whole septic workup, including blood and urine cultures as well as a lumbar puncture ("spinal tap") and a two-day field trip to inpatient peds or peds ICU for IV antibiotics until they are proven to be cute (& not septic.) This little one screams sepsis and, as with adults in recent years, early goal directed therapy during the "golden hour of sepsis" is optimal. As far back as 2006, the Pediatric Advanced Life Support (PALS) guidelines recommended 5 key points for pediatric sepsis

- Early recognition (someone has to think about possible sepsis)

- Vascular access within 1 hour (someone has to place an IV or IO within 1 hour)

- 60 ml/Kg of isotonic fluid within 1 hour (once the IV or IO is in, push <u>up to</u> three 20 mL/kg boluses)

- Antibiotics within 1 hour (even pre-lumbar puncture)

- Pressors within 1 hour (if they don't get better with IV fluid boluses, go straight to pressors)

Interestingly, in a study from a very well respected pediatric ED, they found that even in the really big, famous, we-see-nothing-but children-ED, they only met all 5 criteria within 1 hour in 19% of the cases! Remember - aggressive volume replacement and oxygen to increase perfusion and oxygen delivery are our first priorities!

19) When administering IV fluid boluses (0.9NS or LR) to a 25kg septic child, which of the following is the preferred administration method?

A) IV pump

B) Gravity

C) Pressure bag

D) IV push with a syringe

D – Push it. The "famous" Salt-n-Pepa song summarizes it nicely. Push it. Gravity or pressure bags result in uncontrolled fluid flow and may result in way too much fluid being given. A recent study found that though IV pumps are certainly appropriate for IV boluses for infants and children under 15kg (and for maintenance fluids for all ages), if the child is over 16kg, the maximum flow rate on the IV pump didn't allow for the 60 ml/kg to be given within the first hour. Amazingly, in pediatric sepsis patients, pushing 60 ml/kg of isotonic fluid within 1 hour, dropped mortality rates from 38% to 8%. That's a 30% reduction in deaths just by pushing the fluids. So for those children over 15kg, push it (then put it on the pump!)

20) The five components of the FLACC pain assessment scale include:

A) Face, legs, activity, cry, consolability

B) Fingers, legs, abdomen, capillary refill, constipation

C) Face, legs, abdomen, cry, consolability

D) Fingers, lips, activity, capillary refill, consolability

A – The FLACC scale is intended to assist with pain assessment for patient's 2-months to 7-years of age and is made up of five components: Face, Legs, Activity, Cry, and Consolability. It is sort of like playing detective because you are looking for clues based on how the child looks and acts. Fingers, lips and capillary refill are important assessment criteria, but not for the FLACC. The abdomen is also a useful assessment area, but won't help much when evaluating pain presentation.

- (**F**)ace – What does their face look like? Facial expression, grimacing, squeezing the eyes shut

- (**L**)egs – What are their legs doing? Leg movements, kicking, muscle tension, drawing the knees up

- (**A**)ctivity – How active are they? Restlessness, arching, fidgeting

- (**C**)ry – Are they crying? Characteristics of crying?

- (**C**)onsolability – How easily can they chill out?

I really don't think it's important for the test to memorize the exact scores, i.e. 2 points for this versus 1 point for this. However, it is very important to review the pain assessment/scales section of the ENPC manual to determine which of the commonly utilized pain scales ENA felt were important enough to include in the book, and have a basic idea as to which scale works for what type/age of patient.

	DATE/TIME					
Face 0 - No particular expression or smile 1 - Occasional grimace or frown, withdrawn, disinterested 2 - Frequent to constant quivering chin, clenched jaw						
Legs 0 – Normal position or relaxed 1 – Uneasy, restless, tense 2 – Kicking, or legs drawn up						
Activity 0 – Lying quietly, normal position, moves easily 1 – Squirming, shifting back and forth, tense 2 – Arched, rigid or jerking						
Cry 0 – No cry (awake or asleep) 1 – Moans or whimpers; occasional complaint 2 - Crying steadily, screams or sobs, frequent complaints						
Consolability 0 – Content, relaxed 1 – Reassured by occasional touching, hugging or being talked to, distractible 2 – Difficult to console or comfort						
	TOTAL SCORE					

FLACC Scale

Certified Pediatric Emergency Nurse (CPEN) Review IV

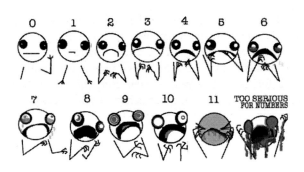

A Better Pain Chart
Courtesy of Allie Brosh - www.hyperboleandahalf.blogspot.com

21) Your facility is utilizing an electronic medical record system but still has paper "code sheets" for use during pediatric codes. You are the designated "scribe" for a pediatric respiratory code and use the paper form for the initial documentation. After the code, you enter the medication administration data into the electronic medical record. You note an error in your original notes and correct that information on the electronic record. Your next action should be to:

A) Include the initial paper documentation "as is" in the limited "paper" chart since you have signed the document
B) Correct the initial paper documentation and add your initials to the corrected portion and include it in the limited "paper" chart
C) Photocopy the original paper document "as is" for your personal records and destroy the original after the data has been transferred to the electronic medical record
D) Destroy the paper documentation and complete an internal "Incident Report" of the error and subsequent correction on the electronic medical record

B - Paper documentation produced during patient care, even with a predominately electronic medical record, is still part of the "chart" and should be treated as such. In the "old days" of paper charting, corrections were made and initialed by the author. That standard has not changed. If you make a correction into the electronic documentation record, but not on the accompanying source record, this discrepancy may be brought into question during a later review. Destroying original documentation should never happen, and an "incident report" is rarely required for corrections in documentation.

22) Parents bring a 6-month old child to the ED because "he hasn't stopped crying for the past 18 hours!" His vital signs are normal except for being slightly tachycardic with a rate of 148. The pediatric assessment triangle reveals this child is "cute and not acutely sick," but he certainly appears to be in pain. Parents report good recent feedings, no change in bowel habits, and that "this is not normal for him." Which of the following actions would the ED nurse anticipate to be a priority?

A) Full septic workup including a lumbar puncture

B) Reporting of the parents to child protective services

C) Instruction about colic symptoms & treatment

D) Examination for a possible hair tourniquet

D – This child looks and acts like they are in pain because when a hair is wrapped around a finger, toe, or even worse, the penis creating a tourniquet, it is a very appropriate reason to scream for 18 hours! A hair tourniquet can be a natural hair, or a thread (often in children from socks or mittens) that wraps tightly around an appendage, potentially resulting in auto-amputation.

The important thing to recognize in this situation is that the child needs a physical examination – which in this case might very well reveal a hair tourniquet. This is a question of elimination. As his vital signs are essentially normal, a septic workup does not seem to be indicated in this case. Without a more thorough history and physical exam, there are no immediately identifiable suspicious findings pointing toward abuse (though it should always be in the differential diagnosis for crying children), so contacting child protective services is probably not warranted. Colic usually begins at 3-weeks of age, peaks between 4-6 weeks of age, and thankfully is gone by 12-weeks of age. By process of elimination we are left with the exam and its findings being the priority.

23) Paramedics are enroute to the ED with a 12-year old female post-minor motor vehicle crash. She was a restrained passenger with no air bag deployment and there was no loss of consciousness. Her only complaint is "being shook up." However, the medics have found that her pupils, while reactive, are of slightly different sizes. The remainder of her neurological exam is reported to be normal. The ED nurse knows that her pupil asymmetry is **most** likely due to:

A) Anasarca

B) Anisocoria

C) Heterochromia iridium (two different-colored eyes within a single individual)

D) Anencephaly

B – Anisocoria is defined as different sized pupils. If this child had been unconscious, had decreasing LOC, or exhibiting any of the "classic" signs of neuro deficits, then the pupil asymmetry would certainly be more concerning. Likely reasons might be a head injury, medications, or drug use. However, in the child who is awake, alert, and neurologically normal (except for different sized (1mm or less difference), but equally reactive pupils,) this is anisocoria. This can be a normal finding in approximately 10-20% of the population (including David Bowie) and this is most likely her baseline. Anasarca is total body edema such as with end-stage liver or renal failure, and anencephaly is a lethal congenital condition neural tube defect in which an infant is essentially born with no forebrain. Heterochromia iridium is the condition in which a single individual has two different-colored eyes, a delightfully intriguing, distinguishing, but non-dangerous abnormality.

Editor's Note: Last time we checked, no extra points were awarded for knowing about David Bowie's anisocoria, but it does make for interesting medical trivia.

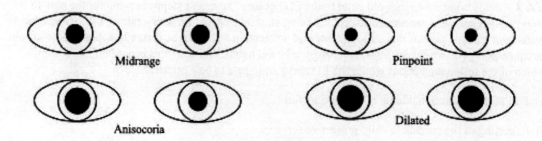

Variations of Pupil Sizes

Illustration Courtesy of My then 14-year Old Aspiring Baker Daughter,

www.ninasbeliciousbakery.com

Certified Pediatric Emergency Nurse (CPEN) Review IV

24) The current recommendations for diagnosis and treatment of intussusception or the "telescoping of the bowel" include....

A) History, physical, KUB radiograph or ultrasound, and barium enema

B) History, physical, KUB radiograph or ultrasound, and air contrast enema

C) History, physical, and laparoscopy

D) History, physical, and laboratory studies

B - Intussusception or the "telescoping of the bowel" occurs when one section of the bowel slides into another. It is commonly diagnosed by history, physical, and ultrasound, and often treated by an air contrast enema. Barium enemas were used in the past; however, if a perforation occurs and surgery is required, barium can mess up the belly, so air contrast enemas are preferred. A peds surgeon taught me the "three strikes rule" for intussusceptions. This means that they get an air enema & hopefully it fixes it – if it comes back (as they can do,) then they get another air enema. However, if it comes back a third time, that's the third strike and they're out (Meaning they get a trip to the OR/theatre!) Air contrast enemas tend to be more successful as a treatment in the infant and toddler population.

25) For patients who are non-English speaking, which of the following translation options are currently recommended and available at all times of day or night?

A) Hospital telephone translation service

B) Staff member from another department

C) Sibling of the child

D) Computer internet translation program

A – Though in real life, options B, C, and D are frequently utilized, the correct answer is to utilize the hospital telephone translation service. The Joint Commission has described the options for "language interpreting and translation services" to include hospital employed language interpreters, contract interpreting services or **trained** bilingual staff. These can be provided in person, telephone or video. In addition to the fact that fluency and knowledge of medical terminology has not been verified, bilingual staff members are not always available. Utilizing non-direct care givers and siblings also raise patient privacy concerns. Though internet translation services are readily available, their ability to correctly translate medical terminology may not always acceptable. When in doubt… Phone a friend (via the language line.)

26) Parents are enroute to the ED with their young child with a clogged gastrostomy tube (G-tube.) Current research-based recommendations include all of the following **except**:

A) Attempt flushing with warm water

B) Attempt flushing with warm water and papain (meat tenderizer)

C) Attempt flushing with Coca-Cola™ or similar product

D) Attempt flushing with thrombokinase (tPA)

D – Over the years, countless therapies and devices have been utilized when trying to unclog G-tubes and as one would expect, with varying degrees of success. Experienced nurses will swear by their favorite tried and true technique, while others will have had less than optimal experiences with that particular option. With that in mind, flushing with warm water, instillation of warm water with meat tenderizer, or Coca-Cola™ are some of the most common ways to unclog a G-tube. According to pediatric surgical specialists, this often involves "old school" vs. "new school" practitioners. (Kind of like Classic Coke™ vs. New Coke™?) There have often been recommendations about Coca-Cola™ and indwelling it within the tube to unclog. However, Coca-Cola™ has a high level of sugar, which may actually cause things to get worse. tPA certainly works great for removing coronary artery clots, but as you can imagine, is not recommended for instillation in a G-tube. If, despite best efforts, the tube is unable to be flushed, or if the G-tube is inadvertently removed, then it should be replaced by the physician or advanced practice provider. Ideally, the same size/same type G-tube should be used, but as a temporary measure, a similar size Foley urinary catheter may be used until the proper G-tube can be obtained and inserted.

27) Three children and their parents present to the ED with a chief complaint of "itchy rashes." Their history is significant for having spent the weekend at a local hotel with a swimming pool and a hot tub. The rash is found to be most prevalent in the areas that were covered by their bathing suits. Probable diagnosis:

A) Allergic contact dermatitis

B) Folliculitis

C) Chicken pox

D) Eczema exacerbation

B – Hot tub + bathing suit + itchy rash = folliculitis (specifically pseudomonas in this case.) Breaking down that word, we have "follicul" referring to a hair follicle and "itis" meaning inflammation, a symptom very commonly associated with infection. Therefore folliculitis is an inflammation or infection of the hair follicles. It usually starts with friction from clothing, shaving or blocking the follicles. But, as in this case, it is also commonly found after swimming in pools or hot tubs that are not properly chlorinated. In most cases, the diagnosis is made by history and physical examination. For uncomplicated superficial folliculitis, use of antibacterial soaps and good hand washing technique may be all that is needed. If oral and/or IV antibiotic therapy is indicated, coverage for icky bugs such as MRSA or pseudomonas is suggested. If patients do not bounce back/get better after initial antibiotic therapy, then a gram stain and culture should be done. Once the diagnosis is made, preventing the spread of the disease is important… the family should wash the linens, wash their bodies, and especially wash their hands! As far as the other possible answers, the essentially isolated location of the rash should help eliminate them.

28) Lead poisoning in children is commonly associated with ingestion of which material?

A) Paint chips

B) Crayons

C) School paste

D) Brussels sprouts

A – On the test, and in real life, if you hear honey, think botulism; and if you hear lead poisoning, think paint chips (or bad plumbing.) Though there is an ongoing documented decline in elevated blood lead levels (BLL) in children around the world, lead is still out there and its ingestion is still causing children to have growth issues and developmental delays. In 1904, lead paint was found to be responsible for poisoning children. Remarkably, it wasn't until 74 years later, in 1978, that lead was banned from American paints. More recently, toys imported from other countries have been found to have dangerously high lead levels. The initial or provisional diagnosis of elevated blood lead levels can be achieved via finger stick (10% false positive rate) and confirmed with a venous stick as needed. Hair sampling, which is commonly done in other countries outside of the United States, has been found to not be as accurate as blood sampling. Lead poisoning more commonly occurs over a period of time, and is more harmful to children than adults because it affects a developing neurological system.

Certified Pediatric Emergency Nurse (CPEN) Review IV

Although children may eat crayons and school paste, there is no known link to lead poisoning. And children may claim that you are trying to poison them with Brussels sprouts, but we know better!

In 2005, the AAP Committee on Environmental Health issued the following guidelines for screening and treatment of elevated BLLs.

BLL less than 10 µg/dL

No action is required

BLL 10-14 µg/dL

Obtain a confirmatory venous lead level within 1 month. If the BLL is still within this range, patient education about lead exposure is needed, and the BLL test should be repeated in 3- months

BLL 15-19 µg/dL

Obtain a confirmatory venous lead level within 1 month. If the BLL is still within this range, patient education about lead exposure is needed, and the BLL test should be repeated in 2- months

BLL 20-44 µg/dL

Obtain a confirmatory venous BLL in 1 week, and if the BLL is still within this range, assess complete medical, nutritional, and environmental hazards. Environmental evaluation by the local health department is also needed.

A large-scale study reported no improvement in neurologic and behavioral test scores after succimer chelation of children with BLL in this range.

BLL 45-69 µg/dL

Obtain a confirmatory BLL within 2 days, and if the level is still within this range, the patient should undergo the same complete evaluation as would patients with a BLL of 20-44 µg/dL. At 45-69 µg/dL, chelation therapy is recommended. Treatment should be in a lead-free environment. If this is not possible, hospitalization is necessary.

Chelation can be started with oral succimer, or if the patient is hospitalized, calcium disodium edetate (calcium EDTA) can be used. These agents have potential toxicities, and monitoring of the CBC count, electrolytes, and liver function test results is necessary.

BLL 70 µg/dL or higher

Hospitalize the patient, obtain a confirmatory venous BLL, and initiate chelation with dimercaprol and calcium EDTA. Because calcium EDTA does not cross the blood-brain barrier, its use as the only agent in this situation is not recommended because of the possibility of lead redistribution from the soft tissues to the central nervous system (CNS). Pretreatment with dimercaprol (which crosses the blood-brain barrier) is recommended.

29) An 8-year-old child is orally intubated with a 6.0 cuffed endotracheal tube. What size catheter should be used to suction the endotracheal tube?

A) 6Fr

B) 8Fr

C) 12Fr

D) 14Fr

C – A 12Fr suction catheter should be used for a patient with a 6.0 endotracheal tube. Crash carts typically hold 5Fr, 6Fr, 8Fr, 10Fr, 12Fr, 14Fr, 16Fr, and 18Fr suction catheters. So, how do you remember which size to use in a child? Simple. Just select the catheter size number (not the actual size…that just wouldn't work!) that is 2X the size number of the ETT. The child is intubated with a 6.0 ETT, so suction with a 12Fr catheter.

30) A 12-year-old child with multi-system trauma is nasally intubated with a 7.0 endotracheal tube. What size catheter should be used to suction the endotracheal tube?

A) 4Fr

B) 8Fr

C) 12Fr

D) 14Fr

D – Use a 14Fr suction catheter. Whether the patient is nasally or orally intubated, the same rule applies. 2X the size number of the ETT is the size number of the suction catheter that should be used. The child has a 7.0 ETT, so suction with a 14Fr catheter.

31) An 8-year-old child is orally intubated with a 6.0 cuffed endotracheal tube. What size nasogastric (NG) tube should be placed?

A) 6Fr

B) 8Fr

C) 12Fr

D) 14Fr

C – The recommended NG tube size in this case is 12Fr. Just as the suction catheter size number should be 2X the size number of the ETT, the same formula is used to determine the suggested size number of the NG tube as well. The child has a 6.0 ETT, so place a 12Fr NG tube and suction with a 12Fr catheter.

32) Your patient has been intubated with a 4.0 endotracheal tube and an orogastric tube has been ordered. What size orogastric tube should be used?

A) 4Fr

B) 8Fr

C) 12Fr

D) 16Fr

B – You should select an 8Fr orogastric tube for this child. As with the suction catheter size, use the same formula (2X the size number of the ETT for the gastric tube) regardless of whether the gastric tube is placed nasally or orally. The infant has a 4.0 ETT, so an 8Fr NG or OG tube is appropriate.

33) An 8-year-old child is orally intubated with a 6.0 cuffed endotracheal tube. What size urinary catheter should be placed?

A) 6Fr

B) 8Fr

C) 12Fr

D) 14Fr

C – A 12Fr urinary catheter should be placed. You may be seeing a pattern here. Once again, the catheter size number is simply 2X the size number of the ETT.

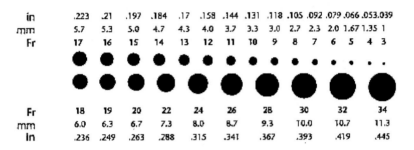

Foley Urinary Catheter Sizes

34) What size urinary catheter should be placed in an infant with an 8Fr nasogastric (NG) tube?

A) 4Fr

B) 8Fr

C) 12Fr

D) 16Fr

B – The NG/OG tube size and urinary catheter sizes will generally be the same for our pediatric patients. This patient has an 8Fr NG tube, so an 8Fr urinary catheter would be selected for insertion.

35) An 8-year-old child is orally intubated with a 6.0 cuffed endotracheal tube. At what centimeter mark should the "lip line" of endotracheal tube be taped?

A) 6cm

B) 8cm

C) 12cm

D) 18cm

D – Generally speaking, the mark at which the ETT should be secured is 3X the size of the ETT. Example: a 6.0 ETT should be taped at 18cm at the lip. Just as a reminder, you should not wait for a chest X-ray to determine tube depth if only unilateral breath sounds are heard and NEVER use a chest X-ray to determine esophageal versus endotracheal tube placement.

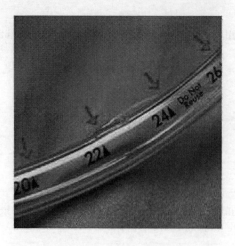

Centimeter Markings on an Endotracheal Tube

36) At what centimeter mark should a 4.0 nasal endotracheal tube be taped?

A) 10cm

B) 12cm

C) 14cm

D) 16cm

C – The nasal 4.0 ETT should be secured at the 14cm mark. Generally speaking, the depth at which the nasally placed ETT should be secured is 3X the size of the ETT + 2. This one is a bit trickier than others, but if you remember that oral ETT is taped at 3X the tube size, just consider that a nasal intubation needs a little more depth. 2cm (like 2 nares) is the additional depth recommended.

37) For management of a pneumothorax, what size chest tube should be anticipated for an infant with a 4.0 oral endotracheal tube?

A) 4Fr

B) 8Fr

C) 12Fr

D) 16Fr

D – Anticipate a 16Fr chest tube in this case. A way to remember the suggested chest tube size is simply to take the ETT size and multiply by 4. The infant is intubated with a 4.0ETT, so placement of a 16Fr chest tube should be anticipated for management of a pneumothorax (air in the chest.)

38) An 8-year-old child is nasally intubated with a 6.0 cuffed endotracheal tube. He requires chest tube placement for a pneumothorax. Approximately what size chest tube should the ED nurse anticipate?

A) 6Fr

B) 8Fr

C) 18Fr

D) 24Fr

D – Don't let the location of the endotracheal tube distract you. Remember that, for management of a pneumothorax, the number of the chest tube size is 4X the number of the ETT size. Thus, a 6.0 ETT would suggest a 24Fr chest tube.

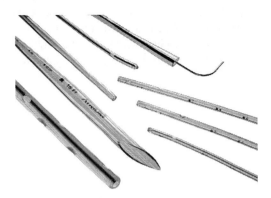

8f-16f Chest Tubes

Courtesy of Atrium Medical - www.atriummed.com

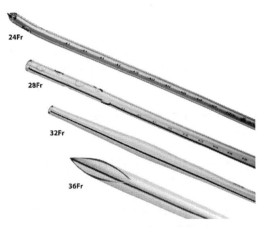

24f-36f Chest Tubes

Courtesy of Atrium Medical - www.atriummed.com

39) An 8-year-old child is orally intubated with a 6.0 cuffed endotracheal tube. He requires chest tube placement for a traumatic hemothorax. Approximately what size chest tube should the ED nurse anticipate?

A) 8Fr

B) 12Fr

C) 24Fr

D) 30Fr

D – In the event of a hemothorax, anticipate a 30Fr chest tube if the patient is intubated with a 6.0 ETT. Evacuating blood, versus evacuating air, calls for a larger chest tube. Look for a chest tube size that is 5X the ETT size to be placed for evacuation of a hemothorax (blood in the chest.)

Certified Pediatric Emergency Nurse (CPEN) Review IV

40) An infant has arrived by ambulance with a police escort. The patient's parent is reported to be inebriated, unavailable for consent and being held in police custody. It is suspected that the patient is the victim of non-accidental trauma. After initial resuscitation efforts have been completed, the infant now has IV access and has been orally intubated with a 4.0 endotracheal tube. Capnography confirms proper ETT placement, and a chest X-ray indicates the ETT tube is in good position. The chest X-ray also reveals a large hemothorax. The attending physician has indicated that a chest tube will be needed due to the hemothorax noted on X-ray. The placement of what size chest tube should be anticipated for this patient?

A) 2Fr

B) 20Fr

C) 32Fr

D) 40Fr

B – A 20Fr chest tube would be anticipated for this patient with a 4.0 endotracheal tube and a hemothorax. This question provided way more information than needed, and sometimes that's how life is. Sift through the data and remember your priorities. 5X the size of the oral endotracheal tube is the suggested chest tube size for management of a hemothorax. The infant is intubated with a 4.0ETT, so a 20Fr chest tube should be anticipated.

41) A child, approximately 4 years of age, is enroute to the ED per ALS ambulance. The child is the only survivor of a head-on motor vehicle crash. He is hemodynamically unstable and the ED nurse correctly anticipates:

A) 4.0 uncuffed ETT, 4Fr OG, 4Fr suction catheter, 4Fr urinary catheter, and 4Fr chest tube – Oral endotracheal tube to be taped at 4cm at the lip

B) 5.0 uncuffed ETT, 10Fr OG, 10Fr suction catheter, 10Fr urinary catheter, and 20Fr chest tube – Oral endotracheal tube to be taped at 15cm at the lip

C) 5.0 uncuffed ETT, 10Fr OG, 10Fr suction catheter, 10Fr urinary catheter, and 10Fr chest tube – Oral endotracheal tube to be taped at 15cm at the lip

D) 4.0 ETT uncuffed, 8Fr OG, 8Fr suction catheter, 8Fr urinary catheter, and 16Fr chest tube – Oral endotracheal tube to be taped at 12cm at the lip

B – When faced with so many items in the answers, it is often easiest to work by process of elimination, starting with whatever known facts are available. In this case, the only "known" is the approximate age of 4. This single fact will help us determine the anticipated ETT size. We should also recognize that once we know the anticipated ETT size, we can determine the sizes of the other pieces of equipment to be used. There are several formulas for determining the correct endotracheal tube size, but the one with the least amount to memorize is: (Age/4) + 4. So in the case of this 4-year-old, 4 divided by 4 = 1, and 1 + 4 = 5. The correct endotracheal tube is a 5. From that point, and remembering the rules of 2X, 3X, 4X, and 5X, answer B shows the correct emergency tube sizes as well as approximately where to tape the oral endotracheal tube.

From the ETT size:
- 2X the size of the ETT is the suggested size of the suction catheter, NG/OG tube and urinary catheters
- 3X the size of the ETT is approximately where the oral ETT should be taped at the lip
- 4X the size of the ETT is the suggested size of the chest tube to be placed for evacuation of a pneumothorax (air in the chest.)
- 5X the size of the ETT is the suggested size of a chest tube to be placed for evacuation of a hemothorax (blood in the chest)

Pediatric emergency medicine and critical care attending physician insights: Remember, the ETT size formulas above are for UNCUFFED tubes. When using a cuffed ETT, most experts suggest ½ size smaller, i.e. 4.5 (uncuffed) vs. 4.0 (cuffed.)

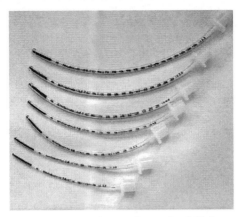

2.5-5.5 Uncuffed Endotracheal Tubes

Photo courtesy of Julie Bacon MSN-HCSM, RN-BC, NE-BC, CPN, CPEN, C-NPT

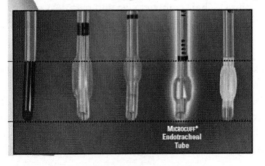

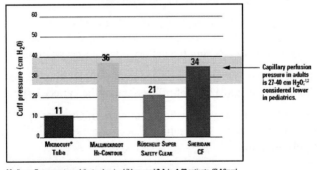

Microcuff Cuffed Pediatric Endotracheal Tubes

Images courtesy of Avanos

www.avanosmedicaldevices.com

Certified Pediatric Emergency Nurse (CPEN) Review IV

Children will eat anything...

Under and including the kitchen sink, that doesn't eat them first

If they have eaten one, assume they have eaten them all!

Jill Glick MD, FAAP

42) Parents arrive at the pediatric ED frantic because their 18-month old child just swallowed a battery. The child is alert, calm, drinking a juice box with no apparent respiratory distress. Radiographs reveal not one, but two button batteries and a dime in the stomach with none in the esophagus. Anticipated management would include:

A) Immediate endoscopy for removal of the items

B) Immediate administration of GoLYTELY® (polyethylene glycol electrolyte solution)

C) Patience and parental reassurance

D) Immediate administration of Syrup of Ipecac

C – Patience and parental reassurance is the first step. Electronic toys and gadgets have become increasingly miniaturized and their power requirements are being met by a new generation of compact, high-performance batteries. These disk or button batteries contain heavy metals such as zinc, mercury, silver, nickel, cadmium, and lithium. Their compact size and harmless appearance hide their true danger. The danger comes when children (and sometimes adults) put these tiny batteries in their mouths and swallow them.

Most swallowed batteries cause no problem (89.9% of the time.) However, batteries lodged in the esophagus must be removed immediately. They can cause tissue ischemia in several ways, including by pressing against the wall of the esophagus, from leakage of caustic alkali and from the electrical current they generate. Injuries can occur in as little as one hour and full-thickness burns can occur in as little as four hours. Once the batteries (or coins) have made it past the esophagus and into the stomach, the vast majority pass uneventfully through the rest of the digestive tract.

Immediate removal of the battery may be indicated in the following cases:

- If X-rays show the battery is located in the esophagus.
- If the child develops abdominal pain or is vomiting blood.
- If the battery is large (15.6 mm in diameter - about the size of a AA battery – or bigger), the child is younger than 6 years of age, and the battery does not pass through the stomach within 48 hours.
- The majority (85.4%) of batteries are passed in the stool within 72 hours, however it may take longer. At home, strain stools to confirm passage of the battery or coin.
- If the battery contains mercury and is found to have fragmented (per X-ray), blood and urine mercury levels are necessary. Medication to decrease mercury levels should be used only when abnormal levels are found.

Radiographic studies of the entire digestive system may be taken. Disk batteries have a characteristic double-density (two-layer) shadow on X-rays. Laterally, their edges are rounded, and they contain a step-off junction at the positive and negative terminal. This can help distinguish them from coins and buttons.

It is possible to accurately find ingested coins and button batteries with a metal detector. It is a safe and radiation-free alternative to diagnose this type of ingestion, but it cannot rule out other co-ingested items. A metal detector also cannot determine the condition of metallic objects, or if shape and texture pose a problem. In those cases, radiographic imaging is still the way to go.

Pediatric emergency medicine and critical care attending physican insights: "You really need not only an AP, but also a lateral X-ray to help determine esophageal vs. tracheal position of the foreign body."

Medical Maladies & Trauma Trivia

Certified Pediatric Emergency Nurse (CPEN) Review IV

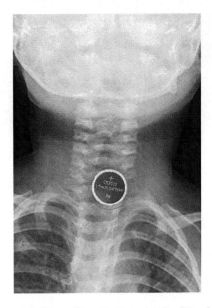

Radiograph Revealing Battery in the Esophagus

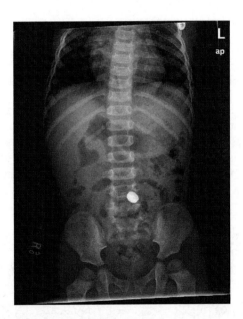

Radiograph Revealing Battery in the Stomach

Images Courtesy of Christopher Straus MD - University of Chicago Medicine

Certified Pediatric Emergency Nurse (CPEN) Review IV

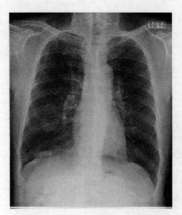 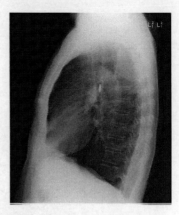

Radiographs Revealing Coin in Right Mainstem Bronchus

Images Courtesy of Christopher Straus MD - University of Chicago Medicine

43) A 15-year-old arrives in the Emergency Department with a swollen ankle. His grandmother is with him and informs you that the patient is hearing impaired, but is fluent in American Sign Language. She states that she can sign "a little bit" to communicate with her grandson. The patient needs to go for an X-ray. What would be the **most** appropriate option to share the plan of care with him?

A) Have the grandmother sign to tell the patient what needs to happen

B) Use hand gestures to communicate the next steps

C) Write down information for the patient, including rationale about what needs to happen

D) The patient is 15 and probably will know about these things so no explanation is needed

C – All teenagers deserve to be included in their plan of care. Giving the patient a way to be in control and ask questions via another form of communication (i.e. writing, typing on a phone or tablet) will provide opportunities for increased compliance and support throughout his stay. In this particular scenario, the patient's grandmother is not sufficiently fluent in the patient's language and probably not be able to communicate all of the medical terms needed. While an interpreter would be the most appropriate option, it doesn't appear to be an option in this case.

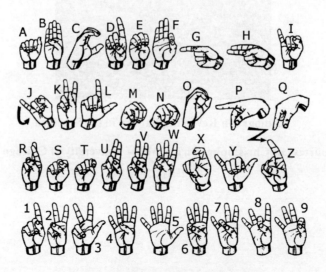

American Sign Language Alphabet

Image Courtesy of Dr. William Vicars - www.lifeprint.com

Certified Pediatric Emergency Nurse (CPEN) Review IV

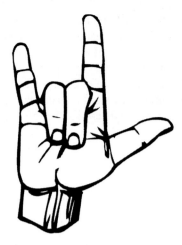

I Love You in American Sign Language

Image Courtesy of Dr. William Vicars - www.lifeprint.com

44) A 6-year-old who is visually impaired needs an IV started. Her mother tells you that this is the child's first experience with an IV, but she typically does "OK" when she gets shots at her doctor's office. Of the following options, which is the **most** appropriate while starting this patient's IV?

A) Get extra hands to help safely hold the patient as this is a new experience for her and you are unsure how she will respond

B) Tell the patient each step of the procedure and allow her to hold materials in her hands to increase her familiarity

C) Have the mother explain the procedure to the patient as you are performing it

D) Tell her it is just like a shot and place the IV quickly before she has a chance to become anxious

B – Many kids in this age group need to engage with materials in multiple ways. Some might need to see the procedure rehearsed, some might need to hear each step, and some might need to hold materials or a combination of the above. In the case of a child having an impairment affecting one of their senses, the other modalities for increased understanding become even more important. Play to each child's strengths. Ask the parents how the child learns best and follow their advice. Kids need to know what is going to happen before it happens. In most cases, being honest with a child will increase compliance and make your job that much easier.

45) A father brings his 18-month old to the emergency department stating, "I think my son ate the magnets off my desk." During the initial triage, he comments; "I'm sure this is nothing – those little magnets can't be strong enough to cause any harm." The triage nurse knows:

A) Desktop magnets are not strong enough to cause harm

B) Desktop magnets can be strong enough to cause harm

C) The danger of desktop magnets is not the strength, but the shape

D) The danger of desktop magnets is not the strength, but the number

B – Rare earth magnets, currently marketed to adults as desk toys, are incredibly powerful. If more than one magnet is swallowed, or if the magnet is swallowed with another metal object, the bowel may be trapped and squeezed between them. There have been multiple published case reports of children with abdominal emergencies due to the strong attraction of these magnets. In 2008 the American Academy of Pediatrics was successful in advocating for safety standards insuring that magnets cannot fall out or become detached from children's toys. Unfortunately, this does not apply to adult magnet desk toys, which often include over 100 small magnets in each toy, and did not appear on the market until the following year. Since 2009, there have been over 1,700 incidents of rare-earth magnet ingestions requiring emergency intervention (including surgery.) Ongoing discussions between the manufacturers and the Consumer Product Safety Commission are taking place to determine the safety of these products, not for adults, but for children.

46) Therapeutic hypothermia has recently evolved as a post-cardiac arrest treatment in both adults with cardiac arrest and newborns after birth asphyxia. Which of the following best explains the rationale(s) for therapeutic hypothermia as a post-cardiac arrest treatment?

A) Therapeutic hypothermia is protective by decreasing cerebral oxygen demand and minimizing the untoward effects of ischemic-reperfusion injury

B) Therapeutic hypothermia increases the therapeutic effect of anti-arrhythmics, thus decreasing the chance of further life-threatening arrhythmias

C) Therapeutic hypothermia decreases blood pressure, thus decreasing preload and providing better cellular perfusion

D) Therapeutic hypothermia is neuroprotective by increasing cerebral oxygen demand

A - Intentional reduction of body temperature can reduce cerebral and myocardial oxygen demands by up to 40%. Therapeutic hypothermia also minimizes the effects of ischemia-reperfusion injury. Hypothermia *decreases* the therapeutic effects of anti-arrhythmics, therefore lidocaine and amiodarone can be *less effective* in the presence of hypothermia. This technique has been used in the neonatal ICU setting for many years for hypoxic-ischemic encephalopathy, and more recently, on the adult side in cardiac arrest as well. While it is estimated that about 16,000 children suffer a cardiac arrest each year, therapeutic hypothermia has not been well studied in children or infants after cardiac arrest. A few individual hospitals have found that therapeutic hypothermia was feasible but requires additional research. The ongoing Therapeutic Hypothermia After Pediatric Cardiac Arrest (THAPCA) study is the first to address the effectiveness of therapeutic hypothermia in pediatrics on a large scale basis. While it would not be surprising to see it used in children routinely in the future, officially, the jury is still out when it comes to therapeutic hypothermia use for pediatric patients.

47) Parents present with their 10-month old child who recently swallowed a "water ball" (also known as water pearls or imbibition balls.) Anticipated intervention(s) for this child include:

A) Syrup of Ipecac

B) Endoscopic removal of the "water ball"

C) Gastric lavage

D) No interventions are needed

B – "Water balls" are commonly used for decoration or hydroponic gardening, but also more recently are marketed as colorful kid's toys as well. They are superabsorbent crystal jelly balls, not visualized on X-ray, and can rapidly swell up to 400X their original size. It is estimated that 80-90% of all objects ingested by little ones are small enough to pass through the pylorus of the stomach and will safely pass through the GI tract spontaneously. The remaining 10-20% of foreign body ingestions require endoscopic removal and less than 1% requires surgical removal. As these expandable toys swell very fast, endoscopic removal before they pass through the stomach is recommended, and if "it has gone below," then surgical intervention may be warranted. Note: As of 2013, this product was withdrawn from the market by the manufacturer, however, they are still available for purchase from various internet sites.

Pediatric emergency medicine and critical care attending physician insights: Of note, syrup of ipecac is no longer commercially available and is NOT recommended for ingestions unless under the guidance of a toxicologist.

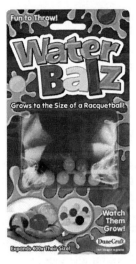

WaterBalz

Photo courtesy of DuneCraft

48) A 4-year old male child is found wandering on the street outside of the local pub. Police bring the child to your ED for evaluation. Shortly after arrival, they are able to identify the child and the parents are contacted. What could the parents be charged with?

A) Neglect

B) Abuse

C) Abuse and neglect

D) Stupid parent syndrome (SPS)

A - Most likely, the charges would involve neglect (and in our ED worlds, just not on the test, SPS - Stupid Parent Syndrome - as well.) The parents in this case did not provide the proper supervision to keep this child safe. A 4-year old alone on the streets (in front of a pub no less) would definitely fall under the 'not safe' rule. Neglect is the most common form of child abuse. The broad governmental definition of neglect is "the failure of a parent or other person with responsibility for the child to provide needed food, clothing, shelter, medical care, or supervision to the degree that the child's health, safety and well-being are threatened with harm." For your everyday practice, verifying your local statutes for specifics are always suggested as there are differences between (and even within) states. Remember that the test is global and there won't be any region-specific questions.

The term "child abuse" has been replaced with the more correct term "non-accidental trauma." This can include striking, kicking, burning, biting, or any action that results in a physical impairment. In many states, this definition also includes acts or circumstances that threatens to or actually puts a child at risk. Abuse can also include actions that cause an injury to the psychological or emotional stability of the child.

If anything in the history or the physical exam "just doesn't fit," one must suspect neglect or abuse and these needs to be reported and investigated by Child Protective Services (or the equivalent in your area).

Why? Not only because it's the law, but also because it's the right thing to do for the child. The safety of the child should always come first; remember the first rule in medicine... Do No Harm!

49) When applying a dressing to a 4-year old with a partial-thickness burn to the right hand, it is important to remember to cleanse the hand with soap and water, apply anti-microbial cream or ointment and:

A) Wrap the hand in dry gauze, keeping the fingers together

B) Wrap the hand in dry gauze, keeping the fingers separated

C) Wrap the non-burned areas in dry gauze and the burned areas in wet gauze

D) Wrap the non-burned areas in wet gauze and the burned areas in dry gauze

B – In addition to cleansing the burn area and applying the ointment or cream, the important consideration here is keeping the fingers separated. As the burns heal, if the fingers are not wrapped with some sort of dressing between them, they can actually start to grow together, which is certainly not the ideal situation.

When a patient with an isolated burn to the hand initially presents to the ED, most burn centers say that either wet or dry dressings are fine. Hypothermia is not typically an issue for a burn only to the hand, and wet dressings feel better to the patient. Check for allergies and choose an appropriate topical dressing and anti-microbial agent. The key is to 1) keep the wound wrapped with a sterile dressing, and 2) keep the fingers separated.

50) A 3-month old infant presents to the ED with weakness, poor head control, increased drooling, history of poor feeding, and constipation. The infant seems uninterested in your attempts to elicit a smile and the eyelids are drooping. The child's mother states that they only feed the baby natural and organic foods. With the infant's age and history, which disease should be seriously considered?

A) Botulism

B) Epiglottitis

C) Guillain-Barre syndrome

D) Respiratory syncytial virus

A – Infant botulism, which is the most common presentation of botulism in the United States, is caused by ingesting botulism spores releasing toxins into the gut. Most times on the test, when you hear baby and honey (note the part of the question that referred to "only natural and organic foods"), the answer is botulism. Interestingly though, honey or corn syrup are the culprits for botulism in only 15% of the cases. The other 85% are unknown. Botulism was first described in healthcare by a German physician in the 1820's when he found that many of his patients developed symptoms after eating improperly prepared sausages, and the Latin translation for sausage is botulus!

Botulism toxin affects the neuromuscular junctions from the **head down**. Patients present with blurred or double vision, along with the much more common symptoms of nausea, vomiting, and diarrhea (then constipation and urinary retention as the motor nerves of the colon and bladder are affected.) Quickly after the ophtho and GI symptoms kick in, then rapid descending weakness or paralysis ensues. Airway management is crucial not only to prevent aspiration, but also to ensure the patient's ability to breathe. Antibiotics are not indicated unless there is a complicating infection and can actually worsen if aminoglycosides are used. Diagnosis is by history, physical, and stool culture (sent to the CDC; in most cases, stool will be positive for toxin or culture for C. botulinum.) Treatment is supportive in nature (think airway!) and it is imperative to initiate treatment upon clinical suspicion without delay for confirmatory testing.

Can Guillain-Barre kick in this young? Anything seems possible, yet the average age for Guillain-Barre is 4-8 years, with cases reported as young as 1-year. A distinct presentation in Guillain-Barre is symmetric, **ascending** weakness or paralysis. Drooling is a classic presentation of epiglottitis, yet this presents with high fever and respiratory distress secondary to stridor from upper airway compromise. RSV is seemingly always the answer in the winter for all things respiratory, yet this infant did not present with pulmonary findings. When you hear honey, corn syrup, or improperly prepared German sausages, think botulism!

51) Law enforcement was called to assist with a fight in which multiple teens were involved. Three 14-year olds are enroute to your ED complaining of severe eye burning after being "Maced." Anticipated initial interventions would include:

A) Intravenous morphine

B) Bilateral eye enucleation

C) Bilateral eye irrigation with normal saline/Morgan lens

D) Bilateral patching of the eyes

C – Mace®, pepper spray, etc. are self defense sprays that commonly, and appropriately cause incapacitating severe eye pain and tearing. In addition, especially in those with a history of asthma or other chronic respiratory diseases, laryngospasm, wheezing, and even respiratory arrest can occur. In most cases however, the effects are self-limiting and resolve after about 20-30 minutes. Immediate irrigation of the eyes with normal saline is the intervention of choice to relieve the symptoms and minimize possible ocular damage. Patching of the eyes for corneal abrasions is not commonly done nearly as often as we used to, and bilateral enucleation (surgically removing the eyes) will certainly remove the eye irritation, but saline irrigation is probably a better choice. Remember that in these patients, skin surface and clothing will still be contaminated, so if the option of decontamination had been offered, it will almost always be the answer!

52) A young child involved in a motor vehicle crash in which the car is "totaled" is ready to be discharged from the ED. The parents ask you if they can have their original car seat returned to them so they can use it in their other car. The ED nurse knows that:

A) The parents should expect to receive a replacement car seat from the ED

B) The parents should be advised that the original car seat is no longer able to be used

C) The parents should be advised to take the original car seat to the local fire department for their evaluation as to suitability of use

D) The parents should be advised that they will be able to take the child home without a car seat as their original one is no longer safe for use

B – If the car is "totaled," then the car seat is potentially damaged as well. The National Highway Traffic Safety Administration (NHTSA) recommends that car seats that have survived moderate or severe crashes be replaced, as the structural integrity cannot be confirmed. Even if there is a certified child passenger safety technician at the local fire department, the fire department does not make the determination whether the car seat is suitable for use, so that is not a correct answer. The recommendations from the child safety seat manufacturer, coupled with NHTSA guidelines, are what should be followed. Some ED's stock extra car seats for situations such as this, but this is a nicety, and not a legal requirement. Lastly, if the child was lucky enough to be doing well enough to be discharged home from the ED after a major crash, don't push your luck and send them back on the road without a car seat!

53) A 16-year-old female reports that she has received the "sex virus" (human papillomavirus or HPV) vaccine. She says that she does not use condoms because she is on oral birth control pills and that the vaccine protects her "from most of that other stuff." What is an appropriate response to this?

A) The vaccine protects against HPV (the most common sexually transmitted disease), and the cervical cancers that it causes, but it does NOT protect against chlamydia, gonorrhea, syphilis, or HIV, which are also <u>very</u> common.

B) While the HPV vaccine protects against most sexually transmitted diseases, it does not protect you from HIV, the virus that causes AIDS.

C) The HPV vaccine protects you from all STD's

D) The HPV vaccine does not prevent genital warts; it only prevents cervical cancer in later life

A – HPV is a common virus that is spread skin to skin during sexual contact. The HPV vaccines protect against the HPV types that cause most genital and oropharyngeal cancers and also against the viruses that cause most genital warts in both males and females. None of the currently available HPV vaccines will treat existing infections, they only help prevent them. They also do not protect against other common sexually transmitted diseases such as chlamydia or gonorrhea. Genital warts from HPV can be treated, but not with antibiotics. Especially in diseases involving cancer and/or genital warts, prevention, or even better abstinence, is the key!

54) The use of high-dose inhaled albuterol (Proventil®) can be useful in the immediate management of what electrolyte imbalance?

A) Hypernatremia

B) Hypercalcemia

C) Hyperchloremia

D) Hyperkalemia

D - While even a normal inhaled breathing treatment of 2.5 mg albuterol can cause a small reduction of K^+, for management of hyperkalemia, much higher doses of 10-20 mg albuterol nebulized over 15 minutes can decrease the serum potassium significantly. The effects begin within 30 minutes of giving albuterol and last about 2 hours. This gives us plenty of time to initiate other therapies or corrective actions to decrease the K^+ long term. So in a known to be hyperkalemic patient, the potassium reduction is certainly a very good thing. However, in patients who "emptied their inhalers" over the past two days, or have received high doses of β-agonists in exacerbations of their asthma or other lung diseases (i.e. continuous nebs,) close monitoring of the patient's potassium level is indicated.

Pediatric emergency medicine & critical care attending physician insights: I use the acronym "C BIG K" to remember the other things that you can give in the management of hyperkalemia: C – calcium gluconate (super important for cardiac stabilization,) B – bicarbonate, I – insulin, G – glucose and K – kayexelate. C BIG K.

55) What is/are the appropriate method(s) for obtaining test samples for pertussis (Whooping Cough)?

A) Nasal swab using a cotton tipped wooden swab and sampling just inside the nares

B) Nasal swab using a synthetic fiber swab with an aluminum or plastic stick to the posterior nasal pharynx

C) Nasal swab using a synthetic fiber swab with an aluminum or plastic stick just inside the nares

D) Routine sputum culture in a "cough cup"

B - Testing is done through Polymerase Chain Reaction (PCR) of the organism's DNA. This is the fastest method of testing. Cultures can be done, but can take up to 7 days for results. PCR testing is most sensitive if samples are collected within the first three weeks of coughing. After that the amount of DNA rapidly declines.

Acceptable sample collection is thru the use of a nasal swab inserted straight back following the floor of the nares until the tip is in the posterior nasal pharynx, rotated several times and withdrawn. Collection should be with a synthetic tipped swab (Dacron, rayon, nylon etc) with an aluminum or flexible plastic stick. Samples obtained from the anterior nares usually produce samples with inadequate amounts of pertussis DNA and cotton tipped swabs with wooden sticks are not appropriate as they have residues present that may inhibit the PCR testing. Once the sample has been collected, the tip of the swab should be place in an empty collection tube and sent to the lab for PCR. Mucous is not collected, and in fact, before testing, the patient should be asked to blow their nose in order to clear unwanted mucous. The preferred sample collection technique for many centers is via nasal aspirate of a saline wash of the posterior nasal pharynx. PCR methods may vary slightly from lab to lab so it is always a good idea to check with your lab prior to collecting a sample.

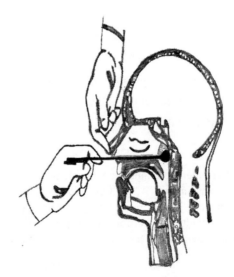

Obtaining a Nasopharyngeal Specimen for Pertussis Testing

Illustration courtesy of my then 14-year old aspiring baker daughter

www.ninasbeliciousbakery.com

56) It is RSV (respiratory syncytial virus) season in your area. Although it is not a standard of care to test ALL patients with upper respiratory infection symptoms for RSV, which of the following patients would you consider testing prior to discharge?

A) 1-year old with history of premature birth

B) 2-year old with history of a heart transplant

C) 3-year old who is normally healthy who also has coarse breath sounds on exam

D) A & B

D - Routine testing for RSV is no longer recommended by the American Academy of Pediatrics. Most children can be diagnosed by symptoms and treatment is usually not affected by the results. Exceptions to this are the high risk groups such as children with a history of prematurity, those who are immunocompromised such as transplant patients, and some patients receiving treatment for cancers.

RSV can be found in just about everybody – including staff during RSV season (October-November through February-March depending on your area in the northern hemisphere.) But less than 2% of people with RSV require hospitalization, and most of these are under the age of six months. Usually treatment of symptoms is all that is required. In most adults and healthy children, RSV may cause mild cold symptoms or sneezing (URI), but it is not an issue as our immune system can fight it off. It is in those who have weakened defenses or increased susceptibility for which we must be concerned.

Testing for RSV has greatly improved over the recent years. Samples are obtained via nasal swabs, nasal aspirate or washes (similar to pertussis.) Testing used to require samples going to the lab with result times of hours to days. Now the point-of-care testing can take place in the ED, with results in as little as 15 minutes by use of a rapid detection test similar to a bedside pregnancy test. This saves time and money, as well as speeding up the appropriate treatment for those high risk patients.

Pediatric emergency medicine & critical care attending physician insights: Although routine testing is not recommended, most hospitals require testing for RSV if a pediatric patient is admitted the hospital with URI symptoms during the RSV season for infection control purposes.

57) A mother brings in her child to the ED after she has had complaints of abdominal distention and pain following gastrostomy feedings. You are concerned that the G-tube may be malpositioned. The **most** definitive diagnostic tool to verify the tube is within the stomach is:

A) Push air through the G-tube and auscultate for sounds over the abdomen

B) Obtain a fluoroscopic contrast study through the G-tube

C) Obtain a plain radiograph of the abdomen

D) Attempt to aspirate gastric contents

B - A contrast study through the G-tube will either show the stomach fill with contrast material, or it will show the contrast escape into the peritoneum. Auscultating for air or aspirating gastric contents cannot confirm the tube is within the stomach. The air may simply be being pushed into the peritoneum or the aspirated contents are coming from within the peritoneum. A plain radiograph of the abdomen may show the G-tube is intra-abdominal on a lateral view, but it cannot confirm the tube is definitively in the stomach.

Certified Pediatric Emergency Nurse (CPEN) Review IV

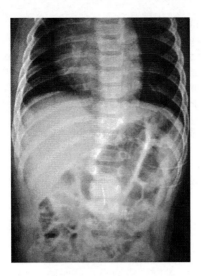

Radiograph Demonstrating Gastrostomy Tube in the Stomach

Image Courtesy of Christopher Speaker RN, MSN, APN - Lurie Children's Hospital of Chicago

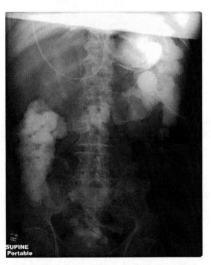

Radiograph Demonstrating Intraperitoneal (not stomach) Gastrostomy Tube

Image Courtesy of Christopher Straus MD - University of Chicago Medicine

58) A 2-year old, 16kg child presents to the ED one hour after ingesting "Grandma's Glucophage®" (metformin) and is found to have a finger stick blood sugar of 22. Intravenous access is obtained and the emergency nurse practitioner requests that 1 g/kg of dextrose be given. As the 50% dextrose box label says 0.5 g/mL (total 25g), how much dextrose should the ED nurse administer?

A) D10W - 16mL

B) D25W – 64mL

C) D25W – 25mL

D) D5W - 25mL

B – This question not only asks you to calculate the appropriate dextrose dose in grams, but also then to take it one step further and calculate the actual amount in milliliters to be administered. First rule of thumb

- when administering IV dextrose boluses to an infant or pediatric patient, simply remember, the older you get, the more concentrated sugar you get. In the neonatal ICU, premature babies frequently get D5W, while bigger sick babies get D10W boluses and maintenance fluids. As 50% dextrose can be very damaging to young children's fragile veins, many experts recommend diluting the D50W ½ and ½ with sterile water to result in a 25% dextrose concentration (if no commercially prepared D25W in the little box is available.) Teens and adults are much bigger and therefore they get the big box straight from the big box, i.e. D50W.

In this case, let's do the math! At 1 g/kg, we can all agree the dosage is 16g of dextrose. Our med box has 50% Dextrose (0.5 g/ml.) To get to our dosage, it would be 16 / 0.5 = 32 ml of D50W (Pancake syrup to the little one's veins.) We need to dilute it to D25W (in half.) So we would add 32 ml of sterile water and hurray! We end up with 64 ml of a D25W solution equaling 16g of Dextrose!

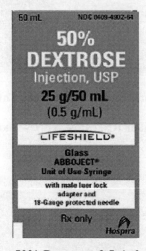

50% Dextrose, 0.5g/ml

Photo courtesy of Hospira - www.Hospira.com

59) The primary social-emotional developmental goal in the adolescent period is:

A) Intimacy

B) Merging of self with their parents

C) Separation of self from parents

D) Socialization

C - The primary developmental goal of adolescence is for the child to separate themselves from their parents in preparation for transitioning to becoming an independent adult. Erikson's theory of psychosocial development refers to this as "Identity vs. Confusion" or what we might call the "Who Am I?" stage. It is a time to explore their independence and establish a sense of identity. Be careful not to confuse the goal of the developmental period with what the adolescent *wants*, which tends to be more primitive in nature!

60) A mother brings her infant to the ED. While assessing the infant, the triage nurse notes which of the following behaviors as a sign of a negative infant-parent attachment?

A) Parent avoids looking at infant

B) Parents calls infant by name

Certified Pediatric Emergency Nurse (CPEN) Review IV

C) Parent holds the infant closely

D) Parent strokes infant head to calm

A - Assessing attachment behavior should include observations as to how the parents look, act, hold, and talk about the infant. Nursing Outcomes Classification defines parent-infant attachment as behaviors that show an enduring, affectionate bond. Any observations of behaviors where the parent avoids the infant, acts with disgust, ignores crying, or talks about how inadequate they are as a parent should raise concerns about the infant-parent attachment.

61) Which of the following is considered a developmental milestone associated with feeding for a 12-18 month old?

A) Begins to hold a fork.

B) Cannot hold cup

C) Distinguishes between finger and spoon foods.

D) Drinks well from a cup

D - Drinking without difficulty from a cup is appropriate for 12-18 months of age. Being unable to hold a cup is appropriate for 8-9 months of age; Distinguishing between finger and spoon foods is appropriate for 24 months old; and beginning to hold a fork is appropriate for 36 months of age. (As a side note, even though it is possible to be asked a question like this on the CPEN exam, the above questions involve feeding children, and if they are well enough to eat, they are probably well enough to go home!)

62) The parents of a 3 ½ yr old tell the ED nurse that their son has an imaginary friend. The mother further explains that she was not concerned until the child asked to set a place for the friend at the dinner table. Which of the following responses would be **most** appropriate for the ED nurse to offer?

A) "Imaginary friends are quite common, and can help your child feel safe in strange situations. Most children grow out of them by kindergarten."

B) "Ignore him when he talks about the imaginary friend. Playing into the child's fantasy could lead to developmental issues later in life."

C) "You should make an appointment with a mental health professional. Children need to develop coping skills when facing the reality of imaginary friends."

D) "You should play with your child more often as it is a sign they miss you. Children turn to the company of imaginary friends when parents are neglectful."

A – This age is a time filled with fantasy and imagination! Imaginary friends often help the preschooler create and explore a make-believe world, and to develop play and social skills with this "friend." These imaginary friends also help out during times of loneliness, and to help children feel safe in strange or new situations. Parents can't make the pretend friend go away, so it may be best to acknowledge the friend without letting the child "get away" with behaviors that they blame on their imaginary playmate!

63) Mannitol 0.5g/kg bolus via IO is ordered for a young child with blunt head trauma and signs of increasing intracranial pressure. The child weighs 40kg and the mannitol bottle is labeled as 25%, 12.5g/50ml bottle (250mg/ml.) How many mL of mannitol would this child receive?

A) 20g

B) 160ml

C) 0.5g

D) 80ml

D – This question not only asks you to calculate the appropriate mannitol dose in grams, but then to take it one step further and calculate the actual amount in milliliters to be administered. First – what is the RIGHT dose for the child? 0.5g for every kg = 0.5g x 40kg = 20 g; Now, its basic algebra coming back from freshman year to haunt us yet again!

- 12.5g/50ml = 0.25g/mL

- The child weighs 40kg and needs 20g

- At 0.25g/ml, the amount needed for 20g = **80ml**

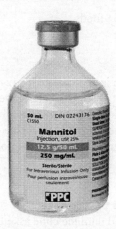

25% Mannitol Bottle, 12.5g/50ml

64) For the previous child with blunt head trauma and increased intracranial pressure, the ED nurse finds no vials of mannitol are available. However, a bag of 20% mannitol (100g/500 mL) is available. At this concentration, what volume (mL) of mannitol would this child receive?

A) 20g

B) 100ml

C) 0.5g

D) 50ml

B – Okay, same formula, but different concentration! But our child still needs 20g of mannitol (we found that out in the last question)

- 100g/500ml = 0.20g/ml

- The child weighs 40kg and needs 20g

- At 0.20g/ml concentration, the amount needed for 20g = **100ml**

Certified Pediatric Emergency Nurse (CPEN) Review IV

This question not only asks you to calculate the appropriate mannitol dose in grams, but also to take it one step further and calculate the actual volume (in milliliters) to be administered. The <u>grams</u> of medication to be administered to the child are the same whether the medication comes from a bottle or a bag. However… it is crucial to note that there are different concentrations between the vial and the bag and therefore the <u>milliliters</u> to be administered to the child are different.

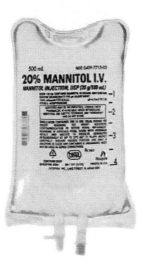

20% Mannitol Infusion, 20g/100mL

65) Prior to initiating an IV infusion of mannitol, the ED nurse finds numerous visible crystals in the bag. The nurse should:

A) Immediately discard the still sealed bag of mannitol into biohazard container

B) Immediately return the bag of mannitol to the manufacturer for their evaluation

C) Immediately see if there is another bag of mannitol available without visible crystals and place the crystallized bag in the blanket warmer

D) Immediately administer the dose from the currently available bag as the crystals are not of clinical concern

C – Crystals in your IV solution are never a good thing! Unfortunately, crystal formation in mannitol bottles and bags is a very common situation, especially when the solutions above 15% concentration are stored at low temperatures. Several methods to rewarm mannitol and allow the crystals to return to solution are described in the literature. In an emergency setting, probably the easiest option is to see if there is another bag or bottle without visible crystals immediately available. If this is not the case, then the bag or bottle may be placed in a dry-heat cabinet, i.e., a blanket warmer, until the solution temperature has increased to the point that the crystals have returned to a liquid state. After the mannitol has returned to room temperature, it can then be administered to the patient. When administering greater than 20% mannitol either as an IV bolus or a continuous IV infusion, a filter needle or filter IV tubing should be used as not all mannitol crystals are visible to the naked eye! Option A may sound inviting because of the specificity of the answer, but that amount of information (and the safety implication) is intended only as a distraction. Returning the bag to the manufacturer does not address the need to care for the patient. Finally, as mentioned above, crystals in an IV solution are never a good thing.

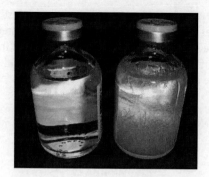

Mannitol Bottles with Visible Crystals

Image courtesy of Springer Images - www.springerimages.com

66) 0.01 mg/kg of 1:10,000 epinephrine (1mg/10ml) is to be given to a 6-week old, 5kg infant in cardiac arrest. What is the correct volume that the peds ED nurse should administer?

A) 0.01 ml

B) 0.05 ml

C) 0.1 ml

D) 0.5 ml

D - 0.5 ml of 1:10,000 epinephrine (1 mg/10mL) will deliver the ordered 0.01 mg/kg for a 5kg child. I wish I could take credit for this truly cool epi trick, but I learned it from a brilliant pediatric emergency medicine physician, Dr. Alson Inaba at Kapi'olani Children's in Honolulu, Hawaii. Here's the summary: Rule 1 - Just about everything in children is something per kilo. Whether it's medications or defibrillation, it's something per kilo. Rule 2 - During the "heat of battle," i.e. during a pediatric resuscitation, all we nurses really care about when it comes to epinephrine is "how many ml's do I need to push?" The other stuff (such as how many mg of epi do I push) is for when we write the chart (remember the good old days when we could actually write vs. click to chart… but I digress.) So combining the two rules, we take the weight in kilograms and push the decimal point one digit to the left to determine how many ml to push during resuscitation. Pushing the decimal point on the weight (in kilos, of course) one point to the left and a 5kg child should receive 0.5ml of epinephrine (5.0kg - decimal one to the left - 0.50 ml. How easy!) A 100kg adult should receive 10ml of epinephrine (i.e. a box of epi,) and a 1kg premature neonate should receive 0.1ml of epinephrine.

Now – let's chart! Remember that charting is RARELY in ml for medications and ALMOST ALWAYS in the unit of measure (like mg, mEq, etc). To quickly and easily figure out the dosage of epi in mg, push the decimal point on the weight in kg TWO points to the left. Our 5kg child should receive 0.05mg of epinephrine. Keep going – a 100kg adult should receive 1.0mg of epi, and a 1kg preemie should receive 0.01mg of epi. ONE decimal place to the left for epi in ml, TWO decimal places to the left for epi in mg.

Change Weight	5.0kg
To	
Volume	0.5ml
To	
Dose to chart	0.05mg

$$5kg * \frac{0.01mg}{kg} \approx 0.05mg$$

$$0.05mg * \frac{10ml}{1mg} \approx 0.5ml$$

Pediatric critical care and emergency medicine attending physician insight: Whenever you give epi in a code, whether it is via ETT (epi 1:1,000 aka. 1 mg/mL) or IV (epi 1:10,000, aka. 1 mg/10 mL) - the dose in mL's is always 0.1mL/kg - hence moving the decimal point one place to the left. And remember that the max epi dose is 1mg.

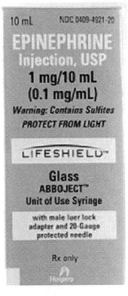

Epinephrine 1 mg/10 mL Injection
Photo courtesy of Hospira
www.Hospira.com

67) It is feared that your unconscious pediatric patient aspirated after a vomiting episode. He has just been intubated and you have placed a colorimetric end-tidal CO_2 device (CO_2 detector) on the endotracheal tube. Immediately after intubation, vomit is found to be in the endotracheal tube. What effect, if any, will the presence of vomit have on your colorimetric device results?

A) False positive reading (positive for CO_2 even if tube is in the esophagus)

B) False negative reading (negative for CO_2 even though tube is in the trachea)

C) True positive reading (positive for CO_2 only if the tube is in the trachea)

D) True negative reading (negative for CO_2 only if the tube is in the esophagus)

A – The presence of vomit (and stomach acids) could cause a false positive reading. Colorimetric devices include a piece of litmus paper encapsulated in plastic. Litmus paper, as you may remember from chemistry class, tests for pH, and most commonly acids. In colorimetric devices, the litmus paper is designed to test for CO_2 which reacts as an acid. These devices work on the principle that there is no *naturally* occurring CO_2 in the stomach. So if the endotracheal tube is in the esophagus, it will not detect any acid, and should not change color (purple detector + purple patient = bad!) If the endotracheal tube is in the trachea, it should change colors (gold detector = gold is good!) reflecting the presence of CO_2, an acidic gas released through the lungs. However, should gastric contents (i.e. vomit) come up the tube and make contact with the device, it can affect the reading. Vomit is acidic, and therefore it will cause the litmus paper to read a positive (acidic) response. The other cause of false positive readings that is frequently described is the presence of soda pop in the stomach. There have also been case reports of false positives after kids ate raw bread dough. False negatives would occur when there is a lack of CO_2 being exhaled from the lungs. This can be from a severe decrease in systemic perfusion (hypotension or cardiac arrest) or pulmonary perfusion (pulmonary hypertension.)

Any of the previously described false positive and false negative readings are minimized if you are using wave-form capnography. This is one of the reasons that the American Heart Association highly recommends use of waveform capnography over the use of colorimetric detectors.

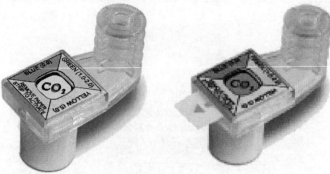

Colormetric End-Tidal CO_2 Detectors Demonstrating Gold and Purple Colors

Images courtesy of Mercury Medical - www.mercurymed.com

68) When evaluating the cuff pressure of an endotracheal tube (ETT) in a child, which of the following represents current best practice?

A) Pushing some air into the cuff and "feeling the balloon"

B) Inflate the cuff only until placement has been verified radiographically and then deflate

C) Attach a device specifically designed to measure cuff pressure

D) Inflate until the cuff pressure is greater than or equal to the mean airway pressure

C – Current best practice calls for the use of cuff pressure monitors, not only in adults, but in children as well. Just placing air into the cuff, without regular monitoring of cuff pressures, is becoming an unacceptable practice not only in the operating room, but in the ED and pediatric ICU as well.

We should always remember that kids are not small adults. The cuff pressure on an endotracheal tube needs to be enough to seal the airway, but not so much as to impair tissue blood flow in the trachea. In the adult population, this is considered around 20-25 cmH_2O. A recent study looked at the current practice of placing air into the child's endotracheal tube pilot balloon (like we do for adults many times) until it "feels right," and measured how much pressure was being exerted on the child's airway. Findings showed tracheal pressures were between 60 -120 cmH_2O! They then looked at how much pressure is required to seal the cuff in the child. The pressure was found to be ≤ 10 cmH$_2$O (versus 20-25cm in adults.) Obviously, much less pressure is required when using a cuffed tube in the child. Option B should be quickly eliminated since the question asks about cuff pressure, and this option doesn't mention pressure at all (And it's just wrong on the concept level.) Option C may sound tempting, but we should easily recognize that there is no connection between cuff pressure and mean airway pressure.

For many years, it was taught that only uncuffed endotracheal tubes should be used in children. The rationales were twofold: 1) Kids' airways are funnel-shaped, and when the right size endotracheal tube just squeaked through the funnel, it created its own natural seal and 2) Cuffed endotracheal tubes caused tracheal ischemia and necrosis. Both of these were true, but as the folk song goes, "times they are a changing." First, the endotracheal tube itself continues to evolve and there are now tubes with "smaller/gentler" (meaning much lower pressure) cuffs that don't cause the damage we used to see. Secondly, we are now keeping kids alive who wouldn't have survived a short time ago (with the evolution of pediatric ventilators, emergency/critical care, etc...) Case in point... A horrible near-drowning kid is in ARDS and requiring airway pressures of "2,000,000 over 1,000,000" to barely make his chest go up and down. With these kinds of pressures and an uncuffed endotracheal tube, even with the best funnel-ETT fit, the air leaks all over the place and the critically ill child may have to be extubated and reintubated with a cuffed ETT. In the most recent PALS guidelines, as well as the author's/editors' experiences, we're seeing more and more pediatric ICUs that are placing cuffed ETTs (usually ½ size smaller than an uncuffed tube) and recommendations that EDs do the same. If you don't need to inflate the cuff - great; but if you are having trouble making air go in and out and all you must do is put a little air into the cuff - even better! Although uncuffed tubes are still commonly used for children in the ED, the change to cuffed ETTs is something you will see more of in the very near future.

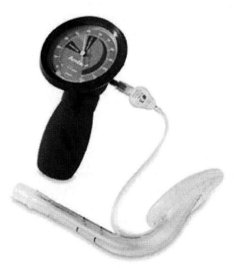

Endotracheal Tube (& King Airway/Laryngeal Mask Airway) Cuff Pressure Monitor

Image courtesy of Ambu USA - www.ambuusa.com

69) Parents arrive to your ED with their 6-year-old daughter who has said that her uncle has been "touching" her where she doesn't like it. What would you expect to find on physical assessment?

A) Genital injuries or tearing

B) Genital or rectal bruising

C) Normal exam

D) Redness or swelling

C - Pedophiles normally make sure that they are not causing trauma or pain to their victims. Pain or discomfort is likely to make the child not want to participate, or more likely to say something to another adult. Abusers tend to be very good at grooming their prey, so it isn't unusual to encounter a normal physical exam in these cases. If possible, it is best that examinations related to possible sexual abuse or assault on children be conducted by a trained Pediatric Sexual Assault Nurse Examiner and the patient should have a forensic interview done by someone specifically trained in this field as well. The appropriate Child Protective Services (CPS) agency should be notified. If the meantime, your priorities will include making sure the child is safe, and accurately documenting any pertinent information.

70) A 2-year-old male is brought into your ED. The child has slurred speech, is unable to stand on his own, and smells strongly of alcohol. Family members state that while they were hosting a party at their home, the child began to vomit uncontrollably. The father says that he thinks the child was probably "ok" and that the child just needed to "sleep it off." When your colleague asks about reporting this situation, your response would be based on which of the following?

A) A report is not needed as this was clearly an unintentional alcohol exposure

B) Any reporting should wait until lab tests rule out diabetic etiology

C) Any reporting should wait until a CT scan rules out head injury

D) A report should be filed with the appropriate agency in this case.

D - Even though each state is ultimately responsible for determining laws related to child abuse, neglect, and endangerment, the federal government has established minimum standard definitions. Permitting a child to use, or giving a child, alcohol or illegal drugs constitute emotional neglect or abuse. Regardless of individual state statutes, this is definitely a case for child protective services! Reasonable precautions should always be exercised to avoid alcohol or drug exposure, so even "accidental" or unintentional incidents will be avoided. There is no reason to delay in starting the reporting process as diabetic etiology doesn't seem likely, and a CT would not be of benefit here.

Medical Maladies & Trauma Trivia

71) A 16-year-old female presents to the emergency department with abdominal pain, vaginal bleeding and passing blood clots. The patient admits to being sexually active without the use of protective measures. Upon further evaluation, the patient is found to have a positive pregnancy test, blood type A negative, and hemoglobin of 14.6. An ultrasound reveals a first trimester intrauterine pregnancy. What would the nurse anticipate the physician to order?

A) Packed red blood cells

B) Rho (D) immune globulin (Rhogam®)

C) CT scan of the abdomen and pelvis

D) Blood cultures

B - Rho (D) immune globulin (Rhogam®) should be given to all Rh negative pregnant patients who present with vaginal bleeding. This includes cases of suspected ectopic pregnancy, miscarriage or any situation where there is a high risk of fetomaternal hemorrhage (entry of fetal blood into the maternal circulation.) Rhogam® prevents alloimmunization (an immune response) and ultimately prevents fetal hemolytic disease. The hemoglobin test result of 14.6 would indicate that a transfusion isn't necessary and a CT is probably not necessary at this stage. Blood cultures would not provide any useful information based on the patient presentation.

72) A 6-year-old Caucasian male presents to the emergency department with a one-week history of cough and congestion. For the last two days he has complained of strong "tummy" pain that comes and goes, as well as pain to hips, knees and ankles. He is eating well, ambulates without difficulty and does not have hematuria. You observe a palpable purpuric rash on his lower extremities. The patient is diagnosed with Henoch-Schonlein purpura (HSP.) The nurse understands that patients with a diagnosis of HSP require:

A) Contact Isolation

B) PICC line with total parenteral nutrition.

C) Pain control with non-steroidal anti-inflamatories (NSAIDS)

D) IV antibiotics

C - Henoch-Schonlein purpura (HSP) is the most common vasculitis of childhood. The course of HSP in children is usually self-limiting, and treatment is primarily supportive with NSAIDs and glucocorticoids. HSP is characterized by four classic symptoms: (1) palpable purpura, (2) arthralgia/arthritis, (3) abdominal pain, and (4) renal disease. HSP occurs primarily in children 3 to 15 years of age, with peak incidence rates seen between 4 and 6 years of age. The underlying cause is unknown, but is thought to be immune-related.

73) A two-week-old infant with a history of prematurity presents to the emergency department with vomiting, diarrhea, abdominal distension and tenderness. You note that he has poor perfusion, hypotension and tachycardia. The patient is intubated for apnea and receives a fluid bolus of 20 ml/kg NS. After these initial treatments, the improvements in the blood pressure and tachycardia are noted. An X-ray is obtained and reveals pneumatosis intestinalis (air within the walls of the small or large intestine.) The **most** likely diagnosis for this infant is:

A) Necrotizing enterocolitis

B) Abdominal trauma

C) Pneumonia

D) Bacteremia

A - Necrotizing entercolitis (NEC) is the most common gastrointestinal surgical emergency in the newborn population, and is even more prevalent with the premature infants. Pneumatosis Intestinalis is caused by bacteria in the wall of the gut producing air, and is a sign of NEC. Necrotizing enterocolitis is characterized by varying degrees of damage to the intestinal mucosa, ranging from mucosal irritation to a full ischemic perforation of the bowel. We know what happens, but there is still argument as to why it happens! Management of NEC is based upon the severity of illness, and may include simple supportive care, antibiotic therapy, close laboratory and radiological monitoring or surgical intervention if needed. In the ER – an infant presenting with NEC may be shocky – get in that IV or IO and start fluids ASAP! Necro means death… entero means in… colitis means unhappy bowel. Anything involving a baby and death in the unhappy bowel can't be good!

Pneumatosis
(Gas in the bowel wall)

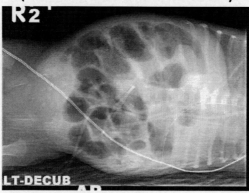

Abdominal Radiograph Demonstrating Pneumatosis Intestinalis

Image courtesy of Terri Russell RN, DNP, NNP

74) Paramedics bring in a five-year-old female victim from a motor vehicle crash (MVC.) She was reported to be a back seat passenger with no booster or child safety seat, and was restrained with only a lap belt. Upon arrival, she is complaining of abdominal and back pain. On exam, she is noted to have transverse ecchymosis on her mid-abdomen near her umbilicus (looking very much like the imprint of a seat belt.) What is the **most** common hollow organ injury associated with seat belt patterns in children?

A) Duodenum

B) Spleen

C) Jejunum

D) Stomach

C - The jejunum is the most common location for a hollow organ injury in a child who was restrained with only a lap belt in a MVC. An ecchymotic seat belt pattern should make you *very* suspicious for spinal cord, vertebral, or hollow viscous injuries. In over 60% of pediatric cases where there is a "seat belt pattern" on the abdomen, there was an injury to one of the hollow viscous organs (small or large bowel, stomach, bladder), with the jejunum being the most common. An automobile lap belt is meant to be worn low over the hips. When a small child wears one without a booster seat, the lap belt tends to slide up over the hip bones and rest squarely over the unprotected abdomen. When a crash occurs, the rapid deceleration "folds" the child over the lap belt, and all the force ends up injuring the organs and bones.

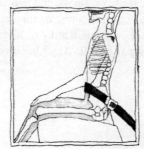 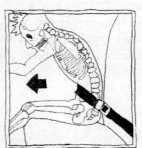

Lap Belt Injuries

Illustrations Courtesy of My Then 14-year Old Aspiring Baker Daughter,

www.ninasbeliciousbakery.com

75) Which of the following is an inappropriate option for pain management prior to intravenous line (IV) placement?

A) Distraction

B) Cold spray

C) Inhaled nitrous oxide

D) Oral acetaminophen at 10-15mg/kg

D – While the dosage for the oral acetaminophen is correct, it is unlikely that acetaminophen would be of any real value for pain management prior to an IV insertion. Distraction has been found to be a simple and effective approach to make the IV insertion process go well. Distraction can be human or even electronic (think smart phones, tablet computers, or electronic book readers.) Emergency departments have used cold spray for years and nitrous oxide continues to be used to facilitate IV placement in anxious children.
Tips for the clinical side: What's the "buzz" about "Buzzy?" There is a relatively new product out there called Buzzy® and it can be used for children as well as adults! It utilizes cold and vibration while working with the "blocking the gate" theory for pain management prior to needle sticks (IVs, lab draws, or injections.) You can find more information at www.buzzy4shots.com

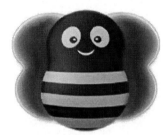

Buzzy
Image courtesy of Amy Baxter MD, FACEP - www.buzzyhelps.com

76) EMS arrives with a 4-year-old male patient. He is complaining of a sore throat, stiff neck and difficulty swallowing. On initial physical exam, you note swollen lymph nodes and difficulty with extension and flexion of the neck. The oral pharynx looks red and swollen and there is no respiratory distress. Vital signs reveal HR 120, RR 24, sats 93% on room air, and oral temperature of 102.5F (39.2C.) The parents state that the child is current with all of his recommended immunizations, but has recurrent ear infections with the last episode treated two weeks ago. What would be the **most** likely diagnosis for this patient?

A) Meningitis

B) Epiglottitis

C) Retropharyngeal abscess

D) Strep throat

C – Pediatric retropharyngeal abscesses (RPAs) are relatively rare, but occur most frequently in the under-five age group. One hypothesis to explain this prevalence is the relatively common occurrence of infections such as otitis media, tonsillitis, adenoiditis, and other upper respiratory infections. The classic pediatric presentation of RPA is an upper respiratory tract infection that spreads to the retropharyngeal lymph nodes.

RPAs can also be caused by trauma to the throat. Yes, there really is a reason why Mom told you not to run with that pencil in your mouth. Procedures such as laryngoscopy, endoscopy and feeding tube placement can all cause traumas leading to a retropharyngeal abscess.

While rare, it is important to recognize and treat RPAs promptly. Left untreated, they can lead to airway compromise, migrate to other nearby tissues, and even spread to the mediastinum with the potential for causing potentially lethal mediastinitis.

The most common symptoms are neck pain, neck stiffness/torticollis, sore throat and fever. One study showed that additional symptoms of wheezing and/or stridor, once thought common for RPA, were actually found in less than 2% of cases.

Even without respiratory distress, the patient should be admitted for administration of IV antibiotics and observation for possible progression to airway compromise. Symptom improvement should be seen within 24-48 hours. Corticosteroids may also be used in conjunction with antibiotics, especially in patients who <u>are</u> experiencing airway compromise. The current trend is to first try medical management (drugs) and if they are not working then add surgical interventions to drain the abscess. Moral of the story… listen to mom about the whole running with pencils thing. She really was smarter than you think!

77) Treatment of a severe reaction from fire ant stings involves all of the following **except**:

A) EpiPen® auto injector

B) Benadryl® (diphenhydramine)

C) Antivenin

D) Corticosteroids

C - Like other hymenoptera (such as bees and wasps,) there is no antivenin for fire ant envenomation. Treatment is supportive, paying particular attention to the risk of anaphylaxis which can be deadly. Swarming of fire ants and multiple sting locations are common as with other hymenoptera. Of note, the queen fire ant may live for 6 to 7 years and can produce up to 3,500 eggs in a single day. That is roughly 9 million in her lifetime. Male fire ants mate with the queen (and do nothing else) for their 4-5 day lifespan. Though short, some (guys) would say that the male fire ant has a good life. On the other hand, consider the very, very busy life of the fire ant OB nurse!

78) The primary concerns with West Nile Virus infection are:

A) End organ failure and renal compromise

B) Pulmonary edema and acute respiratory distress syndrome (ARDS)

C) Endocarditis and pericarditis

D) Encephalitis and meningoencephalitis

D – While 80% of West Nile Virus (WNV) infections are asymptomatic, West Nile Virus is now one of the most common causes of epidemic viral encephalitis in the United States. Symptoms of severe WNV infection commonly include stiff neck, severe headache, and confusion. Just hearing "stiff neck" in the history should certainly make one think of ruling out meningitis. Treatment is supportive as there is no vaccine or specific antiviral medication for WNV infection. Prevention efforts should be community based, focusing on the reduction of mosquito populations and educating the community regarding risks and symptoms. West Nile Virus is a reportable disease under the CDC category of Arboviral diseases. Follow your institutional policy regarding the reporting of diseases to the CDC or state department of health.

79) A 9-year-old male presents to the ER with a laceration to his index finger. His mother states he was reaching into the trash can to get a toy that fell in and cut his hand on aluminum can. The child's finger was bleeding at the time, but the bleeding is easily controlled. He is up to date on his immunizations. The laceration is located between the middle knuckle (proximal interphalangeal (PIP) joint and distal knuckle (distal interphalangeal (DIP) joint) on the palm side of the hand. What is the **most** important clinical finding to document before the repair is undertaken?

A) Identifying whether extension of the finger is intact

B) Identifying whether flexion of the finger is intact

C) Making sure the patient can hold an object with his other fingers

D) Confirming that flexion is intact in the distal phalanx

D - Confirming that flexion is intact in the distal phalanx. With any finger laceration it is critical to determine and document if a flexor tendon injury occurred so appropriate follow up can be made. In order for the fingers to grasp objects they need intact flexor tendons.

Anatomically speaking, the finger tendons insert distal to each joint of the finger. This means that if the distal tendons are lacerated, the finger can seemingly flex normally at the point of injury, but in reality it is the proximal tendons that are flexing the finger. It is critical that each joint of the finger be isolated and independently tested for flexion. Extension is considered less important for the function of the finger. However, if a tendon injury is suspected anywhere in the hand or fingers, prompt follow up should be arranged. Primary repair of the flexor tendons of the hand should done by a specialized practitioner.

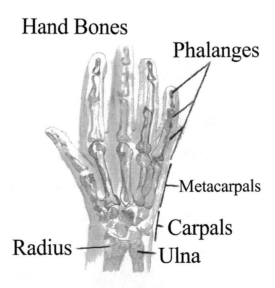

Bones of the Hand

Illustration Courtesy of My Then 14-year Old Aspiring Baker Daughter,

www.ninasbeliciousbakery.com

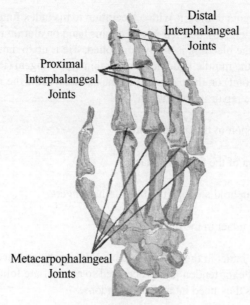

Joints of the Hand

Illustration Courtesy of My Then 14-year Old Aspiring Baker Daughter,

www.ninasbeliciousbakery.com

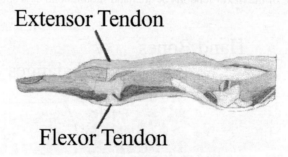

Hand Flexor and Extensor Tendons

Illustration Courtesy of My Then 14-year Old Aspiring Baker Daughter,

www.ninasbeliciousbakery.com

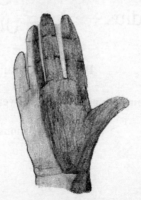

Areas of Sensation: Radial Nerve

Illustration Courtesy of My Then 14-year Old Aspiring Baker Daughter,

www.ninasbeliciousbakery.com

Certified Pediatric Emergency Nurse (CPEN) Review IV

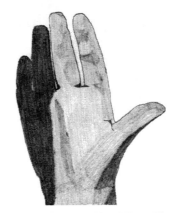

Areas of Sensation: Ulnar Nerve

Illustration Courtesy of My Then 14-year Old Aspiring Baker Daughter,

www.ninasbeliciousbakery.com

80) All of the following statements about alcohol absorption via nebulization or vaporization are true **except:**

A) The consumption will take longer.

B) It is undetectable by breathalyzer.

C) It may be facilitated via atomization or heating.

D) The "buzz" (absorption) is more rapid, compared to oral ingestion.

B - The route of ingestion does not change how the body processes alcohol, so the breathalyzer is still going to detect it. (The breathalyzer doesn't check for odor.) Metabolism is metabolism is metabolism, no matter where the process starts! Nebulization or vaporization are alternative forms of alcohol consumption that bring with them some unique considerations. They take longer to prepare and imbibe than simply "taking a drink," and they are, at least in theory, more dangerous than traditional ingestion. This is allegedly due to two factors: (1) a higher degree of ethanol absorption by nebulization vs. drinking (GI tract); and (2) the fact that the body's natural defense mechanisms against ethanol toxicity (getting rid of the alcohol by vomiting, or stopping the consumption by simply passing out) are bypassed. Also, the slowness of preparation and inhalation often prevents the irritation that alcohol consumption can produce. This, in turn, further encourages overindulgence. Although the Alcohol With Out Liquid (AWOL) nebulizer has been outlawed in 23 states, home nebulizers, such as those used by asthmatics, and vaporization devices remain readily available via the internet.

ABG Normal Ranges	
sPO_2	~95-99%
pO_2	80-100
pH	7.35-7.45
pCO_2	35-45 mmHg
HCO_3	22-26

Normal Arterial Blood Gas Values

Certified Pediatric Emergency Nurse (CPEN) Review IV

81) The following arterial blood gas is observed on a young child following the accidental ingestion of a fentanyl patch.
$pH = 7.25$, $pCO_2 = 55$, $pO_2 = 60$, $HCO_3^- = 25$. The correct interpretation of this blood gas is:

A) Compensated metabolic acidosis

B) Compensated respiratory acidosis

C) Uncompensated respiratory acidosis

D) Uncompensated metabolic acidosis

C – The blood gas indicates uncompensated respiratory acidosis. Now that basic blood gas interpretation has been mastered, let's look at cases of compensated and uncompensated blood gas abnormality. The pH of 7.25 indicates acidosis, and the pCO_2 of 55 is "out of whack" (high) indicating respiratory acidosis. Since the body's metabolic system has not successfully adapted for this situation, we have an example of uncompensated respiratory acidosis.

Medical Maladies & Trauma Trivia

82) Based solely on the above blood gas, patient history, and no other physical assessment data, you recognize that the infant is **most** likely having problems with which of the following?

A) Hypoxia/hyperventilation

B) Hyperoxia/hypoventilation

C) Hyperoxia/hyperventilation

D) Hypoxia/hypoventilation

D – In this case, the infant is most likely having problems related hypoxia/hypoventilation. The PO_2 value corresponds to oxygenation and the CO_2 value correlates to ventilation. A normal PO_2 should be approximately 4 to 5 times the FiO_2. In this example, the infant is breathing receiving room air, (21% FiO_2.) Consequently, we would expect a PO_2 ranging from 80-100 mm Hg, not 60! A PO_2 of 60 or less is generally considered to be indicative of hypoxia and an indication for supplemental oxygen. Normal CO_2 should be between 35-45 mm Hg. The slower and more shallow one breathes, the more CO_2 is retained (hypercarbia or hypercapnia.) Hypoventilation is a common cause of hypercarbia/hypercapnia, and depressed respiratory drive secondary to analgesia/sedation (now you can remember the Fentanyl patch) is a common cause of hypoventilation.

83) The following arterial blood gas is observed on a young patient, who is exhibiting air hunger and hyperventilation:
$pH = 7.55$, $pCO_2 = 30$, $pO_2 = 63$, $HCO_3^- = 22$. The correct interpretation of this blood gas is:

A) Compensated respiratory alkalosis

B) Uncompensated respiratory alkalosis

C) Compensated metabolic alkalosis

D) Uncompensated metabolic alkalosis

B – The blood gas indicates uncompensated respiratory alkalosis. In this case, the pH of 7.55 indicates alkalosis, and the pCO_2 of 30 is "out of whack" (low) indicating respiratory alkalosis. Since the body's metabolic system has not successfully adapted for this situation, we have an example of uncompensated respiratory alkalosis.

Certified Pediatric Emergency Nurse (CPEN) Review IV

84) The previous patient with respiratory alkalosis continues to hyperventilate and deteriorates to the point that a decision needs to be made for assisted ventilation. Which of the following combinations would you anticipate as **most** likely?

A) Shorter Inspiratory Time, Longer Expiratory Time

B) Longer Inspiratory Time, Longer Expiratory Time

C) Shorter Inspiratory Time, Shorter Expiratory Time.

D) Longer Inspiratory Time, Shorter Expiratory Time.

A – In this case, you would anticipate assisted ventilation to provide shorter inspiratory time and longer expiratory time. In addition to blowing off CO_2 and inducing more respiratory alkalosis, this patient's hyperventilation may lead to air trapping and reduced tidal volumes due to incomplete exhalation. Providing a longer time to exhale is the key to correcting any air trapping.

Pediatric emergency medicine and critical care attending physician insights: Note that this will only work if the patient is sedated well and possibly paralyzed. Allowed to spontaneously breathe on the vent, the patient will continue to breathe the same as prior to the intubation.

85) Possible ways to reduce the amount of CO_2 "blown off" include:

A) Decreasing respiratory rate/ Decreasing inspiratory pressure.

B) Increasing respiratory rate/ Increasing inspiratory pressure.

C) Decreasing respiratory rate/ Increasing inspiratory pressure.

D) Increasing respiratory rate/ Decreasing inspiratory pressure.

A - Decreasing respiratory rate/ Decreasing inspiratory pressure will reduce the amount of CO_2 "blown off." (I'm not a Respiratory Therapist, but I DID stay at a Holiday Inn Express last night!) If a patient is ALREADY blowing off CO_2, the LAST thing they need is further alveolar recruitment, which is exactly what increasing inspiratory pressure will produce. Decreasing respiratory rate is the most basic way to increase expiratory time.

Let's take a moment (and a little bit of math) and look at the relationship between rate and time.
Given an respiratory rate (inspiration and expiration) of 20 breaths per minutes and an inspiratory/expiratory ratio (I:E) of 1:2, let's calculate E time:
        60 seconds/minute divided by 20 breaths per minute = 3 seconds per breath. An I:E of 1:2 means that the patient spends ONE second inspiring or inhaling and TWO seconds in the expiratory phase, exhaling.
Now, drop the rate to 10 bpm.
        60 seconds/minute divided by 10 breaths per minute = 6 seconds per breath. An I:E ratio of 1:2 means that the patient spends TWO second inspiring or inhaling and FOUR seconds in the expiratory phase, exhaling.
By dropping the respiratory rate to half of what it was, you have DOUBLED the expiratory time. This will prevent air trapping and help correct the hypoxia seen on the original blood gas. If you are thinking that increased expiratory time may blow off more CO_2 in an already HYPOcarbic patient, you are partially correct. You need to consider the rate as well. 2 seconds of exhalation per breath at 20 breaths per minute and 4 seconds of exhalation per breath at 10 breaths per minute both result in 40 seconds of exhalation per minute at an I:E of 1:2.

Certified Pediatric Emergency Nurse (CPEN) Review IV

86) Your patient is a child with a history of Type 1 diabetes. He presents with altered mental status and the following blood gas: pH =7.25, pCO_2 = 28, pO_2=95, HCO_3- = 15. The correct interpretation of this blood gas is:

A) Compensated metabolic acidosis

B) Compensated respiratory acidosis

C) Uncompensated respiratory acidosis

D) Uncompensated metabolic acidosis

D – The blood gas results indicate uncompensated metabolic acidosis. In this case, the pH of 7.25 indicates acidosis, and the HCO_3 of 15 is "out of whack" (low) indicating metabolic acidosis. Since the body's respiratory system has not successfully adapted for this situation, we have an example of uncompensated metabolic acidosis.

87) An infant is brought to the ER with severe acute diarrhea. This blood gas results are reported as: pH =7.35, pCO_2 = 32, pO_2=75, HCO_3- = 18. The correct interpretation of this blood gas is:

A) Compensated metabolic acidosis

B) Compensated respiratory acidosis

C) Uncompensated respiratory acidosis

D) Uncompensated Metabolic acidosis

A – The blood gas results in this case indicate compensated metabolic acidosis. The pH is in the normal range, but the bicarb (HCO_3) of 18 is still "out of whack." The metabolic acidosis is "compensated" based on the normal pH. Note: A metabolic acidosis can result from HCO_3 loss just as easily as it can result from HCO_3 consumption in neutralizing acids, i.e. CO_2, and is a common finding in gastroenteritis/shock patients.

Medical Maladies & Trauma Trivia

88) The pathologic electrolyte abnormality **most** likely to be seen with the patient experiencing uncontrolled diarrhea is:

A) Hypokalemia

B) Hyperkalemia

C) Hyponatremia

D) Hypernatremia

A - Hypokalemia is the most likely electrolyte imbalance found with patients experiencing excessive diarrhea. GI losses are one of the most common causes of hypokalemia in children. Remember… you lose "P"otassium in the "P"oop.

89) Inhaling fumes resulting from the combustion of synthetic materials is arguably the most common route of cyanide poisoning in children. This is unintentional and may be seen in house fires. Accidental ingestion of what common household substance may also result in cyanide toxicity?

A) Nail polish remover

B) Artificial nail remover

C) Toilet bowl cleanser

D) Grout mildew remover

B –Ingestion of artificial nail remover can result in cyanide toxicity. Cleaning agents, such as offered in choices C and D often contain chlorine bleaching agents, and nail polish remover often contains acetone. Both of these are bad, but they are not cyanide. Some artificial nail removers contain acetonitrile, which is metabolized to cyanide. There have been several reported cases of cyanide toxicity secondary to ingestion of the acetonitrile contained in artificial nail remover. NOTE: There has been at least one case of delayed treatment for cyanide toxicity because the ingestion was reported as "nail POLISH remover" vs. "artificial nail remover." Although the poisonous agent in both starts with "aceto," nail polish remover has NOTHING to do with cyanide poisoning. It is the NITRILE group in acetonitrile that results in cyanide toxicity. Treatment may also be delayed due to the fact that there are no toxidromes (specific set of signs and symptoms) specific for cyanide toxicity. Symptomology reflects the extent of cellular hypoxia and resultant dysfunction of organs with high metabolic oxygen demands, e.g., the central nervous system and the heart.

90) Aside from supporting airway, breathing and circulation, and considering activated charcoal, treatment of cyanide toxicity may consist of administration of hydroxocobalamin and/or thiosulfate and which of the following?

A) Flumazenil

B) Naloxone

C) Glucagon

D) Nitrites

D - Nitrites, in addition to thiosulfate and/or hydroxocobalamin may be administered in cases of cyanide toxicity. These are the ingredients in the commercially available cyanide antidote kit. Note: Nitrites should ALWAYS be followed by thiosulfates and/or hydroxocobalamin. HOWEVER, in the case of smoke inhalation, thiosulfates should be withheld due to the methemoglobinemia that may accompany smoke inhalation. (Administration of thiosulfates can cause a rise in methemoglobin.)

Pediatric emergency medicine and critical care attending physician insights: Victims of fires may be suffering from both carbon monoxide and cyanide toxicity. Carboxyhemoglobin causes the oxygen-hemoglobin dissociation curve to be shifted to the left creating tissue hypoxia. In these patients, the induction of methemoglobinemia could be lethal.

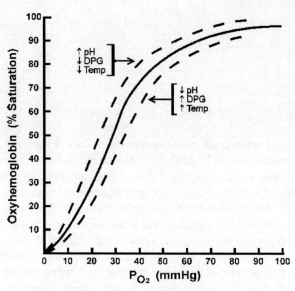

Oxygen-Hemoglobin Dissociation Curve

91) When preparing for High Flow Nasal Cannula (HFNC) oxygen therapy which of the following should be expected:

A) A traditional nasal cannula at flows up to 5 lpm and heated humidification

B) Large bore tubing and short nasal cannulas

C) A traditional nasal cannula with Intermittent Pressure Enhancer (IPE)

D) Large bore tubing with leak-resistant nasal prongs

B - In order to provide High Flow Nasal Cannula (HFNC) oxygen therapy (and reduce resistance to flow) we must couple the use of larger bore tubing, similar to what is used in infant or pediatric ventilator circuits, with shorter nasal cannulas to alleviate the back pressure issue. A review of the current literature for infants (where they have been doing this much longer than in pediatrics) shows that there is no firm consensus as to what flows should be utilized for HFNC therapy. A general guide would appear to be setting the flow at 1-2 liters/kg/min, but use of up to 4-5 liters/kg/min has been reported. So a patient weighing 5 kg would be set at a flow of 5-10 liters per minute (lpm), but based on the literature, it could go as high as 20-25 lpm. The key to HFNC therapy is meet the patient's minute ventilation needs, so these higher levels would be the exception rather than the rule. .

Option A is partially correct in that when using HFNC therapy, the gas must be well humidified. If not well humidified, your patient may end up with drying of the mucosa, along with the potential for cracking, bleeding, and pain. A simple bubble humidifier will not be able to support the humidity required. This type of therapy requires <u>heated</u> humidification. As you increase the temperature, you also increase the relative humidity. Heating the high flows of gas in the small infant is also important to prevent drops in body temperature from breathing in all that cold gas. Now that you have the gas heated, you must keep it warmed as long as possible on its journey to the nose and this suggests the use of a heated circuit as well.

A leak-resistant nasal device would essentially be a CPAP-like system, and that is another discussion entirely.

Test Taker Tips: This question has used a number of common distracter types to watch for. Numbers don't always point to the right answer, so don't let the number 5 lead you astray. Fancy sounding terminology, like Intermittent Pressure Enhancer (IPE), may attract your attention and create a significant distraction. You may be concerned because you aren't familiar with an IPE device. The reason you aren't familiar with it is because it doesn't exist. Don't let fancy sounding terms or numbers fool you!

92) High Flow Nasal Cannula therapy (HFNC) is used for all of the following reasons **except**:

A) To reduce work of breathing

B) Deliver higher FiO_2s

C) Hyperoxygenation prior to intubation

D) Relative comfort for the patient

C - If intubation is imminent, think bagging! All of the other options are real reasons for using HFNC therapy. HFNC can reduce work of breathing the same way CPAP does. In fact, the high flows can potentially create CPAP much like the nasal CPAP used in Neonatal ICUs everywhere. So, you say, why not just put them on nasal CPAP then? Primarily it is a comfort thing. Nasal CPAP uses a circular circuit of large bore tubing right up to and then away from the nasal prongs. This makes for a much stiffer and somewhat cumbersome set-up. Use of HFNC uses only a single segment of large bore tubing. The large tubing goes part of the way to the patient and then connects to a specially made nasal prong interface so it is less bulky near the patient. This can ease parenting in the pediatric ICU or ER by allowing the parent to hold and comfort their child more easily than with a nasal CPAP set-up.

Studies have also shown that HFNC can be used in lieu of a non-re-breather mask for delivering high FiO_2s. Because we are using such high flows, we are meeting the patient's inspiratory minute ventilation needs. The FiO_2 of the delivered gas is not diluted as it would be with lower flow devices. It is often better tolerated by the patient than a mask. Utilizing a gas blender with the set-up will allow the inspired oxygen levels to be titrated to specific FIO_2s.

Moral of the story, HFNCs are excellent in the pediatric population for treating respiratory distress and later for weaning from oxygen support.

Pediatric emergency medicine & critical care attending physician insights: I am a huge fan of HFNC! Particularly for the tachypneic bronchiolitic – clinically often helps significantly with work of breathing.

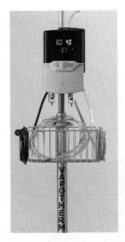
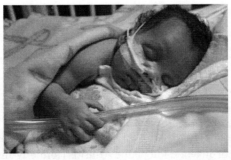
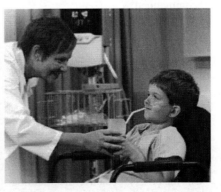

Vapotherm High-Flow Nasal Cannula Therapy

Images courtesy of Vapotherm - www.Vapotherm.com

93) Prior to starting prednisone therapy for a patient with an acute flare-up of symptoms of inflammatory bowel disease, which test should be performed?

A) Clostridium difficile (C. Diff)

B) Comprehensive metabolic panel

C) Complete blood count

D) Coagulation panel

A - Patients with inflammatory bowel disease are at an increased risk for C. Diff infections. Symptoms of this infection can mimic an acute flare up of the patient's inflammatory bowel disease and C. Diff infection should be ruled out prior to beginning steroid therapy. In fact, treatment with prednisone (and without antibiotics) in this situation can cause the patient's condition to deteriorate.

94) Signs and symptoms that you would anticipate noting when evaluating a pediatric patient for celiac disease include all of the following **except**?

A) Abdominal bloating

B) Diarrhea

C) Failure to thrive

D) Jaundice

D – Jaundice, often associated with hyperbilirubinemia, is not an expected sign of celiac disease. Celiac disease is a complex, autoimmune disease that primarily affects the small intestine's mucosal lining. The culprit in celiac is gluten (anything containing wheat, rye or barley.) While the presentation can vary greatly, children most commonly exhibit "classic" signs of gastrointestinal symptoms such as diarrhea, abdominal distention and pain, and weight changes. Recent research has found good evidence that some cases of failure to thrive and stunted growth may be caused by celiac disease. When you think celiac disease, think "can't have breads, pasta, cereals – anything with gluten" since it will have significant and unpleasant side effects!

95) In pediatric patients with Juvenile Idiopathic Arthritis (JIA,) which of the following are **most** often recommended?

A) Long term steroids and bed rest

B) Oral non-steroidal anti-inflammatory medications (NSAIDS) and exercise as tolerated

C) Oral aspirin and bed rest

D) Intravenous steroids, oral aspirin, and exercise as tolerated

B - For the initial symptom management of Juvenile Idiopathic Arthritis (formerly Juvenile Rheumatoid Arthritis (JRA), pediatric rheumatologists now recommend NSAIDS (ibuprofen, etc.) and, in contrast with bed rest, exercise and physical therapy, especially hydrotherapy. These recommendations have been found to be helpful in minimizing flare ups. The use of steroids is typically only as a bridge until other disease-modifying anti-rheumatic medications (such as methotrexate) have kicked in. The ultimate goals in managing this chronic disease are to prevent or control joint damage, to prevent loss of function, and to decrease pain. In the past, strategies such as aspirin, long term steroids, and bed rest were common; but current treatment recommendations have definitely changed over the years. We know that very few good things (and lots of bad things) happen when sick kids remain in bed for too long. So the goals for JIA patients are: More remissions (and hope of permanent remission) and less flare-ups with the least toxicity from medications.

96) Which of the following is the correct initial defibrillation energy in joules for a 10 kg child?

A) 2j

B) 10j

C) 20j

D) 30j

C - The correct initial defibrillation energy for a 10 kg child is 20 joules. With pediatric defibrillation, "pick up your paddles or pads and count them." If you are holding paddles or pads, how many should there be? Two. If there are anything but two, put them down, as another ED nurse should be defibrillating this child. Since just about everything in children's medical treatment is "something per kilo," the first defibrillation attempt is 2j/kg. If that is unsuccessful, 2x2 is 4, so it's 4j/kg for the second and subsequent times. 4j/kg is commonly as high as we go. Though recent resuscitation guidelines indicate that defibrillation attempts up to 10j/kg can be utilized, I've only read of it being done. 2j/kg initially, and then doubling to 4j/kg for subsequent defibrillation attempts is the correct answer for the test. Interestingly, some pediatric centers are not even attempting defibrillation at 2j/kg, but are delivering all defibrillation efforts at 4j/kg with good results. Their rationale is that if 2j/kg doesn't work, then we would have to increase to 4j/kg anyway. So, they are just starting with 4j/kg. But for the test, count your paddles or pads (2j/kg) then double if needed (4j/kg.) Last, but not least, don't forget that if the child is one year of age (>10kg) or older, you should use the "big people" paddles or pads.

97) Which of the following is the correct initial defibrillation energy in joules for a 12 kg child?

A) 12j

B) 20j

C) 30j

D) 48j

C – Two joules per kilogram with a 12 kilogram child means the initial defibrillation attempt should be 24j, but that's not an option here. Most defibrillators increase energy selection by larger increments as the energy level increases, so it we wouldn't expect to find the exact energy level that the formula recommends. Given the choices above, we would round up to 30 joules and not down, even though 20 is closer to 24. It's like a reverse "Price is Right" game where you want to go closest without going under the formula amount.

Pediatric emergency medicine and critical care attending physician insights: Remember to <u>round up</u> to the next highest number on the defibrillator, because in pediatrics, you will often fall between numbers on the dial.

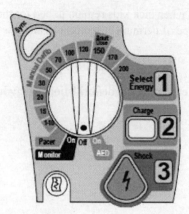

Options for Defibrillation or Cardioversion Energy in Joules
Image courtesy of Philips Healthcare - www.usa.philips.com/healthcare

98) What is the suggested <u>initial</u> synchronized cardioversion energy level (in joules) for an unstable 6 kg infant with palpable pulses in supraventricular tachycardia (SVT)?

A) 3-6j

B) 6-12j

C) 12-24j

D) 50-100j

A – 0.5-1 j/kg is what is currently recommended for <u>synchronized</u> cardioversion of unstable infants and children with tachyarrhythmias. Cardioversion starts at 0.5-1j/kg and then can be doubled to 2J/kg on subsequent attempts if there are no results from the initial attempt. 0.5–1j/kg and then 2 j/kg, but no higher. Cardioversion begins with "C" and it's for patients that are "C"onscious or "C"rashing, but not dead. If your patient is not dead, but only "half-dead," the energy for cardioversion is half that of defibrillation (for death), and that means 0.5-1j/kg. If the patient is stable and cardioversion is necessary, sedation should be considered, especially if a pediatric cardiology/referral center is available. (Yes, babies feel pain and shooting electricity through the chest really does hurt!) Hopefully, synchronized cardioversion will convert the SVT into a NSR.

Because the infant has a perfusing rhythm, you want the electricity delivered at the "right" point of the cardiac cycle to avoid "shocking" the heart into V-Fib (which would be a very bad thing.) **It is crucial to remember to hit the "sync"** button prior to each cardioversion attempt to ensure that cardioversion, not defibrillation, is done. Defibrillation is for people with "deadly" rhythms such as ventricular fibrillation and pulseless ventricular tachycardia. Defibrillation should only be used on a patient that has a disorganized, ineffective electrical impulse. This infant has a pulse and rhythm with a QRS complex; it's just REALLY fast. Defibrillating SVT can disrupt the QRS complexes and cause a full arrest in this patient.

99) What is the suggested intervention for an unstable 20 kg child with palpable pulses in supraventricular tachycardia (SVT)?

A) Age appropriate vagal maneuvers

B) Synchronized cardioversion at 10-20j

C) Adenosine, 2mg IV (0.1 mg/kg)

D) Rapid intubation with a 4.5 mm uncuffed ETT

B – The combination of a pulse and an unstable patient means Synchronized Cardioversion. Vagal maneuvers are only appropriate with stable patients. Unstable also means "do something now" and don't wait for IV access. (In addition, obtaining an appropriate IV for administering adenosine might be even more time-consuming.) Last, but not least, this is a cardiac emergency and not a respiratory one, so don't worry about the ETT at this point.

Remember this basic decision tree when it comes to the majority of cases of SVT:

Pediatric emergency medicine and critical care attending physician insights: Vagal maneuvers in children include: Blowing on a straw, rectal temperature, or evoking the "dive reflex" by placing a bag of ice/water over the face – and not just a small bag, use a BIG bag!!!! (Please remember to keep the nose and mouth open so patient can breathe!) We do not push on eyeballs or the carotids in children anymore!

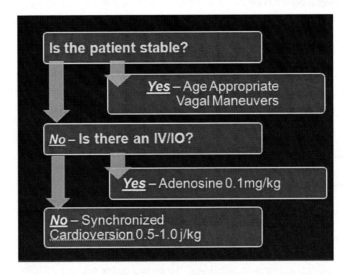

Pediatric SVT Algorithm

Image courtesy of Julie Bacon MSN-HCSM, RN-BC, NE-BC, CPN, CPEN, C-NPT

100) Cerebral perfusion pressure (CPP) is calculated with intracranial pressure and which of the following measurements?

A) Systolic blood pressure

B) Diastolic blood pressure

C) Mean arterial blood pressure

D) Central venous pressure

C – Cerebral perfusion pressure is calculated by subtracting the intracranial pressure from the mean arterial pressure (MAP.) CPP = MAP – ICP. Mean arterial pressure is a calculated measure of the body's blood pressure. Intracranial pressure is a measure of the pressure inside of the skull. CPP relates to the amount of blood perfusing the brain. You must have enough blood pressure to push the blood (supplying oxygen and glucose) into the brain. If the intracranial pressure is rising, the increasing pressure might be enough to keep the blood out. If the child is hypotensive, the MAP may not be adequate to push blood up into the brain. Cerebral perfusion pressure (CPP) is the number representing this important relationship. Body pressure minus brain pressure = how effectively the blood is getting to the brain tissue, and is often associated with changes in the level of consciousness (LOC.)

Pediatric emergency medicine & critical care attending physician insights: CPP is very important to remember in head trauma patients. They may be hypertensive; however this is likely secondary to intracranial hypertension (or elevated ICP.) You do not want to correct the elevated BP in these patients

Certified Pediatric Emergency Nurse (CPEN) Review IV

because it is helping perfuse their brain! Goal CPP's are: infants 40-50, child: 50-60, older teens/adults 60-80. Example: So if the ICP (normal ICP < 20) is suspected to be high, the MAP needs to be at least 40 points higher than ICP in order to maintain a CPP of 40 in an infant.

Basic Blood Gas Reminders

pH 7.35-7.45

pCO_2 35-45 (same numbers as the pH – isn't that handy?)

Bicarbonate 22-26

pO_2, Base Excess, Oxygen Saturations (doesn't matter as it doesn't come into play when interpreting blood gases on the test – In real-life patients, yes they matter; blood gas answers on the test, not so much)

101) A 17-year-old presents the ED after reportedly doing "meth" for the first time. Vital signs are: BP 140/80, RR 36, and HR 140. He states he "feels like he's going to pass out" and has numbness in both of his hands. ABG reveals pH 7.55, PCO_2 18, PO_2 132, Bicarbonate 23. The ED nurse interprets this ABG result as:

A) Metabolic acidosis

B) Metabolic alkalosis

C) Respiratory acidosis

D) Respiratory alkalosis

D – The ABG results indicate respiratory alkalosis. Here is a quick and easy 2-step process to help with ABG interpretation. 1) Look at the pH. Is it normal (7.35 – 7.45), acidotic (< 7.35) or alkalotic (> 7.45)? This pH is alkalotic (above 7.45), so the answer is "something" alkalosis. 2) Is it metabolic or respiratory? Check which of the other values are out of whack? Is it the PCO_2 (respiratory) or the Bicarbonate (metabolic)? In this case the CO_2 is way too low, so the answer is <u>respiratory alkalosis</u>. It's always important to read through the case scenario as well. This one specifically mentions that the teen is hyperventilating (RR 36.) That's a clue that the answer is looking for something respiratory.

102) A 3-week old infant is in the ED for evaluation of intractable vomiting. Your assessment reveals diminished pulses, RR 48, and HR 182. ABG results are: pH 7.50, PCO_2 38, PO_2 140, Bicarbonate 29. The ED nurse interprets this ABG result as:

A) Metabolic acidosis

B) Metabolic alkalosis

C) Respiratory acidosis

D) Respiratory alkalosis

B – The ABG results indicate metabolic alkalosis. Here is a quick and easy 2-step process to help with ABG interpretation. 1) Look at the pH. Is it normal (7.35 – 7.45), acidotic (< 7.35) or alkalotic (> 7.45)? This pH is alkalotic (above 7.45), so the answer is "something" alkalosis. 2) Is it metabolic or respiratory? Check which of the other values are out of whack? Is it the PCO_2 (respiratory) or the Bicarbonate (metabolic)? In this case the Bicarb is too high, so the answer is <u>metabolic alkalosis</u>. Always read through the case scenario. This one specifically mentions that the patient has had intractable vomiting (losing acid from above – resulting in alkalosis.) That's a clue that the answer is looking for something metabolic.

Medical Maladies & Trauma Trivia

Certified Pediatric Emergency Nurse (CPEN) Review IV

103) An 8-month-old ex-preemie with a history of chronic lung disease (Bronchopulmonary dysplasia (BPD)/Chronic lung disease (CLD)) presents to the ED in respiratory failure. He has good peripheral pulses, RR 68, HR 190. The ABG reveals pH 7.15, PCO_2 78, PO_2 52, Bicarbonate 26. The ED nurse interprets this ABG result as:

A) Metabolic acidosis

B) Metabolic alkalosis

C) Respiratory acidosis

D) Respiratory alkalosis

C – The ABG results indicate respiratory acidosis. Here is a quick and easy 2-step process to help with ABG interpretation. 1) Look at the pH. Is it normal (7.35 – 7.45), acidotic (< 7.35) or alkalotic (> 7.45)? This pH is acidotic (below 7.35), so the answer is "something" acidosis. 2) Is it metabolic or respiratory? Check which of the other values are out of whack? Is it the PCO_2 (respiratory) or the Bicarbonate (metabolic)? In this case the PCO_2 is way too high, so the answer is <u>respiratory acidosis</u>. Always read through the case scenario. This one specifically mentions the patient is in respiratory failure – that's a sure fire giveaway that we are looking for something respiratory!

104) A 14-year-old patient with a history of multiple chronic medical issues and severe developmental delay is in the ED with presumed sepsis. The assessment reveals diminished pulses, RR 32, and HR 142. ABG results are pH 7.15, PCO_2 35, PO_2 100, Bicarbonate 17. The ED nurse interprets this ABG result as:

A) Metabolic acidosis

B) Metabolic alkalosis

C) Respiratory acidosis

D) Respiratory alkalosis

A – The ABG results indicate metabolic acidosis. Here is a quick and easy 2-step process to help with ABG interpretation. 1) Look at the pH. Is it normal (7.35 – 7.45), acidotic (< 7.35) or alkalotic (> 7.45)? This pH is acidotic (below 7.35), so the answer is "something" acidosis. 2) Is it metabolic or respiratory? Check which of the other values are out of whack? Is it the PCO_2 (respiratory) or the Bicarbonate (metabolic)? In this case the Bicarbonate is too low, so the answer is <u>metabolic acidosis</u>. Always read through the case scenario. This one specifically mentions the patient has presumed sepsis, which is a clue that we are looking for something metabolic.

105) A patient's ABG results are: pH 7.37, PCO_2 37, PO_2 120, Bicarbonate 24. The ED nurse interprets this ABG result as:

A) Metabolic acidosis

B) Metabolic alkalosis

C) Respiratory acidosis

D) Normal blood gas

D – The ABG results indicate a normal blood gas. Here is a quick and easy 2-step process to help with ABG interpretation. 1) Look at the pH. Is it normal (7.35 – 7.45), acidotic (< 7.35) or alkalotic (> 7.45)? This pH is normal, so the answer is "normal blood pH." 2) Is it metabolic or respiratory? Check which of the other values are out of whack? Is it the PCO_2 (respiratory) or the Bicarbonate (metabolic)? In this case both the CO_2 and the Bicarbonate are both normal also. So our formula is "normal pH + normal CO_2 + normal Bicarb = Normal Blood Gas! Remember, you will most likely never get this type of question on the exam - why would they waste a perfectly good blood gas question asking you to identify a normal blood gas? But... if you know the normal ranges for pH (7.35-7.45), PCO_2 (35-45), and bicarbonate (22-26), and remember the above steps, you can conquer CPEN blood gas questions!

106) The emergency physician has indicated that she wants to use ketamine for a procedure on a child. The emergency nurse should plan care with the understanding that all of the following are commonly considered possible side effects of ketamine **except:**

A) Bronchoconstriction

B) Hallucinations

C) Hypersalivation

D) Laryngospasm

A – Bronchoconstriction is not commonly considered a possible side effect of ketamine.
Ketamine is a PCP derivative, and therefore causes hallucinations, vivid dreams or even delirium (which is why teenagers intentionally abuse it.) Some believe that if you give a pleasant suggestion to the patient as you are administering the ketamine they will have pleasant hallucinations - and vice versa. Most ED nurses have a tendency to talk sweetly and calmly to kids anytime we are doing a procedure or about to do a procedure to them. This may explain why some say that hallucinations are less common in kids. It is not necessarily that the hallucinations are less common, just nicer (like dreams) so they aren't reported. Some practitioners believe that the co-administration of Versed® (midazolam) can decrease the hallucinations, while others feel that this is an urban legend.

Ketamine can cause lots and lots of saliva (spit, goobers, etc.) and bronchial mucous so having suction (that works) is essential prior to administration. Suctioning the back of the throat is good, but remember to not go down the middle or swish the suction back and forth. That can stimulate the gag reflex, lead to a vagal response, and subsequently result in profound bradycardia (which is really bad.) Some practitioners believe that the co-administration of atropine or Robinul® (glycopyrrolate) can decrease the hypersalivation, while others feel that this is an urban legend as well.

Ketamine can cause laryngospasm and some practitioners believe this is more likely in kids, especially after rapid IV push administration versus the recommended IV push over 1-2 minutes. However, a review study looking at ketamine use in over 8,000 kids showed that the incidence was actually only 0.4%. Causality is either idiopathic (medical terminology for "we haven't a clue") or related to the increased secretions and an increased reactivity of the airway caused by ketamine. So keep the airway clear of secretions and this should reduce the risk. But as the bumper sticker says... "S#*! Happens!" So should laryngospasm happen to your patient, open the airway with a jaw thrust and bag, baby, bag.

After the downsides of ketamine, what else do I need to know? This is a question that certification exams love to ask. Ketamine is also a bronchodilator, and can relieve acute bronchospasm. It is often the drug of choice in unstable asthmatics, and may allow us to avoid intubation.

Pediatric emergency medicine and critical care attending physician insights: I would include myoclonic jerking: If you push it too fast this often happens and can be a little unnerving if you aren't aware of this as a side effect. Additionally, I always make sure that residents I work with realize the impact ketamine has on vital signs as well. It is a sympathomimetic causing increased HR and increased BP. Very rare, but a side effect that can happen in patients with poor cardiac function and minimal intrinsic catecholamine response – If you give ketamine to these patients they may arrest because their own intrinsic catecholamines can be depleted after giving ketamine. Just important to remember when choosing a med for sedation – I guess that's more of the physician's job to choose, I just think this is really interesting.

107) An 8-month old child with short gut syndrome and home IV total parenteral nutrition (TPN) presents to the ED because the current bag of TPN is almost empty. The delivery service has not delivered the next bags. Until a replacement bag of TPN can be obtained, which of the following orders would the nurse anticipate?

A) 500ml D50/0.9NS at maintenance rate

B) 500ml D10/0.9NS at maintenance rate

C) 500ml D5/0.9NS at maintenance rate

D) 500ml 0.9NS at maintenance rate

B – A continuous infusion of D10/0.9NS should be started in conjunction with close monitoring of blood glucose levels until a replacement bag of TPN can be prepared by the pharmacy. Total parenteral nutrition (TPN), by definition, means that the child's total nutritional needs are being met via the parenteral, (intravenous) route (typically via a PICC or other central line.) Dextrose concentrations in TPN are commonly up to 25%. If the infusion is stopped, hypoglycemia can quickly occur, especially in infants and young children. D10/0.9NS is obviously not the same as TPN, but in most cases it works just fine to keep the blood sugar at normal levels until "the real stuff" can be obtained. In the event of issues with the PICC or central line, then D10W/0.9NS can be administered via a peripheral IV line.

Our hospital pharmacy reminds us that there is no such thing as a STAT TPN order. Other medications… absolutely. TPN… not so much.

Pediatric critical care and emergency medicine attending physician insights: I would not run plain D10W for very long. If you only have 2 separate bags: One of D10W and one of 0.9NS - I would run them both until you can get a bag that contains both. D10W by itself is just asking for trouble.

108) A 10kg child presents with stable supraventricular tachycardia (SVT) and a heart rate of 238. The advanced practice nurse orders 0.1mg/kg of IV adenosine to be given. Which of the following is the correct dose of adenosine to be administered to this child?

A) 0.1mg

B) 1.0mg

C) 6mg

D) 12mg

B – 1.0mg is the correct dose. For the CPEN exam, it is important to be able to do basic medical math in order to calculate IV fluid boluses and maintenance IV fluid rates. The order for 0.1mg/kg means that the 10kg child should receive 1.0mg of adenosine. The adenosine should be administered via a rapid IV push followed by an equally rapid saline flush. For adults, 6mg and 12mg of adenosine are the common initial and subsequent adenosine doses. With few exceptions, children in emergency situations receive the same medications as their adult counterparts, but dosing, and decimal points really do make a difference!

Tips for the clinical side: Cool trick for administering IV adenosine – Adenosine comes 6mg/2ml in a vial. Mix the 2ml of adenosine with 4ml 0.9NS to make a 6mg/6ml concentration. In this example, the 10kg child will receive 1.0mg of adenosine, so the nurse will push 1ml of the solution.

Attending pediatric critical care and emergency physician insights: Although I realize this question is more about the math, it is also nice to point out that adenosine should be given as "centrally" as possible, so preferable IV placement would be in an antecubital area. Place a 3-way stop cock at the end so that meds and flush can be attached at same time, and then given one quickly after the other.

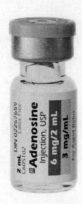

Adenosine 6mg/2mL

109) Intravenous fentanyl is ordered for a 20kg child with an open femur fracture. The dose ordered is 1mcg/kg. What dose of fentanyl should the emergency nurse administer to this child?

A) 20mcg

B) 20mg

C) 200mcg

D) 200mg

A – The ordered dose would be 20mcg. Basic medical math strikes again. But in this case, you not only have to figure out mcg per kilogram, but also recognize that micrograms (mcg) are very different than milligrams (mg.) Fentanyl is a medication that is ordered and given in mcg per kilogram. Morphine, on the other hand, is ordered and administered in mg per kilogram. Big difference in amounts! A 20kg child receiving 1mcg/kg of fentanyl SLOW IV push should receive 20mcg.

If "C" was looking like a good answer to you, it may be helpful to remember that fentanyl comes in 50mcg/ml concentration, and in order to administer 200mcg of fentanyl, it would require the nurse to draw up 4ml of fentanyl. That much volume should be a clue that it's probably way too much medication and you should double check the dose.

Tips for the clinical side: Cool trick for administering IV fentanyl – Fentanyl comes in 50mcg/ml concentration. Mixing 2ml (100mcg) of fentanyl in 8ml of 0.9NS results in a 10mcg/ml concentration. This tends to be much easier to calculate and administer with a 10ml or 1ml syringe to little ones.

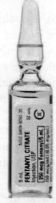

Fentanyl 50mcg/ml

Photo courtesy of Emergency Medical Products - www.buyemp.com

Certified Pediatric Emergency Nurse (CPEN) Review IV

110) Decadron (dexamethasone) 0.6mg/kg IM is ordered for a 10kg child with croup. What is the correct dose for the emergency nurse to administer?

A) 0.6mg

B) 6mg

C) 60mg

D) 600mg

B – At 0.6mg/kg, a 10kg child should receive 6mg. Depending on the concentration of the medication vial, this will commonly result in an IM volume dose of approximately 0.5-1.5ml of medication. If you are going to give what sounds and looks like way too much medication via a particular route, it probably *is* way too much medication and you need to double check your math, decimal points, and route of administration.

111) 0.1mg/kg intravenous Versed® (midazolam) is ordered for an intubated 25kg child in status epilepticus. What is the correct dose of midazolam to be administered to this child?

A) 0.25mcg

B) 0.25mg

C) 2.5mcg

D) 2.5mg

D – 0.1mg/kg for a 25kg patient results in a dose of 2.5mg of intravenous midazolam to be (slowly) administered to this seizing child. Adult emergency nurses may well tell you that the 2.5mg dose sounds like way too much "because we give 0.5mg to a 94-year old and the patient sleeps for three weeks!" Midazolam dosing for children, like many other medications, is dosed at mg/kg and this child should indeed receive 2.5mg to help stop the seizures. Regrettably, research shows that in pediatrics, non-anesthesia providers tend to dramatically underdose children when it comes to sedatives and analgesics. Medication in children is given on a "something per kilo" basis and if the numbers are correctly calculated, many of us may be surprised at the actual dosage that children should receive for seizures, sedation, and analgesics. It may be a bigger dose than we are used to! One drug dose does not fit all patients of all ages and sizes. Figure out the dose, administer the dose, and closely watch the child.

112) An 11-year-old patient presents to the emergency department complaining of a severe headache. He was recently diagnosed with idiopathic intracranial hypertension (pseudotumor cerebri.) The nurse understands that this patient is at risk for what major morbidity associated with idiopathic intracranial hypertension?

A) Diabetes

B) Permanent vision loss

C) Anemia

D) Chronic hypertension

B - Increased brain pressures, from idiopathic intracranial hypertension (pseudotumor cerebri) can lead to swollen optic nerves (papilledema) and in the worst cases can result in visual difficulties and even permanent vision loss. This is a disorder that presents with the classic signs and symptoms of increased intracranial pressure (ICP) including headaches, vomiting, visual changes, and papilledema. By definition, idiopathic means we don't know why it's happening and intracranial hypertension means high pressure within the cranium (not good for the brain and associated organs and nerves.) CT/MRI scans reveal no visible cause for the intracranial hypertension, but when a lumbar puncture is done (both for diagnosis and management of symptoms), the opening pressures reveal increased intracranial pressures. You've probably heard the saying that the eyes are the windows to the soul. Well, in this case, the retinas/optic nerves are the windows to the brain. For chronic cases of this condition, the most common medication treatment is Diamox® (acetazolamide), which is prescribed to help decrease the amount of spinal fluid being produced. Surgical intervention is rarely required if medications are effective, but is certainly an option in cases where medication isn't doing the trick.

113) A child with known Spinal Muscular Atrophy (SMA) Type II presents to your ED with tachypnea, mild nasal flaring, abdominal "see-saw" breathing, and room air saturations of 87%. The preferred treatment would be:

A) CPAP

B) BiPAP

C) Emergent intubation and ventilatory support

D) Immediate albuterol nebulizer treatment

B –Many times BiPAP and suctioning can get children with Spinal Muscular Atrophy (SMA) over their current respiratory "speed bump" and prevent intubation. This is important to recognize because, even more than our "adult COPDers," children with SMA are extremely difficult to wean from mechanical ventilation. SMA is an incurable autosomal-recessive disease and is the most common genetic cause of infant death. There is a mutation in the survivor motor neuron (SMN) gene that usually inhibits apoptosis or "cell death." The mutation results in the destruction of cells in the anterior horn of the spinal cord (motor neurons) and subsequent system-wide muscle wasting and atrophy. SMA manifests itself in various degrees of severity, all of which have general muscle wasting and mobility impairment symptoms in common. The disease spectrum is divided into several types, in accordance with either the age of onset of symptoms or the highest attained milestone of motor development. It is crucial to remember that SMA, like many neuromuscular diseases, only affects the muscles, and not the ability to see, hear, feel, or think. Children with SMA have brains that are fine; the problem is their muscles, and unfortunately this may affect their ability to communicate and tell you how they are feeling!

Type	Usual age of onset	Characteristics
I - Infantile	0-6 months	The severe form manifests in the first months of life, usually with a quick and unexpected onset ("floppy baby syndrome.") Rapid motor neuron death causes inefficiency of the major bodily organs - especially of the respiratory system - and pneumonia-induced respiratory failure is the most frequent cause of death. Babies diagnosed with SMA type I do not generally live past two years of age, with death occurring as early within weeks in the most severe cases (sometimes termed SMA type 0.) With proper respiratory support, those with milder SMA type I phenotypes, which account for around 10% of cases, are known to live into adolescence and adulthood.

II - Intermediate	6-18 months	The intermediate form affects children who are never able to stand and walk, but who are able to maintain a sitting position at least some time in their life. The onset of weakness is usually noticed some time between 6 and 18 months. The progress is known to vary greatly; some patients gradually grow weaker over time while others, through careful maintenance, avoid any progression. Body muscles are weakened, and the respiratory system is a major concern. Life expectancy is somewhat reduced, but most SMA II patients live well into adulthood.
III - Juvenile	>18 months	The juvenile form usually manifests after 18-months of age and describes patients who are able to walk without support at some time, although many later lose this ability. Respiratory involvement is less noticeable, and life expectancy is normal or near normal.
IV - Adult Onset	Adulthood	The adult-onset form (sometimes classified as a late-onset SMA type III) usually manifests after the third decade of life with gradual weakening of muscles – mainly affects proximal muscles of the extremities – frequently rendering the patient wheelchair-bound. Other complications are rare, and life expectancy is unaffected.

Pediatric emergency medicine and critical care attending physician insights: I usually like to try to start with BiPAP, but this requires very close monitoring of the patient's symptoms. Patients with SMA already have decreased muscle tone, and when they are in respiratory distress, their bodies are asking more of the primary respiratory muscles as well as the accessory muscles. BiPAP requires patient effort to be effective and SMA children may tire out more easily because of this.

114) Which of the following treatments should be anticipated when encountering a patient who is positive for smallpox?

A) Utilization of a Mark-1 Kit® (NAAK – Nerve Agent Antidote Kit

B) Multiple atropine boluses

C) Palliative care only as the patient will most likely not survive the hospital admission

D) Supportive care including IV fluids, antibiotics and antivirals

D - While prevention of smallpox infection is certainly preferred, if the patient is now in your ED with signs of smallpox, supportive care is where it's at. After a seven to seventeen day incubation period, the pox-like rash will start to form. The classic rash begins on the head and extremities (as opposed to chickenpox – which starts on the trunk) and is characterized by deep, firm, hard pustules or vesicles. The patient becomes contagious around day fourteen. While not curative, vaccination within three days of known exposure will significantly lessen the severity of smallpox. Management may include ventilator support, wound care and strict infection control measures. Though no medication is currently approved specifically for treating smallpox, studies have suggested that the antiviral drug used in the management of HIV retinitis, Vistide® (cidofovir), might be useful. Smallpox is transmitted via respiratory droplet during close contact, and is considered to be in its most contagious state during the first ten days of the rash. While palliative care (relief of pain) is indicated, the mortality rate is not anywhere near a certainty, but rather around 30%. Large doses of atropine are given for organophosphate (fertilizer) exposure and the Mark-1 kit® (a dual autochamber containing atropine sulfate and 2-PAM) is for nerve gas exposures only.

115) A 15-year old boy has fallen on his outstretched hand while playing soccer. When the wrist is examined there is no gross deformity, but he has mild pain with range of motion. Plain film radiographs are interpreted as normal without fracture. You re-examine the patient and decide to splint the child appropriately even without a fracture. Which physical exam finding would lead you to place a splint on this patient?

A) Mild tenderness in the mid-shaft of the radius

B) Abrasion to the palmar aspect of the hand with bruising

C) Tenderness in the anatomical snuff box

D) Pain at the elbow with hyperflexion of the wrist

C - Snuff box tenderness is critical to evaluate and document on any patient presenting with a wrist injury. The anatomical snuff box is a triangular region at the base of the thumb. Underlying the snuff box is the scaphoid bone (one of the small bones on the thumb side of the wrist.) What makes snuff box tenderness important is the fact that if there is a fracture of the scaphoid (causing the tenderness), blood flow might be cut off from the bone, leading to avascular necrosis. Scaphoid fractures are often diagnosed by X-rays, but not all fractures are apparent at first. Therefore, if there is tenderness over the anatomical snuff box, it is important to recognize this as a possible injury to the bone and splint it and then arrange follow-up with an orthopedic provider. The affected area should be splinted or casted (thumb spica or short arm) from seven to ten days, and followed up with another X-ray. When you hear snuffbox tenderness after a wrist injury, think splinting, follow up X-rays, and possible avascular necrosis (even if no visible fracture.)

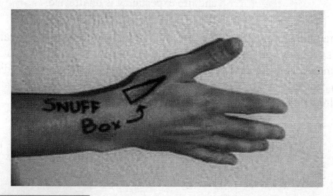

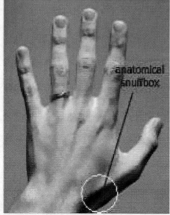

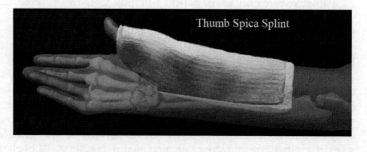

Scaphoid Bone Fractures and Spica Splint

116) Immediately after starting a school tour to the local peanut factory, a 7-year old is enroute to your ED with suspected anaphylaxis. HR 130, RR 36, sats 95% on room air with good peripheral perfusion. He is alert, but in moderate respiratory distress with audible wheezing bilaterally. Current recommendations as to the route for epinephrine (adrenaline) administration:

A) Subcutaneous (SQ)

B) Intramuscular (IM)

C) Intravenous (IV)

D) Intracardiac (IC)

B – Airway, adrenaline, and anaphylaxis! Unlike what many of us were taught in school, current data supports the use of IM epinephrine (this is now taught in PALS as well.) We used to think that the subcutaneous route was best; however, in a recent study it was found that serum epi levels peaked more quickly with IM administration – almost four times faster! Subcutaneous administration relies on blood flow to the skin, and in potential anaphylactic shock the peripheral perfusion might be compromised. In addition, think about epi's local vasoconstrictive properties – again, compromising blood flow to the skin. So here's the latest and greatest for epi and anaphylaxis – IM, not SQ is where it's at!

Pediatric emergency medicine & and critical care attending physician insights: If you are in a pickle to determine dose, although not an exactly accurate weight based dose…..I always just remember that the epi pen Jr. is 0.15 mg and the regular EpiPen® is 0.3mg……..pretty much the EpiPen Jr.® is given for any child < 30 kg because that is the only option as an auto injector.

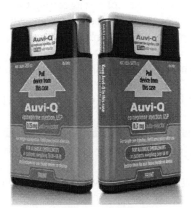

Auvi-Q Talking Epi-Pens

Photo courtesy of Sanofi-Aventis - www.auvi-q.com

117) After a recent outbreak of syphilis among teens, a concerned parent asks, "How exactly do you get syphilis?" The correct answer is:

A) Seats (toilet seats)

B) Soap (bars of soap)

C) Showers (not taking them)

D) Sex (self-explanatory)

D – Transmission of syphilis is through sexual contact, although infants may acquire congenital syphilis from their mothers during delivery. Contrary to urban legend, there is no evidence that syphilis is transmitted through fomites (inanimate objects such as toilet seats, towels, etc.) The use of soap or showering immediately before or after unprotected sexual activities in order to prevent sexually transmitted diseases (such as syphilis) is an urban legend as well. Diagnosis consists of index of suspicion, careful history taking, physical examination and serological testing. Treatment consists of specific types of penicillin depending on the stage/phase. Doxycycline or erythromycin are options for those with allergies to penicillin.

Controlling the spread of syphilis is a concern because people can have syphilis and not know it. Females, in particular, may not notice a problem, especially in the early stages. The first clinical manifestation occurs within three weeks of contact and usually is a painless ulcer at the site of the inoculation. Males are usually aware of this since it is readily noticeable. (Guys tend to notice anything red and icky on their penis pretty quickly.) However, on females it may go undetected since the painless lesions can be on the vulva or inside the vagina. At this stage the infection is called <u>primary</u> syphilis.

<u>Secondary</u> syphilis presents as a diffuse rash, fever, enlarged lymph nodes, and mucous patches. When primary and secondary stage symptoms disappear, syphilis enters a latent phase. During the latent stage, the patient is asymptomatic, but is serologically positive (detectable on blood test.) This latent, "hidden" stage can persist for years.

<u>Tertiary</u> (late) syphilis is not infectious and may affect any organ. Neuromuscular difficulties or CNS deficits such as dementia or altered mental status may be the most obvious signs of tertiary syphilis, and may occur as late as thirty years after the initial infection.

118) A 2-year old child brought in to ED during the warm summer months with complaint of stuffy nose and cough. The child is dressed in tank top and shorts. No obvious signs of respiratory distress are noted. However you do notice that the child has multiple bruises on shins, knees, and elbows, as well as on the chin and forehead. The bruises are various colors suggesting that they are in different stages of healing. A colleague working with you asks about reporting suspected abuse/non-accidental trauma (NAT) in this case. Which of the following would be the **most** appropriate response?

A) No – The parents brought the child in for a non-injury related complaint

B) No – The age and developmental stage of the child is consistent with the bruising noted.

C) Yes – Based on the number of bruises, it is reasonable to assume that abuse or non-accidental trauma has occurred

D) Yes – Based on the different stages of healing, the likelihood of parental misconduct is evident and reportable

B – Toddlers will be toddlers, and accidents will happen. This is where a basic knowledge of child development is important – what is normal for the age? Toddlers are in perpetual motion, and don't have great motor control yet. With active toddlers, it is very normal to have bruising anywhere they have bony prominences, such as knees, shins, elbows, chins and foreheads. Many toddlers are covered in bumps and bruises, from different times and places, because they never, ever stop moving.

That being said, remember the secret to real estate... location, location, location. You should be concerned if the child has bruising over abdomen, back, neck, axillae, or especially the inner thighs. Also be alert if you see identical bruising bilaterally or symmetrically, such as on both hips. Pay attention to patterning as well. Accidental injuries won't usually have a definite pattern. When an object forcefully comes into contact with the skin, blood is pushed out of the area of direct contact and into the surrounding tissue. The "pattern" results from the displaced blood.

Additionally, you should ask yourself – does the injury and the report make sense? Was a sibling blamed for the injury? Is the injury consistent with the developmental level of the child? Is the complaint (and/or the child's clothing) an attempt to "cover" things up?

If something doesn't fit ... whether history, physical exam, or just your gut, it's abuse/non-accidental trauma until proven otherwise and yes – it is your responsibility to report it!

Pediatric emergency medicine and critical care attending physician insights: I am a bit of a pessimist and always keep NAT on my differential when patients have multiple bruises, even if the pattern appears normal for the developmental stage… Up to 30 % of patients with NAT have been previously seen by a physician prior to the diagnosis of non-accidental trauma.

119) Which of the following statements about the Broselow™ Pediatric Emergency Tape is correct?

A) Patients with a suspected spine injury brought in by car seat can be measured in a seated position

B) Patients can be measured from "Nose to Toes" to determine correct color zone

C) The Broselow™ Tape can be used for pediatric patients up to 50 kg

D) The Broselow™ Tape can be used to provide weight-based groupings based on length

D – When used correctly, the Broselow™ Tape will do a really nice job of estimating body weight from the patient's length. Based on the color zone the child falls into, drug dosages and recommended sizes for some specific equipment (endotracheal tubes, suction catheters, mask, etc.) can be determined. On one end of the Broselow™ Tape is a big red arrow and remember "Red goes towards the Head!" Then you can measure to the patient's heels, not their toes. It's all about the Hs – "Head to Heels."

Don't be tempted by that other rhyme about noses and toeses. Think about it… if they point their toes like a ballerina, then they could possibly be bumped up into the next color zone. The tape is designed to be used with the child supine and not in a seated position and only works with children up to 36kg (79lb.) Just remember, red to the head and measure to their heels (not toes to nose.)

With the recent "epidemic" of obesity in children, a question that is frequently asked is "does the tape work with obese kids?" The Broselow-Luten tape suggests that users consider increasing <u>medication</u> doses to the next zone in children that "obviously don't fit." However, <u>equipment</u> sizes should remain consistent with the actual measured zone length/weight.

And as reminder, the Broselow™ Tape is NOT just for resuscitation/cardiac arrest medications and equipment. The Broselow™ Tape also addresses commonly encountered emergencies including:
- Seizures
- Rapid sequence intubation
- Toxicology/overdose
- Increased intracranial pressure
- Fluid management
- Initial ventilator settings
- Cardioversion/defibrillation joules

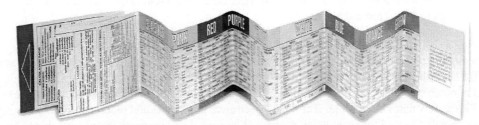

Broselow-Luten Pediatric Emergency Tape

Photo courtesy of Armstrong Medical

www.armstrongmedical.com

120) A 7-year-old child presents to the ED with a chief complaint of "my leg hurts when I walk" for the past two days. Upon physical examination, he is found to have tenderness over the right hip with no history of trauma. Vital signs are stable, and labs reveal a normal WBC, with a mildly elevated C-reactive protein (CRP) and erythrocyte sedimentation rate (ESR.) Comparative extremity X-rays show no fracture, but the radiologist does report a slightly wider joint space on the right hip. A preliminary diagnosis of transient synovitis or toxic synovitis is made. In addition to ultrasound or MRI and possible joint aspiration, the ED nurse would anticipate:

A) Referral to child protective services for evaluation of possible non-accidental trauma

B) Discharge home with anti-inflammatory medications and warm compresses

C) Admission to the hospital for intravenous analgesics

D) Orthopedic consult for spica hip cast placement

B – Transient synovitis is the most common cause of acute hip pain in children from 3-10 years of age. Transient means it is temporary, and it will go away. Synovium are the linings of the joints. The "itis" part of the word means inflammation. So this is an inflammation, usually viral, of the joint lining that in most cases will go away on its own (and usually within the week.)

It is important to differentiate between transient synovitis and septic arthritis, the latter being much worse! In both cases, the patient will have hip pain; but with a classic case of septic arthritis, the patient will not limp. They will be unable to bear ANY weight on the affected leg. Lab results of interest may include slightly elevated WBCs, CRP, and ESR with transient synovitis. With septic arthritis, those results tend to be much higher (It does have septic in the name after all.) Combinations of inability to bear any weight, fever, and markedly elevated ESR/CRP should lead one to think more towards septic arthritis vs. synovitis. Ultrasound and MRI can help with the initial diagnosis and ultrasound-guided joint aspiration can confirm the diagnosis and guide further management.

121) A 14-day-old infant with a distended abdomen and profound jaundice presents to the pediatric ED. In addition to checking the bilirubin levels, other anticipated laboratory studies would include all of the following **except**:

A) Blood cultures x 2

B) Coagulation panel (PT/PTT/INR)

C) Complete blood count (CBC)

D) Electrolytes with liver panel

A – Confession time… yes, this is sort of a trick question. While a single blood culture order might be anticipated, blood cultures x 2 is not a common order for a 14-day-old child. Moral of the story: Read the questions carefully and thoroughly!

Checking a CBC and electrolytes in addition to one blood culture is commonly done in any baby who is sick enough to present to the ED during the first month of life. Additionally, for a child who is specifically noted to have abdominal issues and jaundice (indicating the likelihood that something is not right with the liver,) remember to check the coags as well. This is especially important because as nurses, we want to stick kids as few times as possible. The CBC, electrolyte/liver panel and blood culture tubes are different than the one that is used for coagulation studies. Why stick a child more than once if you don't need to!

Pediatric emergency medicine and critical care attending physician insights: This a fair amount of blood to get from an ill and likely dehydrated baby. You may need to consider an arterial stick or a femoral venous stick by RN if allowed at your institution; if not, may need to be done by the nurse practitioner or physician.

Certified Pediatric Emergency Nurse (CPEN) Review IV

122) What is the correct amount for a 0.9NaCl fluid bolus for a 10kg child?

A) 10 ml

B) 20 ml

C) 100 ml

D) 200 ml

D – The formula to remember is 20 ml/kg as an initial fluid bolus. Want help to remember that? Count the child's fingers and their toes. How many should there be? 20. So it's 20 ml/kg for an initial fluid bolus.

123) What is the correct amount for a LR fluid bolus for a 25kg child?

A) 250 ml

B) 500 ml

C) 375 ml

D) 50 ml

B – 500 ml is a 20 ml/kg bolus of LR. It doesn't matter whether the fluid bolus is 0.9 NaCl or LR, the bolus amount should be 20ml/kg.

124) What is the correct amount of 0.9NaCl or LR for a fluid bolus for a 50kg child with a history of asthma?

A) 50 ml

B) 500 ml

C) 100 ml

D) 1000 ml

D – 1000 ml is a 20 ml/kg bolus of 0.9NaCl or LR. This question is trying to distract you with irrelevant information. Don't be distracted.

125) What is the correct amount of 0.9NaCL or LR fluid bolus for a 15-year-old 72kg child?

A) 150 ml

B) 720 ml

C) 300 ml

D) 1,440 ml

D – 1,440 ml is a 20 ml/kg bolus of 0.9NaCl or LR. Age is not usually a factor, so don't be distracted by another bit of irrelevant information. In reality, any honest ED nurse will tell you: 1) a 72kg child is a really big child and therefore 2) they just get "a liter, and if they are still shocky, they get another liter." Just make sure you can do the math if need be!

Certified Pediatric Emergency Nurse (CPEN) Review IV

126) According to the Neonatal Resuscitation Program (NRP) guidelines, what is the correct 0.9NaCl or LR fluid bolus for a 3kg newborn?

A) 3 ml

B) 30 ml

C) 20 ml

D) 60 ml

B – 30 ml of 0.9NaCl or LR is an appropriate fluid bolus for a 3 kg newborn. From day one in pediatric emergency care, we are taught 20 ml/kg, 20 ml/kg, 20 ml/kg… and for children, that is correct. However, for <u>newborns</u>, the neonatal experts teach that a little fluid goes a long way and you can always give them more (but it's difficult to take it back.) So, PALS is for pediatrics and teaches 20 ml/kg, but NRP is for newborns and teaches 10 ml/kg.

127) According to the Neonatal Resuscitation Program (NRP) guidelines, what is the correct 0.9NaCl or LR fluid bolus for a 500gm extremely premature newborn?

A) 5 ml

B) 10 ml

C) 20 ml

D) 500 ml

A – This very little baby only weighs ½ of a kilogram, so the 0.9NaCl or LR fluid bolus via the IV or umbilical line is only 5 ml! This question hopes to verify knowledge of two concepts regarding fluid boluses and newborns. First, the ability to change grams to kilograms and second, that fluid boluses for newborns (regardless of how small they are) are 10 ml/kg.

128) What is the correct amount of packed red blood cell (PRBC) for a shocky 10 kg child?

A) 1 unit

B) 250 ml

C) 200 ml

D) 100 ml

D – A 10kg child should receive 100 ml (10ml/kg) of packed red blood cells (PRBCs.) Remember, blood is thicker than water (saline or LR), so like newborns, a little goes a long way. For isotonic fluid boluses, such as 0.9NaCl or LR, the bolus amount is 20 ml/kg. But when it comes to packed red blood cells, the amount is 10 ml/kg.

Certified Pediatric Emergency Nurse (CPEN) Review IV

129) What is the correct packed red blood cell fluid amount for a shocky 100 kg child?

A) 100 ml

B) 200 ml

C) 1 unit

D) 1 liter

C – Even though the formula might say 10ml/kg, we need to remember those critical thinking skills. Consider that a 100 kg child is actually larger than many adults. At that size, in most cases, we treat them like an adult when it comes to fluid resuscitation and blood products. When it comes to packed red blood cells, just like adults, they "get a unit," and if they don't get better quickly, then they get "another unit." If the child is bigger than your color coded tape, consider them an adult for resuscitation!

130) What is the correct IV fluid maintenance rate for a 23kg child?

A) 23 ml/hr

B) 36 ml/hr

C) 20 ml/hr

D) 63 ml/hr

D – The correct rate for IV fluid maintenance for a 23kg child is 63 ml/hr. To calculate maintenance IV rates for children go by the classic the 4-2-1 rule:
>0-10kg: 4ml/kg/hr
>10-20kg: +2ml/kg/hr
>\>20kg: +1ml/kg/hr

And therefore:
>4ml/kg for first 10kg (10kg x 4ml/kg = 40 ml)
>2ml/kg for second 10kg (10kg x 2ml/kg = 20 ml)
>1ml/kg for the remainder of the weight (3 x 1ml/kg = 3ml)

For a total maintenance rate of 63 ml/hour

Here's a fun way to remember the 4-2-1 rule:
>The child should have 4 extremities. So the first 10kg are 4ml/kg.
>The next 10kg are half of that amount, so the next 10kg are 2ml/kg.
>The next 10 kg is half again, so for the kilograms over 20 kg, it is half of 2, or 1ml/kg.
>Put it all together, and the total rate for maintenance is 63 ml/hr.

Another way to remember the 4-2-1 rule is to think about a long day of playing golf.
>Start the game with yelling "Fore" (4), so the first 10kg are 4ml/kg.
>You get to play two (2) rounds of golf, so it's 2ml/kg for each of the next 10kg.
>After 2 rounds, you are ready for a frosty cold one (1), so it's 1ml/kg for each of the remaining kilograms.

4-2-1

Certified Pediatric Emergency Nurse (CPEN) Review IV

131) What is the correct IV fluid maintenance rate for a 17 kg child who has received 2 fluid boluses?

A) 17 ml/hr

B) 54 ml/hr

C) 170 ml/hr

D) 340 ml/hr

B – Maintenance fluids for a 17 kg child are calculated to be 54 ml/hour. Whatever method you may use to remember the 4-2-1 rule, remember it and use it. 40ml for the first 10 kg (4x10) and 14ml for the next 7 kg (2x7.) Oh yes, and it is a maintenance rate, so telling you about the bolus was, once again, a distraction.

132) What is the correct IV fluid maintenance rate for a 27kg, 5-year-old male child?

A) 67 ml/hr

B) 27 ml/hr

C) 270 ml/hr

D) 540 ml/hr

A – Maintenance fluids for a 27 kg child are calculated to be 67 ml/hour. Age and sex are important in many considerations, but not typically with maintenance fluid calculations in the emergency department.

133) What is the correct IV fluid maintenance rate for a 37kg child?

A) 370 ml

B) 77 ml

C) 67 ml

D) 740 ml

B - Maintenance fluids for a 37kg child are calculated to be 77 ml/hour. In this example, it is important to remember that the third part of the formula, 1 ml/kg is for every kg over 20. At 37kg, that means 40 (4x10) + 20 (2x10) + 17 (1x17.)

134) What is the correct IV fluid maintenance rate for a 3kg premature infant?

A) 3 ml/hr

B) 9 ml/hr

C) 12 ml/hr

D) 20 ml/hr

C - Maintenance fluids for a 3 kg child are calculated to be 12 ml/hour. Premature or not, it is still the 4-2-1 rule in the ED setting!

Certified Pediatric Emergency Nurse (CPEN) Review IV

135) EMS arrives with a 1-year-old who suffered full-thickness flame burns to his entire head and the front and back of his chest and abdomen. What percentage of body surface was burned?

A) 18%

B) 27%

C) 36%

D) 54%

D – The Rule of 9s teaches that there are two kinds of body parts: Little parts (worth 9%) and big parts (worth twice that amount – 18%). In adults, "little parts" include the arms and head and get 9%. "Big parts" include the entire front of the chest and abdomen or the legs and they get 18%. However, remember that children under the age of two have "big head, little body syndrome." So how much do they get for their big heads? 18%. The front of the chest and abdomen still comprise a big part, so we add another 18% for the front and 18% more for the back. Therefore, 54% is a good approximation of the percentage of the body burned. Burn centers teach that children also have "short little leg syndrome" and they only get 14% for their legs. However, for us in the ED where most of us don't take care of critically ill burn patients every day, simply remembering "big parts and little parts" is much easier. When the patient gets to the burn center, they can more accurately assess the burn percentage using the Lund-Brower chart or other methods.

136) Parents arrive with a 12-year-old who suffered full-thickness flame burns to his entire head. What percentage of body surface was burned?

A) 9%

B) 18%

C) 27%

D) 36%

A – Little children under the age of two have "big head, little body syndrome." However, by the time you are 12-years old, your body proportion has caught up with your head, so the head is no longer a "big part." So if the patient is 12 and the head is the only area burned, we would estimate that the burn covers 9% of the patient.

137) What percentage of body surface was burned in a 4-month old with ½ of their head sustaining deep partial-thickness burns?

A) 4½%

B) 9%

C) 18%

D) 27%

B – This child would be considered to have a 9% burn. At this age, the head is one of the "big parts" and is considered to be 18% for their body surface. This patient is burned on half of the head and half of 18% is 9%.

138) What percentage of body surface was burned in a 4-month old with ½ of their right arm sustaining deep partial-thickness burns?

A) 4½ %

B) 9%

C) 18%

D) 27%

A – This patient would be considered to have a 4½% burn. Whatever the age, an arm is considered a "little" part, or 9%. If the entire arm burn is 9% body surface area, ½ of a whole arm is 4½ %.

139) What is the percentage of body surface burned in a 14-year old with both forearms sustaining deep partial-thickness burns?

A) 4½%

B) 9%

C) 18%

D) 27%

B – An entire arm burn is 9% body surface area, so the forearm (½ of the whole arm) is 4½%. When both forearms are burned, you have 2 times the 4½%, or a total of 9% body surface burn. Arms are always little parts (9%) across the lifespan.

140) In conjunction with airway management and aggressive pain control, fluid resuscitation is vital for a burn patient's survival. Though not universally accepted, the Parkland formula is commonly used in prehospital and emergency department settings to determine the amount of fluids to be administered. Which of the following factors are used in conjunction with a constant (#4) to calculate the correct amount of fluid to give a burn victim in the <u>initial</u> 24 hours of treatment?

A) Age (in years to one decimal point) and % BSA (Body Surface Area) burned

B) Weight in Kg and Age (in years to one decimal point)

C) % BSA (Body Surface Area) burned and elapsed time from burn (in quarter hour increments)

D) Weight in Kg and % BSA (Body Surface Area) burned

D – The Parkland formula uses weight (Kg) and % BSA burn to calculate the fluid volume to be delivered in the first 24 hours. With kids (and in this case adults as well) everything is "something per kg" and the bigger the burn, the more fluid is needed. Age doesn't play a factor. We've all seen patients whose weights are far different than what we would suspect based on age. Quarter hour increments are not a factor in the amount of fluid to be given.

141) According to the Parkland formula, which of the following is the correct amount of fluid to give in the first 24-hours to a 5kg child who sustained 40% BSA burns?

A) 80 ml LR or 0.9NaCl

B) 800 ml LR or 0.9NaCl

C) 1600 ml LR or 0.9NaCl

D) 2000 ml LR or 0.9NaCl

B – A 5kg child with 40% BSA burns should receive 800 ml of LR or NaCl in the first 24 hours. The calculation is 4 (the constant) times 5 (the weight in kg) times 40 (the percent BSA burned). 4 x 5 x 40 = 800.

142) When determining the amount of fluid to be given to a burn patient, we use the Parkland formula to calculate the volume to be given in the first 24-hours. Once the volume is determined, how should the fluid be delivered?

A) Infuse $2/3$ of the volume over the first 12 hours and the remaining $1/3$ of the volume over the next 12 hours.

B) Infuse $1/3$ of the volume over the first 12 hours and the remaining $2/3$ of the volume over the next 12 hours.

C) Infuse ½ of the volume over the first 8 hours and the remaining ½ of the volume over the next 16 hours.

D) Infuse ½ of the volume over the first 16 hours and the remaining ½ of the volume over the next 8 hours

C - The Parkland formula divides the amount of fluid to be given in 24 hours into the first 8 hours and the next 16 hours. One-half of the total calculated fluids are given over the first 8 hours. The remaining amount is then given over the next 16 hours.

143) EMS is enroute with a 40kg child who sustained 30% BSA burns. Though the transport time is only a few minutes, the child was found nearly 4-hours post burn. Using the Parkland formula, which of the following represents the **most** appropriate plan for initial fluid administration? You have calculated that the child in the scenario above should receive 11, 250 ml over 8 hours (1400ml/hour) for the first 8 hours post-burn. However, if the child arrives in your ED four hours post-burn, what is the appropriate fluid rate?

A) 350ml/hour of LR or 0.9NaCl x 8 hours

B) 400ml/hour of LR or 0.9NaCl x 4 hours

C) 600ml/hour of LR or 0.9NaCl x 4 hours

D) 800ml/hour of LR or 0.9NaCl x 8 hours

C – The 40kg patient with 30% BSA burn should receive 4,800ml of LR or 0.9NaCl over the first 24 hours. The calculation is 4 (the constant) x 40 (kg) x30 (%BSA burned.) In addition to knowing the total amount, we need to remember that ½ of the fluid (2400ml) should be administered during the first 8 hours after the burn and the remaining ½ of the fluid (2400ml) should be administered over the following 16 hours. Last, but not least, we need to consider when the burn occurred. In this case, the patient will be arriving 4-hours after the burn occurred, so you now have only 4 hours to deliver the first 2400ml of fluid. Therefore, the initial rate of fluid administration would be 600ml/hr for the first 4 hours after arrival. You can give yourself extra credit if you have already figured out that after the first 4 hours at 600ml/hr, the rate would decrease to 150ml/hr for 16 hours.

When the patient doesn't arrive very soon after the time of the burn, or if access is delayed, you have to play "catch up." The clock starts when they got burned, <u>not</u> when they arrived at the ED. Sometimes we just have to do the math!

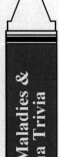

Certified Pediatric Emergency Nurse (CPEN) Review IV

Appendix 11-A: Intraosseous Medications

Excerpts from: 2017 The Science and Fundamentals of Intraosseous Vascular Access

Reprinted with Permission from Teleflex
www.teleflex.com

The infusates listed below were delivered via the IO route and referenced in clinical literature:

- Adenosine[1-6,62]
- Albumin[7,8]
- Alfentanil[9]
- Alteplase[10,11,12]
- Aminophylline[13]
- Amiodarone[13,14,15,16]
- Ampicillin[14,17]
- Anesthetic agents[18,19,20]
- Antibiotics[17,21,22,23,59]
- Antitoxins[24]
- Anti-meningococcal antitoxin[25]
- Anti-pneumococcus serum[25]
- Anti-tetanus serum[26]
- Atracurium besylate[9,27]
- Atropine[13,14,28,29]
- Aztreonam[14]
- Benzylpenicillin (Penicillin G)[59]
- Blood and blood products[7,13,14,18 26,29-33,59]
- Bretylium[34]
- Calcium chloride[14,32]
- Calcium gluconate[35]
- Cefazolin[21]
- Cefotaxime[22]
- Ceftriaxone[14]
- Centruroids (Scorpion) Immune F(ab1)2 (Equine) Injection (Scorpion Antivenom-trade: Anascorp®)[24,36]
- Cisatracurium besylate[37]
- Contrast media[29,38-42]
- Dexamethasone[29,32]
- Dextran[29]
- D5W[9]
- D5 ½NS[14]
- Dextrose 10%[14]
- Dextrose 25%[14]
- Dextrose 50%[13,14]
- Diazepam[34,43]
- Diazoxide[29]
- Digoxin[51]
- Diltiazem[14]
- Diphenhydramine[14]
- Dobutamine hydrochloride[14,21]
- Dopamine[13,14,45]
- Ephedrine[9]
- Epinephrine[13,14,31,59]
- Etomidate[13,14,46]
- Fentanyl[13,14,47]
- Flucloxacillin (floxacillin)[59]
- Fluconazole[14]
- Flumazenil[46]
- Fosphenytoin[14]
- Furosemide[13]
- Gentamicin7[14]
- Haloperidol[37]
- Hartmann's Solution (Compound Sodium Lactate Solution)[29,48,59]
- Heparin[14,15,29]
- Hydroxocobalamin[46,49]
- Hydrocortisone[19]
- Hydromorphone[14]
- Hypertonic saline/dextran (7.5% NaCl/6% dextran)[50]

- Insulin[14,51]
- Isoprenaline[9]
- Ketamine[14,19,47,52,59]
- Labetalol[37]
- Lactated Ringer's Solution[9,13,29]
- Levetiracetam[14]
- Lidocaine[13,14,29,30,56-58,60]
- Linezolid[14]
- Lorazepam[14,37]
- Magnesium sulfate[14,37]
- Mannitol[32]
- Methylprednisolone sodium succinate[14,37]
- Midazolam[13,14,21,59]
- Mivacurium[9]
- Morphine sulfate[14,32,47,53,59]
- Nalbuphine[9]
- Naloxone[13,14]
- Neostigmine[9,19]
- Norepinephrine[13,14]
- Normal saline[13]
- Ondansetron[14]
- Pancuronium[20,21]
- Paracetamol[9]
- Penicillin[21]
- Phenobarbital[14]
- Phenylephrine[14]
- Phenytoin[14,32,54]
- Piperacillin[14]
- Potassium chloride[37]
- Promethazine[13,14]
- Propofol[30,59]
- Recombinant fVIIa[59]
- Remifentanil[9]
- Rocuronium[13,14,30,52]
- Sodium bicarbonate[13,43]
- Standard IV solutions[13]
- Succinylated gelatin solution 4% (Gelofusine®)[55]
- Succinylcholine (suxamethonium)[9,13,27,43,52,59]
- Sufentanyl[46]
- Tenecteplase[15,28]
- Thiamine[13,14]
- Thiopental[27,32]
- Tobramycin sulfate[14]
- Tranexamic acid[18,61]
- Vancomycin[14,17]
- Vasopressin[13,14]
- Vecuronium[14,28,32,59]
- Vitamin K[7]

Appendix 11-B: Intraosseous Samples & Laboratory Results

Excerpts from: 2017 The Science and Fundamentals of Intraosseous Vascular Access

Reprinted with Permission from Teleflex
www.teleflex.com

Laboratory Analysis/Blood Sampling

Are Blood Specimens Drawn Via the IO Route Adequate for Laboratory Analysis?

The most recent clinical studies in healthy volunteers examining IO compared to venous laboratory values demonstrated significant correlation for many commonly ordered lab studies, with some exceptions noted. In these studies, IO blood proved to be reliable for:

- Red blood cell count
- Hemoglobin and hematocrit
- Glucose
- Blood urea nitrogen (BUN)
- Creatinine
- Chloride
- Total protein
- Albumin
- Lactate

Significant correlation was not achieved for sodium, potassium, CO_2, calcium, platelets or white blood cell count. However, sodium and potassium values were clinically similar. [See Laboratory Analysis/Blood Sampling from IO Access on this page for research details.]

From a review of all known published clinical literature examining IO compared to venous laboratory values, the list below summarizes aggregate results of IO correlation with IV blood values.

The following laboratory values have produced significant correlation between IO and IV values in human studies:

- Glucose
- Hemoglobin
- Hematocrit
- BUN
- Creatinine
- Total protein
- Red blood cell count
- Albumin
- Chloride

The following laboratory values have shown mixed results in producing significant correlation between IO and IV values (some values were clinically similar, but not statistically correlated):

- CO_2
- Potassium
- Sodium
- Calcium
- Platelet count
- Phosphorus
- Uric acid/urea
- Total bilirubin
- SGOT
- LDH
- Alkaline phosphatase
- Bicarbonate
- pH
- pO_2 (venous values)
- pCO_2 (venous values)
- Base excess

IO and IV values for white blood count do not correlate in any known study.

Laboratory Analysis/Blood Sampling from IO Access

Based on preclinical and clinical evidence comparing IO and venous or arterial sources a number of common laboratory values correlate well; other values show clinical similarity without statistically significant correlation, therefore caution should be exercised with their interpretation. Certain point of care analyzers have been studied with acceptable results. Check with your laboratory for IO specimen processing capabilities. For more information regarding IO lab analysis, refer to: www.teleflex.com/ezioeducation.

Summary and Recommendations

Overall review of the clinical evidence suggests that early in the resuscitation process, blood gas values derived from IO blood may be used to assess central venous acid-base status, and that a number of blood count and chemistry values will equal venous samples. Other values will approximate venous values; few will not correlate. IO samples should be used with caution after resuscitation efforts beyond the immediate phase. The work of Brickman et al. provides evidence that blood typing and screening can be done accurately and reliably using IO blood.[9] For a tabular summary of laboratory values that have produced statistically significant correlation between IO and IV in human studies, refer to previous section.

Clinical Studies

A small prospective pilot study by Tallman was published in 2016 using a point-of-care analyzer to compare samples from IO and venous samples in the emergency department. With consideration of the study limitations (small subject numbers, inability to obtain venous samples from some patients, limited testable analytes amongst those noted) investigators felt the results were clinically acceptable for pH, bicarbonate, sodium and base excess, and possibly lactic acid.[1]

A prospective study compared IO and venous laboratory values obtained from a point-of-care analyzer (i-STAT) in 20 children. IO blood specimens were collected from the iliac crest; 2 mL were discarded before the sample was collected for analysis. Results showed differences between venous and IO sample were clinically acceptable for pH, base excess, sodium, ionized calcium, and glucose in hemodynamically stable patients. Authors concluded that analysis of IO samples with a bedside point-of-care analyzer is feasible and in emergency situations may be useful to guide treatment.[2]

From a series of healthy volunteer studies conducted in 2012 and 2013, Montez et al. compared IO and venous blood to determine if there is a clinical similarity and/or correlation between samples from the two sources for serum lactate level. From each arm of 15 study subjects, peripheral venous specimens were collected, followed by a proximal humerus IO blood sampling. Each IO and venous sample was analyzed for lactate levels, using the I-Stat point-of-care analyzer. There was a positive correlation between IO blood lactate and venous blood lactate ($R^2 = 0.623$, $n = 23$, $p < 0.001$). Investigators concluded that lactate levels obtained from IO blood appear comparable to lactate levels from venous blood, and those values are reflected in positive correlation. The subjects in this study were healthy and results may not accurately reflect the results that may be seen in patients who are septic or have other illnesses and injuries. Further investigation is needed in patients to determine if the relationship between IO and IV values continues to exist in non-healthy patients.[3]

A 2009 study (unpublished) in healthy volunteers examined the reliability of IO cardiac enzyme and blood gas values.[4] The study compared venous and IO samples of two common cardiac enzymes (Troponin-I and creatine phosphokinase), and also compared venous, arterial and IO samples for blood gas analyses. Values for IO blood gases fell between arterial and venous blood sample values. Results demonstrated a significant correlation between venous and IO blood for creatine phosphokinase, and for pH and base excess. Arterial and IO blood correlated well for pCO_2. Correlation analysis was not possible for Troponin-I. However, results were identical or clinically similar for seven of the ten samples.

A study using adult volunteers conducted in 2009 examined the relationship between IO and venous blood samples for complete blood count and chemistry profile.[5] Researchers concluded that IO and IV laboratory values had statistically significant correlation for many commonly ordered lab studies, with some exceptions noted. The IO space proved to be a reliable source for red blood cell count, hemoglobin and hematocrit, glucose, blood urea nitrogen, creatinine, chloride, total protein, and albumin. No statistically significant correlation was achieved for sodium, potassium, CO_2, calcium, platelets or white blood cell count. However, sodium and potassium values were clinically similar. A 2000 study by Hurren examined IO blood samples for routine blood analysis in pediatric patients.[6] The laboratory values for hemoglobin, hematocrit, sodium, urea, creatinine, calcium were considered to be clinically similar. Potassium levels were elevated in most samples, and study authors recommended "great caution should be exercised in their interpretation." Authors also recommended that blood samples obtained intraosseously may give a useful guide to peripheral blood levels of some hematological and biochemical values, but cautioned the values should be "interpreted with care."

In 1994, Ummenhofer and associates found bone marrow and venous blood samples to be similar in regard to hemoglobin, sodium, chloride, glucose, bilirubin, BUN, creatinine, pH, and bicarbonate in 30 children with blood disorders.[7] IO blood was also moderately accurate for hematocrit, potassium, and total protein, but not for alkaline phosphatase, aspartate aminotransferase, alanine aminotransferase, thrombocytes, pCO_2, pO_2, and leukocytes.

In a 1991, 15-patient study, Grisham and Hastings reported that bone marrow aspirate from the iliac crest was a reliable source for blood gas and serum chemistries.[8] In a 28-patient clinical trial the following year, Brickman et al. compared IO aspirates against standard peripheral IV blood with regard to ABO and Rh typing.[9] Researchers concluded that IO blood can be used for accurate and reliable typing and screening of blood. Their study did not address whether IO blood can be used for cross-matching.

Preclinical Studies

In 1986, Unger and associates reported that electrolytes, calcium, glucose, BUN, and creatinine were not different in bone marrow and venous blood in swine.[10] In a 1989 canine study, Orlowski et al. compared blood laboratory values for IO, arterial, and venous samples. No significant differences were found among the three source sites for most blood electrolytes, chemistry values, and hemoglobin. Results for liver enzymes (lactate dehydrogenase, alkaline phosphatase) varied among the three sites. Blood gases were significantly different among all sites, pH, pO_2, pCO_2, HCO_3, and SpO_2 were consistently intermediate between arterial and venous samples, suggesting a possible correlation with arterialized capillary blood gases.[11] In the 1990s, Kissoon and associates conducted a series of swine studies to determine the relationship between IO and venous blood for determining acid-base values. In a 1993 study the authors reported that acid-base status of IO blood is similar to status of central venous blood, and may be an acceptable alternative to central venous blood gas values in determining central acid-base status during CPR.[11] In a 1994 study comparing pH and pCO_2 values of samples simultaneously obtained from central venous and IO lines, researchers concluded that pH and pCO_2 values were similar.[13] In a 1997 study, Kissoon's group compared the acid-base values of blood obtained through the IO route and mixed venous blood. The authors concluded that IO blood may reflect local acidosis, yield lower pCO_2 and higher pH values than central venous blood as CPR progresses.[14]

A 1999 study by Abdelmoneim et al. examined the acid-base status of blood samples from IO and mixed venous sites during prolonged CPR and drug infusions in swine.[15] The investigators found no difference in pH and pCO_2 levels during the first 15 minutes of CPR. However, this correlation did not continue during resuscitations of longer duration or after bicarbonate infusion. Large volumes of saline infusion and the use of epinephrine did not affect the association in resuscitation times under 15 minutes.

In another 1999 swine study, Johnson et al. found no differences in sodium, potassium, magnesium, lactate, and calcium levels in IO aspirates versus central venous blood samples during the first five minutes of CPR.[16] After 30 minutes, differences were noted in magnesium and potassium values, but the investigators observed no differences in biochemical (i.e. chemistry values) and hemoglobin values if no drugs were given though the intraosseous site.

In a 2011 preclinical study by Strandberg et al., IO and arterial blood samples were collected over a six-hour time period from the tibia of anesthetized swine and analyzed using an i-STAT device to compare values. Results showed compliant values between IO and arterial blood for electrolytes, hemoglobin, pH, and pCO_2. Lactate, base excess (BE), PO_2 and SO_2 were less compliant. There were high correlations between SO_2 and PO_2 although the levels in arterial blood were higher.[17] The same investigator published a 2012 preclinical study with a similar design collecting blood samples from bilateral tibial intraosseous cannulae and an arterial catheter over six hours using an i-STAT point of care analyzer. Authors noted analysis of intraosseous samples with a handheld cartridge based system is convenient and should bypass the potential problem with bone marrow contents damaging conventional laboratory equipment. For most variables, there seemed to be some degree of systematic difference between intraosseous and arterial results; and the direction of the difference seemed to be predictable. Investigators concluded that cartridge based point of care instruments appear suitable for the analysis of intraosseous samples. The agreement between intraosseous and arterial analysis seemed to be clinically useful.[18] In another swine study, several of the same investigators sought to evaluate whether intraosseous blood samples can be used to measure opioids, and if so, to determine the level of accuracy of those measurements. Blood samples were drawn from bilateral tibial IO catheters and from a central venous catheter for six hours. The morphine levels in the CVC samples were higher than those drawn from the IO sites; and authors postulated that morphine has low fat solubility and young swine marrow is rich in fat which may have contributed to the difference in levels. Between IO sites the variability between the two IO ports was less than 10%. The authors concluded intraosseous samples can be used for the analysis of morphine if an IV route is not available.[19] Eriksson et al. conducted a preclinical study in which eight anesthetized swine were put into an induced septic shock state to allow troponin I level measurements to be compared from serial venous plasma, arterial plasma, and intraosseous aspirate specimens collected hourly. Two milliliters of IO aspirate were discarded before collecting each IO specimen for analysis. The levels of IO troponin I increased during the first three hours of shock but then plateaued at a high level while the venous and arterial levels continued to increase. Authors concluded that troponin I can be analyzed in bone marrow aspirates in a shock model and that this information may be useful in medical emergencies where cardiac damage is suspected to be involved.[20]

In 2016 Eriksson compared arterial and intraosseous derived biomarkers to determine if the results would correlate well enough over a period of six hours to consider use of IO derived blood when traditional samples are difficult to obtain. Authors noted there were no clinically relevant average differences between IO and arterial samples for alanine aminotransferase, alkaline phosphatase, aspartate aminotransferase, creatinine kinase (CK), and gamma-glutamyl transferase values; and IO blood may be good enough for initial estimates of these markers in emergencies. However the lactate dehydrogenase levels showed less correlation and for certain tests, the precision of IO samples may be limited.[21]

In Strandberg's 2016 swine study IO and venous samples were analyzed for thromboelastography (TEG), prothrombin time (PT), activated partial thromboplastin time (APTT), and fibrinogen concentration. The IO samples were clinically hypercoagulable, rendering some samples unevaluable; clinically relevant differences were observed for APTT but not for PT and fibrinogen and the TEG demonstrated a shortened reaction time. The ability to use IO drawn blood for coagulation studies may be limited.[22] In 2016 a preclinical swine model study was conducted to compare blood samples drawn from a central venous catheter (CVC) to blood samples drawn from IO catheters. This pilot study had two objectives: determine how long an infusion must be stopped before drawing an IO specimen for analysis; and to determine if there is a difference between IO specimen results when the first 2 mL of IO blood were discarded and not discarded. An i-STAT Handheld point of care (POC) analyzer (Abbott Laboratories) was used to evaluate for sodium, potassium, chloride, TCO2, anion gap, ionized calcium, glucose, urea nitrogen (BUN), creatinine, hematocrit, and hemoglobin. All blood samples were drawn and placed into green top laboratory tubes containing sodium heparin and later the blood was placed into the sample cartridges for analysis. Once initial access was obtained, a baseline sample was obtained at approximately the same time from all access points. For a comparison of IO samples pre- and post- 2 mL discard, the initial 2 mL IO sample was aspirated; then a subsequent 2 mL sample was collected. For the post-infusion wait study, a five minute infusion of normal saline was started to the IO sites and then stopped. The initial post-infusion wait period was five minutes. Time intervals were reduced and results compared to baseline were similar with as little as one minute wait time. A target wait time of two minutes was chosen to stay similar to wait time recommendations in IV lab studies. Authors concluded that if IO vascular access is necessary, and POC samples requested for these specific lab values, the initial specimen drawn from the IO catheter may be considered for sampling. Also, if an IO infusion of saline is occurring, a wait time of two minutes post-stopping the infusion may be adequate for analysis. For these analytes, IO specimen values were comparable to CVC values. Limitations include swine model, sample size, and infusion of one solution. This study is not yet published.[23]

Technical Considerations

Most of the reported study data was based on IO laboratory specimens obtained prior to any infusions or flush, therefore results may differ from samples obtained post-infusions.

It is important to check with your laboratory for specimen processing capabilities. Blood samples for laboratory analysis can be drawn from the EZ-IO® Catheter by connecting a syringe directly to the EZ-IO® Catheter hub. (Note: the only times a syringe should be connected directly to an EZ-IO® Catheter hub is for drawing laboratory samples, for administration of medications that require very small fluid volumes for precise doses to infants and small children, or for catheter removal).

For most laboratory studies, the first 2 mL should be aspirated and discarded prior to withdrawal of laboratory samples. If necessary (e.g. pediatrics), the first 2 mL may be saved for certain tests, such as blood typing or blood cultures.[9,EO] Aspiration of

EO = Expert Opinion

adequate volumes for laboratory samples may vary greatly between patients; and IO blood samples clot more rapidly than venous samples. Therefore, samples should be prioritized in order of importance.

Consider drawing initial blood samples into smaller volume syringes, and placing them immediately into sample tubes. Point of care (POC) analyzers may more easily process IO samples (for available parameters) as they require less volume. Samples must be identified as IO blood so laboratory personnel can determine the suitability of equipment for IO blood lab processing; and accurately interpret results based on the possible presence of stem cells not found in peripheral blood; or cell counts that are known to differ between IO derived blood samples and those from arterial or venous sources.

Questions about the use of results from intraosseous access-derived blood samples were raised in 2008 in two editorial letters; and again in a 2014 letter by Cervinski. Nicoll mentioned possible incompatibilities between the available laboratory analyzers with IO blood that could result in blockage.[24] The recommendation was that laboratory tests only be carried out on either arterial or femoral venous samples during resuscitation. In a letter supporting use of IO derived blood samples, Dr. Salter responded with research supporting several laboratory parameters and stated IO samples were a "legitimate" technique that could guide care especially in consideration of the time delay in gaining venous or arterial access; and stated that IO samples should be appropriately labeled.[25] Cervinski's 2014 letter includes a brief review of the literature, discusses the limitations associated with studies on IO derived blood samples, and recommends IO blood may only be useful in cases of suspected overdose for toxicology.[26] A 2015 article discusses use of bone marrow aspiration fluid using automated blood cell counters and the potential advantages and limitations of this practice. Amongst the key points are bone marrow fluid can be used as a substitute for venous blood in emergency situations, at least for the measurement of red cell parameters; and the complexities of the comparison between the composition of blood aspirated from bone as "bone marrow fluid" compared to peripheral blood, for which most instruments were designed, create difficulties when assessing for hematology.[27]

Appendix 11-C

Alternative Methods for Pediatric Pain Management

Pain Relief Option	Onset (minutes)	Duration (minutes)	Approved Ages	Notes
1% buffered lidocaine & 25-30g needle (1ml 8.4% bicarb & 9ml 1% lidocaine to "buffer")	2-5	30-60	All	Remember max dose of lidocaine 4.5mg/kg without epi (max 300mg) & 7mg/kg with epi (max 500mg) 1% lido is 10mg/ml
EMLA® cream (lidocaine/prilocaine)	60-90	60-120	37+ weeks	Can cause methemoglbinemia Avoid ingestion (as with all topical creams) Dosage & application times differ dependent upon weight
LMX4® cream (lidocaine)	30	60	2+ years	Avoid ingestion (as with all topical creams)
Synera® patch (lidocaine/tetracaine)	20-30	60	3+ years	Don't cut or cover the patch
J-tip® (buffered lidocaine)	1-3	1-3	6+ months	Don't point near the face
"Freeze spray" (ethyl chloride)	Immediate	1	All	Possible frostbite with excess spray

Adapted from: Moisman, W. & Pile, D. (2013). Emerging therapies in pediatric pain management. Journal of Infusion Nursing. 102.

Appendix 11-D

Buzzy & Pediatric Pain Management

How to use BUZZY®... in healthcare settings

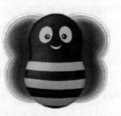
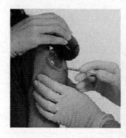
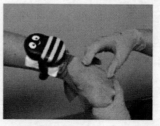

How Does Buzzy® work?

- Uses natural pain relief by confusing your body's own nerves and distracting away from the poke
  - This dulls or eliminates the pain
- Works in the same way as:
  - Rubbing a bumped elbow stops the hurt
  - Running water soothes a burn
  - Putting a hand in ice water lowers pain everywhere else

What procedures can I use Buzzy® for?

- Insertion of IV's
- Venipunctures for lab draws
- Finger sticks for obtaining blood samples
- IM injections to the upper arm
- SQ or Intradermal injection
- On shoulders, sternum, or distant body part for distraction from any procedure

Buzzy needs to go "between the brain and the pain" to be effective.

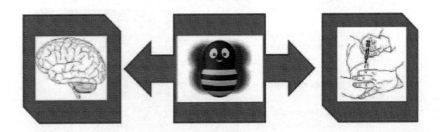

Courtesy of Shriner's Childrens Hospital
Louanne Lunny, MLS(ASCP)cm

IV placement and Venipuncture procedure

- Apply tourniquet if applicable
  - Through Buzzy slot or
  - Prior to placing Buzzy
- Place BUZZY® 2-5 cm proximal to site
- Place wider end of BUZZY® closest to pain. (Head of BUZZY® closer to patient's head during procedures)

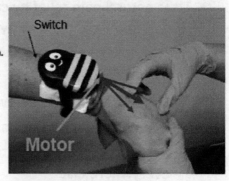

Best numbing is directly distal from the center of the Buzzy where the motor is.

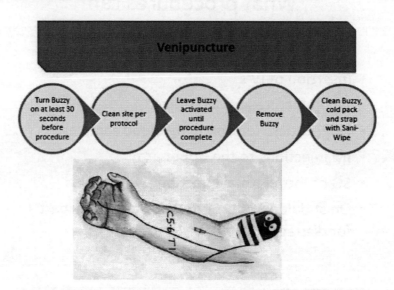

Courtesy of Shriner's Childrens Hospital
Louanne Lunny, MLS(ASCP)cm

Intramuscular Injections in Upper Arm

- Locate site
- 1) Press BUZZY® directly on site and activate vibration. Leave in place at least 30 seconds; for stinging shots or deeper IM, leave on up to 2 minutes for deepest numbing.
- 2) For injection, slide BUZZY® 2-5 cm proximal to site (pressing on bony area if available) for deltoid injections

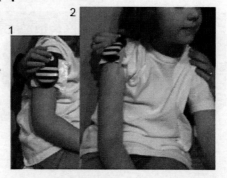

Parent pressing Buzzy using position of comfort. Shot goes where red dot is located. Nurse can reposition so Buzzy's motor is directly above shot.

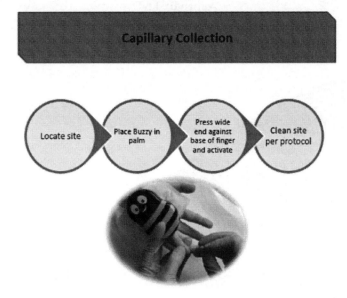

Courtesy of Shriner's Childrens Hospital
Louanne Lunny, MLS(ASCP)cm

 ## Who can use Buzzy®?

- Who can use Buzzy®?
  - Buzzy is an FDA registered Class I device (over the counter)
  - Since Buzzy is over the counter, anyone can use Buzzy.
    - A phlebotomist
    - Child Life
    - A radiology tech
    - A nurse
    - A resident

Certified Pediatric Emergency Nurse (CPEN) Review IV

Appendix 11-E
Hylenex for Subcutaneous Fluids and Medications

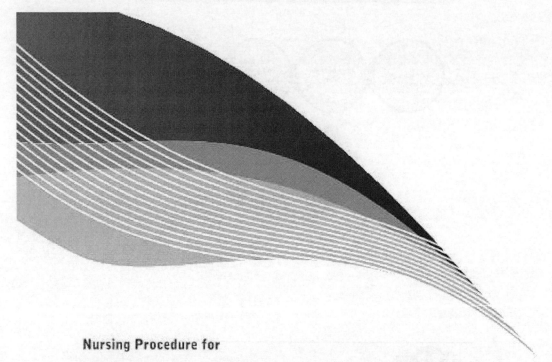

Nursing Procedure for

Initiating Subcutaneous Fluid Administration with *Hylenex*® recombinant (hyaluronidase human injection)

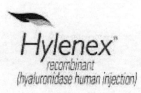

> These draft policies and procedures have been adapted from the Infusion Nurses Society (INS), the Oncology Nursing Society (ONS), and the *Hylenex®* recombinant (hyaluronidase human injection) prescribing information. It is the responsibility of the healthcare organization considering the use of this procedure to conduct an independent review and assessment to determine applicability and appropriateness of this document to their institution and to any particular clinical setting. Infusion therapies present risks; it is the responsibility of the healthcare organization to manage these risks, including the skills and competency validation of personnel.
>
> The healthcare organization that uses these guidelines should be aware that an annual review of organizational policies and procedures should continue to occur in accordance and compliance with regulatory and nonregulatory agencies.

The Purpose of This Guide

To outline nursing responsibilities in providing symptom control and/or fluid and electrolyte replacement by administering fluids subcutaneously.

Policy

Subcutaneous access is utilized to administer fluids via single injection or continuous infusion into the subcutaneous tissue. The fluid is absorbed through both adipose and connective tissue.[1] *Hylenex* recombinant is used for subcutaneous fluid administration, enabling enzymatically augmented subcutaneous infusion.

In subcutaneous fluid administration, a catheter is placed in the subcutaneous tissue.[1] Skilled and competent nurses knowledgeable in subcutaneous administration and the operation of electronic infusion devices may initiate and manage subcutaneous infusions.[1] Some state and facility regulations allow this procedure to be performed by LVNs/LPNs. Please check your state guidelines in regard to administration regulations. The nurse who is administering subcutaneous isotonic fluids and electrolytes should be knowledgeable about the indications for use, appropriate rates of administration, monitoring parameters, adverse effects, stability of infusate, storage requirements, and potential complications.

Fluids given subcutaneously should be isotonic.[2]

Recommended Equipment[1]	
Gloves	Tape
Appropriate antiseptic	Subcutaneous access device (see "Device Selection and Insertion" for options)
Sharps container	Subcutaneous infusion set
Syringe	Extension tubing (optional)
Gauze	Fluid
Transparent semipermeable membrane (TSM)	Electronic infusion device (optional)

Medication

Hylenex recombinant (hyaluronidase human injection)
(1 vial contains 1 mL of 150 USP units/mL)

Procedure

Assessing and Educating Patient[1]

1. Verify patient's identity with them or parent/legally authorized guardian.
2. Obtain and review physician's order for type of fluid, amount, rate, route of administration, frequency, duration, and titration parameters if applicable.
3. Plan patient's care.
4. Per institutional protocol, obtain consent of patient or his/her parent or legally authorized guardian before administering therapy.
5. Educate patient (or his/her parent or legally authorized guardian) as to purpose and anticipated outcome of therapy, site placement, type of fluid, route of administration, adverse effects, and recognition of signs and symptoms of complications. Also educate concerned parties on possible alternatives to this method of fluid administration and possible complications of the alternatives. Include device operation instructions, if applicable.
6. Assess patient according to facility guidelines.
7. Place patient in a reclining, comfortable position based on site selected.

Prior to Beginning Procedure[1]

1. Assemble equipment.
2. Wash hands and dry thoroughly.
3. Put on gloves.
4. Use aseptic technique and observe standard precautions.

Procedure (Cont'd)

Insertion Site Selection
1. Site selection should be based on patient's anticipated mobility and comfort.[1]
2. Assess sites for device placement in pediatric and adult patients[1]:
   a. Scapula region
   b. Anterior or lateral aspects of thighs
   c. Dorsal aspect of upper arm
3. Select insertion site with adequate subcutaneous tissue (a fat fold of at least 1 inch or 2.5 cm when forefinger and thumb are gently pinched together).[1]
4. Avoid areas with compromised integrity, such as, but not limited to[1]:
   a. Edema
   b. Pain
   c. Excoriation
   d. Infection
   e. Bruise or hematoma
   f. Scar tissue

Insertion Site Preparation[1]
1. (Optional Step) Remove excess hair from intended insertion site with clippers or scissors.
2. Wash insertion site with antiseptic soap and water, if necessary.
3. Disinfect insertion site.
4. Cleanse site and allow site to dry. (Do not blow or blot dry.)

Device Selection and Insertion

1. The recommended catheter is a standard 25-gauge butterfly needle. However, 20- to 24-gauge angiocatheters have also been used. Inspect access set for defects.
2. Prepare equipment and prime infusion set.
3. Lift skin into small mound.[1]
4. Insert infusion set/catheter bevel up into prepared site.[1]
5. Secure device and follow facility protocol for dressing.
6. Observe for negative blood return. If blood return is observed[1]:
    a. Remove device and select new insertion site
    b. Prepare new site
    c. Use new sterile infusion set
7. Secure administration-set tubing to skin to prevent accidental dislodgment.[1]
8. Label dressing per facility guidelines.

INFUSE

Hylenex recombinant Administration

Injection before fluid administration:

After obtaining Sub-Q access, inject *Hylenex* recombinant via Sub-Q access device before initiation of fluid administration. Once *Hylenex* recombinant is injected, follow with a 3-5 cc injection of hydration fluid (ie, normal saline or Lactated Ringer's) into the Sub-Q access device to ensure *Hylenex* recombinant is fully administered into the Sub-Q tissue. 150 USP units of *Hylenex* recombinant will facilitate absorption of 1000 mL or more of solution.

Procedure (Cont'd)

Subcutaneous Fluid Administration

The rate and volume of subcutaneous fluid administration should not exceed those employed for intravenous infusion. During subcutaneous fluid administration, special care must be taken in pediatric patients to avoid overhydration by controlling the rate and total volume of the infusion.[4]

1. Deliver isotonic solutions subcutaneously.[2]
2. Inspect fluid container for leaks, cracks, or particulate matter.[1]
3. Initiate fluid administration per physician's orders and monitor patient response.
4. Monitor patient's response and observe for complications at insertion site at regular intervals per facility guidelines.
5. Rotate site per facility policy.
6. Document subcutaneous administration of fluids per facility guidelines.

For Premature Infants/Neonates

For premature infants or during the neonatal period, the daily dosage should not exceed 25 mL/kg of body weight, and the rate of administration should not be greater than 2 mL per minute.

Site Maintenance[1]

1. Observe site per facility policy.
2. Follow facility policy for catheter/needle replacement.
3. Replace catheter/needle if bruising, erythema, or other signs of local irritation or infection appear or if the site is painful to the patient.
4. Change transparent dressing according to facility protocol.
5. Clients, families, significant others, and assistive personnel should be instructed to report any leakage, erythema, edema, or pain at the injection site as soon as possible. Consult the facility's processes and procedures for specific directions.

Device Removal[1]
1. Obtain and review the physician's order for infusion discontinuance.
2. Wash hands.
3. Assemble equipment.
4. Put on gloves.
5. Use aseptic technique and observe standard precautions.
6. Place patient in comfortable position.
7. Clamp administration and stop infusion device.
8. Remove transparent dressing and securement tapes.
9. Remove administration set, activating safety mechanism (if applicable); discard in Sharps container.
10. Apply manual pressure with sterile gauze to prevent bleeding and fluid leakage.
11. Cover site with dry dressing.
12. Discard expended equipment in appropriate receptacle(s).

Documentation
Document the following in the patient's permanent medical record:
a. Date and time of administration
b. Skin integrity and location of access device
c. Number of insertion attempts and location of infusion set

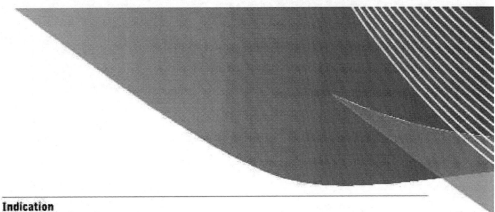

Indication
Hylenex® recombinant is indicated as an adjuvant in subcutaneous fluid administration, and to increase the dispersion and absorption of other injected drugs.

Important Safety Information
- Hypersensitivity to hyaluronidase or any other ingredient in the formulation is a contraindication to the use of this product.
- Discontinue *Hylenex* recombinant (hyaluronidase human injection) if sensitization occurs.
- Hyaluronidase should not be used to enhance the absorption and dispersion of dopamine and/or alpha agonist drugs.
- Hyaluronidase should not be injected into or around an infected or acutely inflamed area because of the danger of spreading a localized infection.
- Hyaluronidase should not be used to reduce the swelling of bites or stings.
- Hyaluronidase should not be used for intravenous injections because the enzyme is rapidly inactivated.
- Furosemide, the benzodiazepines and phenytoin have been found to be incompatible with hyaluronidase.
- Anaphylactic-like reactions following retrobulbar block or intravenous injections have occurred, rarely.
- Hyaluronidase should not be applied directly to the cornea.

The most frequently reported adverse experiences have been local injection site reactions, such as erythema and pain. Hyaluronidase has been reported to enhance the adverse events associated with co-administered drug products.

Patients receiving large doses of salicylates, cortisone, ACTH, estrogens or antihistamines may require larger amounts of hyaluronidase for equivalent dispersing effect, since these drugs apparently render tissues partly resistant to the action of hyaluronidase.

Edema has been reported most frequently in association with subcutaneous fluid administration. The rate and volume of subcutaneous fluid administration should not exceed those employed for intravenous infusion. As with all parenteral fluid therapy, use the same precautions for restoring fluid and electrolyte balance. Special care must be taken in pediatric patients to avoid overhydration by controlling the rate and total volume of infusion. When solutions devoid of inorganic electrolytes are given subcutaneously, hypovolemia may occur.

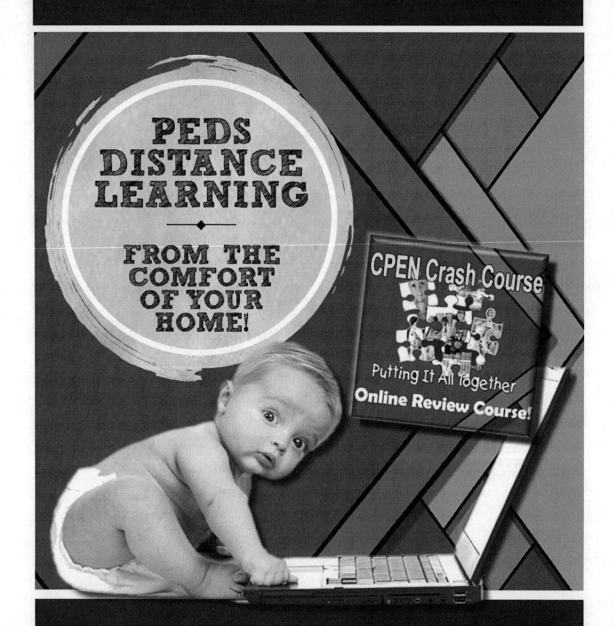

CHAPTER 12

So New... Who Knew? Even More Pediatric Potpourri

Make no mistake about why these babies are here - they are here to replace us.
- Jerry Seinfeld

When your first baby drops her pacifier, you sterilize it. When your second baby drops her pacifier, you tell the dog: 'Fetch!'
- Bruce Lansky

Pertinent Pediatric Ponderings (NOTES)

Certified Pediatric Emergency Nurse (CPEN) Review IV
CHAPTER 12
Sample Test Answer Sheet

1. _____	30. _____	59. _____	88. _____	117. _____
2. _____	31. _____	60. _____	89. _____	118. _____
3. _____	32. _____	61. _____	90. _____	119. _____
4. _____	33. _____	62. _____	91. _____	120. _____
5. _____	34. _____	63. _____	92. _____	121. _____
6. _____	35. _____	64. _____	93. _____	122. _____
7. _____	36. _____	65. _____	94. _____	123. _____
8. _____	37. _____	66. _____	95. _____	124. _____
9. _____	38. _____	67. _____	96. _____	125. _____
10. _____	39. _____	68. _____	97. _____	126. _____
11. _____	40. _____	69. _____	98. _____	127. _____
12. _____	41. _____	70. _____	99. _____	128. _____
13. _____	42. _____	71. _____	100. _____	129. _____
14. _____	43. _____	72. _____	101. _____	130. _____
15. _____	44. _____	73. _____	102. _____	131. _____
16. _____	45. _____	74. _____	103. _____	132. _____
17. _____	46. _____	75. _____	104. _____	133. _____
18. _____	47. _____	76. _____	105. _____	134. _____
19. _____	48. _____	77. _____	106. _____	135. _____
20. _____	49. _____	78. _____	107. _____	136. _____
21. _____	50. _____	79. _____	108. _____	137. _____
22. _____	51. _____	80. _____	109. _____	138. _____
23. _____	52. _____	81. _____	110. _____	139. _____
24. _____	53. _____	82. _____	111. _____	140. _____
25. _____	54. _____	83. _____	112. _____	141. _____
26. _____	55. _____	84. _____	113. _____	142. _____
27. _____	56. _____	85. _____	114. _____	143. _____
28. _____	57. _____	86. _____	115. _____	
29. _____	58. _____	87. _____	116. _____	

CHAPTER 12
Sample Test Answer Sheet

144. _____	173. _____	202. _____
145. _____	174. _____	203. _____
146. _____	175. _____	204. _____
147. _____	176. _____	205. _____
148. _____	177. _____	206. _____
149. _____	178. _____	207. _____
150. _____	179. _____	208. _____
151. _____	180. _____	209. _____
152. _____	181. _____	210. _____
153. _____	182. _____	211. _____
154. _____	183. _____	212. _____
155. _____	184. _____	213. _____
156. _____	185. _____	214. _____
157. _____	186. _____	215. _____
158. _____	187. _____	216. _____
159. _____	188. _____	217. _____
160. _____	189. _____	218. _____
161. _____	190. _____	
162. _____	191. _____	
163. _____	192. _____	
164. _____	193. _____	
165. _____	194. _____	
166. _____	195. _____	
167. _____	196. _____	
168. _____	197. _____	
169. _____	198. _____	
170. _____	199. _____	
171. _____	200. _____	
172. _____	201. _____	

Certified Pediatric Emergency Nurse (CPEN) Review IV

1) A 12-year old with a history of severe developmental delay and cerebral palsy presents unresponsive, hypotensive, and with minimal respiratory effort to the ED. Upon rapid initial physical exam, she is found to have a small round metal device implanted under the skin of her lower abdomen. Her parents indicate the device is a Baclofen pump used to help manage her spasticity. The initial priority is:

A) Establishing an airway with ventilatory support

B) Administration of IV/IO Narcan (naloxone)

C) Disabling and preparing for surgical removal of the Baclofen pump

D) Labs for a full toxicology screen and initiation of the facility's child abuse/endangerment protocol

A - This is an example of a complicated question with an uncomplicated answer. Remember your ABCs! Airway, airway, with a side of airway. The most important part of the child's presentation is the minimal respiratory effort. That means she's barely breathing. So, picking an answer that reflects having a patent airway and adequate breathing is a great choice.

But, what about beyond the ABCs... *What are the Basics of Baclofen?*

Spasticity involves tight, stiff muscles that make movement, especially of the arms and legs, difficult or uncontrollable. It happens when there is an injury to a part of the brain or spinal cord that controls voluntary movements. Baclofen is a derivative of gamma-aminobutyric acid (GABA) and more importantly, is a muscle relaxant with anti-spasticity effects. In children with spasticity from cerebral palsy, multiple sclerosis, or spinal cord injuries, oral Baclofen is commonly tried first. However, when the oral route doesn't bring about the desired effects or produces too many undesired side effects, the intrathecal "spinal" pump has been found to achieve good results.

The Baclofen pump continuously administers the medication directly into the spinal canal which not only treats the issue at the site but allows for a much lower dose. The intrathecal dose of Baclofen is 100-1,000 times **less than** the oral dose. Wow! But, as such, a little difference in dose can make a big difference in symptoms. Baclofen does cross the blood-brain barrier and the associated symptoms of toxicity or withdrawal are actually very similar to opiate overdose or withdrawal.

Too much Baclofen (muscle relaxant) results in children who are way too relaxed. So relaxed, in fact, that they may be unconscious and not breathing very well, if at all. Too little Baclofen results in children who are not nearly relaxed enough and leads to serious spasticity or seizure activity.

In this case, management of presumed Baclofen toxicity first involves what can be immediately treated. Start with "ABC" which means maintaining a patent airway, assistance with breathing, and circulatory support with fluids, pressors, etc. Then, once the ABCs are addressed, steps can be taken to temporarily disable and drain the pump. This is important, but not as important as airway management.

Narcan works great for opiate overdoses, but does not work for Baclofen overdoses. Obtaining labs may be helpful, but should never come before the ABCs, and nothing in this presentation indicates that there would be a high level of concern regarding abuse or maltreatment.

And always remember with healthcare ABCs, *Breathing comes before Baclofen*!

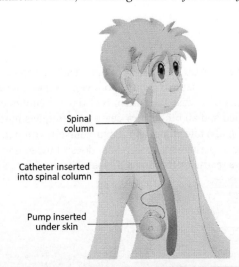

Pediatric Potpourri

2) Which patient would be the best candidate for the application of a tourniquet?

A) 1-year old male with uncontrolled bleeding to the lower leg

B) 5-year old female with uncontrolled bleeding below the knee

C) 9-year old male with uncontrolled bleeding from a groin injury

D) 13-year old female with a deep thigh injury that is controlled with direct pressure

B – The 5-year old patient (regardless of gender) would be the best candidate, even with an injury near the knee. While tourniquets should not be applied directly over joints, the tourniquet can be applied above the knee for this patient.

The 1-year old is likely too small for a commonly available adult tourniquet to be effective and therefore, packing the wound and/or direct pressure would be more appropriate. The 9-year old has a groin injury and a traditional extremity tourniquet would not be able to be applied. The bleeding on the 13-year old patient is being controlled with direct pressure and therefore a tourniquet is not required.

3) You are providing care to a 5-year old with massive bleeding to the right upper leg after being hit by a car. The primary and initial way to help control bleeding in this patient is to:

A) Apply direct pressure to the wound

B) Apply a tourniquet

C) Press on the femoral artery

D) Stabilize using a splint

A – While tourniquet application is appropriate for children and found to be safe, in this question, it was asked what the primary/initial way would be to stop the bleed. Direct pressure should be initiated while someone else obtains and applies a tourniquet.

4) When applying a tourniquet to a child in order to control massive hemorrhage, it is important to:

A) Ensure you don't totally occlude bleed flow

B) Not cause additional pain to the injured extremity

C) Tighten until all the bleeding stops

D) Use only in uncontrolled arterial bleeding

C - Tourniquets are designed to stop ALL blood flow to the area, and can be applied to any major bleed on the extremities. Indications for tourniquet use include both venous and arterial bleeding. All bleeding must stop, not just the venous bleeding, otherwise the patient is at risk for continued hemorrhage. It is important to note that when properly applied and all blood flow ceases, tourniquets hurt! A lot! If you have taken the Stop the Bleed course and have had a tourniquet applied to yourself, you will never forget this. They hurt. But temporary pain is preferable to permanent death. Pain doesn't mean that it was applied incorrectly or it's not working, it just hurts. Be ready for this and anticipate the need for pain meds.

Certified Pediatric Emergency Nurse (CPEN) Review IV

5) While doing community outreach at a local high school, a teacher asks you if, in an emergency, an improvised tourniquet should be used to stop bleeding. Which of the following would be the **most** appropriate response?

A) It would depend on what you were using. Belts are not generally effective, but a necktie, if available, is recommended

B) No, those only work in the movies. They should never be attempted on someone who has massive bleeding

C) They may be effective. You could try it, but it would be best to have a backup plan in case it doesn't work

D) While you may hear about an improvised tourniquet working, research shows these are not reliably effective at controlling bleeding

D – The American College of Surgeons does not recommend the use of improvised tourniquets. The key here is the word "improvised." While it is possible these could work, it is risky to try. They may stop some bleeding, but not all the bleeding. It may be tight enough to cut off venous bleeding (great), but not tight enough to stop arterial bleeding (not so great). If you do not have a commercial tourniquet available, it's best to apply direct pressure and pack the wound if appropriate. Applying an improvised tourniquet can waste valuable time and has been shown NOT to be effective.

6) "Stop the Bleed" is an international program designed to teach the lay public the skills necessary to provide potentially lifesaving treatments in an emergency. This is based on the fact that:

A) Active shooter incidents are a leading cause of injury

B) If someone helps and has not been properly trained, they are legally at risk

C) Many EMS systems have slow response times

D) Uncontrolled bleeding is the leading cause of preventable death after injury

D – Uncontrolled bleeding is the leading cause of preventable death after injury, so being able to stop life-threatening bleeding can be incredibly important. While active shooter incidents are a horrible tragedy, they are not a leading cause of injury. There are many far more common causes of pediatric injuries, including falls, automobile vs. pedestrian collisions, and motor vehicle crashes. These can all cause life-threatening bleeding, which is the leading cause of preventable death after injury. This bleeding can occur within minutes, meaning someone needs to be able to provide immediate assistance while EMS is en route. "Stop the Bleed" saves lives!

7) If a teen is driving at 55 mph (89 kph) and takes her eyes off the road for five seconds to read/respond to a text message, how far has she traveled during those five seconds?

A) 1 yard (0.9 meters)

B) 25 yards (23 meters)

C) 50 yards (46 meters)

D) 100 yards (91 meters)

D - Five seconds of texting while driving translates to over 100 yards of driving essentially with your eyes closed. That's more than the length of a football field. Wow! A lot can happen in that much space. Texting while driving causes a 400 percent increase in time spent with eyes off the road. Of all cell phone related tasks, texting is by far the most dangerous activity. In fact, texting while driving is six times more likely to cause an accident than driving drunk.

The following is reprinted with permission from *DigitalResponsibility.org*

Teens are the age group at the highest risk for texting-related accidents. On average, teens are the most inexperienced drivers out there, and they are also the most addicted to texting. That can be a lethal combination.

The risks:

- Want to become 23 times more likely to crash with just the flick of a finger? Text while driving. A Virginia Tech Transportation Institute study of commercial drivers revealed that texting while driving was the riskiest type of driver distraction, making drivers 23 times more likely of getting into a "safety-critical event." (Virginia Tech Transportation Institute (VTTI) 2009)

- If you are driving at 55 mph and take your eyes off the road for the average amount of time it takes to text, five seconds, you will have zoomed the length of a football field without looking at the road. (VTTI) 2009)

- The CDC reports that a distracted driver was a factor in 18% of all injury-causing accidents in 2010.

- The 2012 NHTSA study on distracted driving classified drivers as "distraction-prone" or "distraction-averse." Fewer than half of respondents under 35 qualified as "distraction averse," while the majority of those over 35 fit that category.

- According to the VTTI, teens are four times as likely to get into crashes or near misses due to cell phone distractions than older drivers.

The following is reprinted with permission from *ArriveAliveTour.com*

Texting While Driving Facts for Teens

- 40% of teens say they have been a passenger in a vehicle where the driver was texting and driving.

- Every day, 11 teens die from texting while driving accidents.

- According to a AAA poll, 94% of teen drivers acknowledge the dangers of texting and driving, but 35% admitted to doing it anyway.

- A teen driver with only one additional passenger doubles the risk of getting into a fatal car accident. With two or more passengers, they are five times as likely.

- Teen drivers are four times more likely than adults to get into car crashes or near-crashes when talking on their cell phone or texting while driving.

- Of all the teen drivers involved in fatal accidents, 21% of them were distracted by their cell phones.

- Peer pressure? 90% of teens expect a response to their text message within five minutes, so if someone is driving and gets a text, then they feel the need to respond quickly and texting while driving issues arise.

- 75% of teens say their friends text and drive.

- 77% of teens say their parents text and drive.

Certified Pediatric Emergency Nurse (CPEN) Review IV

8) A 3-year old is being discharged from outpatient surgery after a tonsillectomy. A common, easy-to-follow, recommendation for Tylenol® (acetaminophen) and/or Motrin® (ibuprofen) pain medication dosing is:

A) Alternate Tylenol® every 6-8 hours and Motrin® every 4-6 hours prn for 3 days

B) Alternate Tylenol® and Motrin® every 3-4 hours around the clock for 3 days followed by alternating every 3-4 hours prn

C) Alternate Tylenol® every 6-8 hours and Motrin® every 4-6 hours for 3 days followed by the same dosing prn for 10 days

D) Alternate Tylenol® and Motrin® every 3-4 hours around the clock for 3 days beginning 7 days post-op

B – Alternating Tylenol® and Motrin® every 3-4 hours around the clock for 3 days followed by alternating every 3-4 hours prn is a very common recommendation for children post-tonsillectomy. This type of question requires careful analysis and thorough reading of all of the options that seem to be overflowing with numbers. Options "A" and "C" have the normal frequencies reversed and would require a complex schedule of administration and the question does suggest that the answer would be "easy to follow."

It should be easy to rule out option "D," as decades of studies have shown that babies and kids, just like adults, feel pain and should receive appropriate post-op analgesics right away (not a week post-op). Pediatric tonsillectomy is one of the most common pediatric surgical procedures performed and it is also one of the <u>most painful</u>. With that in mind, here are a few things to help ensure the kids (and parents) post-procedure experiences are much more pleasant:

- Remember, pain is expected, especially during the first week post-op. For most children, the pain is gone by 2-3 weeks. The day after surgery is bad, but the next 2-3 days tend to be even worse. That's really important for parents to know. After 3 days, the honeymoon phase kicks in and the pain tends to get a whole lot better. But right around the corner are days 7-10 when the scab falls off. Though usually not nearly as painful as the initial post-op period, when the scab falls off, it can hurt, and it's important for parents to know about, and anticipate, this second period of pain.

- The throat is not the only place that hurts! Ear pain, especially with swallowing, is common. This is not due to an ear infection, but is referred pain from the surgery.

- For the first few days after surgery, Tylenol® and/or Motrin® are recommended. In many cases, especially for the first day or two, some sort of liquid narcotic analgesic is prescribed as well. When it comes to Tylenol® and/or Motrin®, many ENT surgeons recommend these medications be alternated and given every 3 hours around the clock for 3 days. That translates to each medication every 6 hours, which is a very good combination/compromise between Tylenol® which is commonly given every 4-6 hours and Motrin® which is commonly given every 6-8 hours. Trying to calculate medication times is difficult enough in the best of times, and even worse by a stressed parent. To help with these situations, some facilities now have templates for a variation of the "Tylenol®/Motrin® Clock." This way, when a parent is home at 3 AM, they don't have to try to remember what med to give. They can just look at the clock. The clock helps with avoidance of accidental "overdoses" as well.

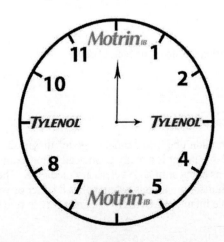

- Drink, drink, and then drink: Not surprisingly, post-tonsillectomy kids don't want to drink because their throat hurts. But dehydration is what will really get these kids into trouble. So, many ENT surgeons simply recommend that whatever the kid will drink (as long as it's not red in color) is great. Can they have all the juice they want? Sure. (Apple or white grape are probably your best bets because it's a good idea to avoid orange or grapefruit as the citrus juices may hurt). Can they have all the ice cream they want? Sure. Can they have all the non-red popsicles they want? Sure. Can they have all the Kool-Aid, or even better, Gatorade, they want? Sure. Can they have all the slushies they want? Sure. If it melts to a liquid at room temperature and it's not red in color, go for it!

- Medicate before you hydrate: Giving the child pain meds 30-minutes or so prior to trying to eat or drink just makes sense.

- Cold packs on the neck and/or forehead can be helpful for throat pain, while a heating pad on the ear can be helpful for referred ear pain.

Did you know that tonsillectomies have been performed for over 3,000 years? Wow! We can be pretty sure that they hurt a lot back then, and we know that they hurt a lot now. But, if you can keep the pain under control and keep the patients drinking (anything cool and not red), you're helping make the situation more tolerable.

Additional Insights from a Pediatric Post-Anesthesia Care Unit (PACU) & Peds ER Nurse: There are several other CPEN questions and rationales that specifically address post-tonsillectomy bleeding. For the test, but more importantly, for your patients, please, please remind parents that "anything more than a teaspoon" of bleeding is worth an immediate call to 911 or a trip to the ER. This is one time that it is far better to overreact than to wait. Post-op tonsillectomy bleeding is one of anesthesia's nightmare scenarios. Scared kid + stomach full of swallowed blood + potential hypovolemia from blood loss and poor PO intake + active bleeding in the same place they want to place an endotracheal tube = the perfect storm for an airway nightmare!

9) An infant has been brought in by parents due to being "inconsolable" for several hours. When considering the mnemonic, "IT CRIES." what does the "C" stand for?

A) Colic

B) Cold

C) Cardiac disease

D) Colon distention

C – The mnemonic, "IT CRIES" can be helpful when evaluating the inconsolable child. The mnemonic stands for:

    I = Infections

    T = Trauma

    C = Cardiac disease

    R = Reaction to meds, reflux (gastric), or rectal fissure

    I = Intussusception

    E = Eyes

    S = Strangulation, surgical processes

Colic is always a possibility, but shouldn't be the automatic "go to" diagnosis – you might miss something important! The key to an inconsolable infant is a really good head to toe examination. Remember that caring for babies has best been described as being similar to veterinary medicine. The patients are unable to verbalize and can't describe what hurts, how it feels, what makes it better or worse, etc. Crying is their only language. So in a truly inconsolable infant, "IT CRIES" is a great way to rule out reasons why "IT CRIES!"

Pediatric Potpourri

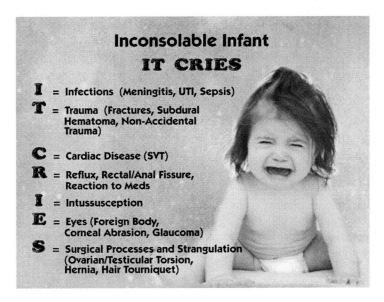

TIM'S CRIES from Life in the Fast Lane (litfl.com)

T - Trauma (accidental and non-accidental injuries) and bites (e.g. insects), tumours

I - Infections (otitis media, herpes stomatitis, urinary tract infection, meningitis, osteomyelitis)

M - Maternal/ parental stress, anxiety or depression

S - Strangulation (hair/fiber tourniquet)

C – Cardio-respiratory disease

R - Reflux, reactions to medications, reactions to formulas, rectal (anal fissures)

I - Intracranial hypertension, immunizations, intolerance of lactose or cow's milk allergy

E - Eye (corneal abrasions, ocular foreign bodies, glaucoma, retinal hemorrhages)

S - Surgical (volvulus, intussusception, inguinal hernia, testicular torsion)

10) In the emergency nursing care of a child with Duchene's Muscular Dystrophy, the priority assessment should be:

A) Deep tendon reflexes

B) Pulmonary function

C) Cardiomegaly

D) Swallow study

B – Pulmonary failure is a primary driver of morbidity in patients with Duchene's Muscular Dystrophy (DMD). Care should be centered on assessing and providing adequate support for their ability to breathe. Deep tendon reflexes are lost in these patients at an early age and will no longer be a useful assessment tool once the child is confined to a wheelchair. While cardiac complications, including cardiomyopathy and cardiomegaly are a significant concern and increasingly a primary cause of death for these patients, airway (and breathing) is the greater priority in the emergency department. These children will eventually have decreased oral intake necessitating a gastronomy tube, but a swallow study is not a priority assessment in the ER. Remember, the American Lung Association slogan... If you can't breathe, nothing else matters!

11) A 16-year-old male with a history of Duchene's Muscular Dystrophy presents to the emergency department. After the initial assessment is complete, the patient is found to have suffered a right ulnar fracture as a result of falling out of his wheelchair. In preparing for procedural sedation, special consideration must be given to avoid:

A) Cardiac arrest

B) Hypotension

C) Hypothermia

D) Respiratory arrest

D – In this special population, respiratory considerations are of vital importance, and BiPAP or CPAP are the preferred ventilatory support options in cases of procedural sedation with Muscular Dystrophy. As one of the biggest concerns with Muscular Dystrophy is respiratory failure, and one of the biggest concerns with procedural sedation is respiratory depression, picking an answer that involves respiratory is probably a good choice.

12) While providing care for a patient with Duchene's Muscular Dystrophy, you note an apparent nutritional deficiency, a state of uncleanliness, and a lack of consistent and ongoing medical care. Child Protective Services should be called due to a suspicion of:

A) Neglect

B) Physical abuse

C) Emotional abuse

D) Sexual abuse

A – Neglect is defined as the lack of attention to basic needs required to sustain life or health of the child. While the different types of abuse are always matters of concern, there is nothing in this scenario that points in that direction. Physical abuse results in substantial physical harm to the child secondary to injuries sustained as a result of assault. Emotional abuse is an observable and material impairment in a child's growth, development, or psychological functioning. Sexual abuse is unwanted sexual contact or activity, with perpetrators using force, making threats, or taking advantage of victims not able to give consent.

13) A patient with confirmed Duchene's Muscular Dystrophy is found to have a Creatinine Kinase (CK) of 35,000 IU/L. Normal lab value is 60 IU/L to 180 IU/L. Appropriate medical treatment to correct this value includes:

A) Lactated Ringers (LR) 20 mL/kg per hour until corrected

B) Normal Saline (NS) 20 mL/kg per hour until corrected

C) Plasmalyte 20 mL/kg per hour until corrected

D) No action is needed

D – Duchene's Muscular Dystrophy (DMD) involves the progressive atrophy/destruction of muscular tissue. An elevated Creatinine Kinase (CK) is a diagnostic tool to help confirm the diagnosis of DMD. Unfortunately, attempts to "flush it out" with IV fluids do not work and there is no corrective action currently available to reverse these extremely high CK levels.

Certified Pediatric Emergency Nurse (CPEN) Review IV

14) Hypotension in children 1-10 years of age is defined as:

A) Systolic BP < 70 + (2x age in years)

B) Systolic BP < 90 + (2x age in years)

C) Systolic BP < 70 + (4x age in years)

D) Systolic BP < 80 + (2x age in years)

A - When it comes to blood pressures, adults are easy as we're taught that hypotension is anything less than 90 mm Hg. But when it comes to kids, it's not that simple. The classically taught peds formula for minimum acceptable systolic blood pressure is 70 + (2x age in years). For the CPEN exam, that's the answer. But honestly, midway through a hectic, stressful shift, who wants to depend on remembering this? Why would you try to remember that formula when there are cheat sheets and apps that remind you what normal vitals are for various age groups? So for real life: 1) Don't stress over memorizing formulas; 2) Use a cheat sheet or app; 3) Check the feet... if the feet are pink, warm, and happy, chances are the child is pink, warm, and happy.

15) Signs of possible fluid volume overload in children include all of the following **except**:

A) Crackles/rales

B) Hepatomegaly

C) Extremity edema

D) Hypotension

D – Hypotension is not a sign of possible fluid overload in pediatric patients. In fact, just the opposite is true. Fluid volume deficit, like hypovolemic shock, is evidenced by hypotension. But, what about the opposite situation in which a child has way too much fluid? Then, just like adults, all that fluid has to go somewhere. In children, the extra fluid tends to go is the lungs, liver, and eventually the extremities. If there is extra fluid in the lungs, crackles/rales, can be heard on auscultation, and imaging (through X-ray or, even faster, through ultrasound), can show signs of too much fluid. Beyond the lungs, one of the easiest and earliest ways to find extra fluid is to feel the liver. Outside of liver failure, palpating a big, congested, swollen liver (hepatomegaly) is an early sign of heart failure and/or volume overload. Later, just like adults, the fluid will find it ways to the extremities and eventually everywhere else. But long before there is 4+ pitting edema of the legs, listen to the lungs and feel the liver. To determine if a child is dehydrated with poor perfusion, feel their hands and feet. Just as with adults, poor perfusion means that the blood that is available goes to the core (heart, lungs, and brain). It is shunted away from everywhere else, notably the hands and feet. Assessment of a child's hands and feet are a great non-invasive way to evaluate perfusion without any fancy formulas, numbers, or monitors.

16) Which of the following represent current pediatric fluid bolus recommendations for poor perfusion with no rales or hepatomegaly?

A) Push a 20mL/kg isotonic fluid bolus over 5-10 minutes and reassess/repeat up to 60mL/kg total in first hour

B) Push a 10mL/kg isotonic fluid bolus over 5-10 minutes, and reassess/repeat up to 40mL/kg total in first hour

C) Place on an IV pump and infuse a 10mL/kg isotonic fluid bolus over 1 hour

D) Place on an IV pump and infuse a 20mL/kg isotonic fluid bolus over 1 hour

A – A handy tip that we have shared over the years is that when it comes to fluid boluses and kids, "count their fingers AND their toes, there hopefully should be 20 of them, so a fluid bolus is 20 mL/kg." After the first bolus, if perfusion is still crummy, then reassess and repeat up to two more times. If the child still looks crummy after the third bolus, they probably need something else. That something else depends on the situation. If its trauma, think blood products. If you suspect sepsis, pressors make sense.

Normally, when giving IV fluids to a kid, we instinctively put everything on a pump as we don't want to give way too much fluid accidentally. This is generally a good idea, but the problem is that in a "shocky" kid, running a pump at 999 mL/hour (the fastest it will go), may not be fast enough to give the fluids needed. This is especially true with hypotension when we really want to give a fluid bolus immediately. Consider using push-pull with a syringe and stopcock or using a pressure bag (extra advantage – frees up your hands!). There are also rapid infusion devices on the market, such as the Life Flow, that will also work for the really sick patient.

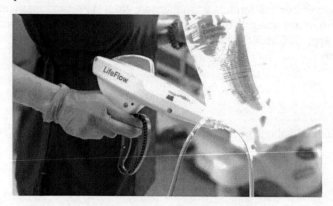

LifeFlow Fluid Resuscitation Device
Image courtesy of 410 Medical
www.410medical.com

17) Which of the following **best** describes the group of patients for which video laryngoscopy equipment is currently available and recommended?

A) Newborns to adults

B) 4-years of age and older

C) 20 kg or greater

D) 32 kg or greater

A – Video laryngoscopy is available and recommended for all ages. Think about automatic external defibrillators (AEDs) for a minute. Remember when all we had available was adult-size pads and the only people that we could use the AED on were adults? After a while, it was determined that we could use the AEDs (with the adult pads) on children 8-years old and older. Then we moved on and could use the AED on kids 1-year old on up. And now, AEDs are okay for any age. The same idea now applies to video laryngoscopy (VL), which, per many airway experts, is the preferred method of intubation for ALL age groups.

These video scopes not only provide a clearer view of the airway and with some practice improve first-pass success, but also have the advantage of allowing others to simultaneously view the screen to confirm tube placement or help with tasks like suctioning. They can also allow more experienced colleagues to "coach" trainees to the right spot. Taking that one step further, many of these scopes now allow for screen shots and video recording of the intubation, providing images which can be included in the medical record. In court, when there is a question as to where a tube was placed, if a picture is worth a thousand words, a video is worth a million!

You may have read somewhere that with pediatric patients; seemingly everything is something per kilo. You may have seen it once or twice in this book. Important for medications, but not so much when it comes to whether or not you can use video laryngoscopy (or an AED).

18) Your patient has presented to the Emergency Department with a lower airway foreign body obstruction. Which of the following is the **most** acceptable intervention when ventilation is unable to be achieved?

A) Intubation and positive pressure ventilation in the hope it will force the item deeper and out of the way

B) Continuous blind deep tracheal suction until the obstruction clears

C) Continue to make removal efforts with Magill Forceps

D) Intubation and positive pressure ventilation in the hope it will force item up and out of the airway

A – This is an emergent, last-ditch effort to achieve ventilation in an aspiration case where a lower airway foreign body obstruction is about to become the cause of death. This is obviously not an ideal intervention, but it can provide a means to ventilate one good lung while stabilizing the child and preparing for a bronchoscopy in the operating room to remove the foreign body.

Foreign body aspiration is not an uncommon issue in children, especially in those 1 to 3 years of age. These little ones are very mobile and still quite low to the ground where they can find all sorts of things. Not only do they find things, but they tend to put everything they find into their mouths. And in addition to non-food items, it's important to remember that these young ones don't yet have molars, so food may be not chewed completely. Of note, over 3,000 children die every year from foreign body aspiration, and food products (peanuts, hot dogs, etc.) are the most commonly aspirated objects.

The basic intervention in an aspiration event is the abdominal thrust, previously known as the Heimlich maneuver, a term which is no longer used per Dr. Heimlich's own request. The abdominal thrust has been around for many years and in many cases, really does work. If it is unsuccessful, then removal with Magill forceps may be attempted if the foreign body is able to be visualized.

Unfortunately, aspirated foreign bodies lodge in a bronchus in 80-90% of cases. In this particular question, we are told specifically that ventilation is not possible; you can't make air go in and out. That makes this a very different story. Given this situation, where nothing else has worked to remove the obstruction, intubation, bagging, and hoping the foreign body goes deeper into one lung is the best answer. The majority of children have two lungs and can live with only one, especially if just for a short time. Rigid bronchoscopy can then be performed in the operating room to remove the foreign body and allow breathing with both lungs to resume. Remember, the American Lung Association motto reminds us... If you can't breathe, nothing else matters!

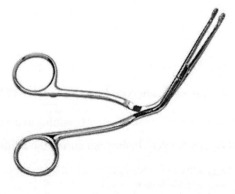

Pediatric Magill Forceps

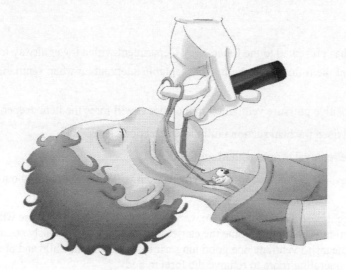

Removal of airway foreign body with Magill forceps

19) Which of the following interventions can **best** help to improve oxygenation during an emergency intubation situation?

A) High-flow O_2 via nasal cannula before the intubation

B) High-flow O_2 via non-rebreather mask during the intubation

C) High-flow O_2 via non-rebreather mask before the intubation

D) High-flow O_2 with a non-rebreather mask before and a nasal cannula throughout the intubation

D – Originally utilized with adult patients, the technique of providing high-flow O_2 with a non-rebreather mask before and a nasal cannula throughout the intubation is now also used with pediatric intubations. The goal is to allow as much oxygen as possible to be given to the patient before oxygen delivery is interrupted during the intubation attempt(s). The more oxygen reserve they have, the more time is allowed when trying to successfully place the artificial airway.

So, what does this involve? Placement of a non-rebreather mask with high-flow O_2 has been done for years, but when the laryngoscope goes in the mouth, the mask must get out of the way. Recently a relatively big change has involved not only using a non-rebreather mask, but also placing (*and leaving*) a nasal cannula in place before and during the intubation procedure. It doesn't get in the way of the intubation procedure and allows some oxygen to continuously flow downstream while intubation is being attempted. Again, the more oxygen your patient has equals more time to find the airway.

A useful acronym to remember this is "ENTAPS"

"Emergency Nurses Train And Practice Safely" (ENTAPS)

E - Elevate the head of the bed 30 degrees (Provides better breathing and better visualization of airway.)

N - Nasal Cannula High-flow (Oxygen delivery before and during the intubation.)

T - Two People Bagging (Unless you are anesthesia, have one person place and hold the mask on the face and the other person gently squeeze the bag.)

A - Alternate Airways (Nasal airway, oral airway, or one of each. That means at least two holes are patent and makes bagging with air going in and out much easier.)

P - PEEP (Use a bag-mask with a PEEP valve set at 5 cm. This helps to keep the bagged airways open.)

S - Suction (Suction that actually works with a big catheter like a Yankauer, Ducanto®, etc.)

20) For tracheal intubation, what is the primary difference between an intubation stylet and a bougie?

A) Bougies are flexible, while stylets are stiffer

B) Bougies are stiff, while stylets are more flexible

C) Bougies are always blue, while stylets are always white

D) Bougies only are available in adult sizes, while stylets are available from baby to big people sizes

A – Bougies are more flexible than stiffer stylets, which will bend and hold the bent shape. Though used by anesthesia for over 70 years, the gum elastic bougie has now become an essential part of the airway tool kit, especially in the adult Emergency Department. These devices may at first glance look relatively similar to a stylet, but they are completely different devices with different purposes. Intubation stylets are typically metal, relatively stiff but bendable, and placed inside of an endotracheal tube to allow the bending of the tube to the desired shape prior to intubation.

When using stylets, it is crucial to remember a few key points:

- Stylets can be very helpful, but as they are made of metal, they can cause injury to the airway.

- The stylet should be placed nearly, but NOT all the way though the endotracheal tube (ETT). The goal is to add stiffness to the endotracheal tube so that it can be easily guided to the right place, aka., the trachea. But, if the stylet is advanced too far into the ETT, then the metal will stick out of the bottom end of the tube and can easily cause trauma to the airway during intubation. Once the stylet is advanced to the correct depth into the tube, it is suggested to "bend it" (like Beckham) in <u>two</u> places. First, at the top of the tube, as bending the stylet will help prevent the stylet sliding down even further through the tube or through the tube and into the lungs. The second bend is near the bottom of the tube where the cuff begins. At that location, an additional 30-degree bend is recommended. Once the tube is placed in the trachea, remember to HOLD THE TUBE when removing the stylet. Otherwise when you pull out the stylet, you will pull out the tube as well. Not a good two for one special!

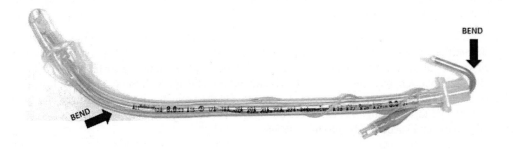

Stylet and ETT resulting in "hockey stick" shape

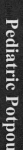

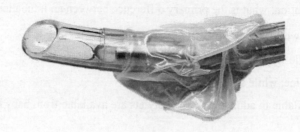

Stylet in proper position
NOT protruding past the tip of the ETT

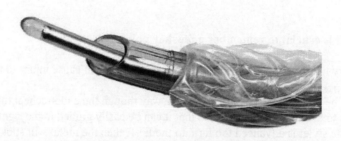

Stylet NOT in proper position
Protruding WAY past the tip of the ETT
The stylet can easily cause significant damage to the airway

Stylets are used to make the ETT less flexible and allow the practitioner to bend it into a shape more conducive to intubation. Bougies are used to assist the person performing the intubation in putting the tube into the right hole. Imagine bougies as being an intubation placeholder. Remember, anatomically, the trachea is in the front (anterior) and the esophagus is in the back (posterior). Because of the normal angle of approach, and especially in difficult intubations, the tube tends to take the path of least resistance and go into the esophagus. Obviously, a situation we wish to avoid.

Bougies are kind of like a coude urinary catheter. Coude catheters are often used with adults with big ol' prostates. The stiffer catheter with the curved tip allows for easier passage through the prostate. Bougies, with their curved tip, allow the practitioner to "hook" under the epiglottis that is guarding the entry to the airway. If during intubation, one can see vocal cords and put the tube through them, great. But, with difficult airways, this is not the case. The trachea is up top and the bougie, with its curved tip, can be gently guided into the top spot, the trachea. Once the bougie is in place, the endotracheal tube can be threaded over the top and successfully into the trachea.

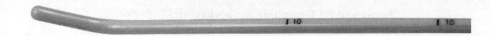

Bougie airway catheter
Courtesy of SunMed Medical
www.sunmedmedical.com

But, how do you know the bougie is in the trachea versus the esophagus? The key is remembering a few anatomical details. The trachea has cartilaginous rings that go almost, but not all the way, around. When a bougie is introduced into the trachea, if the pointed tip remains pointed up or towards the trachea, "clicks" may be felt as the bougie is advanced. In little ones, these clicks may, or may not be felt. And contrary to urban legend, they will not be audible. In addition to the "clickety clack of the railroad tracks," the other finding commonly described is the "hold up." This occurs when the bougie encounters resistance when bouncing off the carina or mainstem bronchi. Current research indicates that feeling for clicks may be overrated and advancing until the "hold up" is felt with a bougie may be potentially dangerous. So when checking for either finding, the key is to be gentle to avoid possible tracheal trauma.

What if the bougie is inadvertently placed into the esophagus? Two key findings will be present. First, as the esophagus does not have any cartilaginous rings, there will be no "clicks." Second, if the bougie is advanced, and then advanced some more, and then advanced even more, no resistance will be felt as the bougie, like a sword-swallower's sword, has a final destination of the stomach.

Up until recently, many practitioners only utilized bougies for difficult airways. However, that is changing as more and more airway experts are recommending their use for every intubation, especially in bigger kids and adults. Rationale: Seemingly, 99 times out of 100 intubations, you don't need it. But, if you've used the bougie 99 times with "easy airways," you've had a whole lot of practice and are probably good at using it. So, when you confronted with time 100, when you are staring into the airway and "can't see squat," your chances of success are a whole lot better.

Bougies are now available in baby, peds, and adult sizes. Though very rarely used in babies, especially in neonatal ICU and pediatric anesthesia, they are an option. In children, they are very rarely used as well, but again, with difficult airways, are certainly an option. In adults, they are now being used more and more for routine and difficult airways. Interesting side note: On the adult side, bougies are now being used for more than just intubations. They are also being used to aid in chest tube placement and surgical crics as well. What's the take-away thought? Bougies have been in use for over 70 years, and it appears that they will be used even more in the next 70.

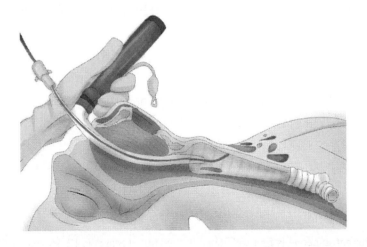

Oral Endotracheal Intubation Using a Pediatric Bougie

Additional Insights from a Pediatric ICU Attending Physician:

As a disclaimer, my bias is that we don't need bougies in kids. And as someone who has done hundreds of intubations, many in super difficult situations, I have never felt the need to use one, nor have I ever used one.

The theory is that the bougie allows easier and more reproducible passage of something into the airway. In the case of the bougie, the "something" is the tool over which you will then blindly thread the ETT. This makes sense for adults and adolescents with adult anatomy, but I think less so for smaller kids.

The bougie was designed to overcome some of the problems with direct laryngoscopy (DL), which has now been superseded by video laryngoscopy (VL), thereby removing the need for a secondary tool like a bougie. With VL, a properly styletted ETT is all you need (in addition to some practice, of course).

A few additional thoughts:

- The pediatric bougies are by definition softer and more flexible than adult bougies, and therefore possibly more difficult to aim and manipulate
- The tracheal rings are softer and less well defined, and will less reliably produce the "clicks" that are felt in adults
- The greater flimsiness of the pediatric bougie will further reduce the click sensations
- The softness of the pediatric bougie will not reliably allow blind ETT passage, as the bougie may instead bend into the retropharynx (much like the pediatric central venous lines (CVL) guide wires may bend in the subcutaneous soft tissue rather than reliably guiding the CVL into the vein)
- The time required to place the bougie, slide the ETT over, then remove the bougie and attach to oxygen source is probably too long in many cases to prevent significant O_2 desaturation, and what if ETT passage is then not possible?

Video laryngoscopy on the other hand overcomes direct laryngoscopy drawbacks and obviates the need for a bougie. Instead, a sufficiently stiff and properly bent stylet works better to guide the tube through the cords.

21) At what age does the typical human trafficking victim become "trafficked" in the United States?

A) < 12 years old

B) 12-16 years old

C) 16-18 years old

D) > 18 years old

B – The average age that someone is first trafficked in the United States is 12-16 years old. Traffickers often choose victims that are perceived as vulnerable. Children are often preyed upon as they are less likely to recognize they are being trafficked and exploited. Poverty, isolation, drug addiction, family history of violence, family dysfunction, school failures, history of sexual abuse and history of criminal behavior also make individuals appear more vulnerable.

22) From what region of the world do the majority of United States human trafficking victims come?

A) South America

B) Asia and the Pacific Islands

C) Eastern Europe

D) The United States of America

D – Although the underground nature of human trafficking makes it difficult to track statistics, data indicates that nearly 80% of victims in the United States are U.S. citizens. High-risk populations include runaway/throwaway teens and homeless youth. A multi-city study in 2017 surveyed 300 homeless youth and found that 17% of those surveyed were victims of sex trafficking. Two-thirds of homeless females reported being offered money for sex.

23) The passage of the Trafficking Victims Protection Act of 2000 (TVPA) officially delineated trafficking in the United States into these two categories:

A) Sex trafficking and sexual slavery

B) Labor trafficking and prostitution

C) Sex trafficking and labor trafficking

D) Labor exploitation and sexual slavery

C – The passage of the TVPA of 2000 officially delineated human trafficking in the U.S. into two categories: Sex trafficking and labor trafficking. Trafficking occurs when people are seen as commodities and have been victimized by force, fraud, or coercion for the purpose of physical or sexual exploitation. The A-M-P model is a tool used to articulate the federal definition of human trafficking. A-M-P stands for Action, Means, and Purpose. When at least one element of all three categories are present, a potential human trafficking case has occurred. This excludes minors where force, fraud or coercion is not required in order to be charged for trafficking; Only an action and purpose are required.

- Action: Acting so as to induce, recruit, harbor, transport, provide or obtain a person
- Means: By means of force, fraud, or coercion
- Purpose: For the purpose of commercial sex (sex trafficking) or labor/services (labor trafficking)

24) According to the Trafficking Victims Protection Act of 2000 (TVPA), which example is **not** a case of human trafficking?

A) A 16-year old runaway who chooses to sell herself for sex to buy food and shelter

B) An 18-year old who sells sex to pay for college tuition and rent

C) A 25-year old who sells sex, keeps some of the profit, but is abused by a pimp

D) A 19-year old who moves to America and stays with family, but his passport is held until he pays off debt related to his travel

B – An 18-year old who sells sex to pay for college is at risk for being trafficked, but this does not meet the requirement for a trafficking case. Willing participation in prostitution is a difficult reality and some consenting adults may choose a life in the sex industry. While the 16-year old chose to sell herself, as a minor, she is still considered a victim of human trafficking. The 25-year old chose prostitution as a means of income, but is controlled and threatened by a pimp, making her a trafficking victim. The 19-year old willingly moved to America, but is trafficked as he is being forced to work off a debt.

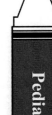

Certified Pediatric Emergency Nurse (CPEN) Review IV

25) Statistics on survivors of trafficking indicate that many received medical treatment at some point during their captivity. Most survivors receive care within what setting?

A) Urgent care

B) Primary Care

C) Planned Parenthood

D) Hospital/Emergency Department

D – One study surveyed trafficking survivors and found that of those who received medical care, 63% received care within a hospital/emergency department setting. Survivors also reported receiving care with urgent care, primary care, and Planned Parenthood.

26) A non-English-speaking teen arrives in the emergency department via ambulance after becoming dehydrated while working outdoors. He does not have identification and is accompanied by an English-speaking work supervisor who consistently speaks on behalf of the patient. The nurse should prioritize which action:

A) Remove the coworker and triage patient using facility approved interpreter service

B) Triage patient for medical complaint using the assistance of the supervisor

C) Alert social worker to the situation following triage process

D) Request assistance of a hospital employee who speaks enough Spanish

A – The priority is to adequately assess the patient and obtain information directly from the patient by utilizing approved interpreter services (**TIP**: Approved interpreting service vetted by the hospital is always the answer to interpreting questions). Separating the patient from the controlling person may also help ensure the patient's safety. Lack of identification and being accompanied by a controlling figure who insists on answering questions for the patient are red flags for a potential trafficking case.

27) A 15-year old girl presents to the emergency department for treatment of frequent and recurrent urinary tract infections. During the physical assessment, bruising and burn marks are noticed on the patient's thighs. Which of the following should the nurse do **first**?

A) Alert the parent(s) or legal guardian(s) of the findings

B) Document the suspicion of abuse for referral to a social worker

C) Follow mandated reporting laws regarding suspected abuse or neglect

D) Call the local Human Trafficking hotline

C – After ensuring the patient's immediate safety (**TIP**: Safety is always the right first step if given as an option), the registered nurse should be trained and prepared to follow mandated reporting law. An underage girl with suspected signs of abuse or neglect necessitates a report. The patient may be a trafficking victim as well, but an official child abuse report has precedence over a human trafficking hotline call.

28) A patient presents to the emergency department with multiple red flags pertaining to human trafficking. Which of the following is **not** a typical indicator of trafficking?

A) Patient works and sleeps in the same place

B) Patient appears malnourished and fatigued

C) Patient is open about discussing his/her injuries

D) Patient admits to using drugs or shows signs of drug use

C – A patient is typically hesitant to discuss his/her injuries obtained during captivity. It is important to take time and develop a rapport with a patient who you suspect may be trafficked prior to probing for additional details. The remaining answers are all possible indicators for trafficking. The following findings may also be considered red flags:

- Patient has no identification documents and/or the documentation is in the possession of an accompanying party
- Accompanying party insists on answering/interpreting for patient
- Patient is reluctant to explain his/her injuries
- Patient has someone speaking for him/her
- Patient is unaware of his/her location
- Patient exhibits fear, anxiety, depression, submission, tension, or nervousness and avoids eye contact
- Patient has no money or has no control over money
- Patient shows signs of a lack of regular health care, dental care, and/or hygiene
- Patient shows signs of physical and/or sexual abuse, or physical restraint

29) A 16-year old female checks into the emergency department for suicidal ideation and reports she is seeking placement for drug rehab. Following evaluation and medical treatment, it is determined that the patient is a human trafficking victim, and she is requesting assistance. The treatment team should do the following:

A) Call a local victim services organization

B) Call the National Human Trafficking Hotline

C) Call the local police department

D) Call a local anti-trafficking organization

B – While reaching out to the other options may be beneficial, the first call should be to the National Human Trafficking Hotline at 1-888-373-7888. The hotline will contact the appropriate authorities and other local services to provide comprehensive victim services. The National Human Trafficking Hotline is a nationwide anti-trafficking hotline and resource center serving victims and survivors of human trafficking and the anti-trafficking community in the United States. Callers can speak with the hotline in English, Spanish, or in more than 200 additional languages using a 24-hour tele-interpreting service. When you call the hotline, an advocate will speak with you about needs, options, and the resources available to help. The hotline can also be reached by texting "info" or "help" to 233733.

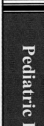

30) Casey, an adolescent sex trafficking survivor, is meeting with police investigators who are gathering evidence for a case. Police notice changes in the story as aspects of the experience are being described. When asked to give further details, Casey does not remember some of the specifics and is unable to confirm some of the things that were previously reported. Casey appears to be disconnected, passive, and has poor eye contact. Which of the following is an appropriate trauma-informed intervention for addressing Casey's memory gaps and disconnected presentation to police?

A) Provide written information to help Casey follow verbal requests and validation of feelings that might be affecting the situation

B) Question the memory gaps Casey has expressed

C) Suspect Casey may not have been truthful previously and demand that the law enforcement officers obtain further detailed responses

D) Ask why Casey is presenting the relevant information differently than before

A – Check in to make sure Casey is hearing and understanding verbal statements. Information and circumstances can be overwhelming; thus, providing written instructions and questions may be particularly helpful for trafficking survivors who struggle to process the details of the situation due to trauma. Be aware that changes in memory do not necessarily indicate falsehood or storytelling, but may be evidence of a trauma response.

31) A person is a victim of human trafficking if which of the following actions occurs?

A) A minor travels or is transported across state or national borders without the knowledge and consent of a parent or guardian

B) A person is seen as a commodity and has been victimized by force, fraud, or coercion for the purpose of physical or sexual exploitation

C) An immigrant is smuggled to another country and accepts sub-standard wages or compensation

D) An adult chooses prostitution as a means of income and unknowingly contracts or transmits a contagious disease

B – Human trafficking involves commercial sex acts or labor services that are induced by force, fraud or coercion, regardless of whether transportation occurs. Human trafficking violates an individual's human rights while human smuggling violates the country's immigration laws. Although smuggling is illegal, an adult can consent to be smuggled into a country. The term "trafficking" implies movement, but victims do not have to be moved across physical or political borders to be "trafficked." Victims can be trafficked out of the home they are living in by parents or relatives. Willing participation in prostitution is a difficult reality for millions globally. Men and women living in poverty turn to prostitution due to few economic opportunities elsewhere. Prostitution becomes a viable option because of the ability to make fast money, misconceptions of a glamorous lifestyle, and pressure to provide for their family or other expenses.

32) Most sex trafficking victims that enter the hospital or healthcare facility while in captivity will:

A) Immediately ask for help or assistance and will self-identify as a victim of trafficking

B) Quickly seek to develop a dependent relationship with a compassionate healthcare professional and request additional services in order to expose their traffickers to authorities

C) Not seek immediate help or self-identify as victims of a crime

D) Be grateful that you are treating them and finally feel safe and secure

C – Victims of human trafficking often do not immediately seek help or self-identify as victims of a crime. They may not seek help due to a variety of factors. These factors can include a lack of trust, self-blame, or specific instructions by the traffickers regarding how to behave when talking to law enforcement or social services. Avoid making snap judgments about who is or who is not a trafficking victim based on first encounters. Trust takes time to develop. Continued trust-building and patient interviewing is often required to get to the whole story and uncover the full experience of what a victim has experienced.

33) You are caring for a hemodynamically unstable 12-year old with suspected multiple traumatic injuries after an ATV crash. There is no obvious uncontrolled external hemorrhage. Which of the following is the **highest** priority for you?

A) Prompt primary survey and focus on life-threatening injuries

B) Prompt establishment of IV or intraosseous access

C) Prompt evaluation by the pediatric/trauma surgery service

D) Stat CT of the head, neck, chest, abdomen, and pelvis

A – This is not a trick question. While all the above interventions are important, the primary survey must be completed and all life-threatening injuries addressed prior to moving to the other tasks. The mnemonic of "ABCDE" is still commonly taught in many emergency and trauma courses, however, there's a new game in town. The "XABC" algorithm, which places treatment of life threatening "X'ternal" hemorrhage before airway management in the treatment protocol, is something now being adopted by many facilities.

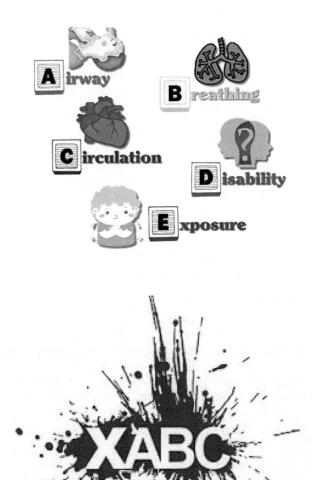

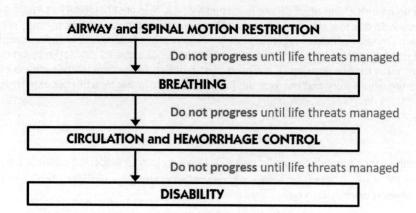

34) The trauma nurse understands which of the following to be correct about the Focused Abdominal Sonography for Trauma (FAST) in pediatrics:

A) FAST is rarely useful in trauma decision making

B) FAST indicates the need for immediate operative intervention

C) FAST has important limitations as a screening tool in pediatric trauma

D) FAST has higher sensitivity in pediatric trauma than adult trauma

C –FAST exams can be user dependent, lack sensitivity in children, and can miss smaller amounts of blood. Given these limitations, should trauma services remove this practice from routine use? Should a negative FAST give the trauma team an absolute sense of security? Recent research says probably not. Are FAST exams perfect? Of course not. They are only as good as the person performing and interpreting them. Should they only be used for unstable patients? Of course not.

Not so FAST... Where FAST really appears to have a role in pediatric trauma care is two-fold. First, it can help in the decision making process when you have a multi-trauma patient where a determination of priorities must be made rapidly. With a grossly negative FAST exam, which takes only a few minutes at the bedside, the "badness" is probably not in the belly. If there is a grossly positive FAST exam and the patient is hemodynamically stable, then off to CT they go. This is important as most blunt abdominal injuries in children are managed without surgery. However, if the FAST is grossly positive and the patient is trying to die, going immediately to the OR (and not to CT for multiple imaging exams which may result in death by diagnostics) is a very good possibility and plan.

The second more recent use of the FAST exam involves its evolution from FAST to eFAST. This stands for Extended Focused Abdominal Sonography for Trauma. This is a FAST exam with a fast look at the lungs as well. In expert hands, bedside ultrasound has been found to spot a pediatric pneumothorax faster, and in some cases, better than standard chest X-rays, without the radiation exposure.

One becomes an expert at doing FAST exams (or taking care of pediatric patients) by doing it a whole lot. Recent research currently tells us that FAST is not harmful, but that we definitely need more practice!

Certified Pediatric Emergency Nurse (CPEN) Review IV

35) Which statement made by a new emergency department (ED) nurse demonstrates an understanding of ED triage?

A) "Each patient is assessed in the order that they arrive to the department."

B) "My priority is to perform a brief, rapid assessment on all incoming patients and to prioritize each patient accordingly."

C) "Each patient needs a rapid, comprehensive assessment immediately upon arrival."

D) "All patients receive a comprehensive assessment based on their pain at arrival."

B – Key among the responsibilities of the Triage Nurse is to do a brief rapid triage assessment on all incoming patients and to prioritize those patients accordingly. For pediatric patients, the use of the Pediatric Assessment Triangle helps the nurse determine if the patient is "sick" or "not sick" or, as recently modified in the ENPC course (and probably the CPEN exam), "Sick, Sicker, or Sickest." By performing a rapid triage assessment, the patients of highest acuity can be quickly identified, and appropriate care initiated. Some patients will never receive a comprehensive triage assessment during the initial intake. The triage nurse must constantly prioritize and re-prioritize the incoming patients, often in a truly short period of time.

36) Triage is not a place, it is a:

A) Process

B) Program

C) Training Assignment

D) Treatment decision

A – It is critical for nurses in the emergency department to understand the concept that triage is not a place, it is a *process*. Triage can occur anywhere with only a moment's notice. It might begin before the patient arrives in the ambulance bay, as the patient rolls through the emergency department's doors, or walks into the waiting room. It is crucial to get beyond thinking that "triage" needs to occur in a designated location, as triage occurs in many places (urgent care facilities, areas of disaster, in the field, etc.) and is not limited to a single nurse. Anytime a patient is re-evaluated, there is an opportunity to re-triage. Are they getting sicker and need to be moved up the priority list to go to the ICU or to CT? Is it time to jump the patient ahead of others if the wait to see the provider is long?

37) Triage comes from the French verb "trier" which means to:

A) Sanction

B) Select

C) Share

D) Sort

D – Triage comes from the French verb "trier" which means "to sort." The earliest use of the word was in 1918, during World War One. It is believed to have originated as a way of describing the sorting of different types of coffee beans, and it now continues to work pretty well for the sorting of patients as well.

Pediatric Potpourri

38) Which behavior demonstrates best practice at triage?

A) Performing a rapid triage assessment on every patient

B) Triaging five patients quickly and maintaining their original order of arrival

C) Performing a complete medication reconciliation list for each incoming patient

D) Initiating an immediate bed assignment on every patient

A – Performing a rapid triage assessment, beginning with the across-the-room assessment on every patient as they arrive, is important to assess for a potential or actual life-threatening condition. Patients should not be triaged in order of arrival, but rather in order of need or priority. Although securing an immediate bed assignment is appropriate for some patients, it's important that there is an open bed and available staff to care for the patient. The triage nurse should not necessarily obtain a complete medical history and/or a complete medication list on all arriving patients. Patients with potentially life-threatening conditions should not have their care delayed in order to obtain such information.

39) Two hours ago, a patient was triaged and appropriately assigned a Level 3 acuity. The patient continues to wait in the waiting room until a treatment area room becomes available. Which statement demonstrates an appropriate understanding of the triage nurse responsibilities?

A) The patient can be reassessed once they are in the treatment area

B) The patient will let me know if their condition changes

C) Reassessment of the patient is necessary in order to identify a change in condition

D) The house nursing supervisor will let me know if the patient condition changes

C – Any patient, regardless of the initial acuity assessment is still at a risk for deterioration. Regularly reassessing the patient (in accordance with facility policies) is the best way to ensure early identification of a change in the patient condition. Once in the treatment area, the patient should be reassessed by the primary nurse, but there may be times when the wait times prior to moving to a treatment area will be lengthy and the triage nurse cannot leave reassessments solely to the treatment team. This time frame is a period of danger for the patient. Although some patients may let the triage nurse know if their perceived condition seems to change, often patients will not speak up for fear of bothering the staff. True, we hate being bothered, but if patients are getting sicker, it's probably a good thing to be interrupted! The house nursing supervisor likely does not know about the patients waiting in the waiting room and should not be counted on for this role.

40) A 2-year old patient arrives in the emergency department from a house fire. The triage nurse finds reddened areas on the face, neck, and hands with scattered intact blisters. Which assessment finding is of **most** immediate concern for the nurse?

A) Yellowish color of fluid under the blisters

B) Coughing, increased work of breathing, and vocal changes

C) Absence of urinary output since arriving in the emergency department

D) Bilateral hand and finger edema

Certified Pediatric Emergency Nurse (CPEN) Review IV

B – Exposure to smoke during a house fire, especially with a visibly reddened face, always puts the patient at risk for airway edema. The assessment findings of coughing, increased work of breathing, and vocal changes, moves the patient from being simply at risk to a near (non-visualized) confirmation of airway involvement. Protecting this patient's airway is the most immediate concern for the nurse.

It's crucial to remember that once the airway edema has gotten to the point of causing audible voice changes, we've pretty much missed the boat! The edema has been brewing for quite a while by this point and you may need to secure the airway quickly. With few exceptions (safety and uncontrolled major, active external bleeding), airway trumps everything!

41) An 8-year old patient presents to triage from a house fire with partial thickness burns to the face and hands. Which assessment finding requires priority intervention?

A) Blisters to the face
B) Erythema to the chin and cheeks
C) Sputum with presence of dark particles
D) Bruises to the legs and thighs

C – Presence of dark particles in the sputum is evidence of smoke inhalation, which should certainly raise your concern level regarding the potential for the patient to deteriorate. This finding says that not only is the patient burned on the outside, but very likely on the inside as well! Although blisters, bruises, and erythema elsewhere on the body should get our attention, these would not prompt a priority intervention.

42) A 5-year old patient presents to triage with his distraught parent who states that the boy had a witnessed fall from a bunk bed. Which assessment finding is concerning for an **early** sign of increased intracranial pressure?

A) Change in level of consciousness
B) Hypothermia
C) Bradycardia
D) Dilated pupil(s)

A – Changes in level of consciousness are an early sign of increased intracranial pressure. Any indication that the child's mentation is different from baseline requires immediate intervention, and in this age patient, it's crucial to listen to the parent/caretaker's assessment of whether the child is "acting normal." Other common signs of increased intracranial pressure include headache (difficult to assess in an infant), nausea, and vomiting. Although a person with increased intracranial pressure may present with one/both pupils dilated or may develop bradycardia, those are really, really late signs.

43) An 18-month-old patient is being seen in the emergency department after sustaining a burn to the corner of his lip from "biting an electrical cord." Which of the following is the highest priority for this patient?

A) Monitor the airway
B) Start an intravenous line
C) Clean the wound
D) Draw labs

A – Evidence of an electrical injury to the mouth should lead the nurse to think about the potential of the electrical energy traveling from the mouth through the airway. And we know that airway is always a top priority. Don't be distracted by the mechanism of injury, the "distraught" caregiver, or even suspicious circumstances. If you lose the airway, you can forget everything else. It is likely that an intravenous line, labs, and cleaning of the wound will all occur, but airway remains the priority.

Additional Insights from a Pediatric Emergency Medicine Attending Physician:

Cord bites by children are low voltage exposures. The literature supports not doing EKGs on all these kids as long as there was no history of a loss of consciousness or other significant physical findings. By the way, the greatest danger is actually 7-10 days down the line when the eschar from the burn at the corner of the lips comes off and exposes (and sometimes disrupts) the labial artery, causing significant bleeding. I think giving parents this guidance is an extremely important aspect of the care for this patient!

44) A 14-year old female presents to triage complaining of the sudden onset of severe, lower right-side abdominal pain. Her last menstrual cycle was two weeks ago, but she acknowledges some scant vaginal bleeding. Gravida 0, Para 0. What is the **most** likely source of the pain?

A) Mesenteric ischemia

B) Ruptured ectopic pregnancy

C) Renal aneurysm

D) Aortic aneurysm

B – Being a young female of childbearing years should cause the triage nurse to consider the real possibility of a ruptured ectopic pregnancy. The classic triad of an ectopic pregnancy includes abdominal pain, vaginal bleeding, and a missed menstrual cycle. One must remember that the reported last menstrual cycle at triage must not be taken as an absolute, as women who are indeed pregnant can have spotting and/or may be off on the reported dates. Also, don't rely on getting an accurate history of presence or absence of sexual activity. A ruptured ectopic pregnancy is one example of an "acute abdomen" that requires surgical intervention.

Mesenteric ischemia is more common in the older adult and has a classic triad of abdominal pain, gastrointestinal emptying (vomiting/diarrhea), and an underlying cardiac disease. A renal artery aneurysm is more commonly associated with flank pain and hematuria. A classic aortic dissection involves sudden onset of sharp back pain radiating to lower extremities, although the patient can have chest pain or abdominal pain. While these other problems could be possible (very, very rare, but possible), on the CPEN exam, the combination of teenage girl and anything involving abdominal pain/vaginal bleeding, screams "I have an ectopic" until proven otherwise!

45) A mother brings in her 8-week old infant to triage and describes projectile vomiting and constant hunger. The infant is found to have an olive-shaped abdominal mass upon palpation. What condition do you suspect?

A) Pyloric stenosis

B) Intussusception

C) Appendicitis

D) Peptic ulcer disease

A – An olive-shaped abdominal mass in a child 3 to 12 weeks old is considered to be indicative of pyloric stenosis. Research now shows that the classic sign of an "olive shaped abdominal mass," as a result of a thickened pylorous, is far rarer than previously thought. So, while the terminology is still out there in teaching and testing, finding this occurring in actual practice seems to be pretty unusual. A delay in the diagnosis and treatment of this obstruction can lead to severe dehydration from the persisting projectile vomiting.

Intussusception signs and symptoms include vomiting, "red currant jelly" stools, and episodic abdominal pain. This condition is from strangulation of the small intestine when it gets stuck as it telescopes into an adjacent segment of bowel. Appendicitis is more common in the school-age and teenage years and tends to be associated with right sided abdominal pain (although not always) and a low-grade fever. Peptic ulcer disease is very rarely a condition of infants. Just as severe abdominal pain and a female teenager should prompt you to think about an ectopic pregnancy, when you hear Persistent Projectile Puking in a child less than 3-months of age, always think about pyloric stenosis.

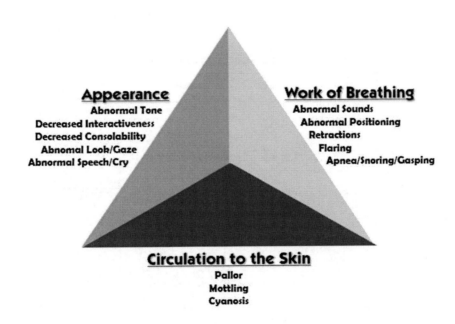

46) In pediatric assessment, the first impression of the child's physiologic stability is by evaluating which of the following factors?

A) Activity, breathing, circulation

B) Airway, breathing, circulation

C) Appearance, work of breathing, circulation

D) Attentiveness, work of breathing, circulation

C – The first step in the assessment of a pediatric patient is the use of the Pediatric Assessment Triangle (Appearance, Work of breathing, Circulation to the skin), and can even be done from a reasonable distance as the patient approaches. The airway may be more difficult to assess initially, and activity and attentiveness may be factors that contribute to appearance assessment.

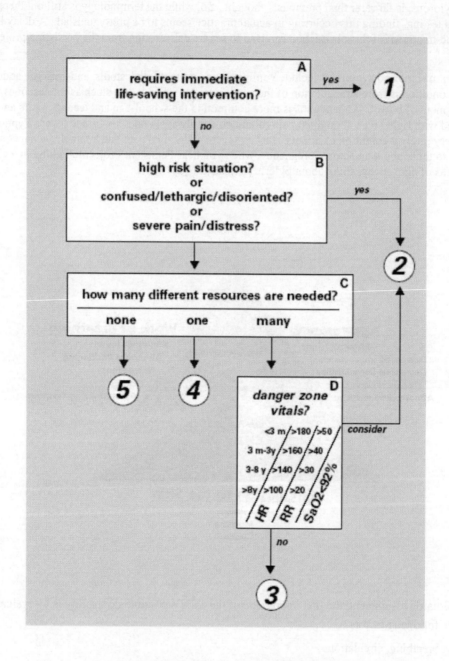

Emergency Severity Index (ESI)

Adapted from: Gilboy, N., Tanabe, T., Travers, D., & Rosenau, A. (2011). Emergency Severity Index (ESI): A Triage Tool for Emergency Department Care, Version 4. Implementation Handbook 2012 Edition. AHRQ Publication No. 12-0014.

Agency for Healthcare Research and Quality

www.ahrq.gov

Certified Pediatric Emergency Nurse (CPEN) Review IV

NOTES:

A. <u>Immediate life-saving intervention required</u>: airway, emergency medications, or other hemodynamic interventions (IV, supplemental O2, ECG or labs, DO NOT count); and/or any of the following clinical conditions: intubated, apneic, pulseless, severe respiratory distress, SPO2 < 90, acute mental status changes, or unresponsive.

<u>Unresponsiveness</u> is defined as a patient that is either:
(1) nonverbal and not following commands (acutely) or
(2) requires noxious stimulus (P or U on AVPU scale)

B. <u>High risk situation</u> is a patient you would put in your last open bed.

<u>Severe pain/distress</u> is determined by clinical observation and/or patient rating of greater than or equal to 7 on 0-10 pain scale.

C. <u>Resources</u>: Count the number of *different types* of resources, not the individual tests or x-rays (examples: CBC, electrolytes and coags equals one resource; CBC plus chest x-ray equals two resources).

Resources	*Not Resources*
• Labs (blood, urine) • ECG, X-rays • CT-MRI-Ultrasound-Angiography	• History and Physical (including pelvic) • Point-of-Care Testing
• IV Fluids (Hydration)	• Saline or Heplock
• IV or IM or Nebulized Treatments	• PO Medications • Tetanus Immunization • Prescription Refills
• Specialty Consultation	• Phone Call to PCP
• Simple Procedure=1 (lac repair, foley cath) • Complex procedure=2 (conscious sedation)	• Simple wound care (dressings, recheck) • Crutches, splints, slings

D. <u>Danger Zone Vital Signs</u>
Consider uptriage to ESI 2 is any vital sign criterion is exceptional

<u>Pediatric Fever Considerations</u>
- 1 to 28 days of age: assign at least ESI 2 if temp >38.0 C (100.4 F)
- 1-3 months of age: consider assigning ESI 2 if temp > 38.0 C (100.4 F)
- 3 months to 3 years of age: consider ESI 3 if temp >39.0 c (102.2 F), or incomplete immunizations, or no obvious source of fever

Emergency Severity Index (ESI)

Adapted from: Gilboy, N., Tanabe, T., Travers, D., & Rosenau, A. (2011).
Emergency Severity Index (ESI): A Triage Tool for Emergency Department Care, Version 4.
Implementation Handbook 2012 Edition. AHRQ Publication No. 12-0014.

Agency for Healthcare Research and Quality

www.ahrq.gov

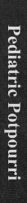

47) A cute 14-day old infant presents to triage. The parents state "He just doesn't seem well." Rectal temperature reads 100.5 F (38.1 C). All other vital signs are within normal limits and no rash or petechiae are noted. What Emergency Severity Index (ESI) acuity should you assign this patient?

A) 2

B) 3

C) 4

D) 5

A – According to the Emergency Severity Index for pediatric triage, an infant less than 60-days old with a confirmed fever of 100.4 F (38 C) or greater is at "high risk" for a bacterial infection and should be triaged at least a Level 2. Certainly, you would want to consider a Level 1 acuity if you deem the patient requires immediate life-saving interventions.

As infants move from "life is good inside of mom" to "the harsh outside world," their chance of catching something icky is really good. Infants with a fever most often get the whole kit and caboodle of diagnostics, including a lumbar puncture, blood and urine cultures, chest X-ray, and a field trip to a pediatric unit for IV antibiotics until the cultures come back showing that the cute baby really is cute, not septic!

Moral of the story, nothing good comes of a little one (under 60-days old) with a fever.

48) You are called to assess a 3-year old patient who just arrived by private vehicle. The parent states the child has "been shaking" for 15 minutes and you find the child actively seizing. What ESI acuity should you assign this patient?

A) 1

B) 2

C) 3

D) 4

A – According to the Emergency Severity Index for pediatric triage, active seizures are Level 1 acuity. The patient requires immediate, potentially life-saving interventions.

49) A 10-year old patient presents with stridor and audible wheezing. The parent states the child was playing outside with friends when a bee nest got disturbed. What ESI acuity should you assign this patient?

A) 1

B) 2

C) 3

D) 4

A – This patient is an ESI Level 1. Your concern should be anaphylaxis. According to the Emergency Severity Index for pediatric triage, a patient exhibiting respiratory compromise with stridor, wheezing, dyspnea and/or hypoxemia is Level 1 acuity. The patient requires immediate, potentially life-saving interventions. Wheezing and bees are bad, but wheezing, and stridor, and bees….oh my! Airway trumps just about everything!

Certified Pediatric Emergency Nurse (CPEN) Review IV

50) A 15-year old male brought in by his mother reports hearing voices telling him to kill himself. He has a history of suicide attempts. What ESI acuity should you assign this patient?

A) 1
B) 2
C) 3
D) 4

B – According to the Emergency Severity Index for pediatric triage, a suicidal patient is Level 2 acuity. This patient is high risk. Your role is to provide safety for the staff, the patient, and their family (in that order)! A healthcare worker injured on the job is unavailable to help patients. Safety first...

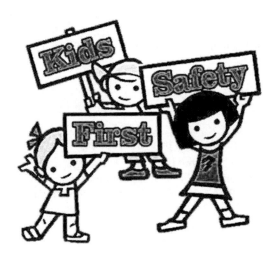

51) A 7-year old patient arrives at the triage area. The parent states the child has a known history of seizures and had a 5-minute generalized seizure at home about 20-minutes prior to arrival in the emergency department. The patient remains confused with unlabored respirations. Skin color is pink. What ESI acuity should you assign this patient?

A) 1
B) 2
C) 3
D) 4

B – According to the Emergency Severity Index for pediatric triage, a patient with a prolonged postictal period and an altered level of consciousness is a high-risk patient and should be assigned level 2 acuity. Actively seizing gets a 1. Not seizing, but not quite right yet, gets a 2.

52) A 16-year old did a spectacular double flip off a diving board, and then struck her head on the side of the pool. The ambulance was called, and the patient was placed into spinal motion restriction precautions. She was initially unconscious for a few minutes, but now is awake, alert, and moving all extremities. Vital signs are temperature 98.6 F (37C), heart rate 80 beats per minute, respiratory rate 14 and unlabored, blood pressure 112/76, and pulse oximetry 99% on room air. What ESI acuity should you assign this patient?

A) 1

B) 2

C) 3

D) 4

B – According to the Emergency Severity Index for pediatric triage, a patient with a significant mechanism of injury is a high-risk patient and should be assigned Level 2 acuity. If life-saving interventions are needed, the patient would be Level 1 acuity. However, in this scenario, there is no indication that life-saving measures are needed at this time.

53) A 5-year old child complains of abdominal pain and vomiting. The parent states that the patient isn't interested in playing which is very much not his norm. Vital signs are temperature 100.5 F (38.1C), heart rate 90 beats per minute, respiratory rate 24 breaths per minute and unlabored, blood pressure 100/56, and pulse oximetry 99% on room air. Pain 5/10. What ESI acuity should you assign this patient?

A) 1

B) 2

C) 3

D) 4

C – According to the Emergency Severity Index for pediatric triage, a patient with abdominal pain at a minimum will require two resources (lab work up and an ultrasound or CT scan), thus making the patient Level 3 triage acuity.

54) A 5-year old patient is carried to triage. The child appears weak and confused with labored respirations and a visible, purple, non-blanching petechial rash. What ESI acuity should you assign this patient?

A) 1

B) 2

C) 3

D) 4

A – According to the Emergency Severity Index for pediatric triage, a patient with altered mental status and a petechial rash is Level 1 acuity. The patient requires immediate, potentially life-saving interventions. This scenario just screams badness! 5-year olds (like 55-year olds) should not be confused and labored breathing only makes things worse. But if that's too much to remember, just remember B5 - Big Blue Blotches that don't Blanch are Bad!

Certified Pediatric Emergency Nurse (CPEN) Review IV

55) A 10-year old child tripped and struck his right forearm on a table. There is no obvious deformity and vital signs are within normal limits. Pain is a 2/10. What ESI acuity should you assign this patient?

A) 3

B) 4

C) 5

D) 6

B – According to the Emergency Severity Index for pediatric triage, a patient needing an X-ray to rule out a fracture (with no severe pain) uses one resource, making the patient an ESI Level 4. Ruling out D as an answer should not be difficult as the ESI scale goes from 1 to 5, and there is no ESI Level 6.

56) An 8-year old patient fell while running and suffered a minor laceration to her right elbow. Based on the Emergency Severity Index (ESI), how many resources will this patient require?

A) 0

B) 1

C) 2

D) 3 or more

B – According to the ESI, a patient with a simple laceration that requires suturing will utilize one resource, making the patient a Level 4 triage acuity.

57) An 18-month old presents pulling on her right ear. The mother states there is a known history of multiple ear infections and "she always pulls on her ear when she has an ear infection." The child is playful and vital signs are within normal limits. Based on the Emergency Severity Index (ESI), how many resources will this patient require?

A) 0

B) 1

C) 2

D) 3 or more

A – This patient will most likely not require any resources as defined by the ESI. All that is expected is an exam and discharge instructions (possibly with a prescription), neither of which is considered a resource according to ESI guidelines.

58) A 12-year old suffered a scratch to his left hand on a rusty nail. Bleeding is controlled and vital signs are within normal limits. Based on the Emergency Severity Index (ESI), how many resources will this patient require?

A) 0

B) 1

C) 2

D) 3 or more

A – This patient will most likely only require a tetanus injection and then be discharged. By ESI standards, those actions utilize no resources. The key here is the word "scratch" and not "laceration." A simple tetanus immunization is not a resource according to ESI.

59) A 15-month old patient had a ground-level fall. The parent reports that the child "doesn't seem to be using her right arm." Upon assessment, there is an obvious deformity of the extremity and you anticipate the need for procedural sedation to reduce the extremity. Based on the Emergency Severity Index (ESI), how many resources will this patient require?

A) 0

B) 1

C) 2

D) 3 or more

D - Using the ESI, treatment for this patient will most likely require 3 or more resources. A complex procedure such as procedural sedation is two resources. In addition, the patient will require IV, IM, or IN (intranasal) medication administration which is an additional resource.

60) A 4-year old says she was playing with some small beads and put one into her ear. No bleeding or drainage is noted and vital signs are within normal limits. Based on the Emergency Severity Index (ESI), how many resources will this patient require?

A) 0

B) 1

C) 2

D) 3 or more

B – This patient will most likely require irrigation of the ear which, based on ESI guidelines, is the use of one resource.

61) Using the Emergency Severity Index (ESI) to determine the triage acuity level for each patient, which patient will be your first priority for placement in a treatment bed?

A) A 2-year old who complains of ear pain after a week of swimming lessons. Vital signs stable.

B) A 6-year old with an itchy rash to face and neck with swelling to eyes, face, and lips, worsening over the last 3 days. Unlabored respirations but some difficulty swallowing fluids. Vital signs stable.

C) 10-year old with a fever of 101.4 F (38.6C). Other vital signs stable. Unlabored respirations. Family member recently diagnosed with strep.

D) A 12-year old was running and twisted her ankle. Slight swelling is noted to the foot and ankle with minimal pain with weight bearing. Vital signs stable.

Pediatric Potpourri

B – Based on the ESI, the 6-year old should be the priority as this child will require two or more resources – likely an intravenous line for hydration and medications to reduce inflammation and itching – making the child Level 3 triage acuity. The 2-year old patient likely does not require any resources (a prescription is not considered a resource). Although we don't know for certain, we must consider that the 10-year old child has been exposed to strep and will likely require one resource, a rapid strep and perhaps a strep culture. The 12-year old child will probably require an X-ray which uses one resource.

62) Using the Emergency Severity Index (ESI) to determine the triage acuity level for each patient, which patient will be your first priority for placement in a treatment bed?

A) An 18-month old in severe respiratory distress.

B) A 12-year old with facial swelling and audible wheezing after eating shellfish.

C) A 6-month old with a fever, vomiting and cough. Skin is hot to touch and slightly sunken fontanelle.

D) A 10-year old who complains of weakness and vomiting for 4 days. The child states he is urinating often and thirsty all the time.

A – The 18-month old patient is the priority and should be placed in a treatment bed before the other patients. He is in severe respiratory distress and requires life-saving interventions to manage the airway. Using the ESI, a patient requiring life-saving interventions such as this child is Level 1 acuity. The other patients are certainly all high risk, which would likely make them Level 2 acuity. The 12-year old requires airway monitoring, the 6-month old is at high risk for dehydration and sepsis and will likely require a septic work up, and the 10-year old patient may be in diabetic ketoacidosis.

63) Using the Emergency Severity Index (ESI) to determine the triage acuity level for each patient, which patient will be your first priority for placement in a treatment bed?

A) A 3-week old infant with a rectal temperature of 100.6 F (38.1C), heart rate 150, respiratory rate 40, pulse oximetry 100% room air. Infant acting appropriately. No delivery complications.

B) A 16-year old restrained driver involved in a high-speed motor vehicle accident. Temperature 98.1 F (36.7C), heart rate 76, respiratory rate 16 and unlabored, BP 124/82, and pulse oximetry 99%.

C) A 17-year old with sudden onset shortness of breath for 3 hours. Temperature 98.2 F (36.8C), heart rate 110, respiratory rate 30, BP 118/64. Smoking history and takes birth control pills.

D) A 15-year old who is "confused and acting wrong" according to parent. Self inflicted cuts on wrists noted and suspicion of a medication overdose. Temperature 98.1 F (36.7C), heart rate 124, respiratory rate 10, BP 111/78 and pulse oximetry of 84% on room air.

D – The 15-year old patient is the priority and should be placed in a treatment bed first as this patient has a depressed respiratory rate, an abnormally low pulse oximetry level, and cannot reliably protect their own airway. Immediate life-saving interventions, potentially involving endotracheal intubation may be necessary, making this patient Level 1 triage acuity. The 3-week old is high risk as an infant less than 28-days old with a temperature above 100.4 F (38C) is considered high risk, even if the infant looks good and is acting appropriately for age. The 16-year old restrained driver has stable vital signs, but due to the mechanism of injury, this patient will require an evaluation by the trauma team. The 17-year old patient should raise a suspicion for a pulmonary embolus. All these patients are "high risk," but there is one "risk" to rule them all. (Apologies to Mr. Tolkien)

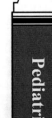

64) Using the Emergency Severity Index (ESI) to determine the triage acuity level for each incoming patient, which patient will be your first priority for placement in a treatment bed?

A) A 14-year old with a mental health history complaining of paranoia and states, "They are trying to kill me."

B) A 13-year old with a syncopal episode. Alert and oriented now.

C) A 12-year old who was skateboarding and struck his head on a pole. Intubated in the field by EMS for unresponsiveness.

D) A 10-year old immunocompromised patient with a temperature of 102.4 F (39.1C).

C – The 12-year old patient is the priority as a patient requiring intubation in the field requires life-saving interventions and would be Level 1 triage acuity. According to pediatric ESI psychiatric guidelines, the 14-year old is high risk and needs to be placed into a safe environment to prevent the potential of self harm. While the 13-year old with a syncopal event and the 10-year old immunocompromised child with a fever are both considered high-risk, they present less sick than the other two patients

65) Using the Emergency Severity Index (ESI) to determine the triage acuity level for each incoming patient, which patient will be your first priority for placement in a treatment bed?

A) A 5-month old with petechiae scattered all over the body and not acting normally. Vital Signs: Temperature 102.3 F (39 C), heart rate 192 beats per minute, respiratory rate 60 breaths per minute, pulse oximetry 88% on room air.

B) A 10-year old was playing tennis and complained of immediate severe 9/10 pain to the right shoulder. Shoulder appears dislocated. Neurovascular status intact.

C) A 17-year old breastfeeding young mother complains of continued left breast pain with a fever after 3-days on antibiotics.

D) An 8-year old diabetic child presents with right foot redness and swelling with an open wound for 5-days. No fever. Other vital signs are within normal limits.

A – The 5-month old is the first priority because this child requires life-saving interventions (Level 1) due to acute mental status changes, pulse oximetry less than 90%, not to mention the concerns for meningitis and bacteremia. The 10-year old with a dislocated shoulder in severe pain and distress is high risk (Level 2) according to ESI, because the patient's pain will not be able to be adequately treated at triage. This patient will require ice, a sling, IV pain medication, and sedation to reduce the shoulder. The 17-year old young mother will require two or more resources (likely labs, IV fluids, antibiotics) making her a Level 3 acuity. The 8-year old likely requires two or more resources (Level 3) due to the diabetic history and apparently infected foot. This patient will likely require an IV with labs, radiology, and IV antibiotics.

66) The FOUR score is utilized as a way to:

A) Remember the beginning of President Lincoln's famous Gettysburg Address

B) Remember the name of a famous kids game from the 70's

C) Remember what you called kids who wore glasses in elementary school

D) Assess a patient's neurologic status

D – The Full Outline of Unresponsiveness (FOUR) score was created by Dr. E. Wijdicks and colleagues at the Mayo Clinic in 2006 and is considered by many to be more accurate than the Glasgow Coma Scale (GCS). Prior to 2006, the GCS (introduced in 1974) was the most common measure for evaluating changes in a patient's level of consciousness.

Certified Pediatric Emergency Nurse (CPEN) Review IV

The FOUR score, as luck would have it, has 4 components which, with a little practice, are easy to REMBr: (R)espiration, (E)ye response, (M)otor response, and (Br)ainstem Reflexes. The examiner rates each component on a 0-to-4 scale, with 0 signifying complete lack of response and 4 indicating a normal or expected response. Each component is scored individually, for example, R1, E4, M3, or B4; and unlike the Glasgow Coma Scale, the four components are NOT all added up and totaled. With the Glasgow Coma Scale, each of the 3 components have a different scoring scale. Motor response is measured on a 6-point scale, verbal response on a 5-point scale, and eye-opening response on a 4-point scale. But trying to remember which gets 6, or 5, or 4 is way too difficult. With the Four Score, to no surprise, each of the FOUR components gets FOUR possible points.

Here are some tips for working with the FOUR Score Coma Scale:

- To evaluate breathing (versus verbal responsiveness with the GCS) with an artificial airway (endotracheal tube, cric, or trache) in place, the FOUR Score respiration component specifically takes into account whether the patient is intubated. Intubated patients may receive a score of either 0 or 1, depending on whether they're breathing at or above the preset ventilator rate. An artificial airway makes it exceedingly difficult to assess the VOICE component of the GCS as there is plastic in your airway. So, with the GCS, tubed patients get a V1.

- To test eye response, evaluate the patient's eye opening <u>and</u> tracking. Assessment of tracking may help reveal "locked-in" syndrome.

- To test motor response, ask the patient to make a fist or to give a "thumbs up" or peace (aka., "V" for victory) sign. A patient who is able to perform these actions demonstrates the ability to respond to a command with a voluntary motor action. The reason for this type of command, as opposed to "squeeze my fingers" is that squeezing fingers that contact the palm of a patient's hand can be either from a voluntary command or a simple grasp reflex. If you've ever heard a family member of a really sick patient exclaim, "He squeezed my hand, he squeezed my hand... That means he's going to wake up...", you know just how important that distinction is. Remember, the worse the head or brain injury you have, the more like a baby you act. Babies reflexively squeeze a person's fingers, but only as the brain matures do they squeeze on command (responsively). Why do head injured patients squeeze fingers? It could be voluntary, or it could be a reflex – it's crucial to determine real vs. reflex.

- To test brainstem reflexes, the nurse checks the patient's pupillary response (do they react?), corneal response (do they blink?), and cough reflex (do they cough with suctioning?) To reduce the risk of corneal damage from testing, instead of using a cotton tip swab to brush the cornea, use a drop of saline solution in the eye. Brainstem reflex testing, which is <u>not</u> included in the GCS, may promote earlier recognition of progression to brain death. When such progression cannot be prevented, early recognition can help the family prepare for the patient's imminent death and consideration of organ donation.

Respiration (R)

4	Not intubated, regular breathing pattern
3	Not intubated, Cheyne-Stokes breathing pattern
2	Not intubated, irregular breathing pattern
1	Breathes above ventilator rate
0	Breathes at ventilator rate or apnea

Eye Response (E)

4	Eyelids open or opened, tracking or blinking to command
3	Eyelids open but not tracking
2	Eyelids closed but open to a loud voice
1	Eyelids closed but open to pain
0	Eyelids remain closed with pain

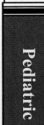

Pediatric Potpourri

Motor Response (M)

4 Thumbs up, fist, or peace sign to command
3 Localizing to pain
2 Flexion response to pain
1 Extensor posturing
0 No response to pain or generalized myoclonus status epilepticus

Brainstem Reflexes (B)

4 Pupil and corneal reflexes present
3 One pupil wide and fixed
2 Pupil or corneal reflexes absent
1 Pupil and corneal reflexes absent
0 Absent pupil, corneal, and cough reflex

67) Which of the following is **NOT** utilized while calculating your patient's FOUR score?

A) Eye Response

B) Verbal Response

C) Motor Response

D) Brainstem Reflexes

B – Verbal response is not a component of the Full Outline of Unresponsiveness (FOUR). The FOUR components of FOUR should be easy to remember as "REMBr" – (R)espiration, (E)ye response, (M)otor response, and (Br)ainstem Reflexes. Each category has assigned values ranging from 0 to 4 with 0 indicating nonfunctional state and a score of 4 indicating normal functioning. The FOUR Score assess FOUR domains of neurological function and grades the severity of coma. Decreasing FOUR scores signal a worsening level of consciousness.

GCS	FOUR score

• Three major components
  • Eye—4 points
  • Motor—6 points
  • Verbal—5 points
• Limited utility in intubated patients and children with limited language development
• Key component of other ICU severity of illness scales such as acute physiology and chronic health evaluation II score (APACHE-2)
• Widely used and validated for more than 30 years
	• Four components (E_4, M_4, B_4, R_4) with maximum score of 4 points each
	  • Eye response
	  • Motor response
	  • Brainstem reflexes
	  • Respiratory pattern
	• Includes testing for intubated patients and brainstem reflexes
	• Useful in detecting patients with locked-in syndrome and VSs
	• Multicenter trials and validation are pending

Glasgow Coma Scale (GCS) versus FOUR score

68) Which of the following questions is **NOT** part of the initial stroke screening for a teenager presenting with a possible stroke?

A) Is there a focal neurological deficit?
B) Did the problem begin or worsen suddenly?
C) What is the patient's current FOUR Score?
D) Has the problem been present for less than 5 hours?

C – While the FOUR (**F**ull **O**utline of **U**n**R**esponsiveness) Score is being used more and more frequently with neurologically injured patients, determining a FOUR Score is not part of the initial stroke screening questions in the pediatric acute stroke guidelines.

Some of the common (and crucial) questions to be asked with a stroke screening include:

- Is there a focal neurological deficit? This can consist of unilateral weakness or sensory changes, vision loss or double vision, speech difficulty, trouble walking or dizziness, or new onset of seizures with focal findings.

- Did the problem suddenly begin or worsen? These should be pretty self-explanatory questions and may help differentiate between a stroke, a bleed, or a tumor.

- Time of symptom onset and when the child was last seen symptom free. Though thrombolytics such as tissue plasminogen activator (tPA) or endovascular clot removal may be options, just like with adults, determining when they were "last normal" is absolutely crucial. When it comes to strokes, time is brain.

- Last time the child ate or drank anything. Just like adults undergoing any major procedure (thrombolytics, airway management, surgery), potential for aspiration is a big concern.

- Does the child have any dental hardware or appliances (fillings, spacers, retainers, or braces)? This is not much of an issue with CT scans, but it can be a significant concern for MRIs, depending on the nature of the dental work in place. Orthodontic appliances using stainless steel brackets seem to pose the greatest likelihood of significant artifact. Importantly, YES, you can still perform the MRI, and NO, the braces or fillings will not come flying out of the child's mouth during imaging. However, the amount of artifact and distortion caused by the braces or fillings and seen on a brain MRI is different for each kid. Either way, CT scans are great initially to see big tumors, big bleeds, and big strokes (and determine hemorrhagic vs. ischemic). But MRIs are also performed for additional info and treatment guidance. Distortion and/or artifact may happen, but the bigger issue is that the kid needs an MRI for a reason. So, get the MRI and see what they can see. And remember... Silly rabbit, "Trixs are for kids," but strokes are for adults AND kids!

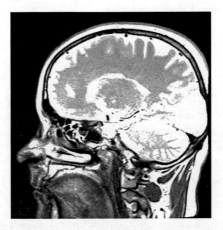

Brain MRI

69) Requiring helmet use for anyone under age 18 using an electric scooter is an example of what category of injury prevention?

A) Primordial

B) Primary

C) Secondary

D) Tertiary

C– Secondary injury prevention practices aim to minimize the severity of injuries that occur during incidents that cannot be primarily prevented. Wearing a helmet won't stop someone from crashing an electric scooter (or a bicycle for that matter) into a parked car, but it might limit the injuries to minor bumps and bruises, scrapes and scratches, instead of a traumatic brain injury. Other examples of secondary injury prevention practices include mandating seatbelt use, providing trigger locks for firearms, and locking access and/or covers for swimming pools.

Prevention has "prevent" at its root, indicating a desire to prevent something from happening. In the realm of healthcare, the goal of all levels of injury prevention is injury control, meaning the attempt to either prevent something bad from happening or if that is not possible, at least to mitigate or minimize the impact of that bad thing happening. The American College of Surgeons Committee on Trauma's Subcommittee on Injury Prevention and Control has stated that injury prevention and injury control are not synonymous terms. There are categories of injury PREVENTION, all of which, taken as a whole, comprise injury CONTROL!

Primary injury prevention activities rarely occur because they would involve inhibiting or eliminating the possibility of the injury incident from even occurring. The goal would be to avoid the emergence of risk factors leading to an injury through actions and measures affecting social, cultural, economic, and behavioral conditions and patterns of living. Doing away with certain organized sports might be an effective method of preventing a certain type of injury, but it is not likely to see bowling outlawed as a method of controlling sprained thumbs.

Tertiary prevention activities include programs and practices that will optimize the outcome from injury, regardless of injury severity. Examples of tertiary prevention programs include the development of trauma programs, rehabilitation facilities, and support groups.

Remember... "Know safety, no injury. No safety, know injury." ~ Author unknown

70) A child involved in an auto vs. pedestrian collision may be anticipated to present with which of the following recognizable triad/combination of injuries?

A) Bilateral wrist fractures and single kidney lacerations

B) Blunt chest trauma, C-spine injury, and ankle fracture

C) Head injury, splenic laceration, and femur fracture

D) Spinal fracture, pelvic fracture, and sternal fracture

C – Many children who have been the unfortunate pedestrian in an auto vs. pedestrian collision have been seen to present with head injuries, splenic lacerations, and femur fractures. This is common enough to be referred to as Waddell's Triad and is caused when the child:

1. Turns toward the oncoming car and is struck fracturing the femur

2. Hits the hood causing chest and abdomen injury

3. Is thrown away the car by the impact, injuring their head and cervical spine

Though all the above injuries are certainly possible in a pedestrian vs. auto accident, here are some tips to remember when encountering a child vs. auto question on the CPEN exam.

1. Waddell's sounds like waddle which is how little kids may appear as they walk (waddle) across the street.

2. Triad means three which means the answer must involve three injuries, or even better, three different areas of injury.

3. Remember the obvious and think about the size of a little kid vs. the size of the much bigger car. What's going to happen first, second, third, and where it's going to happen? In most cases, there is a split second just prior to the collision when the child sees or hears something and turns toward the vehicle, presenting the femurs as the initial point of contact. Next, as the movement of the vehicle continues and the child's body bends forward, the chest and belly impact the bumper or another part of the car. Finally, the transfer of energy and motion causes the child to be thrown up, up, and away from the initial point of contact and the head hits either the car or the ground. Why the head? Simply remember that the younger the child, the greater the head to body ratio, aka., "Big Head, Little Body" syndrome.

Research has shown, as you can imagine, that these injuries are not always found with all pediatric-pedestrian versus car collisions, but Waddell's triad and the three areas of anticipated injury are great classic CPEN questions.

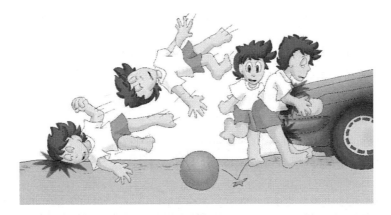

Waddell's Triad

71) You have been tasked with creating a community-wide injury prevention initiative for your department. The suggested **first** step in that project would be to:

A) Choose an injury category project for which you are uniquely qualified

B) Collect data on the most common injuries in your area

C) Create meaningful partnerships within your community

D) Provide overall safety teaching to children at time of discharge

B – The nursing process applies just as much to starting a project, as it does to treating a patient. The assessment and collection of data should be your first step. To know where you are going, you have to first know where you are. To hit a target, you must first know where you are shooting.

With that in mind, just as every Emergency Department, every shift, and every child is different, the most commonly encountered injuries can be different depending on your area. As such, understanding the specific needs of children in your community can help you hit a bull's eye with targeted injury prevention initiatives.

72) Which of the following are indicated for the management of North American rattlesnake envenomations?

A) CroFab® (Crotalidae Polyvalent Immune Fab) or Anavip® (Crotalidae Immune F(ab')$_2$

B) Anascorp® (Centruroides Scorpion Immune F(ab')$_2$

C) HDCV vaccine (Imovax®) or PCECV vaccine (RabAvert®)

D) Lactro Mactans Antivenin

A – Different strokes for different folks, and different antivenins for different envenomations. For many years Crofab has been, and continues to be, commonly utilized for rattlesnake bites. However, Anavip is the "new kid on the block" when it comes to rattlesnake bites. While Crofab is derived from sheep, Anavip is derived from horses, which for reasons only understood by really smart people, may result in less risk for serum sickness. Another significant benefit of Anavip is its much longer half-life which helps reduce the risk of late coagulopathy (bleeding several hours after the bite) and need for repeat dosing of the antivenin.

Anascorp, as the "scorp" part of the name alludes to, is for Bark Scorpion stings, while RabAvert ("avert rabies") and more recently, Imovax (they need an easier to identify name?), to no surprise are for rabies. Antivenin Lactro Mactans is for black widow bites (another one that could use an easier to remember name). Different strokes for different folks, and different antivenins for different bites

73) When administering antivenin to a patient who has been bitten by a North American Rattlesnake, which of the following are possible signs of a hypersensitivity reaction?

A) Bleeding from the ears, nose, and mouth

B) High fever, increased blood pressure, and aphasia

C) Urticaria, rash, tightness of the chest, wheezing, and hypotension

D) Severe abdominal pain, paralysis, and muscle fasciculations

C – These are the common signs and symptoms of hypersensitivity related to antivenin administration. They sound remarkably similar to the symptoms of any allergic reaction (because they are) and conveniently, the management is essentially the same as other allergic reactions. Bleeding from lots of body sites is a sign of severe coagulopathy from the venom, but not a reaction to the antivenin. Severe abdominal pain, paralysis and fasciculations can be a result of the venom, but not a reaction to the antivenin. High fevers, labile blood pressure or trouble speaking can be symptoms of many bad things from sepsis to stroke, but are not associated with reactions to the antivenin. If, shortly after initiating a medication, in this case, antivenin, the patient has symptoms that sound like an allergic/hypersensivity reaction and look like an allergic/hypersensitivity reaction, treat it like an allergic/hypersensitivity reaction!

74) Common symptoms of a scorpion sting can include:

A) Decreased salivation and dry mouth

B) Redness and swelling at the sting site

C) Immediate local pain and burning sensation

D) Temporary blindness

C – Scorpion stings are <u>extremely</u> painful and may require the administration of narcotic analgesics.

"Patients stung by the bark scorpion (*Centruroides sculpturatus*) experience immediate burning and stinging sensation at the sting site. Following the pain, bark scorpion envenomation produces a pattern of neurotoxicity with a spectrum of severity ranging from trivial to life threatening. Severe envenomation, more common in small children than adults, may involve loss of muscle control, roving or abnormal eye movements, slurred speech, respiratory distress, excessive salivation, frothing at the mouth, and vomiting. Overall, 95-100% of patients were relieved of systemic signs associated with scorpion envenomation in less than four hours after initiating *Anascorp* treatment. In the historical control database, *meaning no Anascorp*, only 3.1% of patients experienced relief of symptoms within 4 hours of hospital admission."

(**anascorp-us.com**)

75) In addition to neurotoxicity, scorpion venom is known for which of the following toxicities?

A) Cardiotoxicity and hepatotoxicity

B) Cerebrotoxicity and hepatotoxicity

C) Nephrotoxicity and hepatotoxicity

D) Nephrotoxicity and cardiotoxicity

D – Drop for drop, scorpion venom is potentially more life threatening than rattlesnake venom as it is not only a neurotoxin (brain) and nephrotoxin (kidneys), but a cardiotoxin (heart) as well!

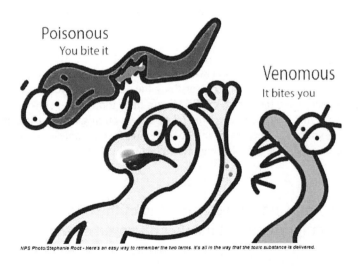

Poisonous versus Venomous Bites & Stings

76) Capnography is utilized in place of, or in conjunction with, arterial blood gases in patients with all of the following conditions **except**:

A) Cardiac arrest

B) Reticular Erythematous Mucinosis

C) Diabetic ketoacidosis

D) Asthma

B - Reticular Erythematous Mucinosis may sound nasty and dangerous and has lots of parts of words that look familiar, but what it is has nothing to do with capnography. In case you were wondering, it actually is a condition characterized by persistent, mildly pruritic, reticulated erythematous macules, papules or urticarial plaques that most often occur on the upper back and chest. It falls into the category of dermatology and as opposed to the other options; it has nothing to do with breathing (or the lack thereof).

As far as this question goes, waveform capnography is a great diagnostic tool. Although no single vital sign is definitive as a simultaneous measure of metabolism, ventilation and perfusion, capnography reliably provides information about all three. In addition to being a great way to initially and continuously confirm airway device placement and monitor ventilation, capnography can do so much more! Carbon dioxide (CO_2) is a product of cellular metabolism, transported around the body via perfusion, and later removed through ventilation. End-tidal carbon dioxide ($EtCO_2$) waveform monitoring allows measurement of all three simultaneously, making it one of the most important diagnostic tools available, especially to emergency providers.

Capnography comes from the Ancient Greek, *kapnós*, meaning smoke. The use of capnography to verify endotracheal tube placement has been the standard of care for years. Capnography can be attached to an endotracheal tube, a nasal cannula, or a mask, and its uses continue to evolve and expand for patients across the lifespan and with a wide variety of conditions. From babies to big people, from sedation to sepsis, emergency professionals are always looking for a non-invasive, reliable, bedside instrument to detect life-threatening conditions in patients. Capnography is one such tool.

Testing tip: When you know something about most of the options and nothing about one of them, and if the question asks for an exception, go with what you know. If it were reasonably important, you probably would have heard about it.

[*Editor's comment*: A clever test question writer will often take an answer designed to be implausible and make it seem possible for those who are prone to over-think the question. If you over-think "Reticular Erythematous Mucinosis" and make the acronym "REM" out of it, it might cause you to associate that answer with "REM" sleep. Once you start down that rabbit hole, you might spend valuable time and mental energy questioning yourself. Keep calm and go with your instinct unless you have hard evidence or a truly compelling reason to change (like having misread something).]

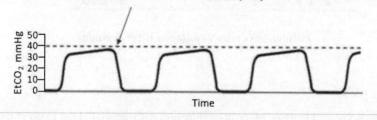

The arrow is pointed to the end of the tidal wave.
This point represents the number displayed on the monitor.

A "normal" capnogram waveform has a regular up and down pattern with a "sloping square" shape. The normal $EtCO_2$ range is 30-45 mm Hg

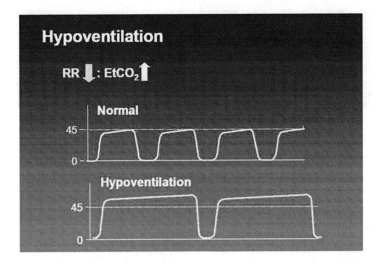

A "hypoventilation" capnogram has a regular waveform, but the $EtCO_2$ levels get progressively higher. When the patient is not breathing often enough, not as much CO_2 is removed from the lungs, so the concentration of carbon dioxide in the exhaled air is higher.

Additional Insights from a Pediatric Emergency Medicine Attending Physician:

I would add that it's also possible to have a rapid respiratory rate and still hypoventilate if the breathing is very shallow. It's more likely to happen in kids than in adults due to the higher baseline respiratory rates in infants and younger kids. In that case, it would look like this tracing, but the peaks would be above the 45 line.

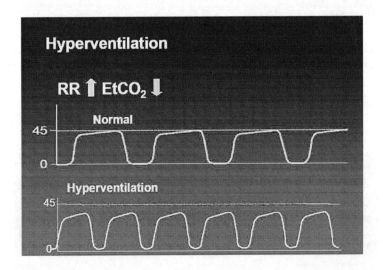

A "Hyperventilation" capnogram has a regular waveform, but way too many waves and low $EtCO_2$ numbers. Hyperventilation can occur as a result of DKA, ingestion of some drugs, anxiety, etc.

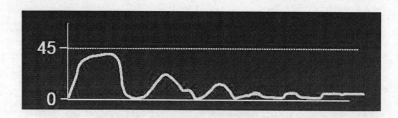

An esophageal intubation will produce a capnogram waveform that is irregular and has significantly and rapidly decreasing CO_2 values.

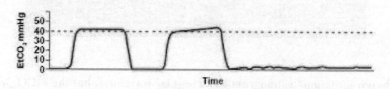

The sudden loss of a recognizable capnogram waveform followed by sudden flat waveform can be caused by extubation, cardiac arrest, apnea, etc.

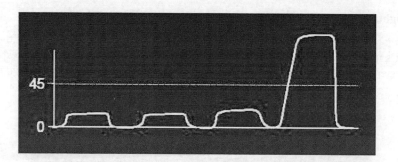

Capnography during CPR that results in a "Return of Spontaneous Circulation" (ROSC) is characterized by a regular (but significantly low) waveform matching compressions and ventilations, followed by a sudden INCREASE in waveform size indicating probable ROSC

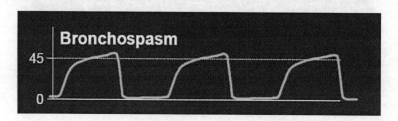

A "Shark Fin" capnogram waveform has a more distinctive upward slope and is often seen with patients that are being treated for really bad asthma, COPD, or other conditions which might cause bronchospasms. This waveform might also be caused by an endotracheal tube which is too small, kinked, or otherwise obstructed, aka., crud encrusted

Certified Pediatric Emergency Nurse (CPEN) Review IV

Capnography has been described as "the 12-lead for the lungs." If your department has it, use it. If your department doesn't have it, get it. Capnography is an invaluable tool for everything from treating tiny tots to terrible traumas.

For additional capnography education, we highly recommend the following websites:

www.capnography.com

www.capnoacademy.com

www.respironics.com

77) A 4-year old presents to the emergency department (ED) with a complex laceration requiring suture repair. What would be considered the **least** invasive form of sedation for this procedure?

A) IV procedural sedation

B) Nitrous oxide

C) Topical analgesics

D) Distraction

B – Whether in the ED or the surgical arena, nitrous oxide sedation is generally considered safe for use in the pediatric population. Adverse effects are rare as long as the use is limited to less than three hours. (And let's be honest, if your sedation is over three hours long, other discussions should probably take place.) Alternative practices include oral medications (midazolam) or IV sedation on toddlers and young children, but this question specifically asks for the least invasive, and oral medication was not an option. And since the question asked about sedation, distraction and topical analgesics, while helpful in many situations, can be eliminated.

At this stage in their psychosocial development, toddlers have common fears of separation from caregivers and loss of control. Utilizing a non-invasive approach to sedation, i.e. nitrous oxide, allows parents and caregivers to stay present during the procedure. This results in the child (and the caregivers) staying calmer.

Nitrous oxide, (also referred to as N_2O, "nitrous," or even "laughing gas") was first discovered in 1793 by the English scientist Joseph Priestly and has been used medically (and socially?) ever since. It is colorless, odorless, and tasteless. Nitrous oxide also provides analgesia (not a lot), amnesia, and it relieves anxiety. All 3 things...and no shot. That's an amazing combo for the EMS/ED environments, especially with children.

Most commonly, nitrous oxide is administered in a 70:30 mix (70% nitrous and 30% oxygen) or a 50:50 mix. That's not a lot of oxygen, but think about it, 30-50% is more than room air (21%) and unless nitrous is mixed with opiates (morphine, fentanyl, etc.), it rarely causes respiratory depression. After the procedure is complete, giving 100% oxygen for 5 minutes will wash out any residual nitrous and quickly return the patient to baseline.

Contraindications to nitrous in the ER are few, but important to keep in the back of your head (and in preparing for a test). Nitrous can enter air-filled cavities 34 times faster than nitrogen found in room air. As a result, nitrous is contraindicated for patients in whom expansion of air-filled cavities could result in profound badness. This includes patients with an actual or suspected pneumothorax (trauma), pulmonary blebs (Marfan's), air embolism (divers), bowel obstruction (lots of reasons), and those undergoing surgery of the middle ear (not performed in the ED.)

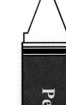

Pediatric Potpourri

Certified Pediatric Emergency Nurse (CPEN) Review IV

Here are a few neat tricks from anesthesia for the ED:

1. Stickers are your best friend. Have the child pick their favorites and cover the mask in them.

2. They make pediatric nitrous masks that are pre-impregnated with aromatherapy scents. You can ask your patient if they want a bubble gum or strawberry mask (or other flavor).

3. Be like Bath and Body Works... For years, anesthesia has used a few drops of "aromatherapy scents" onto the mask before beginning nitrous to allow the child a choice in "sleepy smells."

4. And yet another anesthesia and nitrous mask trick comes from the "Dollar Store." Pick up a multi-pack of flavored Chap Stick and ask the child what their favorite flavor is. Smear a small amount onto the mask and off they go (to sleep, that is).

N_2O – No smell, no taste, no color... No wonder it's still around and helping with pain, anxiety and amnesia!

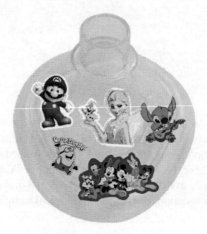

Stickers and Nitrous Oxide Mask
Photo courtesy of Michelle Webb RN, MSN, CRNA

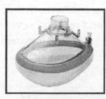
Unscented Size 5

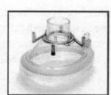
Fresh Scent

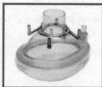
Strawberry

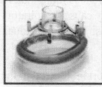
Cherry

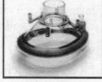
Bubble Gum

Aromatherapy Nitrous Oxide Masks
Photo courtesy of Ambu
www.AmbuUSA.com

78) The most common adverse effect of nitrous oxide is:

A) Nausea/vomiting
B) Sleepiness
C) Headache
D) Hallucinations

A – Nausea and vomiting are the most common adverse effects, occurring in just up to 2.4% of patients. Note: Giving 100% oxygen post-procedure not only helps to "flush out' the nitrous, but also helps with "nitrous nausea" as well. Children may also rarely experience headaches, excessive sweating, or shivering. Hallucinations can be seen with medications such as ketamine, but not typically with nitrous oxide. Sleepiness, feelings of euphoria, relaxation and calmness are the intended, not adverse, effects of nitrous oxide.

79) Advantages of nitrous oxide use with the pediatric patient include all of the following **except**:

A) No need for IV access
B) Short onset of action
C) Not associated with malignant hyperthermia
D) Provides several hours of analgesia and anxiolysis in the pediatric patient

D – Unlike other anesthetics used in the operating room, nitrous oxide sedation is not associated with malignant hyperthermia. When used for pediatric procedural sedation, nitrous oxide has several advantages, including no need for IV access, rapid onset (30-60 seconds) and rapid recovery. An additional benefit is that there have been no reported allergies to nitrous oxide.

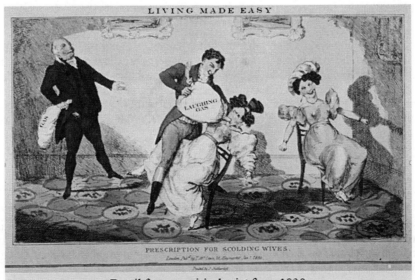

Detail from a satirical print from 1830 depicting Humphry Davy administering a dose of Laughing Gas to a woman while Count Rumford looks on.

80) Cystic fibrosis is suspected in a six-week old infant undergoing genetic testing. What additional test should be the priority to verify the diagnosis?

A) Stool fecal fat testing

B) Sweat chloride test

C) Amylase and lipase levels

D) Chest radiography

B – The sweat chloride test, while rarely if ever performed in the emergency department, remains the primary test for verification of cystic fibrosis in babies over 2-4 weeks of age. A painless electrical current stimulates sweat production in the patient, which is collected on a filter paper. The amount of chloride is then measured. Sweat chloride test results of greater than 60 mmol/L are abnormal, and with a confirmed second test, is enough to verify the diagnosis of cystic fibrosis. Interesting bit of medical trivia– experienced (aka., older) neonatal nurses remember (or at least hearing about) the times when licking the skin of babies who were suspected as having cystic fibrosis was not uncommon. If they tasted salty, the diagnosis was informally confirmed. You can't make this stuff up!

Stool fecal fat testing can be used to evaluate a patient for malabsorption, a condition where the body either isn't absorbing nutrients properly or isn't making the enzymes or bile needed to digest food effectively. Amylase and lipase level testing is useful in diagnosing pancreatic diseases. Chest radiography is generally considered insensitive to the early changes caused by cystic fibrosis.

81) Infants and children diagnosed with cystic fibrosis (CF) commonly present with any/all of the following symptoms **except**:

A) Respiratory symptoms

B) Abnormal renal function

C) Failure to thrive

D) Meconium ileus

B – Interestingly, for a condition in which salt transport is a primary abnormality, patients with CF have apparently normal renal function. While the majority of newborns are diagnosed with cystic fibrosis through the newborn screening process, the clinical presentations shown by infants and children with CF typically include respiratory symptoms (no surprise there), failure to thrive (priority of breathing vs. eating), or a meconium ileus (blockage in a part of the small intestine). These symptoms typically present within two months to two years of age. Think "problems with secretions" – in particular mucous, sweat, and digestive juices.

82) A 3-month old presents to the emergency department extremely irritable without a known cause, beyond being three-months old. The patient's mother explains that last evening she gave the patient a bath and then put him in bed in his full-length pajamas. The patient then woke up fussy and is inconsolable upon arrival to the ER. Vital signs, including rectal temperature, are normal. The nurse should suspect which of the following:

A) Hair tourniquet

B) Hunger

C) Dehydration

D) Allergic reaction

A – Hair tourniquet is a condition that is most commonly found on toes, but can also involve fingers or genitalia. (Anything involving tourniquets and genitalia would make any man scream!) In young infants, a loose hair or thread may wrap around an appendage and become constricting as movement occurs in a confined area (especially socks, gloves, diapers, or full-length pajamas). Discomfort from the tourniquet may lead to additional movement, causing further constriction. Hair that falls into bath water may easily attach to an appendage. Wet hair stretches and is typically loosely attached, but may become more constrictive as it dries. Nothing in this scenario indicates feeding issues or an allergic reaction.

83) Following the removal of a hair tourniquet from an infant, the nurse should provide the parents/guardians each of the following recommendations **except**:

A) Check the child's extremities and genitalia after each diaper change and bath for possible loose hairs/threads

B) Inform the mother that hair loss is increased in postpartum period and advise her to brush hair often

C) Recommend that only the father bathe the patient

D) Wash the child's clothes inside-out

C – While a postpartum mother can have increased hair loss and should certainly be aware of loose hairs, it is not appropriate to exclude her from the bonding and baby bathing process. All of the other options will help reduce the likelihood of a hair tourniquet occurring.

84) After the removal of a hair tourniquet or other constricting band, which of the following should be the nurse's **priority** action?

A) Apply heat to the affected area

B) Ready the patient for surgery

C) Elevate the affected region if possible

D) Provide a prophylactic antibiotic

C – Elevation of the affected area, if possible, should be the priority to promote a more rapid decrease in swelling. Applying heat would likely increase swelling, antibiotics are typically unnecessary, and a surgical consultation may only be required if swelling is unchanged or worse several hours after initial tourniquet removal.

85) A 10-year old boy presents to the emergency department with a straddle injury following a fall on monkey bars while at school yesterday. Which finding is **most** concerning for a bladder rupture?

A) Testicular pain

B) Perineal swelling and ecchymosis

C) Hematuria

D) Persistent abdominal pain

D – Irritation from leaking urine related to a bladder rupture can lead to persistent abdominal discomfort, peritonitis, and possible sepsis. As opposed to a urethral injury, bladder rupture is characterized by one or more of following: the inability to void, suprapubic discomfort, persistent abdominal pain (caused by peritoneal irritation), and a palpably distended bladder. All these signs are near the bladder and therefore probably involve the bladder. Hematuria can indicate injury to any part of the genitourinary tract (i.e. kidney, bladder, ureter, or urethra). Blood at the meatus and perineal swelling/ecchymosis is more indicative of urethral injury. Again, especially with test questions, signs and symptoms around the urethra should lead you to think issues with the urethra on the test. Testicular pain is a concerning finding, especially in women, but not necessarily related to bladder rupture.

86) The provider order indicates "80 mg Lovenox® (enoxaparin) given sub q nightly." Which part of the order should the nurse identify as an inappropriate documentation?

A) 80

B) mg

C) sub q

D) nightly

C – "Sub q" has been listed as an "Error-Prone" abbreviation by the Institute of Safe Medication Practices (ISMP), and therefore should not be used. The term "sub q" has been mistaken for "sublingual" or "sub every." It should be replaced with either "subcut" or "subcutaneously." The term "nightly" is preferred, as "qhs" should not be utilized. 80 and mg are currently approved terminology.

87) The nursing student is reviewing medication orders and notes the following: "4 U insulin given per sliding scale t.i.d." Which portion of the documentation should be identified as an incorrect use of abbreviations/medical terminology?

A) 4

B) U

C) sliding scale

D) t.i.d.

B – The use of "U" has been identified as an error-prone abbreviation by the Institute of Safe Medication Practices (ISMP) and is on the official "Do Not Use" list published by The Joint Commission (TJC). Both groups have deemed the use of "U" as unsafe and recommend using the term "units" in its place. Numbers should have no trailing zeroes after a whole number, i.e. 4 is correct whereas 4.0 is incorrect because it can easily be confused with 40. "SS," "SSRI," or "SSI" should not be used to denote the use of a sliding scale. TID or t.i.d. are currently approved abbreviations.

88) The provider order writes ".4 mg Narcan PRN NAS." Which part of the order should the nurse identify as an example of unsafe documentation?

A) .4

B) mg

C) PRN

D) NAS

A – ".4" without a "0" before the decimal point is considered an error-prone dose designation by the Institute of Safe Medication Practices (ISMP). A zero should always be placed in front of the decimal point when the value is less than a whole number, i.e. 0.4. The use of "mg" and "PRN" are currently approved abbreviations. For nasal medications, the ISMP recommends "intranasal" or "NAS" as safe abbreviations. "IN" should not be used for intranasal as it can be confused for IM or IV.

89) The nurse sees a medication order for "5,000 units Heparin subcutaneously qd" on the list of "new orders" for a patient. Which portion of the documentation is inappropriate per the Institute of Safe Medication Practices (ISMP)?

A) 5,000

B) units

C) subcutaneously

D) qd

D – The use of "qd" has been identified as an error-prone abbreviation by the ISMP and therefore should not be used in any order, old or new. The abbreviation "qd" has commonly been confused with "qid." The acceptable term to use is "daily." "5,000" is correct, as large doses at or above 1,000 units should either utilize commas or utilize the long form wording (i.e., five thousand). "Units" and "subcutaneously" are currently approved per the ISMP.

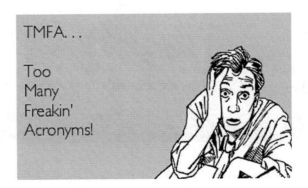

90) During a hazardous materials incident, which control zone would require the highest level of personal protective equipment (PPE)?

A) Exclusion Zone ("Hot Zone")

B) Contamination Reduction Zone ("Warm Zone")

C) Support Zone ("Cold Zone")

D) Danger Zone ("Dead Zone")

A – Anyone in the Exclusion Zone, also known as the Hot Zone, requires the highest level of personal protective equipment (PPE) because of the potential concentration of materials present. This zone is immediately around the incident and has the highest risk for exposure to or contact with any hazardous materials present.

Determining the level of protection needed is based on many factors including location, occupancy, and what specific hazardous materials are present, if known. An enclosed location that can cause entrapment of hazardous materials would require a higher level of PPE versus an open location such as a field. Occupancy refers to the nature and/or purpose of the location. For example, a chemical plant would have far more dangerous materials than a daycare facility.

If the material is known, one can refer to the "Safety Data Sheet" (formerly referred to as the Material Safety Data Sheet or "MSDS") for a great deal of specific information. The Occupational Safety and Health Administration (OSHA) of the United States Department of Labor outlines the required information in the Safety Data Sheets. Section 8 covers "Exposure Controls/Personal Protection" and includes recommendations for personal protective measures to prevent illness or injury from exposure. These recommendations include personal protective equipment (PPE) such as the appropriate types of eye, face, skin, or respiratory protection needed based on hazards and potential exposure.

If the material is unknown, then the highest level of PPE would be required.

And just in case you were wondering, "The Dead Zone" is not a control zone. It is a 1983 horror thriller film based on the 1979 novel of the same name by Stephen King. It is not necessarily the place where one hears a child saying, "I see dead people."

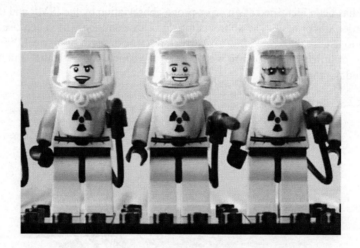

91) At a hazardous materials incident, the decon corridor is set-up in which zone?

A) Exclusion Zone ("Hot Zone")

B) Contamination Reduction Zone ("Warm Zone")

C) Support Zone ("Cold Zone")

D) Decontamination Zone ("Decon Zone")

B – The Contamination Reduction Zone, otherwise known as the Warm Zone, contains the decon corridor and is preferably upwind of the Hot Zone. This corridor allows victims and responders to egress from the Hot Zone, undergo decontamination and then be allowed into the Cold Zone. The Support Zone is the Cold Zone, while the Exclusion Zone is the Hot Zone. There is not a Decon Zone. Hot, to warm, to cold. Exclusion to Contamination Reduction to Support. Just about everyone except the patient is "excluded" from the Exclusion "Hot Zone." Reducing the amounts of contamination is the goal of the Contamination Reduction "Warm Zone." Support for the now hopefully not grossly contaminated patients begins in the Support "Cold Zone."

Certified Pediatric Emergency Nurse (CPEN) Review IV

Treatment Performed By Zone	
Zone	**Treatment**
Hot	Opening airway; inserting oral or nasal airway(s); tourniquet application; IM antidote injections
Warm	Everything performed in Hot Zone; administer oxygen or nebulized medications; supraglottic airways; Bag-mask ventilation
Cold	Any additional treatment needed for patient not provided in Hot or Warm Zones

Hazmat 101 for Pediatric ED Nurses: Additional Insights from EMS

Decontamination is required when a liquid, solid or gaseous substance of unknown or suspected hazardous properties potentially contaminates victims.

Routes of Exposure:

There are four main routes that hazardous materials or poisons can enter the body.

Inhalation – The most frequently encountered route of exposure, materials or poisons enter through the inhalation of gases, vapors, smoke, fumes, dusts, mists or fogs. A vapor is the gaseous state of a chemical usually found in liquid or solid state at standard temperature and pressure. Smoke, fumes, and dust are airborne suspensions of solid particles. Mists and fog are airborne suspensions of liquid particles.

Transdermal and transmucosal – Absorption can be through the skin, eyes, or mucous membranes. Lipid (fat) soluble chemicals absorb through the skin easily. Hospital providers should not assume these patients are thoroughly decontaminated and need to ensure that all areas of the skin have been decontaminated, especially genital areas and between folds of skin.

Ingestion – Ingestion is NOT a common route of exposure for hazardous materials. Most ingestions are usually either intentional during a suicide attempt or accidental by younger children. This route can be potentially dangerous for medical personnel caring for victims of ingestions because of a phenomenon called "off-gassing." Off-gassing is vapor released from the product that is still on or inside the patient. Usually residual product around the mouth, vomit from the patient or in rare cases, ingested or aspirated product can still release vapors from inside the patient and find its way out through the esophagus or trachea and to medical personnel. This last route is very uncommon, but is possible with a large ingestion or in the event of aspiration or regurgitation after ingestion.

Injection – Not a typical route of exposure, injection can occur from accidental high-pressure contact from paint guns or hydraulic lines. During explosions, injections can occur from contaminated debris that is turned into projectiles which then penetrate the body.

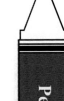

Certified Pediatric Emergency Nurse (CPEN) Review IV

Decontamination Goals:

There are two important goals of decontamination: (1) Altering absorption and (2) preventing secondary contamination.

Altering absorption – Remove the victim from the poison and the poison from the victim. In all instances, except known biological warfare incidents, remove all victims' clothing (including diapers or underwear) and provide gross decontamination of patient with copious amounts of water. Modesty and prevention of hypothermia are certainly a concern, but adequate decontamination is the key. Flush, flush, flush, flush, flush.

Reduce/Avoid secondary contamination – Avoid the transfer of the poison from the victim to the medical provider. Secondary contamination can occur from improper gross decontamination, a contaminated victim treated before decontamination, or "off-gassing" of poison from vomitus or respirations. Vapors from a toxic chemical ingestion can still be released by the patient if there is a route available, such as the esophagus for ingested chemicals or trachea for inhaled/aspirated chemicals. Additional decontamination steps may be necessary to ensure prevention of secondary contamination.

Gross or Emergency Decontamination

This type of decontamination is used when circumstances exist that require <u>immediate</u> decontamination of victim(s).

Ideal Procedure:

- The victim moves from the contaminated area to the gross decontamination area independently or with the assistance of properly attired and trained responders.
- Properly attired responders remove the victim's clothing or victim removes their own clothing.
- The victim proceeds through the decon line and is flooded with copious amounts of water, until thoroughly rinsed.
- The victims receives cover or clothing after flush, flush, flush...
- The victim is assessed for any residual contamination and if none, proceeds to triage.
- If contamination is still present, the victim goes through decontamination again. Flush, flush, flush...

Removing <u>all</u> clothing can remove up to 80% of the icky substance from the victim!

Personal Protective Equipment

The US Environmental Protection Agency (EPA) has defined four levels of protective clothing for anticipated contact with chemical hazards:

Level A

    Fully encapsulated vapor resistant suit; self-contained positive pressure breathing apparatus (SCBA); chemical resistant outer gloves and boots

Pediatric Potpourri

Level B

Chemical resistant splash suit; SCBA; chemical resistant outer gloves and boots

Level C

Chemical resistant suit; full-face cartridge respirator (gas mask); chemical resistant outer gloves and boots

Level D

All other clothing, including structural firefighting gear, medical scrubs, EMS uniform and flip-flops, tank top and shorts. They are all considered level D, as they provide NO protection against chemical contact

Levels of Personal Protective Clothing			
Level Type	**Respiratory**	**Chemical Barrier**	**Notes**
A	SCBA*	Vapor Protective Clothing	Highest level of respiratory and chemical protection
B	SCBA*	Liquid/Splash Protective Clothing	Highest level of respiratory protection and only splash chemical protection (not vapors)
C	APR**/ PAPR***	Liquid/Splash Protective Clothing	Same level of skin protection as B, lower respiratory protection
D	None	None	No protection from either

* Self-contained breathing apparatus; ** Air-purified respirator; **
*** Powered air-purified respirator ***

Hazmat Zones

The pre-hospital management of a hazardous materials incident will involve the identification of different areas of the incident. Within these zones, a decon corridor is used that allows for entry and exit of hazmat operators and for decontamination of victims.

These different zones:

- Specify the type of operation to occur in each zone
- The degree of hazard within each zone
- The areas of the incident where no entry should occur without authorization

Usually, the incident is broken down into three zones: Hot, warm and cold.

The Hot Zone (exclusion zone)

This area contains the incident or hazard and is restricted to those personnel with a specific activity and ONLY AFTER donning proper personal protective equipment (PPE). Access to this zone is tightly controlled and entry/exit is restricted to one location, the decontamination corridor.

The decontamination corridor is the only point of entry/exit from the hot zone. This corridor allows for decontamination of hazmat team personnel, equipment, and victims.

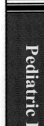

The Warm Zone (contamination reduction zone)

This area surrounds the hot zone and is restricted to those personnel with a specific activity and ONLY AFTER donning proper PPE. The PPE required will usually be one level less than required for the Hot Zone.

This zone contains the decontamination corridor, with entry into and out of the Hot Zone. All personnel, victims, equipment, evidence, etc. must pass through the decontamination corridor from the Hot Zone. Any personnel or equipment entering the Hot Zone must pass through this decontamination corridor.

If required, hazardous materials trained medical personnel (tox or haz mat medic) may perform limited medical treatment to victims in the Warm Zone.

The Cold Zone (support zone)

This zone is the safe area beyond the warm zone and is essentially the rest of the world. This area is safe and no hazmat specific personal PPE is required to remain in the Cold Zone. Personnel here are in normal uniform with standard biological precautions (gloves, face mask/shield, etc.) Patients here have been decontaminated and can be transported to the appropriate facility without any additional hazardous material precautions. Only authorized personnel should be allowed in the immediate area surrounding the Warm Zone. Medical triage, on scene treatment and transport of victims occur in this zone. Non-hazardous materials trained medical personnel can provide treatment only in this zone.

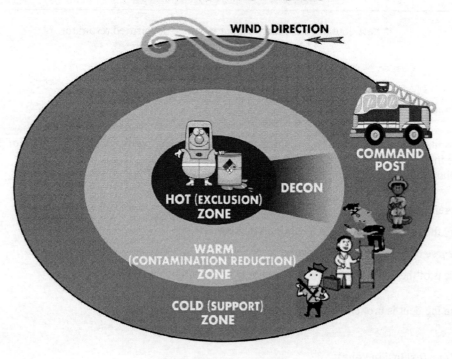

Hazmat 101 for Pediatric ED Nurses: Additional Insights from EMS
Courtesy of Michael Austin EMT-P, FP-C

Certified Pediatric Emergency Nurse (CPEN) Review IV

92) All of the following are considered elements of the primary management of chemical burn injuries EXCEPT:

A) Irrigation

B) Removal of clothing

C) Brush off powdered chemicals

D) Induce vomiting

D - Vomiting should not be induced in these cases as if it burned on the way down, it will most certainly burn on the way back up. If post-vomiting aspiration occurs, that just makes the situation even worse! The primary management of chemical burns includes procedures designed to stop the burning process while maintaining safety... for both the healthcare professional and the patient. Safety first. In addition to the understood need for the use of protective gear, the first line of management with chemical burns means that we do what we can to stop the burning process (remembering safety first.) This includes removal of all patient clothing, brushing off powdered chemicals, and if the patient is stable, irrigation of the affected area. If it's icky... flush, flush, flush. Then flush, flush, flush some more. Remember, with most burns from chemical exposures, dilution is the solution to the task of stopping the burn process!

Attempts at "neutralization" should only be attempted with poison center guidance and/or clear instructions from industry sources such as the Material Safety Data Sheets (MSDS). Adding water to many dry chemicals will cause an exothermic reactions, resulting in additional burning if the chemical is still on the patient or the patient's clothing. When it comes to chemical exposures, always safety first and with few exceptions, **dilution is the solution**!

93) What is the **most** common route of laundry detergent pod toxicity?

A) Ingestion

B) Eye exposure

C) Skin exposure

D) Inhalation

A - Ingestion remains the most common route for toxicity followed by exposure to the eyes, skin, and finally, in rare cases, inhalation. Laundry detergent pods were first introduced to the market in 2012, but it wasn't until early 2018 that the "Pod Challenge" became a viral internet sensation. (Gotta love the cultural effects of "YouTube!") Now little ones eat them because they come in bright colors, shapes, sizes, and textures which all resemble a bite-sized snack. Teens ingest them because they are teenagers and honestly, who can really determine why teenagers do 99% of what they do?

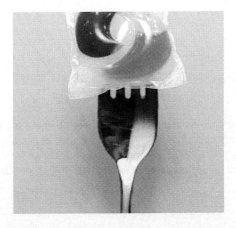

Certified Pediatric Emergency Nurse (CPEN) Review IV

94) A pediatric patient presents with an eye injury related to direct contact with the ingredients in a laundry detergent pod. The child's eye is swollen, red, and draining clear fluid. Which of the following is the **most** important action to be undertaken?

A) Visual acuity assessment

B) Assessment and examination of the cornea and sclera

C) Copious irrigation with normal saline (NS) or Ringer's Lactate (LR)

D) Slit lamp examination

C – When the contents of a laundry detergent pod (or any other common commercial detergent product) make contact to the eye, the result is an alkaline chemical burn injury. The most important initial action to be taken is to begin irrigation of the affected areas with copious amounts of normal saline (NS) or Ringer's Lactate (LR). The goal of the irrigation is to neutralize the pH of the eye. Acidic or alkaline substances in your eyes are really icky, so flush, flush, flush, flush, flush! Assuming no immediate life-threatening injury exists, further assessment and examination of the eye can wait until the chemical burn has been stopped and the pH of the eye has returned to normal.

95) What is the normal pH of the eye?

A) 1.5-3.5

B) 7.0 to 7.3

C) 4.5-8

D) 7.35-7.45

B - The normal pH of the eye is 7.0 to 7.3. Normal and Neutral both begin with the letter "N". And we should all remember what we learned in basic high school chemistry, that a Neutral pH is 7. So, as you don't want your eyes to be anything but Normal, pick a pH close to Neutral, i.e. around 7. When dealing with toxic exposures to the eye, it is essential to quickly attempt to return the pH to neutral to avoid further injury. When it comes to chemical burns, acid is bad, but alkali is worse. And for the physiology geeks out there, the other answers involving normal pH, but not for the eye: 1.5-3.5 is the normal pH of the stomach, 4.5-8 is the normal pH of the urine, and 7.35-7.45 is the normal pH of arterial blood.

96) A 17-year old male presents to the ER with body aches, fever, and jaundice. His past medical history is unremarkable except for receiving a tattoo "by a buddy" a few weeks ago. With these particular symptoms, what is the likely diagnosis?

A) Influenza

B) Hepatitis

C) HIV

D) Gastroenteritis

B - The key to this question is the specific mention of jaundice. Without the jaundice, either flu or gastroenteritis would be likely considerations. HIV is a possibility, especially with non-professional tattoos; however, it is unlikely to present with symptoms this quickly after exposure. So, that leaves hepatitis as the most likely culprit, especially since "buddy" rarely has sterilized equipment with which to perform the tattoo procedure.

Pediatric Potpourri

Certified Pediatric Emergency Nurse (CPEN) Review IV

Body piercings and tattooing have been performed around the world for well over 5,000 years. Complications such as infections, scars, etc. have been documented in medical journals and other publications. However, when one compares the thousands and thousands of body art procedures performed around the world each year to the number of published case reports, the incidence of complications is relatively rare.

The keys to body art (piercings and/or tattoos) are essentially two-fold. First, the person should have the procedure performed by a professional piercer or tattoo artist. If the experienced artist uses sterile equipment, jewelry, ink, etc., the complications immediately after the procedure are rare. However, research shows that the initial procedure is only one chapter of the story. The remaining chapters involve aftercare, i.e. how to properly care for the new piercing or tattoo. This is a huge deal as many piercings take weeks, if not months, to completely heal. In teens with the attention span of a doorknob, this can be big deal. Getting the art is easy... Caring for it is a whole different story!

Type of piercing (Top to bottom and everywhere between!)	Anatomically Where Does the Jewelry Go?	Approximate Healing Times	Common Types of Jewelry Placed
Ampallang	*Horizontally* through the glans (spongy head of the penis) and ± through the urethra	4-6 months	Barbell
Apadravya	*Vertically* through the glans (spongy head of the penis) **and** urethra and out on the head in front of the coronal ridge – you get a free Prince Albert with every apadravya	4-6 months	Barbell
Branding	You name it, it's been branded	First: Red, nasty phase – The cauterized tissue will come off in about 2 weeks. Second: A second scab will form, and this will come off 4-8 weeks into the healing process. Full healing: 1 year	N/A
Cheek	Self-explanatory (through the buccinator muscle, between the facial artery and vein)	2-3 months	Barbell with a disc back on the inside
Chest (surface)	Usually between the jugular notch and superior to the xiphoid process (front of the chest)	6-12months	Surface barbell
Christina	Vertically just below the mons pubis, superior to the anterior commissure of labia majora (on the pubic mound and above the vagina)	6-8 months	Barbell
Clitoral hood (vertical)	Vertically through the prepuce (thin bit of tissue) above the clitoris (<u>not</u> through the clitoris itself)	4-6 weeks	Bent barbell or ring

Pediatric Potpourri

Type of piercing (Top to bottom and everywhere between!)	Anatomically Where Does the Jewelry Go?	Approximate Healing Times	Common Types of Jewelry Placed
Clitoris	Self-explanatory and *very rare*	4-6 weeks	Ring
Cutting	Through the epidermis and dermis into the subcutaneous tissue	4-6 weeks	N/A
Dydoe	Top and sides rim of glans (spongy head of penis) through the coronal ridge (commonly done in pairs)	2-3 months	Curved barbell
Ear (daith)	Through the crux helix or innermost ridge of cartilage above the tragus (cartilage in front of the ear canal opening)	2-6 months	Ring
Ear (cartilage)	Commonly refers to the helix of the ear. Conch, daith, rook and tragus are all cartilage piercings.	2-6 months	Barbell, ring, or circular barbell
Ear (conch)	The concha (shell of the ear) may be pierced in many different directions	2-6 months	Barbell, ring, circular barbell, plug, or eyelet
Ear (head)	Juncture of the ear and head in the cartilage	2-3 months	Ring, barbell, or mini barbell
Ear (lobe)	Lobule (traditional) or transverse lobe piercing	4-8 weeks	Transverse barbell or ring
Ear (rook)	Crura of antihelix, opposite of the crus of the helix – through the antihelix (upper ridge of cartilage in the ear)	2-3 months	Barbell or ring
Ear (tragus)	Through the prominence of cartilage in front of the opening of the ear canal	2-3 months	Barbell or ring
Earl (mid brow)	Below the glabella and above the nasal bone (middle of an eyebrow)	2-3 months	Barbell
Etching	Anywhere on the skin	2 weeks	N/A
Eyebrow	Through the soft tissue, behind the eyebrow ridge	6-8 weeks	Barbell or ring
Foreskin	Self-explanatory	6-8 weeks	Barbell or ring
Fourchette	Vertical perineum piercing from the vestibular fossa to the posterior commissure of the labia majora (Female Guiche)	4-6 weeks	Bent barbell
Frenum	Loose piece of flesh between the head and shaft of the penis – Not through the shaft itself – Anywhere on the shaft where it is possible to pinch up the tissue – Your imagination and pinchability factor of the tissue are the main limitations	2-3 months	Barbell, rows of jewelry, or a large ring that fits snugly around the erect head of the penis (once fully healed)

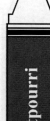

Certified Pediatric Emergency Nurse (CPEN) Review IV

Type of piercing (Top to bottom and everywhere between!)	Anatomically Where Does the Jewelry Go?	Approximate Healing Times	Common Types of Jewelry Placed
Guiche	In the urogenital triangle, behind the pubic symphysis near the prostate (Inseam of flesh between the scrotum and anus)	2-3 months	Ring or curved barbell
Hafada	Anywhere on the scrotum, typically near the top and in pairs	2-3 months	Barbell or ring
Hand (web)	Self-explanatory – Between the fingers	6-9 months	Barbell or ring
Implants	Facial, sternal, arms, and genitals	4+ weeks	Titanium, Teflon, silicone, pearl, stainless steel implants (shapes, horns, etc)
Labia (inner)	Labia minora	4-6 weeks	Rings
Labia (outer)	In the pudendal cleft, behind the labia majora	2-3 months	Captive rings, bead rings, or circular barbells
Labret	Through the inferior part of the orbicularis oris muscle (below the lower lip and above the chin)	6-8 weeks	Disc back barbell or fishtail
Lingual frenulum	Laterally, through the frenulum (web under the tongue)	6-8 weeks	Barbell or ring
Lip (side)	Just above or below the tubercle of the lip (side of the lip)	6-8 weeks	Ring or circular barbell
Lorum	Like a frenum, but "lower-um" (juncture of penile shaft and scrotum in the center)	2-3 months	Ring or barbell
Madison (mid-neck)	Superior to the jugular notch (front of the neck) near the insertion of the sternocleidomastoid muscles	6-12 months	Surface barbell or Tygon
Nape (back of neck)	Between the external occipital protuberance and the spinous process of the vertebrae (back of the neck)	6-12 months	Surface barbell
Nasal septum	Between the major alar cartilage and the nasal septal cartilage (in the middle of the nose)	4-6 weeks	Barbell, circular barbell, ring, plug, septum spike or tusk
Navel	Usually above, but not through the umbilicus (bellybutton)	4-12 months	Curved barbell, circular barbell, or ring
Nipple	Between the nipple and the areola (vertically or horizontally)	2-3 months	Barbell, circular barbell, or ring
Nostril	Between the greater and lesser alar cartilage (outside of the nose)	2-3 months	Nostril screw, nose bone, or ring

Pediatric Potpourri

Type of piercing (Top to bottom and everywhere between!)	Anatomically Where Does the Jewelry Go?	Approximate Healing Times	Common Types of Jewelry Placed
Prince Albert	In the underside of the glans (spongy head of penis) and out through urethra	4-6 weeks	Captive ring, circular barbell, or curved barbell
Princess Albertina (Female Prince Albert)	Through the lower portion of external urethral orifice, resting within the vagina	4-8 weeks	Barbell or ring
Pubic (male)	Placed in the natural juncture where the pubic mound and the shaft of the penis meet	2-3 months	Ring
Reverse Prince Albert	In the top of the glans (spongy head of penis) near the center and out through the urethra	4-6 months	Ring or circular barbell
Surface	You name it, something can go under it – Also see implants	6-12 months	Surface barbell or Tygon
Tattoos	You name it, it's been inked	2-3 weeks	N/A
Tongue	Vertically through the midline groove and lateral fold of the tongue, although some get venoms or snake bites through the sides of the tongue	4-6 weeks	Barbell
Tongue (tip)	Vertically through the apex (tip) of the tongue	4-6 weeks	Ring or barbell
Triangle	Horizontal piercing behind the nerve bundle of the clitoris at the base of the hood tissue where it forms from the body	2-3 months	Circular barbell, barbells, bent bars, or rings
Uvula	Thing hanging down in the back of the throat	6-8 weeks	Barbell or rings

Thanks to Elayne Angel from Rings of Desire, Yucatan, Mexico and Troy Amundson from Apocalypse Piercing, Seattle, Washington for their invaluable help with the creation of this chart

97) Which of the following BEST describes CPAP (Continuous Positive Airway Pressure) therapy?

A) CPAP therapy involves the use of a pressurized mask or nasal pillows that are secured to the patient's face and can be used to assist oxygenation and ventilation for the spontaneously breathing patient

B) CPAP therapy involves the use of a pressurized mask or nasal pillows that are secured to the patient's face and can be used to assist oxygenation and ventilation for the apneic patient

C) CPAP therapy involves the use of a non-pressurized mask or nasal pillows that are secured to the patient's face and can be used to assist oxygenation and ventilation for the spontaneously breathing patient

D) CPAP therapy involves the use of a non-pressurized mask or nasal pillows that are secured to the patient's face and can be used to assist oxygenation and ventilation for the apneic patient

A - CPAP (continuous positive airway pressure) therapy involves the use of a pressurized mask or nasal pillows that forms a seal around the patient's mouth and/or nose. The flow of air then increases the pressure in the airways and alveoli. CPAP can be used to overcome a pulmonary shunt in patients that are not being adequately oxygenated by devices such as a nasal cannula or non-pressurized mask (non-rebreather, etc.).

It is important to remember that CPAP only works if you are breathing, so if you aren't providing the ventilatory effort (breathing), CPAP won't do that for you. Ventilation is a two-way street; CPAP is a one-way delivery. If you are apneic, dead, etc., CPAP will not help you.

CPAP delivers a set, constant pressure and doesn't change no matter what the respiratory status is. The pressure helps the alveoli stay open and allows the oxygen enriched air to flow in.

You probably saw that the term CPAP has the word "pressure" in it, so any choice that includes "non-pressurized" probably isn't a correct answer! Many people struggle to understand the difference between CPAP (Continuous Positive Airway Pressure) and BiPAP (Bi-level Positive Airway Pressure), so we offer the following explanation from Kristin Ireland, RRT.

> "Imagine that you are a friendly, happy puppy dog. We are driving in a car, and you have your head stuck out of the passenger window looking forward, and feeling the air blow past. We are driving at 30 miles an hour, but, every time you breathe in, I accelerate to 60 MPH in a split second. When you go to breathe out, I slam on the brakes and go back down to 30 MPH. Repeat to infinity. That's how BiPAP works. It's like CPAP on steroids. When the patient breaths in, the machine increases the pressure to help the air get in, then goes back down when they breathe out."

The alternating pressure creates a pressure variant which assists the inspiratory as well as the expiratory phases of ventilation. Thus, it helps both the oxygenation and ventilation.

98) For a child, having a CPAP/BiPAP mask placed on them can be a scary experience, especially if they are not familiar with the therapy. Which of the following strategies will likely prove **most** effective in getting cooperation from your young patient?

A) Try to convince the patient that the mask won't be uncomfortable at all

B) Explain the procedure, have them gently hold the mask to their face at first, but do not try to tighten and secure the straps immediately

C) Administer Ativan® (lorazepam) prior to initiating therapy

D) Place the mask on yourself first, to show the patient that there is nothing to fear

B - Someone once said, "Honesty is the best policy" and that is certainly the case here. Honest explanations with time to get to know the equipment works well in most cases. For some of us, if we're honest, the Ativan answer may be attractive, but remember that choosing the least invasive option first (if appropriate) is a better choice in real life and on tests! Trying to convince a patient of something that is not true is a sure-fire way to never having that patient trust you or your colleagues again. It may work for Fleetwood Mac's song "Little Lies," but our patients are not thinking "Tell me lies, tell me sweet little lies." Kids can smell insincerity, BS, and lies a mile away.

The technique of placing a mask on yourself to show that there is nothing to be scared of might seem attractive at first. However, this means you have now contaminated the mask with ER nurse cooties. Be honest with the patient and let them know you're just going to trial it for a few seconds, perhaps at some very low settings, at first. It might take a few tries, but once the patient feels the relief from the mask, you can move on to securing the straps and adjusting the settings. Getting a pediatric patient to accept a new form of therapy is more like a marathon than a sprint.

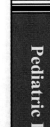

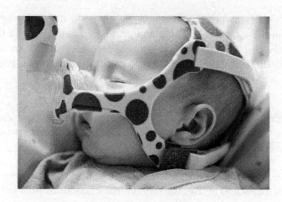

Fitting guide for Wisp pediatric patients
Achieving the right fit with Wisp pediatric is easy. Simply follow the instructions below.

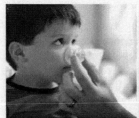 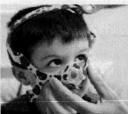 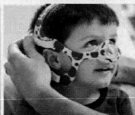 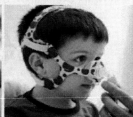

1. The mask cushion should fit the width of the nose without blocking the nostrils.
2. Pulling the headgear over the child's head, gently hold the cushion over the nose.
3. Reconnect the clips by pushing them into the mask frame.
4. Connect the Wisp pediatric tubing and elbow swivel to the front of the mask.

Three cushion sizes (SCS, SCM, SCL) are available. Please read the Instructions for Use for additional fitting information.

Infant & Pediatric CPAP Masks
Photos Courtesy of Philips Respironics
www.usa.philips.com

99) After successful placement of the non-invasive therapy CPAP therapy, you notice that your initially lethargic child is now whining and getting restless. You readjust the mask and adjust settings to optimize comfort, but neither of these things appears to make any difference. What would be your next step in obtaining ongoing cooperation from your patient?

A) Administer sedation

B) Administer analgesia

C) Provide distraction

D) Remove the mask

C – The key to this question is identifying that the patient's change in mental status, from lethargic to restless is actually an improvement, and we want to encourage that to continue.

So in this case, distraction is our best (and safest) option. Parents often have tablet or phone devices that children love to watch or play games on, and just as in the operating room with anesthesia, many providers have had huge success with this. Another option for kids, depending on your available equipment, is to have the patient play a game with the $EtCO_2$ monitor. Place either a nasal cannula $EtCO_2$ monitor under the mask or the one that goes on the endotracheal tube usually works great on the CPAP/BiPAP mask as well. Then, have the child watch their waveform and respiratory rate. Give them a goal to work towards, perhaps something like a set respiratory rate or number of 'bumps' on the waveform. Without distraction, the uncomfortable mask becomes the child's entire world, but having some "screen time" or watching the waves is far more fun!

Sedatives and/or analgesics, i.e. low dose ketamine, Ativan (lorazepam), etc. may sometimes be necessary to allow patients to tolerate non-invasive therapy. However, these medications come with a huge risk and are not attractive first choice options in children with respiratory distress. Removing the mask is rather instinctual since we hate to see pediatric patients be uncomfortable. But remember, they are on non-invasive oxygen therapy for a reason, therefore, it is not recommended to remove the mask (for more than a very short period of time) without consulting the physician and/or respiratory therapy first.

100) Which of the following would be an appropriate method of coaching a child's breathing while they are receiving nebulizer treatments for their asthma?

A) 'Take a quick breath in, then nice and slow on the way out.'

B) 'Everything is going to be okay, just slow down, slow down, slow….'

C) 'One second in, one second out.'

D) 'Take a nice slow deep breath in, then let it go.'

D – We want this patient to take a nice deep, slow, and controlled breath in, followed by a relaxing exhalation. This will allow for the best deposition of medication into the lungs. Embrace your inner "Frozen" and after a nice slow deep breath, let it go!

Additional Insights from a Pediatric Respiratory Therapist: In real life, we tend to gravitate towards giving generalized advice like: 'slow down', 'everything is okay', or 'just calm down.' However, we need to be more specific and provide instruction as well as encouragement. Patients with asthma or other respiratory ailments probably cannot accomplish a one second in, one second out breathing pattern, and this option wouldn't optimize the effect of the medication. The other option is also inappropriate because the faster this patient inhales, the more of the nebulized medication will impact their mouth, throat, tongue, and face, but never reach the lungs.

101) You are caring for a 14-year old who suffered a significant amount of blood loss from bilateral open femur fractures after being struck by a vehicle. The decision has been made to activate your facility's Massive Transfusion Protocol (MTP). This protocol reflects administration of Red Blood Cells (PRBCs), Plasma, and which of the following?

A) Cryoprecipitate

B) Platelets

C) Tranexamic acid (TXA)

D) White blood cells

B – While research continues regarding massive transfusion protocols in the pediatric (and adult) populations, current recommendations include transfusing Red Blood Cells, Plasma, and Platelets at some sort of a ratio of between 1:1:1 to 2:1:1. This ratio should be followed until the attending physicians no longer considered the bleeding to be life threatening. The goal of administration of the blood products in the protocol is to avoid the lethal triad of trauma-related bleeding: Coagulopathy, Hypothermia, and Acidosis.

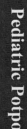

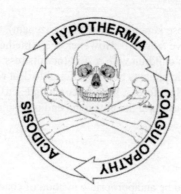

Massive transfusion protocols (MTPs) are based on the recently developed concept of damage control resuscitation, which advocates for early blood component therapy (with minimization of crystalloid use) combined with rapid surgical control of hemorrhage. This is a fancy way of saying "give lots more blood stuff and lots less saline." But, it's not just the red stuff. The protocols also describe the need for plasma and platelets as well. That's important as red cells are invaluable for carrying oxygen round and round, but the other two are needed to help the bleeding actually stop.

Massive transfusion protocols are designed to provide the right amount and balance of blood products, mimicking 'whole blood', to critically injured patients in order to prevent and treat hemorrhagic shock and coagulopathy. Not only does MTP guide resuscitation; it facilitates communication and logistical support between treating clinicians, blood bank, and support staff.

What constitutes the need to activate the Massive Transfusion Protocol? In big people, it has been defined as giving 10 units or more of red cells in 24 hours. More recently, the definition has been adjusted to include the need for three units of red blood cells over one hour or any four blood components in 30 minutes. What this means in far easier language is simply this: Something really bad is going on and the patient is anticipated to need not only surgery, but a whole lot of blood products right now and for an extended period of time until the problem can be fixed.

Great, but what about kids? Pediatric massive transfusion differs from adult massive transfusion because children are better able to tolerate blood loss due to their relatively bigger and better physiologic reserve. That means they compensate better, and longer, than big people do. As such, pediatric massive transfusion may require a greater percentage of overall blood loss before initiating a massive transfusion protocol.

Some of the published "triggers" for initiating massive transfusion protocols in kids include:

- Need to transfuse > 50% total blood volume in 3 hours
- Need to transfuse > 100% total blood volume in 24 hours
- Need to transfuse to replace ongoing blood loss of > 10% total blood volume/minute
- Need to transfuse over 40 mL/kg of PRBCs in 24 hours
- Need to transfuse over 20 mL/kg of PRBCs in 2 hours with ongoing losses anticipated

That means that if four 10 mL/kg blood boluses are needed over 24 hours or two 10 mL/kg blood boluses are needed within 2 hours, something really bad is going on and it's time to seriously consider activating the MTP. The above amounts of blood don't sound like a lot of blood for an adult, but remember these guidelines are for normal circulating blood volumes in children:

- ~90 mL/kg in infants <3 months of age
- ~80 mL/kg in young children
- ~75 mL/kg in school-age children (65 mL/kg in obese children)

That means that if a little kid received 4 blood boluses over 24 hours, those boluses account for approximately 1/2 of their blood volume. That's a lot!

When it comes to the ratio of blood products to give (red stuff to platelets to plasma), again, the jury is still out. For adults and more slowly for children, we are seeing the adoption of "prescription transfusions" in the ED, ICU, OR, with the use bedside or lab tests including Thromboelastography (TEG) and Rotational Thromboelastometry (ROTEM). These tests allow for additional specific insights as to what the patient really needs. Do they just need more red stuff? More platelets? More cryo? More FFP? More fibrinogen? This means not just dumping in lots of stuff, but actually figuring out what the patient really needs. That is "prescription transfusion" medicine.

MTPs don't only involve "getting all hands-on deck" for the administration of blood products, they also come with reminders to regularly monitor calcium levels and give calcium boluses as needed. Blood products in the blood bank refrigerator have preservatives that bind calcium. Giving lots of blood can quickly drop a child's calcium level. This not only affects cardiac activity and the ability for blood vessels to clamp down, but also the ability to clot. That's a big deal as the MTP was being initiated because of uncontrollable bleeding. Interfering with the clotting process is a bad idea!

Finally, in the Trauma Triad of Death... we don't want to overlook hypothermia. If at all possible, we should warm all IV fluids (using an approved fluid warmer, **not** a microwave) to avoid hypothermia. And, if at all possible, we should warm just about all blood products (again using an approved blood warmer, **not** a microwave). Notice we said, "just about all." Platelets should not be warmed! Platelets should be administered at room temperature.

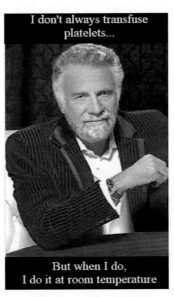

102) Testicular torsion has a peak incidence in what age group?

A) 2-6 years

B) 5-10 years

C) 7-12 years

D) 12-18 years

D - There are two peaks of incidence in testicular torsion. The first peak is during the first year of life (first peak, first year), and the second peak occurs from 12-18 years of age. In the ER setting, with teenage guys who are worried enough (or in enough pain) to actually admit to the nurse that they have a problem "down there," torsions are at the top of the list.

103) Which of the following is a classic finding in testicular torsion?

A) Absent or diminished cremasteric reflex

B) Bilateral testicular pain

C) Abdominal pain

D) Swelling and non-tender unilateral testicle

A – An absent or diminished cremasteric reflex on the affected side is part of the classic presentation of testicular torsion. Additional classic findings include <u>unilateral</u> testicular tenderness <u>and</u> swelling (the testicle is twisted after all), along with nausea and vomiting (but not necessarily abdominal pain). But what is the cremasteric reflex, and how do we tell if it is absent or diminished? The reflex is elicited by stroking, pinching, or poking the skin on the superior medial (upper inner) aspect of the thigh, near the testicles. This can be done using a tongue depressor, either end of a cotton swab, or the back of a gloved hand. The normal reaction is an activation of the cremaster muscle which causes the testicle to elevate. If that doesn't happen, it might just be that the twisted testicle is sick enough to not withdraw, and that's never a good sign!

104) The TWIST score is utilized when evaluating patients with possible:

A) Testicular torsion

B) Torsional nystagmus

C) Torticollis

D) Tinnitus

A – The TWIST score is for evaluating patients (primarily teenagers or pre-toddlers) with possible testicular torsion. You may have been thinking about a dance contest with the band singing Chubby Checker's hit song, "Come on, let's twist again, like we did last summer..." and you know you wanted to sing along! And in case you were wondering, the TWIST score is not utilized to evaluate, an abnormality in eye movement, a "twisting" of neck muscles, or even ringing in the ears. Though the full genital exam will be performed in the ED by the advanced practice provider or physician, here is a short and sweet summary of the TWIST score.

The TWIST (*Testicular Workup for Ischemic and Suspected Torsion*) score consists of the following five clinical variables:

- Presence of testicular swelling = 2 points
- Presence of hard testicle = 2 points
- Absence of cremasteric reflex = 1 point
- Presence of high riding testicle = 1 point
- Presence of nausea/vomiting = 1 point

The total score is used to identify the risk involved using the following parameters:

- High risk = score of 6 or 7
- Intermediate risk = score of 1 to 5
- Low risk = score of 0

Pediatric Emergency Medicine Morsels (pemmorsels.com) provided a great review of the TWIST score with the following summary and recommendations:

High Risk = Score of 6 or 7
- Consider NO imaging and possibly only *using TWIST Score in pubertal males*
- Convey this high-risk score and help expedite surgical exploration with urology

Intermediate Risk = Scores of 1 to 5
- Obtain scrotal ultrasound
- Consider alternative diagnoses (ex, epididymitis) and obtain additional testing as warranted (i.e., U/A, STD screen)

"Low" Risk = Scores of 0
- In the original TWIST score paper, "Low Risk" was not associated with torsion and avoiding ultrasound in this group was advocated for…. but, torsion can be deceptive and present atypically. They still recommend a low threshold for obtaining an ultrasound, even though an alternative diagnosis is more likely.

Remember, intermittent torsion, detorsion, and re-torsion can and does occur. 50% of patients diagnosed with torsion have had a prior episode of intermittent torsion that had spontaneous resolution.

> "If your history, for instance, is concerning for possible intermittent torsion with de-torsion, then your TWIST score when you are evaluating the patient may not be a 6 or 7, warranting bypassing the imaging and going directly to the OR…. but you should still be mindful of your history and your exam and convey your concerns to the urologist (even if the TWIST score is lower). The TWIST Score is most helpful when it is HIGH… you should not use it to "Rule-out" torsion just because the score is low." **(Sean M. Fox in pemmorsels.com)**

Similar to the mantra that with heart attacks, that time is muscle, and with strokes, time is brain, and when it comes to torsions, time is testicles!

- Salvage rates are very good for torsion lasting < 6 hours (90-100%)
- Salvage rates are not as good between 6-12 hours (20-50%)
- Salvage rates are really, really low after 12 hours (<11%)

105) A 4-year old child presents to the Emergency Department with a cough, swollen and reddened eyes, and stuffy nose. Also noted is a scaly red rash reported to have "started at the face and spread all over." At triage, his medical history is significant for **not** being up to date on any vaccinations. Given this presentation, the triage nurse should be especially concerned for which of the following conditions?

A) Measles
B) Seasonal allergies
C) Chickenpox
D) RSV

A – Everything about this presentation screams "measles." In addition to the rash, we have a classic triad of symptoms mentioned here; The 3 Cs of (C)ough, (C)onjunctivitis, and (C)oryza (stuffy/swollen nose). If that's too much to remember, any child with a history of not being up to date on their "shots," (aka., immunizations) should raise a huge red flag at triage.

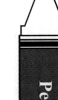

Certified Pediatric Emergency Nurse (CPEN) Review IV

Let's take this opportunity for a quick, but crucial, history lesson. Despite being considered primarily a childhood illness, measles (rubeola) can affect people of <u>all ages</u>. That's important to remember because measles is one of the most contagious infectious diseases, with at least a 90% secondary infection rate in <u>susceptible</u> contacts. "Susceptible" is a particularly important word here. The practice of administering two doses of live-attenuated measles vaccine to children to prevent school outbreaks of measles was implemented when the vaccine was first licensed in 1963. The immunization program resulted in a 99% decrease in reported cases.

From 1989 to 1991, a major resurgence occurred, affecting primarily unvaccinated preschoolers. This measles resurgence resulted in 55,000 cases (wow!), 130 deaths and prompted the recommendation that a second dose of measles vaccine be given to preschoolers in a mass vaccination campaign that led to the effective elimination of measles in the United States.

By 1993, vaccination programs had interrupted the transmission of measles virus in the United States; since then, most reported cases of measles in the United States have been linked to international travel. By 1997-1999, the incidence of measles had been reduced to a historic low (< 0.5 cases per million persons).

In the United States, measles was declared eliminated in 2000, and really, up until 2013, was rarely seen. In 88% of the cases reported between 2000 and 2011, the virus originated from a country outside the US, and 2 out of every 3 individuals who developed measles were unvaccinated. However, in 2013, US measles cases increased threefold to 175 cases. Most of these cases were outbreaks in children whose parents had refused recommended, customary pediatric immunizations. Since 2014, with the continued expansion of international travel, the outbreaks continue to escalate across the US, especially in those not immunized.

Now, onto the medical stuff: The onset of measles is commonly 10-12 days after exposure to the virus. That's important to remember because if the measles vaccine is given within 3 days of known exposure, measles can be prevented. After known or suspected exposure, and without vaccination, if you see a patient with a high fever (104F (40C), that lasts for 4-7 days, accompanied by feeling crummy, anorexia, and the 3 Cs – the culprit is probably measles!

More cool stuff to know... In addition to the 3 Cs, two other symptoms classically associated with measles are:

Koplick spots: Koplick spots are bluish-gray specks or "grains of sand" on a small red base on the inside of the cheeks. They appear 1-2 days before the rash and last for 3-5 days. Not all kids with measles have these spots, but <u>if they are present, so is measles</u>.

The rash: For many practitioners, this is the memorable part of a measles presentation. Developing 14-days after exposure, these red macules (flat and < 1cm) and papules (raised and < 1 cm) often begin at the hairline. Within 48 hours they turn into patches that spread from the head down to the rest of the body (including the palms of the hands and soles of the feet). Kids tend to look sickest during the first or second day of getting the rash, which then after 5-7 days, slowly turns brown, fades, and goes away.

Although the diagnosis of measles is usually determined from the classic clinical picture, laboratory identification and confirmation of the diagnosis are necessary for public health and outbreak control. Immediately reporting any suspected case of measles to a local or state health department is imperative.

The US CDC clinical case definition for reporting purposes requires only the following:

- Generalized rash lasting 3 days or longer
- Temperature of 101.0°F (38.3°C) or higher
- Cough, coryza, or conjunctivitis (3 Cs)

Pediatric Potpourri

For reporting purposes for the CDC, cases are classified as follows: (www.cdc.gov)

- Suspected: Any febrile illness accompanied by rash
- Probable: A case that meets the clinical case definition, has noncontributory or no serologic or virologic testing, and is not epidemiologically linked to a confirmed case
- Confirmed: A case that is laboratory confirmed or that meets the clinical case definition and is epidemiologically linked to a confirmed case; a laboratory-confirmed case need not meet the clinical case definition

Pneumonia and encephalitis are the most common causes of death associated with measles. Another rare, but serious complication is measles encephalitis, which has a 10% mortality rate. Simply put, measles is not to be messed with!

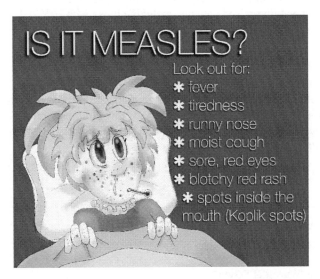

106) Which type of mask is recommended for healthcare professionals treating a patient with a suspected or confirmed case of measles?

A) Surgical mask

B) Halloween mask

C) N95 respirator mask

D) Non-rebreather mask

C - Healthcare professionals should wear an N95 mask whenever caring for the child with suspected or confirmed measles and the patients themselves should have a surgical mask any time they are outside of a negative pressure room. A non-rebreather mask is used for oxygen delivery and a Halloween mask is just an easy option to discard.

Measles is one of the most contagious of all infectious diseases as up to 9 out of 10 susceptible persons with close contact to a measles patient will develop measles. Measles is caused by a highly contagious virus which is spread through close personal (direct) contact with secretions produced when the patient coughs, sneezes, or simply breathes. The infectious droplets can remain infectious in the air for up to two hours after an infected person leaves an area. Ideally, the patient will be placed in a negative pressure room as quickly as possible. If that is not possible, the patient should be in a private room and not in the waiting room. Airborne precautions are indicated for hospitalized children during the period of communicability. For otherwise healthy children, that would be from 3-5 days before the appearance of a rash to 4 days after the rash develops. For patients who are immunocompromised, airborne precautions are recommended for the duration of illness.

107) Risk factors for measles infection include all the following **except**:

A) HIV

B) Leukemia

C) International travel

D) Recent MMR immunization

D – Rather than being a risk factor, the MMR (measles-mumps-rubella vaccine) has been proven to be 93% effective at preventing measles after a single dose (and up to 97% effective with 2 doses). Not being immunized, or being under-immunized (not having all the shots), are actually among the primary risk factors for measles. Immunocompromised patients, including those with HIV/AIDS or leukemia, and patients undergoing chemotherapy, or corticosteroid therapy are also at higher risk. This is true regardless of immunization status.

In addition to disease or medication induced immunosuppression, little babies who lose passive antibodies from mom before being old enough to receive their first immunization are at high risk if exposed. Lastly, despite the highest recorded immunization rates in history, young children who are not appropriately vaccinated may experience more than a 60-fold increase in risk of disease due to exposure to imported measles cases from countries that have not yet eliminated the disease.

108) In healthcare, PEWS is the acronym for:

A) Pediatric Endoscopic Warning System

B) Predictable Emergency Warming Scheme

C) Pediatric Early Warning Score

D) Potential Emergency Weather Siren

C – PEWS stands for Pediatric Early Warning Score and was originally developed in 2005 (a year after Rapid Response Systems became a hospital standard). The purpose of PEWS is to provide a practical and objective method to identify inpatient pediatric patients at risk for cardiac arrest. Since its introduction, it has been used not only by inpatient staff, but more recently in emergency departments as well. Some Emergency Departments score children prior to sending them up to the floor to give clarity as to the current level of illness. Ideally, PEWS can be used in conjunction with the clinical status of the patient by providers of all levels (nursing, physicians, etc.) to escalate care, much the same as with a Rapid Response Team, for sick patients long before a cardiac arrest ensues.

Most commonly, the Pediatric Early Warning Score is a tool used to trend the patient at the time of admission and then to regularly monitor throughout an in-patient stay. It provides a common language used in pediatric healthcare to express patient observations and serves as a predictor for clinical deterioration. Individual pediatric organizations determine their local score threshold that will trigger an escalation of care such as a Rapid Response Team or a Code Blue. The key to PEWS is to determine a baseline and then regularly reassess. If the score is staying the same or decreasing, then the child is most likely getting better. If the score is going up, that's not a good sign! It provides guidance as to suggested interventions, and in many facilities, also how often to reassess, what level of provider should see the patient (intern vs. attending), etc.

Pediatric Potpourri

Certified Pediatric Emergency Nurse (CPEN) Review IV

In teaching hospitals with medical students, interns, residents, fellows, and attendings, it can be difficult for everyone to know and understand each other, not to mention trust each other. Experienced physicians know to trust their nurses, especially when they say; "My gut says something isn't right with the kid." But, when physicians aren't used to working with other staff members, communication of "gut feelings" can be challenging. With PEWS, everyone, from nursing to respiratory therapy to physicians are making the same observations and relaying those findings with common terms and scores. In that regard, it's similar to the Glasgow Coma Scale (GCS). Across the world, if someone hears that a patient has a GCS of 3, we know it's really bad. And the same idea occurs with PEWS. Across the world, if someone hears that a kid has a PEWS score of 9, we know it's really bad. Initial and repeated PEWS scores of 0-4 are good... anytime the PEWS score is ≥ 7, that's really bad. And even at 2 AM, it makes it far easier for everyone to speak the same language and know how sick the kid currently is.

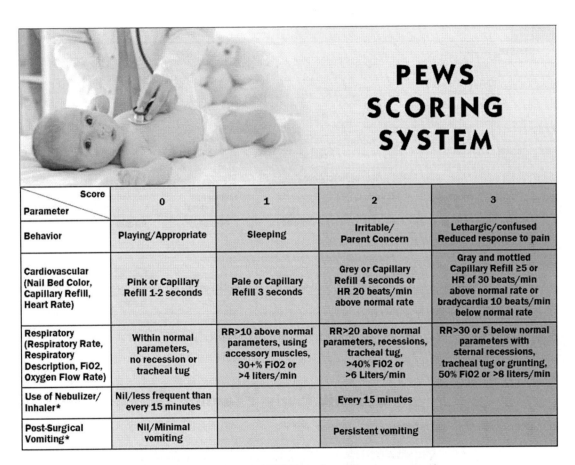

Parameter \ Score	0	1	2	3
Behavior	Playing/Appropriate	Sleeping	Irritable/ Parent Concern	Lethargic/confused Reduced response to pain
Cardiovascular (Nail Bed Color, Capillary Refill, Heart Rate)	Pink or Capillary Refill 1-2 seconds	Pale or Capillary Refill 3 seconds	Grey or Capillary Refill 4 seconds or HR 20 beats/min above normal rate	Gray and mottled Capillary Refill ≥5 or HR of 30 beats/min above normal rate or bradycardia 10 beats/min below normal rate
Respiratory (Respiratory Rate, Respiratory Description, FiO2, Oxygen Flow Rate)	Within normal parameters, no recession or tracheal tug	RR>10 above normal parameters, using accessory muscles, 30+% FiO2 or >4 liters/min	RR>20 above normal parameters, recessions, tracheal tug, >40% FiO2 or >6 Liters/min	RR>30 or 5 below normal parameters with sternal recessions, tracheal tug or grunting, 50% FiO2 or >8 liters/min
Use of Nebulizer/ Inhaler*	Nil/less frequent than every 15 minutes		Every 15 minutes	
Post-Surgical Vomiting*	Nil/Minimal vomiting		Persistent vomiting	

PEWS Practice

The following chart can be used to complete the PEWS calculations for simulated patients. Apply the appropriate score for each row using the values at the top of the column. Total all rows to determine each child's PEWS score. A typical score to initiate a rapid response team alert is 4 or greater.

Certified Pediatric Emergency Nurse (CPEN) Review IV

	0	1	2	3	SCORE
Behavior "Cute vs Coma"	Playing/ Appropriate	Sleeping	Irritable	Lethargic/Confused or Reduced response to pain	
Cardiovascular "Cute vs Crashing"	Pink OR Capillary Refill 1-2 seconds	Pale OR Capillary Refill 3 seconds	Grey OR Capillary Refill 4 seconds OR tachycardia of 20 above normal	Gray or mottled OR Capillary Refill ≥5 OR tachycardia of 30 bpm above normal rate OR bradycardia	
Respiratory "Cute vs Crummy"	Within normal parameters, no retractions	>10 above normal parameters, using accessory muscles, OR 30% FiO2 OR 3+ liters/min	>20 above normal parameters, retractions, OR 40% FiO2 OR 6+ liters/min	5 <u>below</u> normal parameters with retractions and/or grunting, OR 50% FiO2 OR 8+ liters/min	
Add 2 additional points for interventions or conditions, i.e. continuous nebs, O2 changes, persistent post-op vomiting, multiple IV attempts, frequent suctioning, or positioning				TOTAL SCORE	

STABLE → CRITICAL

SCORE 0-2: Vitals and Reassess Q4H; Regular Charting and Updates; Continue Current Plan of Care

SCORE 3-4: Repeat PEWS in 60min; Vitals Q2H; Ensure Pediatrician Response within 60min; Plan of Care May Change

SCORE 5: Repeat PEWS in 30min; Vitals Q2H; Ensure Pediatrician Response within 10min; Plan of Care Will Change

SCORE 6+: Repeat PEWS in 20min; Vitals Every Hour; Immediate Pediatrician Response; Possible Transfer To PICU

Normal Heart Rate Ranges By Age Group

Infant (<1 year)	Toddler (1-3 years)	Preschool (3-4 years)	School Age (5-12 years)	Adolescent (13-16 years)
100-160	85-150	75-140	60-115	60-100

Normal Respiratory Rate Ranges By Age Group

Infant (<1 year)	Toddler (1-3 years)	Preschool (3-4 years)	School Age (5-12 years)	Adolescent (13-16 years)
24-60	22-30	22-30	16-24	16-22

PEWS Summary for Healthcare Professionals

Pediatric Early Warning Score

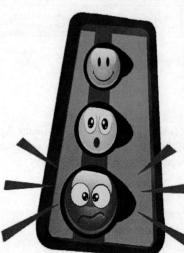

Green
- There has been no change in your child's status
- Your child's vital signs will be checked every 4 hours
- Your child's status will be reassessed every 4 hours
- Your child is stable and we will continue with their current plan of care

Yellow
- There has been a change in your child's status; your nurse will give you more information. The charge nurse and resident have been notified
- Your child will be reassessed in 2 hours, or sooner, if needed
- Your child's plan of care may change

Red
- There has been a significant change in your child's status; your nurse will give you more information. The charge nurse has been notified and will come assess your child
- The resident will be notified and will assess your child; the attending doctor will be notified
- Your child will be reassessed within 1 hour, or sooner, if needed
- We may ask other experts to come assess your child
- Your child's plan of care may change

PEWS Summary for Families

Pediatric Potpourri

Certified Pediatric Emergency Nurse (CPEN) Review IV

Each of these children are about to be admitted to inpatient units from the Emergency Department. Prior to transfer, you will need to calculate the PEWS score by adding the points for the physical findings of behavior, cardiovascular, respiratory, and the additional points for interventions or conditions such as: continuous nebs, O_2 changes, persistent post-op vomiting, multiple IV attempts, frequent suctioning, or positioning.

Harper: A 2-year old, 14.6 kg child admitted for vomiting and fever for the past three days. Vital Signs: T 101.2 F (38.4 C), HR 160, R 30, BP 76/52. Skin is pale, warm, and patient is refusing PO intake and is irritable. Tylenol (acetaminophen) given rectally. PIV to left wrist with maintenance fluids. Dad at bedside. Admit to observation unit.

Seth: A 5-day old, 3.46 kg infant admitted for hyperbilirubinemia. Vital Signs: T 97.9 F (36.6 C), HR 174, R 58. Physical findings include brisk capillary refill, jaundice, icteric sclera. Difficulty feeding is reported and appears sleepy in mom's arms. Bili-lights ordered with admit to infant unit.

Connor: A 14-month old, 9.4 kg child admitted for decreased urine output and influenza. Vital Signs: T 101.2 F (38.4 C), HR 115, R 26, BP 116/58. There is brisk capillary refill, non-labored breathing, but appears irritable. Parents report no wet diapers for >20 hours. Resting in dad's arms. Gave 188 mL bolus of saline, drew a BMP, and respiratory panel. No void after bolus. Admit to general pediatrics.

Ashton: An 8-year old, 21.4 kg oncology patient presented with pain upon urination. Vital Signs: T 102.9 F (39.4 C), HR 106, R 24, BP 74/47. Appears lethargic and the capillary refill is 3 seconds. There is redness and swelling to port site. Tylenol (acetaminophen) given, blood culture obtained from port and PIV, urine cultures, CBC, and BMP sent. Admit to oncology department to rule out sepsis. Parents present.

Owen: A 15-year old, 78.6 kg child presented awake and alert with an asthma exacerbation. Vital Signs: T 97.9 F (36.6 C), HR 112, R 28, BP 107/73, 100% SaO_2, on continuous albuterol nebs with 60% FiO_2. Mild intercostal retractions, bilateral rhonchi, nonproductive cough, color pink, NPO, PIV to right antecubital with maintenance fluids. Grandmother and three siblings at bedside. Admit to intermediate care unit.

PEWS Score	Behavior	Cardiovascular	Respiratory	2 Extra Points
Harper 3	Irritable = 2	Pale = 1	WNL = 0	N/A
Seth 1	Sleepy = 1	Brisk Cap refill = 0	WNL = 0	N/A
Connor 2	Irritable = 2	Brisk Cap refill = 0	WNL = 0	N/A
Ashton 4	Lethargic = 3	Cap refill 3 seconds = 1	WNL = 0	N/A
Owen 5	Appropriate = 0	Pink = 0	60% FiO2 =3	Continuous Nebs =2

Scores of 0-4 are "green" and essentially the kid is "holding his own."
Scores 5-6 mean the kid is sick and you should keep a close eye on them.
Scores ≥ 7 mean that something really bad is likely going on.

Obtaining an initial baseline score is crucial, because you don't know where you're going unless you know where you've been. Once the starting point has been established, regular reassessments will tell you if things are getting better, staying the same, or getting worse. If Harper had a score of 3 at 0200, and then at 0400 it was 5, that's not the way we want the scores to be going and something bad is going on. If at 0200, Owen had a score of 5 and then at 0300 his score was 3, that is reassuring. PEWS isn't perfect... it just allows everyone to speak the same language and helps get kids where they need to be before they code!

Pediatric Potpourri

109) The outcomes associated with thoracotomy and open cardiac massage after pediatric blunt traumatic arrest are:

A) 15% survival to discharge

B) 10% survival to discharge

C) 5% survival to discharge

D) 0% survival to discharge

D – In two published studies looking specifically at pediatric patients, none of the pediatric patients who presented with a blunt traumatic arrest survived despite thoracotomy and open chest cardiac massage. Emergency department thoracotomy, aka., "cracking the chest," is very, very rarely indicated in the pediatric victim of blunt traumatic arrest. Research shows that adolescents and adults who present with traumatic arrest from **penetrating** trauma (shot or stabbed) **may** benefit if a thoracotomy is performed immediately after arrest. Once the chest is open, then hopefully one can plug the hole, clamp the aorta, and/or relieve a tamponade. However, for children with multiple trauma and blunt traumatic arrest, outcomes are regrettably and predictably dismal.

110) In a pediatric trauma patient where shock is suspected, an initial warmed fluid bolus should be:

A) 20 mL/kg of isotonic crystalloid

B) 20 mg/kg of isotonic crystalloid

C) 20 l/kg of isotonic crystalloid

D) 20 g/kg of isotonic crystalloid

A - 20 mL/kg of an isotonic crystalloid solution, typically normal saline (NS) or Lactated Ringers (LR), is the initial recommended dosing for a "shocky" pediatric patient. After the first 20 mL/kg bolus, reassess, and then just as with washing your hair, "rinse and repeat." In a trauma patient, if you are giving a second bolus, then it's time to think about, or even better, call for blood products as well.

In the above question, there are two key points. First is the amount of fluid. 20 mL/kg... Not mg/kg, g/kg, and certainly not l/kg. Decimal points are important, and milligrams vs. grams and milliliters vs. liters really do make a difference. Second is specifically the mention of *warmed* fluids. This is an intervention that, if forgotten, can have huge negative repercussions. If fluid boluses are required, using a fluid warmer (Belmont®, Level One®, QinFlow®, etc.) should be your standard procedure. Infusing kids with cold fluids, and don't forget that room temperature is cold compared to your patient's core temperature, results in cold kids. And cold kids quickly become really sick kids!

111) The trauma team is considering the administration of Tranexamic Acid (TXA) for your pediatric patient. What information would be **most** important to help the team with the decision?

A) Blood products administered

B) Current blood pressure

C) Estimated amount of blood loss

D) Time injury occurred

D – Tranexamic Acid (TXA) should be administered within three hours of injury. This means when the injured occurred, not when EMS arrived, or the patient arrived at the emergency department. Giving TXA **within three hours** of the injury reduces mortality from bleeding (that's great!), but giving it after three hours can actually increase mortality (that's really bad!)

Interestingly, while relatively new to the pediatric trauma world, TXA administration is nothing new in pediatric medical care. It has been used safely and successfully in pediatric cardiac, orthopedic, and craniofacial surgeries for several decades. TXA inhibits the body's natural fibrinolysis (the process of breaking down clots) thereby reducing bleeding and decreasing the need for blood transfusions. In a multi-trauma patient, all of those are certainly desirable outcomes.

Think of TXA for trauma as the opposite of tPA (tissue plasminogen activator) for strokes. Less than a few hours = Possibility for good things. More than few hours = Bad things (i.e. bleeds) happen. Same idea applies for TXA. Sooner is better. Current recommendations are for it to be given within 3 hours of the injury. In some parts of the world, the first bolus dose of TXA for trauma patients can be given in the EMS/prehospital arena. More and more research supports the practice of giving TXA for bad bleeding associated with trauma. But remember, it must be given early!

The dosing recommendation for adults is simple; they get 1 gm IV/IO over 10-15 minutes. And yes, intraosseous TXA works just fine. The initial bolus is typically followed by an infusion of one gram of TXA over the next 8 hours or until the bleeding stops. The pediatric dosing, as with most meds, is "something per kilo," and the most common initial dosing recommendations seem to be 10-20 mg/kg over 10-15 minutes, followed by a drip (commonly 2 mg/kg/hr) for at least the next 8 hours or until the bleeding stops. Remember, fluid boluses (normal saline or LR) in babies and kids are **10-20** mL/kg. So, when giving TXA, the initial bolus dose is **10-20** mg/kg.

Let's look at LVADs...

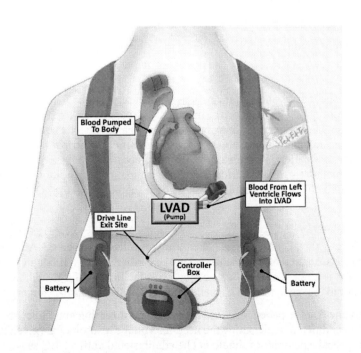

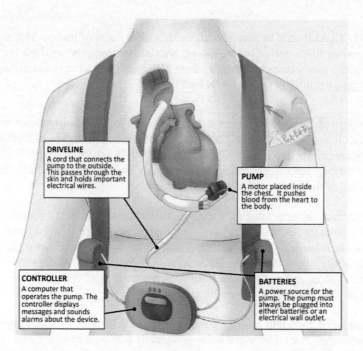

112) An awake and alert 14-year old female presents to the Emergency Department (ED) triage nurse with complaints of a fever and states that the skin around the driveline exit site of her Left Ventricular Assist Device (LVAD) is reddened. She points out there has also been some yellowish drainage from the site. The patient says she has had some vomiting recently and really hasn't felt well the last several days. The blood pressure from the automatic cuff reads 60/55. The nurse is unable to palpate a peripheral pulse and the patient shows sinus tachycardia on the monitor. What is the **first** step the ED nurse should do after assessing the airway?

A) Start CPR as the patient has no palpable pulse

B) Begin the process for an immediate transfer to the adult ICU

C) Obtain a blood pressure with a manual cuff and a Doppler

D) Prepare to immediately administer antibiotics since she is obviously is septic with hypotension and tachycardia

C – This question is all about assessment of the patient. In that respect, the focus needs to be on the patient, not on the extraneous information, and not on the numbers. To paraphrase a familiar admonition, assess the patient, not the numbers. The patient is walking and talking. That alone tells you a lot. So, in this case, it's important to know that an automatic blood pressure reading may not be terribly meaningful on a patient with a LVAD. To assess the patient's circulatory status more accurately, take a manual blood pressure with a Doppler. Additional methods to assess perfusion include evaluating skin color/temperature and end-tidal CO_2 (which can be monitored via nasal cannula even without supplemental oxygen being administered).

While the patient has no palpable pulse, this does not mean the patient is in cardiac arrest and CPR should not be started. Continuous flow LVAD device patients are most likely pulseless. Additionally, remember that she is awake and alert, so therefore (most likely) not in cardiac arrest! Although admission to an ICU is certainly a possibility, it is not the immediate action. Most facilities prefer to admit (or transfer when appropriate) a 14-year old to a pediatric ICU, ideally one with pediatric cardiac surgery/VAD services.

It is reasonable to assume that the patient may be septic, but administering antibiotics should not be the first option. In this case, in addition to anticipating the need for volume resuscitation (given the history of vomiting and possible sepsis), antibiotics should not be administered until a CBC as well as blood and wound cultures have been obtained. *Note: Topical antibiotic ointments such as Betadine, Neosporin, etc. are not routinely recommended by cardiac surgery as these ointments can injure the tissue adjacent to the driveline exit site.*

This patient has a continuous flow LVAD which, generally speaking, pulls blood from the failing left ventricle (LV) through a continuous flow pump and pushes the blood out of the pump and into the aorta. Patients with an LVAD have a seriously sick left ventricle and the LVAD may be providing a large majority of the patient's cardiac output. As such, there will be little to no pulse pressure (difference between systolic and diastolic BP). This is why palpating a pulse on these patients can be nearly impossible and the pulse pressure tends to be really small.

To understand this patient situation more fully, we must understand that the important blood pressure number is not the systolic or diastolic pressures, or even the pulse pressure mentioned above. Since the heart is not creating pressure through pumping, the pressure we are most concerned with is the mean arterial pressure (MAP) which is being maintained by the LVAD.

Unless an arterial line is in place (rarely seen at triage) and with automatic blood pressure machines not always being much help, what's an ED nurse to do? Go back to basics and take a good old-fashioned manual blood pressure (**but with a Doppler**). For a patient with a LVAD, a manual Doppler BP reflects the patient's mean arterial blood pressure. The RN should place an appropriately sized BP cuff on the patient's arm and place the Doppler on the same spot as they would place a stethoscope, over the brachial artery in the antecubital fossa. Inflate the cuff until the Doppler pulse is no longer heard. As the pressure on the cuff is slowly released, the first sound the nurse hears will be the Doppler BP. For the LVAD patient, this is the MAP. With the newer generation of LVADs, it is recommended to perform two doppler blood pressures and then get an average. This is because some newer LVADs (like the Heartmate 3) have alternating rates of RPMs (revolutions per minutes for the LVAD pump). So, in summary for BPs... Use a Doppler and take two BPs. One is good... Two are better... and the average of the two is both the MAP (mean arterial pressure) and the MAP (most accurate pressure)!

In the event that a doppler is not available, an automatic non-invasive blood pressure machine (NIBP) may (*or may not*) provide a relatively accurate estimation of the MAP.

$$MAP = \frac{SBP + (2 \times DBP)}{3}$$

MAP = mean arterial pressure

SBP = systolic blood pressure

DBP = diastolic blood pressure

113) A 15-year-old female with a history of viral cardiomyopathy and a continuous flow Left Ventricular Assist Device (LVAD) presents to the Emergency Department complaining of a three-day course of nausea, vomiting, and abdominal cramping. Her temperature and respiratory rate are normal. The patient reports that it is frequently difficult to obtain BP readings with a non-invasive BP (NIBP) automatic blood pressure machine and recommends using a Doppler. The patient is subsequently diagnosed with gastroenteritis. When the nurse returns to the room, a red flashing alarm has been activated on the LVAD and the words "**low flow**" are noted on the screen. What is the first intervention that the ED nurse should anticipate?

A) Change the controller

B) Administer a heparin bolus and start at drip based on the patient's weight

C) Initiate a 0.9% NS or LR bolus

D) Check the patient's blood pressure

D - This is a low flow state alarm (less than 2.3 liters/minute), so a blood pressure, specifically the MAP (mean arterial pressure) should be obtained first. The MAP will direct you into which treatment path to follow. If the MAP is greater than 90, consult the VAD coordinator and anticipate an order for a vasodilator to decrease the systemic vascular resistance (SVR). The blood pressure is high enough to cause a low flow state. If the blood pressure is low, volume is the answer.

To help you remember some of the common causes of low flow states, consider the following mnemonic that is described in several textbooks:

SHABDORC

  S – Sedation or Sepsis
  H – Hypertension
  A – Arrhythmia
  B – Bleeding (25% are GI in nature)
  D – Dehydration
  O – Overdrive (LVAD speed is too fast)
  R – Right Heart Failure
  C – Clot

*** Or same info – Just in an order that may be far easier to remember ***

BOD CRASH

  B - Bleeding (25% are GI in nature)
  O – Overdrive (LVAD speed is too fast)
  D – Dehydration
  C – Clot
  R – Right Heart Failure
  A – Arrhythmia
  S – Sedation or Sepsis
  H – Hypertension

Regardless of the cause or your preferred mnemonic, if the MAP is less than 70, volume is required. **LVADs love volume** and preload is the key.

114) A 17-year old male with a continuous flow Left Ventricular Assist Device (LVAD) presents to the Emergency Department complaining of two days of malaise. He states that he has been trying to increase fluids because he thought he was dehydrated. The LVAD device now has a "**High Power**" alarm on the controller. The patient's vital signs: Temperature = 99.1 F (37.3 C), HR by auscultation = 88, Respiratory Rate = 16, manual BP with Doppler mean arterial pressure (MAP) = 62, SpO$_2$= 97% on room air. Which of the following interventions would be the **highest** priority?

A) Call the LVAD coordinator and inform them that the patient now has a "High Power" alarm

B) Draw a full set of labs including coagulation studies

C) Start arranging for transfer to the tertiary facility that cares for the patient's LVAD

D) Change the battery

Certified Pediatric Emergency Nurse (CPEN) Review IV

A – The priority action in this scenario is to call the LVAD coordinator and inform them that the patient has a "High Power" alarm. This is the most important priority because the patient has signs of a possible thrombosis in his LVAD, the signs and symptoms of which include the high power/watts alarm, low flow, borderline or low MAP, and malaise. The reference to "watts" in this case relates to HeartWare's™ (a specific type of VAD) power reading. If the pump is requiring increasing numbers of watts to continue circulating blood, then it's likely the pump is trying to push against something that was not there previously, and probably shouldn't be there now. If the LVAD completely clots off, the patient is likely to go into cardiac arrest quite quickly. Once the initial call is made, the LVAD coordinator can triage the situation, assist with a transfer to a tertiary facility, and provide recommendations regarding anticoagulation therapies.

Call in the cavalry for this sick patient, and don't try to everything yourself. This is why LVAD coordinators exist! While it is important to expedite transfer to a VAD implantation center where the clot can be treated and/or the LVAD exchanged, and though coagulation studies are certainly appropriate in an anticoagulated patient (as LVAD patients generally are), the LVAD coordinator can be of immense assistance and may request additional specific labs to be done.

Alarm Type	Alarm Display	Meaning	Potential Causes	Actions Required
Hazard / Critical	Pump Off / VAD stopped	Pump has stopped. Pump is not operating correctly. Pump flow < 2.5 L/min. Percutaneous lead is disconnected	- Driveline disconnected - Driveline fracture - Connector malfunction/breakage - VAD electrical failure	Check connections from driveline, controller and power source. Change controller.
Hazard / Critical	Critical battery / Low voltage	<5 minutes of battery power remaining. Controller receiving inadequate power.	- Limited battery time - Battery malfunction	Replace battery. Connect to alternate power source. ** Do not remove both batteries simultaneously - VAD will stop **
Hazard / Critical	Controller failed	Controller component failed	- Controller component failed	Change controller.
Advisory / Medium	Controller fault	Controller fault. Alarms disabled.	- Controller component malfunction - Electrostatic discharge	Change controller. Review alarm thresholds.
Advisory / Medium	High watts	High power condition in running VAD pump	- VAD thrombus - High RPM - High flow - VAD electrical fault	Assess & optimise preload/afterload. Assess for thrombus
Advisory / Medium	Low flow / Suction	Pump flow < 2.5 L/min. Average flow dropped below threshold	- Suction event - Poor VAD filling - Elevated BP/afterload - Outflow graft kink - RPM too high or low	* Ensure adequate preload/filling. * Treat dysrhythmias. * Investigate for VAD occlusion (inflow and outflow tracts). * Consider afterload reduction or decreasing pump speed
Advisory / Low	Low battery / Low Voltage	<15 minutes of battery power remaining.		Replace battery. Connect to alternate power source.
Advisory / Low	Power cable disconnected	Power cable disconnected		Ensure all connections intact.
Advisory / Low	Replace system controller	System controller is operating in backup mode		Replace system controller.

www.thebluntdissection.org

Additional Insights from Pediatric/Adult Cardiovascular Surgery ICU and Transport Nurses:

Remember:

- If the LVAD is alarming – Check the connections first!
- Just say "Yes"
    - Yes, you can give ACLS medications
    - Yes, you can cardiovert
    - Yes, you can defibrillate
    - Yes, you can externally pace

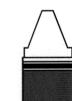

When the device is working, LVAD patients may not have a palpable pulse, even if they are sitting up talking to you. But when the LVAD is not operating, due to pump or power failure (no hum able to be auscultated) the patient will appear dead, with a monitor showing V-fib or asystole, with no spontaneous breathing, and with no exhaled $EtCO_2$ on capnography. If this happens, treat this patient as you would any other with the same presentation. Initiate chest compressions, secure the airway, and provide the medications and therapies per protocols. Once return of spontaneous circulation (ROSC) is achieved, an appropriate cardiology consult should be called immediately to evaluate the LVAD. Among other things, when doing compressions, there is a significant risk of the dislodging the device and causing bleeding.

The LVAD is working if you see a green light or hear an audible mechanical hum over the heart. Obviously, you would expect the hum to be loudest in the area of the left ventricle, however, it is very loud and easily audible if your stethoscope is pretty much anywhere on the chest. VADs are very "high tech" today and have digital screens with constant readings (lots of numbers) and visible as well as audible alarms. HeartMate 3™ and HeartWare™ are currently the two most common LVAD types implanted in the U.S. They are nothing like the old first and second generation VADs, most of which have been changed out due to device age or the patient has expired. There are likely still a few older generation VADS out there, but they wouldn't be in the pediatric population.

Thanks to flight nurse educator Allen Wolfe, some (but regrettably not all) areas "color code" the VAD. That way an EMS service or ED can call the VAD coordinator and simply tell them the patient has a "purple" VAD. Coordinators know which color corresponds with which type of VAD and can immediately lend guidance. Outside of color coding, the device names are very clearly branded today on the VAD controller.

Most common ER issues:
- Thrombosis/clot
- Dehydration/hypovolemia
- GI bleed
- Brain bleed
- Drive line infection
- Pump failure/got unplugged/battery died (leading to asystole)

Power, driveline, power... *Repeat after me*... **Power, driveline, power**... If you need to change a LVAD controller, it must always, ALWAYS remain attached to at least one battery. Change one battery while still attached to the other battery. Very quickly attach the driveline to the new controller while still attached to one battery. Then you can change the second battery. Power, driveline, power...

Do you know what "Dinamap" means? It is an acronym for "Device for Indirect Non-invasive Mean Arterial Pressure." If you are using any sort of device to monitor non-invasive blood pressure (NIBP), it *may* detect a blood pressure (usually with a really narrow pulse pressure) and a MAP i.e. 72/68 (69). But it will only do so if the heart is able to pump stronger than the LVAD flow. Most of the time, automatic BP machines will only give a MAP reading or no reading at all, due to the lack of strong pulsatile flow. This is why the gold standard recommendation is to check at least one, or even better average of two manual/Doppler BPs initially to verify correlation with the MAP on a NIBP.

Reminder: As above, with the newer generation of LVADs, it is recommended to actually perform two doppler blood pressures and then get an average. This is because some newer LVADs have alternating rates of RPMs and the first MAP may be different than one taken shortly after. So, in summary for BPs... Use a Doppler and take two BPs. One is good... 2 are better... and the average of the two is the MAP (mean arterial pressure) or MAP (most accurate pressure!)

Pulse oximeters may or may not work. Regrettably, it's as easy as that. Why, you might ask? Well, most LVAD patients don't have a pulse, so getting a pulse ox to work accurately can be difficult. So, here's the scoop. If a pulse ox is picking up and appears to be "good," i.e. normal, then it probably is correct. However, if the pulse ox is not picking up well or is "bad" (low or really low), it may or may not actually be accurate.

VADs love volume!

The local tertiary (really big) hospital VAD coordinator can be your best friend. Call them early and often!

Look
 ## Listen
Feel

Approach to the LVAD patient...

LOOK: At ALL the connections & controller
Battery life & hopefully green lights

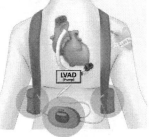

Approach to the LVAD patient...

LISTEN: Hum versus no hum

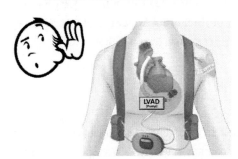

Approach to the LVAD patient...

FEEL: The controller box
Hot = Big clot

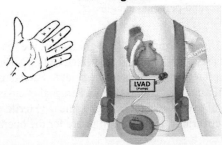

Great LVAD Resources

www.rebelem.com
www.emcrit.org
www.myLVAD.com

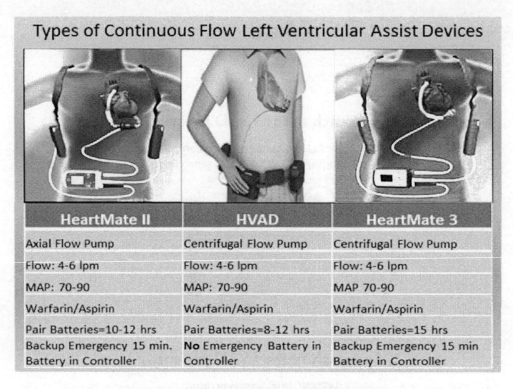

Revised from VAD Community CPR Guideline
University of Rochester Advanced Heart Failure Program
www.urmc.rochester.edu

115) The nurse is about to enter an emergency department (ED) examination room to care for a child with suspected COVID-19 (novel coronavirus 2019). What personal protective equipment (PPE) should the nurse wear?

A) Gown, clean gloves, N-95 respirator mask, and face shield/eye protection

B) Gown, sterile gloves, face mask, and head covering

C) Gown, clean gloves, N-95 respirator mask, and shoe coverings

D) Gown, sterile gloves, face mask, and personal eyeglasses

A – According to the Centers for Disease Control (CDC) guidelines, the recommended PPE for health care team members caring for patients with known or suspected COVID-19 include a gown, clean gloves, an N-95 respirator mask, and eye protection, such as a face shield. Face masks, such as surgical masks, are only indicated if N-95 respirator masks are unavailable. Personal eyeglasses are not enough because they don't provide the same level of eye protection as a face shield. Sterile gloves or a second set of gloves, head coverings, and shoe coverings, though appropriate for the operating room/theatre, are not indicated under the CDC guidelines.

Certified Pediatric Emergency Nurse (CPEN) Review IV

116) The nurse caring for a child with confirmed COVID-19 understands that mild symptoms of COVID-19 may include which of the following?

A) Persistent chest pain/pressure and fever
B) Circumoral cyanosis and fever
C) Non-productive cough and fever
D) Altered mental status and fever

C – COVID-19 is primarily a respiratory disease and as such, symptoms reflect respiratory issues. Mild symptoms of COVID-19 include a non-productive cough, fever, and shortness of breath. Severe symptoms of COVID-19 include persistent chest pain or pressure, circumoral cyanosis, altered mental status, and severe difficulty breathing associated with hypoxia and respiratory failure.

117) When providing discharge instructions to the care giver of a child with suspected COVID-19, what information should the emergency department emphasize regarding the **primary** mode of transmission of the virus?

A) The virus is spread by direct contact only, so don't touch the patient, clothing, or bed linens
B) The virus is spread through urine, so clean the toilet after every time the patient uses it
C) The virus is spread through mosquitoes, so keep the patient indoors and clear potential mosquito breeding grounds like pools of standing water
D) The virus is spread by respiratory droplets, so adhere to the elements of respiratory hygiene and cough etiquette

D – The Centers for Disease Control (CDC) has identified that COVID-19 is *primarily* transmitted through respiratory droplets when the infected person coughs or sneezes. It is also possible that COVID-19 can spread when a person touches a surface or object that has the virus on it, and then touches his or her mouth, nose, or eyes, but this is not thought to be the primary way the virus spreads. Though the virus has been found in feces, thus far, COVID-19 is not currently thought to be spread via urine, blood, or mosquitoes.

The elements of Respiratory Hygiene, aka., Cough Etiquette include:

1. Education of healthcare facility staff, patients, and visitors
2. Posted signs, in language(s) appropriate to the population served, with instructions to patients and accompanying family members or friends
3. Source control measures (e.g., covering the mouth/nose with a tissue when coughing and prompt disposal of used tissues, using surgical masks on the coughing person when tolerated and appropriate)
4. Hand hygiene after contact with respiratory secretions
5. Social distancing, ideally > 6 feet (2m), of persons with respiratory infections in common waiting areas when possible.

118) While the Broselow-Luten system determines pediatric weights using length, the Handtevy system uses:

A) Age
B) Head Circumference
C) Age or length
D) Arm

C - Introduced in 1986, the Broselow-Luten color coding has been successfully used around the world as a way to help take the terror out of pediatric emergency equipment sizing and medication calculations. However, the "New Kid on the Block" (ahh… such 80's memories), the Handtevy system arrived on scene in 2010 and continues the tradition of minimizing the terrors associated with tiny tots and traumas. So, here are some of the key features and differences when it comes to Handtevy vs. Broselow-Luten.

- Broselow-Luten system primarily uses a length-based tape with "red to the head" and "head-to-heel" measurements to determine the approximate ideal body weight.

- Handtevy also has a length-based tape with "red to the head" measurements for ideal body weight, but it also allows users to approximate the weight using the child's age. The tape is only recommended to be used if the age of the child is not known and/or the child is larger or smaller than their stated age.

- Broselow-Luten system determines ideal body weight by head-to-heel length. The child's weight as well as all corresponding medication dosing and equipment sizing can be found on each color zone section.

- Handtevy system determines ideal body weight by age or length. Medication dosing, equipment sizing and electrical values can be found: 1) In a printed guide or 2) In the Handtevy Mobile app. All dosing information in Handtevy is customized to the EMS agency or hospital using it.

- Remember that the Handtevy system uses <u>exactly</u> the same colors as Broselow-Luten and the tapes reflect <u>exactly</u> the same lengths.

Disclaimer: None of the authors or editors of this 4th Edition CPEN Review Book have any conflicts to disclose. We don't work for either the Broselow-Luten or Handtevy systems, but we do strongly recommend the use of their systems.

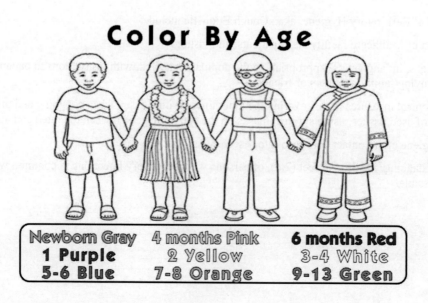

1 YEAR

EQUIPMENT	
BVM	Child or Adult
Blade	1 - 1.5 Straight
ETT Size	4.0 Uncuffed or 3.5 Cuffed
Stylet	10 French
Suction Catheter	10 French
ETCO2 (Colorimeter)	Pediatric
ETT @ Gum or Teeth	11 - 12 cm
OPA (Teeth to Angle Jaw)	60 mm (Size 1)
NPA (Nostril to Earlobe)	18 French
i-gel Supraglottic Airway	Size 1.5
King Laryngeal Tube Airway	Size 1
IV Catheter	20 - 24 Ga
EZ-IO — Place needle on bone → 5 mm line should be visible before drilling	25 mm
NG Tube	8 - 10 French

Emergency Pediatric Equipment from Printed Guidebook
Courtesy of Dr. Peter Antevy & Pediatric Emergency Standards
www.Handtevy.com

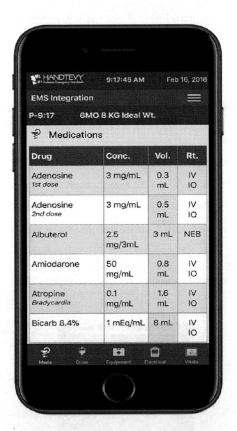

Emergency Pediatric Medications from Handtevy app
Courtesy of Dr. Peter Antevy & Pediatric Emergency Standards
www.Handtevy.com

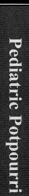

Pediatric Potpourri

119) Using your understanding of pediatric development, which patient could most likely have their cervical spine cleared <u>without</u> imaging after a motor vehicle crash?

A) 4-year old with a suspected broken femur

B) 6-year old who appears tired and confused

C) 9-year old who is awake and has no neck pain or neuro deficits

D) 12-year old with neck pain and numbness in the arms

C – This patient has no neuro deficits or neck pain and is very likely to have their C-spine clinically cleared. Child "A" has a distracting injury (a broken femur), which may mask any immediate mention of neck pain. Even though neck injuries certainly hurt, chances are the femur hurts a whole lot more. Child "B" has an altered mental status which, to no surprise, makes clinical clearance of a C-spine not an option. Lastly, not a trick question, but Child "D" has not only neck pain, but specifically post-trauma neck pain, so imaging and more imaging is in this child's immediate future.

Fortunately, while possible, spinal cord injuries are rare in children. That being said, 60-80% of pediatric spinal injuries involve the cervical spine. That means that 20-40% of the time, there's an issue with the some other part of the spine. In the neck, most injuries are between the skull and C4. That's really important because "C3, C4, C5 Keeps the Diaphragm Alive." So, injuries to C5 (or above) are a huge red flag for issues with the ability to breathe either immediately post-trauma or a few hours later when the edema kicks in!

There are several "rules" for clinically clearing C-spines in the big people population such as the NEXUS criteria and the Canadian C-Spine Rule. However, when it comes to kids, the "jury is still out" as to how well these rules apply. Recent Pediatric Emergency Care Applied Research Network (*PECARN*) publications are showing great promise with guidance as to who gets what, i.e. no imaging/clinical clearance, plain films, CT, or MRI. Bottom line… Since there is currently no research validated strategy for clearing children's C-spines, it is good to have an institutional plan!

120) While working in the Emergency Department, you notice a suspicious man trying to gain access to a secure area. As you approach him, he states he is brand new, shows you his badge, and just needs to get through the door. You should:

A) Use your badge and let him into the restricted area

B) Get more information from him before allowing him through

C) Welcome him to the team and invite him down to lunch with the rest of the crew

D) Get his name and advise him you will call security to come assist him with getting into the area

D – He could be a new employee, or he could be an imposter with a fake badge and a lab coat purchased at a costume store. Certainly, follow your hospital protocols, but if you don't recognize him and something doesn't feel right, stay calm and call security to assist him. Remember the airport TSA motto... If You See Something, Say Something™!

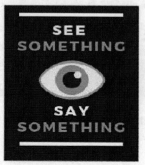

121) Local EMS units are transporting a group of teenage patients to your Emergency Department after a shooting incident at a local high school. As you assist with the placing of ambulatory patients, you see a backpack that apparently was left near the door. You should:

A) Pick it up and open it trying to find if it belongs to one of the ED patients

B) Ask the unit secretary to immediately notify security of a suspicious item inside the ED

C) Leave it there because the owner will probably be back to retrieve it

D) Ask an environmental services worker to take it to the security office when time permits

B – Anyone of those patients could be the attacker – or an accomplice. The book bag is probably just that, a kid's book bag. However, it could also be explosives wired to a timing mechanism or set to be activated remotely. All unknown or suspicious items found during or after an active attacker event need to be reported and dealt with immediately by proper authorities.

122) You are working in the Emergency Department when a patient suddenly becomes violent and pulls out a gun. You have escaped the room, but have not yet left the building. Law enforcement officers arrive and the one nearest you tells you to walk towards them and exit the building. You should:

A) Run as fast as you can in the direction the officer is pointing

B) Tell the officer you need to get your computer as you turn and head back to the locker room

C) Put your hands straight up in the air with outstretched fingers to show the officer your palms and walk quietly toward him making no sudden moves

D) Lie flat on the ground with your hands behind the back of your head

C – The officer does not know if you are a good guy or a bad guy. In high stress situations such as this, you really want to make it clear that you are one of the good guys. Follow the directions given. If told to walk, walk, don't run, and don't lie flat on the ground like you are a bad guy who's just been apprehended. And don't even think about going back into the area of danger. Even if you have your computer bag near you, trying to exit the scene with it just is not smart. The law enforcement officers don't know if you are carrying a laptop or a bomb (big difference)! Follow his/her orders, do not reach out and hug or kiss the officer (you can do this later), answer any questions only when asked, and always let him/her see your empty and open hands. In particular, a cell phone in your hands may look very suspicious, so empty means EMPTY!

123) We will never be able to fully stop active attacker events, so we need to be prepared. All of these are sound examples of preparation **except**:

A) Know your lockdown plan and practice it on a regular basis

B) Establish a process for staff to report persons of concern to security for monitoring, additional scrutiny or intervention

C) Pre deploy medical supplies, Active Attacker Trauma/Stop the Bleed kits in multiple areas of the facility

D) Train all staff to wait until the charge nurse gives the "all clear" before leaving the area

D – For every minute you do nothing, you increase your chances of being in the "kill pool" by 70 percent. Proper planning prevents...

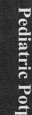

Certified Pediatric Emergency Nurse (CPEN) Review IV

Active Shooter
RUN. HIDE. FIGHT.

Be Informed

- Sign up for an active shooter training.
- If you see something, say something to the authorities right away.
- Sign up to receive local emergency alerts and register your contact information with any work-sponsored alert system.
- Be aware of your environment and any possible dangers.

Make a Plan

- Make a plan with your family and make sure everyone knows what to do if confronted with an active shooter.
- Wherever you go, look for the two nearest exits, have an escape path in mind and identify places you could hide if necessary.
- Understand the plans for individuals with disabilities or other access and functional needs.

During

RUN and escape if possible

- Getting away from the shooter or shooters is the top priority.
- Leave your belongings behind and get away.
- Help others escape, if possible, but evacuate regardless of whether others agree to follow.
- Warn and prevent individuals from entering an area where the active shooter may be.
- Call 9-1-1 when you are safe and describe the shooter, location and weapons.

HIDE if escape is not possible

- Get out of the shooter's view and stay very quiet.
- Silence all electronic devices and make sure they won't vibrate.
- Lock and block doors, close blinds and turn off lights.
- Don't hide in groups. Spread out along walls or hide separately to make it more difficult for the shooter.
- Try to communicate with police silently. Use text message or social media to tag your location or put a sign in a window.
- Stay in place until law enforcement gives you the all clear.
- Your hiding place should be out of the shooter's view and provide protection if shots are fired in your direction.

FIGHT as an absolute last resort

- Commit to your actions and act as aggressively as possible against the shooter.
- Recruit others to ambush the shooter with makeshift weapons like chairs, fire extinguishers, scissors, books, etc.
- Be prepared to cause severe or lethal injury to the shooter.
- Throw items and improvised weapons to distract and disarm the shooter.

Pediatric Potpourri

After

- Keep hands visible and empty.
- Know that law enforcement's first task is to end the incident and they may have to pass injured along the way.
- Officers may be armed with rifles, shotguns or handguns and may use pepper spray or tear gas to control the situation.
- Officers will shout commands and may push individuals to the ground for their safety.
- Follow law enforcement instructions and evacuate in the direction they come from unless otherwise instructed.
- Take care of yourself first, and then you may be able to help the wounded before first responders arrive.
- If the injured are in immediate danger, help get them to safety.
- While you wait for first responders to arrive, provide first aid. Apply direct pressure to wounded areas and use tourniquets if you have been trained to do so.
- Turn wounded people onto their sides if they are unconscious and keep them warm.
- Consider seeking professional help for you and your family to cope with the long-term effects of the trauma.

RUN. HIDE. FIGHT.

www.ready.gov/active-shooter

124) When troubleshooting respiratory issues with intubated patients, it is helpful to consider which of the following mnemonics?

A) SAMPLE

B) FAST

C) PQRST

D) DOPE

D – The DOPE mnemonic is commonly used (and taught) as an easy way to remember the crucial troubleshooting tips for mechanically ventilated patients.

> **D- Dislodged tube -** Reposition or replace the endotracheal or tracheostomy tube
>
> **O- Obstruction or Oxygen** – Suction or change the endotracheal or tracheostomy tube and ensure oxygen is flowing and attached
>
> **P- Pneumothorax** – Needle decompression and/or chest tube
>
> **E- Equipment or Error** – Something is messed up with the ventilator or bagging technique

This is sometimes expanded and becomes DOPES by adding:

> **S - Stacked Breaths** – The patient may need to be off the vent for a few moments to allow for full exhalation

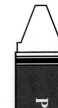

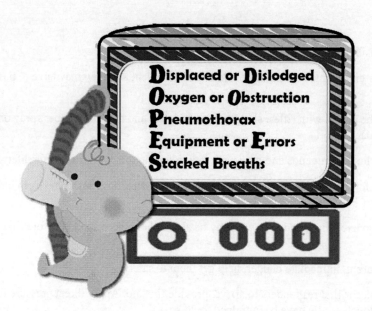

(D)isplaced or (D)islodged: There is a reason that the DOPE mnemonic begins with this one. If the tube (ETT or trache) is no longer in the right spot, bad things will happen. Before all other interventions, verify that the tube/trache is in the right place first! With this in mind, remember breath sounds aren't a reliable way to confirm tube or trache placement. The standard of care, when assessing the initial tube placement or when things are not going well is end-tidal CO_2 (colorimetric or capnography) verification.

(O)bstruction or (O)xygen: Air has to be able to go in, before it can come back out. So, if you can't easily pass a suction catheter all the way down the tube or trache, then an obstruction may be the problem, and a tube/trache change in the near future is a very real possibility. As far as the other "O" – Oxygen, well this part of the DOPE mnemonic should be self-explanatory. If the oxygen is disconnected, kinked, empty, etc., then ventilated patients tend not to do very well.

(P)neumothorax: If you hit the "P" level in the mnemonic, it's time to assess for a pneumothorax; essentially air where there shouldn't be air and no air where there should be air. And what's worse than a pneumothorax? How about having the "mother" of all "pneumos," i.e. a tension pneumothorax. This can quickly result in not just respiratory issues, but death. So, just like adults, if the child is trying to die and a tension pneumo is the suspected culprit, needle decompression, aka., "needling the chest" is the next step! This will allow the trapped air to get out and keep the child alive until a chest tube or pigtail catheter can be placed. But... especially in little ones, before sticking a needle in their chest, make sure the tube is not down too far, i.e. in a mainstem bronchi. Right mainstem intubation is the most common pediatric ETT "poor placement." Recently, in addition to breath sounds and X-rays, bedside ultrasound has become very useful in assisting with rapid diagnosis of mainstem intubation vs. pneumothorax.

(E)quipment Failure or User (E)rrors: Simply, something's not working properly. So, if the patient is on a vent, take the vent out of the DOPE equation and "bag" the patient. That way, only DOP remains and respiratory therapy can quickly work to fix the vent while you make sure your patient is breathing. If the patient is being bagged but still having problems, consider the other equipment being used. Do you have the correct size bag and mask and are they connected properly? Is the bagging at the appropriate rate and depth? The error may be with the user. Back to basics... Airway and breathing come before vent. Not only in the alphabet, but in patient care as well.

(S)tacked Breaths: For many years, the DOPE mnemonic has been used with great success. Recently however, it has been expanded from DOPE to DOPES, to reflect the potential problem of Stacked Breaths. For example, in asthma, one of the many problems is not necessarily getting the air in, but getting the air back out. If a child is sick enough that they are intubated for their asthma, "breath stacking" or a breath being given by the ventilator before the previous breath has had time to exhale, is a real concern. So, especially with kids who might be considered "bad wheezers," if they suddenly crash, and after troubleshooting with DOPE, taking them off the vent for a few seconds (or longer) and allowing them additional time to exhale can be lifesaving.

Pediatric Potpourri

Certified Pediatric Emergency Nurse (CPEN) Review IV

The other mnemonics in the question are explained below (and there is a special 2 for 1 with FAST).

PQRST: Mnemonic for a complete pain history

P3 = Positional, palliating, and provoking factors

Q = Quality

R3 = Region, radiation, referral

S = Severity

T3 = Temporal factors (time and mode of onset, progression, previous episodes)

SAMPLE: Mnemonic for a focused history in traumatic or emergency medical conditions

S = Signs and symptoms

A = Allergies

M = Medications

P = Pertinent past medical and/or surgical history

L = Last oral intake

E = Events leading up to

FAST: Mnemonic for a thoracic/abdominal ultrasound exam after trauma

F = Focused

A = Assessment with

S = Sonography in

T = Trauma

FAST: Mnemonic to help educate the public on detecting symptoms of a stroke

F = Facial drooping: A section of the face, usually only on one side, that is drooping and hard to move. This can be recognized by a crooked smile.

A = Arm weakness: The inability to raise one's arm fully.

S = Speech difficulties: An inability or difficulty to understand or produce speech.

T = Time: If any of the symptoms above are showing, time is of the essence; call emergency medical services and go to the hospital immediately.

125) Which of the following is a significant indicator of the possibility a tension pneumothorax in an intubated child?

A) High airway pressure alarms

B) An enlarged cardiac silhouette

C) Absent breath sounds bilaterally

D) Low airway pressure alarms

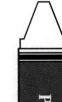

A – It is a really good habit in the Emergency Department and Critical Care worlds to consider a tension pneumothorax when the high pressure alarm starts. Do not EVER let yourself become the nurse who later hears there was a massive tension pneumothorax discovered during a post-mortem examination. Diagnosis and treatment for a tension pneumothorax should be based on clinical assessment, and possibly, if time permits, supported by a bedside ultrasound. It should never be made by waiting for a chest x-ray or even worse, autopsy!

Another significant indicator of a possible tension pneumothorax would be worsening tachycardia (early sign) OR bradycardia (really late sign), but neither of these options were offered (but might have been).

An enlarged cardiac silhouette (seen on X-ray) may be associated with cardiomegaly, pericardial effusion, or even the technique used for the x-ray, but isn't considered an indicator of a tension pneumothorax.

Low air pressure alarms are usually caused by leaks or disconnects in the tubing, or "circuit."

Absent breath sounds unilaterally would be a significant indicator of a possible pneumothorax, but absent breath sounds bilaterally is something completely different. When preparing for a certification exam, train yourself to fully read the question and answers before making your selection.

126) What is the normal end-tidal CO_2 ($EtCO_2$) range for pediatric patients?

A) 35-45

B) 25-35

C) 30-40

D) 30-50

A - 35-45... Exactly the same as with adults. Nothing tricky, just basic, <u>must have</u>, knowledge.

127) When suctioning an infant's endotracheal or tracheostomy tube, suction should be applied:

A) Only during insertion of the suction catheter

B) Only during removal of the suction catheter

C) During both insertion and removal of the suction catheter

D) Only during the exhalation phase of breathing

B – What is the goal of suctioning a tube or trache? To remove boogers, blood, bugs, etc. Suction is only applied on the way out, otherwise you are shoving the stuff further downstream. And yes, they make suction catheters for all sizes of human patients, from preemies (2.5 ETT, use a 5 Fr suction catheter) to big 'ol adults (8.0 ETT, use a 14 Fr suction catheter.)

128) In contrast to the Glasgow Coma Scale (GCS), GCS-P, Four Score, and AVPU neuro assessment scales, the Simplified Motor Score (SMS) only involves assessment of:

A) Motor

B) Verbal

C) Pupils

D) Overall level of consciousness

A – The Simplified Motor Score (SMS) is exactly as advertised. It is a simple motor assessment. Nothing tricky and nothing meant to distract you on this question. Sure, we could have offered an option something like "auto mechanic knowledge" or "method of measuring the power of your riding lawnmower," but beyond giving you a chuckle, what good would that have done? Some questions are just straightforward, like this one.

So now you might want to know more assuming you "guessed" correctly in answering this question. Well, first introduced in 2006, the "new neuro kid on the block" is the Simplified Motor Score or SMS. As opposed to the ever popular Glasgow Coma Scale (GCS), which may require a score sheet (paper or digital) to remember the components and their respective values, enters the SMS. For several years, especially in prehospital emergency care, the Simplified Motor Score has been utilized with very nice results. Simply, for an initial, critical evaluation, just knowing that the patient is not following commands (indicating a GCS motor component score <6) works well to predict significant injury

Calculating coma scores is not something many ED nurses do on a daily basis, and for prehospital professionals, this can be even more true. A study found that when two professionals performed a simultaneous and independent GCS assessment on a patient, the calculated scores differed by at least 2 points in 30% of the cases. That's a huge amount of variability. So when it comes to neuro assessment scales and scores, Option 1: Practice, practice, and practice, or Option 2: Make an easier scale.

Researchers are finding that use of the Simplified Motor Score could drastically simplify prehospital assessment of trauma patients for determining which patients need to go to what level of trauma center. Is the patient able to follow commands? Yes = lower risk. No = higher risk. It's hard enough to rescue a patient from a horrible motor vehicle accident. Trying to work out the GCS in your head at 3 AM in a rainstorm is even tougher. Several studies have found that the most important part of the GCS is the motor part. Patients who are not following commands are sick and need a trauma center. How Simple!

[**Editor's note**: SMS also stands for "Short Messaging Service" which is a fancy way of saying "Texting." You're not likely to need to know that for CPEN.]

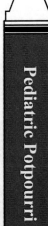

BEHAVIOR	RESPONSE	SCORE
Eye opening response	Spontaneously	4
	To speech	3
	To pain	2
	No response	1
Best verbal response	Oriented to time, place, and person	5
	Confused	4
	Inappropriate words	3
	Incomprehensible sounds	2
	No response	1
Best motor response	Obeys commands	6
	Moves to localized pain	5
	Flexion withdrawal from pain	4
	Abnormal flexion (decorticate)	3
	Abnormal extension (decerebrate)	2
	No response	1

Traditional Adult Glasgow Coma Scale (GCS)
Versus

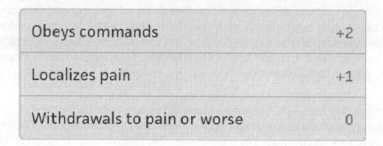

Simplified Motor Scale (SMS)

129) Which unit of measure is recommended for documenting the weight on patients of **all** ages in the emergency department?

A) Pounds

B) Kilograms

C) Milligrams

D) Instagrams

B – When it comes to documenting (and communicating) the weight of patients in the ED, the Emergency Nurses Association recommends that kilograms be the only unit of measure used. Why so much attention to kilograms instead of the commonly used measure of pounds? Simple…studies have shown that over 25% of medication errors are due to confusion over pounds vs. kilograms. This is unacceptable and preventable. National recommendations state that all scales used for patient weights: infant, standing, wheelchair, integrated, bedside, etc. should only display weights in kilograms (or grams). If the only weight shown on the scale is in kilogramic and the electronic medical record (EMR) only displays weights in kilograms, the chance for weight-based medication errors is much less.

If you chose option D, "Instagrams," we applaud your sense of humor.

Remember the famous line from the original Karate Kid movie... "Fear does not exist in this dojo... Pain does not exist in this dojo..." and when it comes to weighing patients, "Pounds do not exist in this ED!"

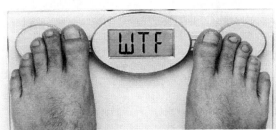

130) What is the currently recommended **best** method to confirm proper placement of an alternative/backup airway, such as a laryngeal mask airway, King airway, or i-gel?

A) Auscultation of bilateral breath sounds

B) Observation of chest rise and fall

C) Auscultation of the epigastric area

D) Observation of end-tidal carbon dioxide

D – Confirming that an alternate/backup airway is properly placed should involve end-tidal CO_2 monitoring: colorimetric (change colors), capnometric (displays a number), or ideally, capnographic (displays a number and a waveform). That shouldn't come as a surprise because alternate airways, just like endotracheal tubes, allow air to go in and out of the same place (the lungs) through the trachea. All of the other techniques may be helpful, but the bottom line is, just as with endotracheal tubes, verification of proper placement with end-tidal CO_2 monitoring is not only highly recommended, it is the standard of care.

131) All of the following are true about the placement of an alternate or backup airway in infants, children, or adults **except**:

A) Does not require interruption of CPR

B) Decreases the risk for gastric insufflation and aspiration as compared to bag-mask ventilation

C) Must be immediately replaced by an endotracheal tube (ETT) upon return of spontaneous circulation (ROSC)

D) Bypass the common challenges for achieving a tight bag-mask seal

C – Alternate airways do not need to be replaced immediately upon the return of spontaneous circulation, although in many centers, that would be the common practice. If a patient regains circulation, respirations, and is conscious and able to protect their own airway, it might not be appropriate to "replace" the alternate airway with an ETT. Alternate airways are easily placed during CPR and do not require interruption of continuous chest compressions. They decrease, but do not completely eliminate, the risk of gastric insufflation, aka., "bagging the belly," and subsequent aspiration potential. And lastly, they bypass many of the common challenges for achieving a tight mask seal. Remember, performing really good bag-mask ventilation is not nearly as easy on humans as it is on the PALS or ACLS manikins. Alternate airways just make the basics of bagging much easier!

Testing Tip: Watch out for absolutes; words like always, never, and must are usually red flags that should attract your attention. There are very few "musts" when it comes to emergency medicine.

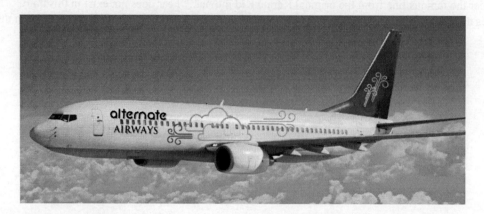

132) An 8-month old child presents to the ER with intermittent episodes of drawing her knees up to her chest and refusing to eat for the past 24 hours. An ultrasound is performed that shows a target sign (doughnut sign or bull's eye sign). What diagnosis do you suspect?

A) Intussusception

B) Appendicitis

C) Mid-gut volvulus

D) Gastroenteritis

A – Intussusception is a condition where the intestine slides or telescopes into an adjacent part of the intestine causing an obstruction. It occurs most commonly in children ages 6-months to 3-years and is the most common cause of obstruction in patients less than three years of age (but it can occur in older kids and even adults). Ultrasound may show a bull's eye or doughnut of intestine within the intestine. The classic presentation is <u>intermittent irritability</u> with <u>intermittent cramping</u> pain (their intestines are intermittently where they shouldn't be after all). They will <u>intermittently</u> cry while drawing their knees into their chest. Diagnosis is by history and physical exam (do they have an intussusception?), ultrasound or CT (confirm they have an intussusception), and eventually barium, or now more commonly, air enema (yep, they definitely have an intussusception). In addition to its diagnostic value, the enema can be successful in correcting the problem. (Reports show upwards of 80% successful reduction of intussusception non-surgically.) If the enema is unsuccessful at resolving the problem, it's off to the OR for surgical intervention and restoration of blood flow to the intestines before a perforation occurs.

Although the books describe "Currant jelly stools" as a classic sign of intussusception, real life experience and research reveal that is a late, and rare, sign. Intermittent irritability (with knees into the chest) = intussusception!

Hallmark signs of appendicitis include periumbilical or lower right quadrant abdominal pain, fever, and nausea. Infants with mid-gut volvulus typically present with abdominal pain and vomiting, which may occasionally be bilious. Gastroenteritis patients typically present with diarrhea and vomiting, along with abdominal pain, fever, and chills.

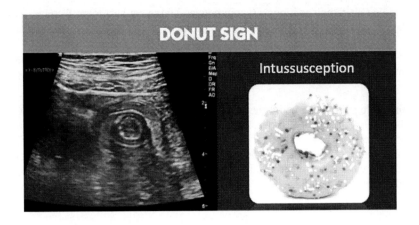

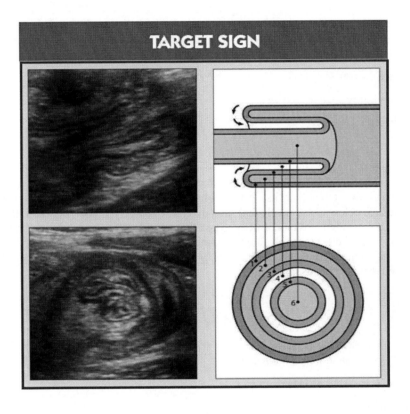

Donut, Target, or Bull's Eye Signs on Abdominal Ultrasound

133) As part of your discharge teaching for an 11-month old, you educate the family on proper use of an appropriately sized infant or convertible car seat. In addition to checking that the straps are tight enough so they cannot be pinched, the car seat should be:

A) Rear-facing with the chest bar at the bottom of the rib cage

B) Forward-facing with the chest bar at level of the armpits

C) Forward-facing with the chest bar over the abdomen

D) Rear-facing with the chest bar at level of the armpits

D – Children should be rear-facing as long as recommended by the car seat manufacturer, and the chest bar should be at the chest (armpit level) and not at the bottom of the rib cage (abdomen level). This is important because 80% of care seats are <u>improperly</u> installed and used (wow!) Most state laws require children to be rear-facing until they are a <u>minimum</u> of 12-months old, and, several states require children to be positioned that way until they are 2-years of age.

Remember the vulnerable points on a pediatric patient – the abdomen is one! The chest bar should be placed at the level of the armpits so that it overlays the rib cage (i.e. the chest), protecting the abdominal organs. If the chest bar overlays the abdomen, damage to the abdominal organs can occur not only from the motor vehicle accident, but from the car seat itself. The straps should always be tight enough so that excessive strap webbing cannot be pinched and no more than one finger (adult finger!) fits under the harness strap. And remember, car seats should be checked by a certified child passenger technician.

134) Your 6-year old patient was involved in a motor vehicle collision. The patient was wearing a seatbelt, but was not secured in a booster seat. What would you anticipate being the **most** common presenting injury in this patient?

A) Aortic arch tear

B) Coup contrecoup injury

C) Abdominal injuries

D) Pelvic fracture

C - Studies have shown that the use of booster seats in young children reduces the risk of abdominal injuries by improving how the seat belt fits. Automobile safely belts are made to protect the wearer by fitting low over the hips below the stomach, and snug over the shoulder. In the "big head, little body" population, the seat belt is often worn incorrectly, typically over their large abdomen, and the shoulder belt isn't worn at all! Seat belts are invaluable for young kids, but they are not enough. Whether for teaching or reminding yourself, remember: <u>B</u>oosters, <u>B</u>ack seats, and <u>B</u>elts (**B₃**) are the keys for little kids! **B₃ <u>before</u>** you drive with kids in the car.

135) A 7-year old patient has presented for acute ethanol intoxication. Administration of which of the following medications should be anticipated?

A) 10% or 25% Dextrose (D10 or D25)

B) Narcan® (naloxone)

C) Antizol® (fomepizole)

D) Romazicon® (flumazenil)

A – Administration of a dextrose solution should be anticipated because hypoglycemia frequently occurs in younger children with alcohol intoxication. The metabolism of alcohol impairs gluconeogenesis (synthesis of glucose). During an episode of acute alcohol intoxication, it is critically important to closely monitor the patient and take steps to prevent secondary complications such as hypoglycemia and resulting hypoglycemic seizures. Just as with adults, these children may also require an antiemetic as well as IV fluid hydration during their course of treatment. And, just as with adults, the infamous "banana bag" (0.9NS or LR with thiamine, folic acid, ± magnesium, and multivitamins) is no longer routinely recommended.

Just as a reminder, Narcan (naloxone) is used for opioid reversal and Romazicon (flumazenil) reverses benzodiazepines. Antizol (fomepizole) is used to treat methanol and ethylene glycol (antifreeze) poisoning.

136) Which intramuscular site is preferred for a 6-month old infant?

A) Deltoid muscle
B) Anterolateral aspect of the thigh
C) Gluteal muscle
D) Upper-outer triceps

B - In infants and toddlers, the anterolateral aspect of the thigh (vastus lateralis muscle) is the preferred site for IM injections. Extreme care should be taken to avoid possible nerve injury when using the gluteal muscle. For little ones, make your life easy and just pinch an inch of the thigh!

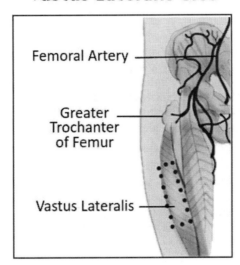

137) Your patient is in status asthmaticus. Ketamine has been ordered. You can anticipate that the medication will have all of the following effects on the respiratory system **except:**

A) Decreased airway resistance
B) Bronchodilation
C) Improvement in hypercarbia
D) Decreased lung compliance

D - Ketamine has been shown to have several beneficial effects when used in status asthmaticus patients. It leads to smooth muscle relaxation and bronchodilation, as well as decreased airway resistance and improved (not decreased) lung compliance (good things). Some studies have also shown some improvement in oxygenation and hypercarbia after administration (2 more good things). In addition to the benefits to breathing, low-dose ketamine also helps really sick children tolerate being placed on BiPAP with nebs. Intubation is sometimes required in these cases, but if it can be avoided, all the better. Ketamine is becoming a first-line choice not only for pediatric sedation and pain management, but now for really sick "wheezers" as well.

138) A 2-year old presents with audible wheezing and mild intercostal retractions. As the child sits in his father's lap, he is unwilling to accept the nebulizer mask on his face, pushes it away, and cries and screams as you attempt to place the mask closer. The child's father, who happens to be a local surgeon, states; "He's fine, just give a blow-by neb. He will still get the medication. Look at how deep he is breathing with crying." The **most** appropriate response by the nurse caring for the child would be something similar to:

A) "Good idea. Let's not upset him further and his good inspiratory efforts will allow the medication to work just fine."

B) "Okay." Then hand the father the nebulizer and teach him how to draw pictures in the air using the mist to keep the child from crying.

C) "Let him play with the mask and get used to it because he will need to have the mask directly on his face to encourage better distribution of the medication in his lower airways."

D) Smash the mask onto the face and don't let go. His increased amount of screaming will help with deeper deposition of the medication.

C - You should politely explain that crying actually <u>reduces</u> aerosol delivery to the lungs and so does the blow-by technique. Research has consistently shown that, in many cases, blow-by nebs just spray the patient's face with medication and incredibly little medication reaches the lower airways. Interestingly, even though the effectiveness of blow-by nebulizers has been considered sub-optimal, respiratory therapy research has not universally supported that conclusion. At the end of the day, efficacy depends not only on the child, but also the type of nebulizer, compressor, and face mask, and, of course, the experience of the individual administering the treatment.

Crying often results in faster and deeper breaths, but calm children with calm breathing tend to have significantly better airflow. Laminar flow is when air has an easy time going in and out. Turbulent flow can occur with obstructions or higher flow rates (i.e. crying or screaming.) The bottom line is that whether in the air or on the ground, when administering nebulized medications, avoiding turbulent airflow makes everything better.

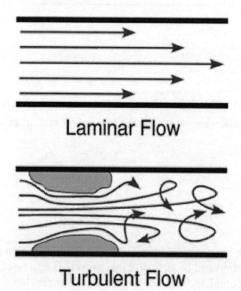

Next, we can take that one step further. Correct placement of the face mask is imperative for getting the medication where it will do some good. If you can take the time to make them comfortable, reducing the distance between the child and the mask will administer medication more effectively and reduce medication loss. When it comes to blow-by, closer is better. And if the child won't tolerate direct placement of the mask on the face, something is better than nothing.

Certified Pediatric Emergency Nurse (CPEN) Review IV

Additional Insights from a Pediatric Transport Respiratory Therapist:

Here are a few short additional items:

1. Previously published research using a nebulized radiopaque fluid produced an excellent example of an esophagram in a crying patient; meaning that it appears most of the aerosol went <u>to the stomach</u>, not the lungs, with crying.

2. A well-fitting mask can also act as a medication reservoir, as the volume of space inside the mask will fill with aerosolized medication. So, when the patient takes their next breath, the medicated air in the mask will minimize medication lost to the outside air and also minimizing entrained room air (similar to the reservoir bag on a non-rebreather mask) and thus increase the medication delivery.

3. Finally, if the child is hypoxic, use oxygen to power the neb. But, in other cases, try running the nebs with compressed air instead of oxygen. That way, if there is an increase in the O2 sat, it probably was from the nebulizer working, and not just from the supplemental oxygen. I've done countless nebs powered by oxygen and the sats (no surprise here) went up. Then, shortly thereafter, my patient was on Q2 hr nebs to "increase oxygenation." With the next neb, I dragged the physician into the room, powered the neb with compressed air and showed that there was no change in sats. The order was then changed to continuous low-flow nasal cannula oxygen, and nebs only prn!

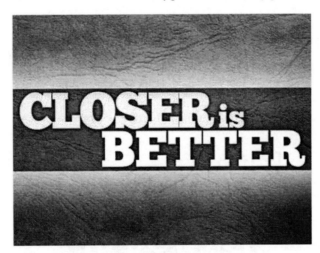

139) You are caring for a 10-year old patient who came into the ED by ambulance with severe shortness of breath. EMS initiated BiPAP and administered a nebulizer treatment in route. You have now transferred the patient to the hospital BiPAP machine with a new BiPAP mask and you see the "LOW PRESSURE" alarm on the ventilator. What is a likely cause of this alarm?

A) The patient is not breathing at an adequate rate

B) The patient is experiencing severe bronchospasms

C) There is a leak somewhere in the circuit or around the mask seal

D) The patient is breathing too quickly for the ventilator

C - Leaks in the circuit (from a loose connection or something being broken) or a leak around the mask (from poor fit or not being tightened properly) will cause pressure to leak out of the circuit. The ventilator will sense that it is not maintaining the desired pressure and begin to alarm. There is not enough pressure in the circuit, hence the LOW PRESSURE alarm.

If a patient has severe bronchospasms, potentially brought on by high airway pressures, this will commonly cause a HIGH PRESSURE alarm, as air is having a hard time getting in and out. Breathing at an abnormal rate (fast or slow) will trigger a breath rate alarm. Unlike many things in medicine, sometimes the alarms (and test questions) are not trying to trick you.

Low pressure = low pressure. High pressure = high pressure. Breath rate = breath rate.

140) A teenage patient is brought back into an ED room from triage. The patient is currently on their own BiPAP home device and is accompanied by a neighbor who is not trained in its use. The patient does not appear to be in any respiratory distress at this time. What should your next action be?

A) Page the respiratory therapist

B) Remove the device from the patient

C) Remove the device and place the patient on hospital CPAP

D) Remove the device and place the patient on a nasal cannula at 2 LPM.

A - When your patient is being supported by a respiratory device that no one in the room is trained on, it is best to quickly get respiratory therapy involved. Continuing therapy using home device (assuming it is currently working fine) is sometimes done, but only after consultation with respiratory therapy. As soon as safely possible, this patient should be transferred to a device that the hospital staff is familiar with, knows how to use, and has been "blessed as safe" (checked out) by the hospital biomedical staff. But remember, you do not want to remove the device before respiratory therapy has the appropriate replacement equipment prepared and at the bedside. In an emergency, if it ain't broke, don't fix it!

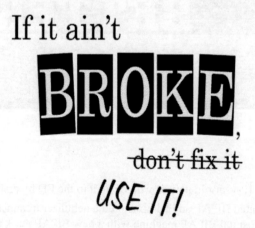

141) You are assisting the respiratory therapist in applying Nasal CPAP. You note that the tubing is pulling the nasal prongs/pillows up into the patient's nares and are secured high on the patients face. You should:

A) Secure the tubing lower on the face so that it does not pull up into the patient's nares

B) Place the patient on a full-face CPAP mask instead

C) Place the patient on a nasal cannula instead

D) Do nothing, as this is appropriate placement for nasal CPAP prongs/pillows

D - Even though it may appear uncomfortable for the patient at times, this is the way the device is meant to be fitted. There must be slight pressure exerted up into the nares for the prongs to form an adequate seal and provide pressure support. This means that the tubing must be secured high on the face to achieve this.

Test Taking Tip 1: Sesame Street had a segment about "one of these things isn't like the others" and that often holds true with standardized tests. In this case, there are three choices suggesting that you do something and one that specifically says don't do anything. In other words, one of those choices isn't like the others, and if you aren't sure, you may want to pick that one.

Test Taking Tip 2: Don't over-think the question and don't change your mind just because of a Sesame Street game. Studies have shown that when you change an answer without 100% clarity, you probably changed from the correct answer to the incorrect one. Read carefully, but don't over-think.

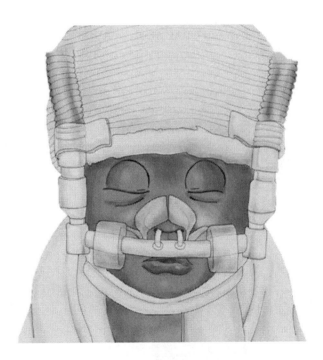

Nasal CPAP Prongs

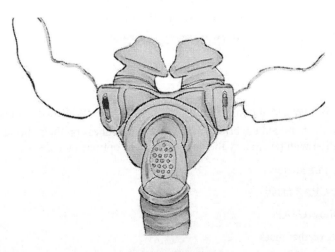

Nasal CPAP Pillows

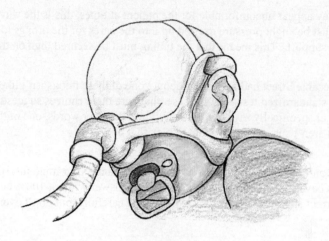

Nasal CPAP Mask

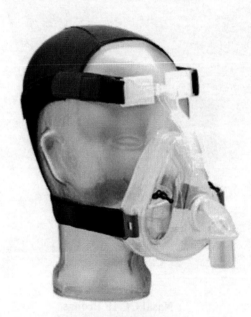

Full Face CPAP Mask
Photo courtesy of Mercury Medical
www.mercurymedical.com

142) Your patient is managed at home on full-face mask CPAP. While assessing the patient, you note that there is skin breakdown around the bridge of the nose and redness on their cheeks along the borders of the mask. In consultation with respiratory therapy, anticipated options include?

A) Remove the mask immediately

B) Trial with a bigger CPAP mask

C) Trial with nasal pillow CPAP

D) Trial with a non-rebreather mask

C – Try a nasal pillow device. This patient clearly has been wearing a mask too frequently, too tightly, or both. A larger mask will not likely fit properly and probably won't create an adequate seal. A non-rebreather mask will not provide the pressure support the patient needs. We also do not want to remove the mask immediately without a backup device ready to support the patient's breathing. This leaves us with nasal pillow CPAP, a good alternative in this circumstance because it will remove the pressure from the areas on the face that are damaged from the mask. If nasal pillows don't work or are rejected by the patient, hydrocolloid dressings such as DuoDERM® can placed to protect the skin under the pressure areas.

143) You and a respiratory care provider are placing a patient on BiPAP therapy. You know that forming a secure and comfortable fit can be a challenging part of the process. While your colleague holds the mask on the patient's face, forming a satisfactory seal, you are asked to tighten the straps of the mask. What is the **best** process for securing the BiPAP mask on the patient?

A) Tighten each of the four straps individually in a clock-wise rotation starting with the strap at the top right of the patient's face and ending with the strap at the top left of the patient's face

B) Tighten both of the bottom straps simultaneously, followed by the top straps one by one

C) Tighten both of the top straps simultaneously, followed by the bottom straps one by one

D) Tighten both of the bottom straps simultaneously, followed by the top straps simultaneously, then assess for proper fit and adjust as needed

D - Fitting a mask can be the hardest part of applying any kind of CPAP or BiPAP. Placing the mask on straight and then keeping it secure as the straps are positioned can ease this process. For this reason, it is recommended that you first tighten both of the bottom straps at the same time and then tighten both of the top straps. Once that is done, assess or evaluate. If minor leaks are detected during the assessment step, this would be when you should either straighten the mask and start over or make independent adjustments to each strap.

A good test taker will get this question correct without even knowing what a BiPAP mask is or how it is applied. The question asks for the best "process" and all you have to remember is the nursing process to spot the correct answer. The last step in the nursing process, after an intervention, is always "evaluate" and another word for evaluate is assess. (Assess is the first step in the nursing process, which is what you would do before making any adjustments.) So read the question carefully and remember the basics of the nursing process!

144) You are in the process of placing a respiratory distress patient on BiPAP therapy. You have been adjusting the straps and placement of the mask for several minutes, but still haven't achieved a satisfactory seal. What is the **most** likely cause of this problem?

A) You have chosen the wrong mask size

B) The pressure on the BiPAP machine is set too high

C) The patient is not adequately sedated

D) The pressure on the BiPAP machine is set too low

A - Given the very limited information presented in the question, it is most likely that the wrong mask size was chosen. There is no indication that the patient requires sedation, or that there is any problem with the machine.

145) You are assessing a pediatric patient whose parents report an acute onset of vague complaints. Which assessment finding would be **least** concerning?

A) Nasal flaring

B) Grunting sounds

C) Thoraco-abdominal muscle retractions

D) Pale yellow-orange discoloration to the distal phalanges bilaterally and circumorally

D – Given vague complaints and no other information from which to work, it is not unreasonable to attribute the appearance of orange colored fingertips and lips to a snack-size or larger bag of Cheetos® (preferably the flaming hot variety). All of the other findings are significant indicators of respiratory distress in children. Nasal flaring indicates that the child is trying to increase air flow by increasing the diameter of the nasal airway. Grunting means the child is attempting to generate positive end-expiratory pressure (PEEP) by creating pressure as they breathe out. PEEP improves gas exchange in the lungs by decreasing the shunting of blood. Retractions mean that the patient is using accessory muscles to improve inhalation. These signs can present independent of each other, and when they occur together, it is a very bad sign.

146) You are caring for a 10-year-old patient with respiratory distress and a high respiratory rate. The patient was placed on BiPAP therapy 10 minutes ago, and the patient states, "I don't like this mask thing." The patient appears uneasy, visibly tachypneic, and the BiPAP machine is alarming. Upon inspection, all of the equipment seems to be working appropriately. Which of the following should be considered at this time?

A) Anxiolysis

B) Analgesia

C) Intubation

D) Arterial blood gas analysis

A - Based on the information given, the patient seems to be having anxiety about the BiPAP mask. There are many patients, pediatric as well as adult, who seem to feel that they can't breathe when a respiratory mask is applied to their face. If these patients cannot be calmed down by therapeutic communication, which should be tried first, careful and cautious anxiolysis may be indicated to increase compliance with the therapy.

If you have a respiratory therapist who is very comfortable with peds CPAP or BiPAP, and who has the time to talk the child through having the mask on their face, the results can be absolutely amazing. If despite attempts to calm the patient through calm communication and reassurance, the patient really needs BiPAP therapy but won't tolerate the BiPAP equipment, some facilities have had very good results with small, titrated, doses of IV medications for anxiolysis.

Pediatric Potpourri

147) Your pediatric patient on BiPAP therapy now is in worsening respiratory distress. You note an oxygen saturation of 88% despite 100% oxygen and you are concerned that the patient may need to be intubated. While preparations are being made for intubation, what BiPAP setting could you change that may help improve the O_2 saturation?

A) Increase the FiO_2 (increase the percent of oxygen)

B) Increase the EPAP (Expiratory Positive Airway Pressure)

C) Decrease the EPAP (Expiratory Positive Airway Pressure)

D) Increase the set respiratory rate

B – In this situation, increasing the EPAP (Expiratory Positive Airway Pressure) is the option most likely to produce an improved level of oxygenation. In this case the patient is already receiving 100% oxygen, so there is no way to increase the FiO_2. Decreasing the EPAP is not likely to help because that would most likely decrease the alveolar gas exchange and oxygen saturation. Since no information has been given about the respiratory rate being insufficient, increasing the BiPAP rate (if it was even being used) is not the most likely solution.

Just because the patient is receiving 100% oxygen, it does not mean that the lungs can get the oxygen into the bloodstream through the alveoli. If the patient has pulmonary edema, the alveoli tend to collapse due to the dilution of pulmonary surfactant and the high surface tension of water. What does this mean? It means that the alveoli collapse, leading to pulmonary shunt (a ventilation/perfusion mismatch). Blood is flowing by the alveoli, but the alveoli have no oxygen in it - only water.

IPAP (Inspiratory Positive Airway Pressure) is the first number you hear in BiPAP settings and EPAP (Expiratory Positive Airway Pressure) is the second number. For example, with a BiPAP setting of "15 over 5" the IPAP is 15 and the EPAP is 5. The IPAP is the pressure pushing air into the lungs. EPAP is the pressure that stays in the lungs after exhalation. Increasing the baseline pressures (both IPAP and EPAP) can help open the alveoli and help them stay open. That way, as blood flows by the alveoli, the lungs actually have some oxygen to give the blood. PEEP / EPAP / CPAP are all just as important to oxygenation as the actual percent of oxygen you are delivering - the alveoli cannot accept oxygen if they are not open in the first place.

148) A small volume nebulizer treatment has been running for approximately 10 minutes. You return to the patient to assess their response to the treatment. You note that there does not seem to be any significant volume gone from the nebulizer. Which of the following would **NOT** be a reason for this problem?

A) The nebulizer was not upright (45°)

B) The oxygen was not turned on

C) The patient was breathing against the treatment

D) The oxygen was not attached

C – Visualize the nebulizer treatment as it is designed to work. Whether held in one's hand or administered through a mask, the patient should be breathing throughout the treatment. The flow of oxygen going through the nebulizer is constant. Constant airflow and a patient actively breathing means that part of the time the patient will be exhaling, and in that sense, breathing against the treatment. It is unlikely that your patient is exhaling quickly enough and with sufficient pressure to push the medication back into the chamber.

Small volume nebulizers are also called handheld nebulizers or T-piece nebulizers. For them to work properly, they should be positioned like a "T," i.e. upright. We need to ensure the nebulizer is upright, attached to oxygen, and that the oxygen is actually turned on to an adequate flow rate. Although they differ in recommended flow rates by manufacturer and protocol, a flow rate of 5-12 LPM is a generally required for adequate nebulization of medication.

149) What does ECMO stand for?

A) Extracapillary membrane oxygenation

B) Extracorporeal membrane oxygenation

C) Extracorporeal maximized oxygenation

D) Extracapillary mandatory oxygenation

B – ECMO stands for extracorporeal membrane oxygenation. It is also known as extracorporeal life support (ECLS).

150) ECMO is a potentially life-saving therapy that is indicated for:

A) Hepatic failure refractory to other customary treatment methods

B) Renal failure refractory to other customary treatment methods

C) Intracranial pressure refractory to other customary treatment methods

D) Respiratory and/or heart failure refractory to other customary treatment methods

D – ECMO is a form of therapy that can be used when a patient is in respiratory and/or heart failure and other forms of customary treatment methods are not effective. Blood is removed from the body through cannulas that are placed in large vessels in the body, pumped through an artificial lung or oxygenator, and returned back to the body. ECMO is a form of heart lung bypass that can be initiated in the operating room or ICU, and more recently, in the ER and even prehospital settings as well.

Forms of ECMO:

Veno-venous (V-V), veno-arterial (V-A), and more rarely, (veno-venoarterial) V-V-A, are the most common forms of ECMO utilized in pediatric emergency and critical care.

V-A, or veno-arterial ECMO, requires the cannulation (with really big catheters) of <u>both</u> an artery and a vein. The cannulas are much larger than traditional central lines in order to handle the blood volume that would allow for heart-lung bypass. The deoxygenated blood is drained from a large central vessel such as the femoral vein or jugular vein, oxygenated outside of the body, and then the oxygen rich blood is returned to the body via a centrally located artery such as the femoral artery or common carotid artery.

V-V, or veno-venous ECMO, involves the placement of either one *really big* double-lumen cannula or two *big* cannulas. If a double-lumen catheter is used, it is inserted into a large vein that allows the pump to draw deoxygenated blood out of one of the channels and replace oxygen rich blood through the other channel of a double lumen catheter. When two catheters are used, one cannula will be placed in a femoral vein and advanced to the level of mid-IVC (inferior vena cava) to drain the deoxygenated blood. The second cannula will be placed into the other femoral vein, advanced to the RA (right atrium) to pump in the oxygen rich blood.

Pediatric Potpourri

Other evolving options include VV-A or veno-venoarterial ECMO which is a hybrid of V-V and V-A ECMO. This process drains oxygen poor blood from the venous system and returns oxygen rich blood into both the venous and arterial sides.

Commonly utilized for many years in the neonatal ICU for respiratory failure and in the adult ICU for ARDS and/or cardiac failure, remember, "Silly Rabbit, Trix Are For Kids" and ECMO is not just for babies.

151) What type of pediatric patient should be considered for V-A (veno-arterial) ECMO?

A) A patient in respiratory failure

B) A patient in renal failure

C) A patient in cardiac failure and respiratory failure

D) A patient with a traumatic brain injury and associated intracranial hemorrhage

C – A patient in both cardiac and respiratory failure would be placed on V-A ECMO to provide support for both the heart and lungs. In other words, V-A ECMO is used when a patient not only requires help with oxygenation and ventilation (lungs), but also with perfusion (heart). Assistance with both issues is only possible with V-A ECMO as this method oxygenates the blood and pumps the blood as well. This can only be done if arterial and venous access for ECMO is obtained.

A patient in respiratory failure alone may only require support for their lungs, and not for the heart. In that situation, V-V ECMO can be a more appropriate option. However, the choice as to V-A versus V-V ECMO is very surgeon, intensivist, and facility-dependent.

A patient in renal failure would utilize modalities such as continuous renal replacement or emergent hemodialysis. A patient with intracranial bleeding would not be considered a candidate for ECMO. When patients are placed on ECMO, they require intense anticoagulation to prevent clotting as the blood goes out of the body, into the ECMO circuit, and back to the body. If the patient has a traumatic brain injury, heparin + head bleeds tends to be a really bad combo.

152) What type of patient would be considered for V-V (veno-venous) ECMO?

A) A patient only in respiratory failure

B) A patient in renal failure

C) A patient in cardiac failure and respiratory failure

D) A patient who has suffered from a hemorrhagic stroke

A – V-V ECMO is used for patients who are in respiratory failure and only require lung support. The patient requires normal heart function because V-V ECMO will only provide support for the lungs. V-V ECMO is less invasive as it *only* requires cannulation of big veins, and doesn't mess with the big arteries. However, it only can be used for assistance with oxygenation and ventilation. If the only issue is the lungs, V-V ECMO can be lifesaving. If support for the lungs and the heart are needed, then V-A (not V-V) ECMO is indicated.

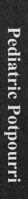

153) ECMO may be considered for which type of pediatric patient in the emergency department?

A) A patient who presents to the emergency department in asystole after 20-minutes of prehospital ALS care

B) A patient who presents to the emergency department in septic shock with a pulmonary hemorrhage and bleeding from the IV sites

C) A patient who has a witnessed arrest while in the emergency department, received immediate high-quality CPR with minimal interruptions, and can be placed onto ECMO within 30-minutes

D) A patient who presents with stage IV cancer and heart failure

C – A patient who has a witnessed arrest, immediate initiation of high-quality CPR, and is able to be placed onto the ECMO circuit within 30-minutes is likely to have the best neurological outcome. In the neonatal and pediatric ICU settings, ECMO has been successfully utilized for respiratory/cardiac failure, sepsis, and more. However, in the ED setting, eCPR (aka., ECMO CPR) is a rapidly evolving and expanding practice, especially in cases of severe hypothermia and/or cardiac arrest.

A patient who presents to an emergency department in asystole after 20-minutes of prehospital ALS care is likely to have a poor outcome and ECMO would typically not be considered an option. ECMO should only be considered on patients who are likely to return to baseline, or near baseline, functional status. A patient who presents with evidence of active internal bleeding is not going to be a candidate for ECMO due to the need for systemic anticoagulation. The goal of ECMO therapy is to return the individual to their baseline or close to baseline. *Remember, ECMO doesn't cure death. It just is an option, in certain patients, to help keep them alive until something reversible can be reversed!*

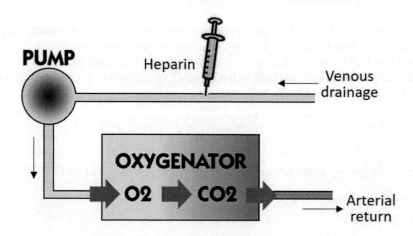

ECMO Pump Components
Pump (helps the blood go round and round)
Heparin (self-explanatory)
Oxygenator (O_2 in and CO_2 out)

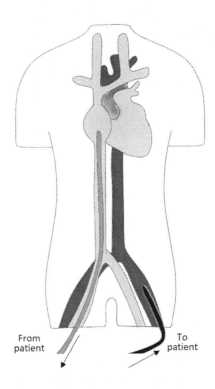

Veno-Arterial (V-A) ECMO (Femoral)
Venous cannula is placed into a femoral vein and drains blood from the vena cava.
Arterial cannula is placed into a femoral artery and returns blood to the aorta.

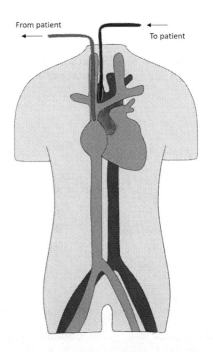

Veno-Arterial (V-A) ECMO (Jugular/Carotid)
Venous cannula is placed into an internal jugular vein
and drains blood from the vena cava.
Arterial cannula is placed into a carotid artery and returns blood to the aorta.

Certified Pediatric Emergency Nurse (CPEN) Review IV

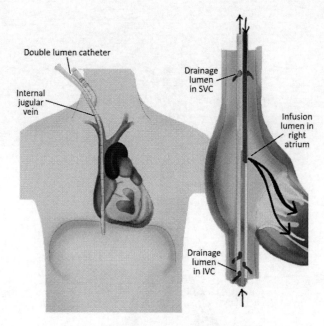

Veno-Venous (V-V) ECMO (Jugular)
Single catheter placed into an internal jugular vein
and advanced into the inferior vena cava.
Blood is drained from lumens in the superior and inferior vena cava
and then returned via the infusion lumen into the right atrium.

Common Indications for ECMO in Pediatrics

Erdil, T., Lemme, F., & Schweiger, M. (2019). *Extracorporeal membrane oxygenation support in pediatrics.* Annals of Cardiothoracic Surgery. 8(1). 109-115.

Indications	**Neonatal**	**Pediatric**
Cardiac	Congenital heart defects: ❖ Hypoplastic left heart syndrome ❖ Left ventricular outflow obstruction ❖ Right ventricular outflow obstruction ❖ Septal defects Cardiomyopathy (bridge to recovery, transplant or long-term mechanical support (VAD, etc.) Myocarditis	Congenital heart defects: ❖ Left ventricular outflow obstruction ❖ Right ventricular outflow obstruction ❖ Septal defects Cardiomyopathy (bridge to recovery, transplant or long-term mechanical support (VAD, etc.) Myocarditis

Indications	Neonatal	Pediatric
Respiratory	Meconium aspiration syndrome	Pneumonia (viral/bacterial/aspiration)
	Persistent pulmonary hypertension of newborn/ persistent fetal circulation	Acute respiratory distress syndrome (ARDS)
	Respiratory distress syndrome (RDS)	
	Congenital diaphragmatic hernia	
	Pneumonia (viral/bacterial/ aspiration); Sepsis	
Other indications at any age	Transplantation: ❖ Pre-transplantation as bridge to transplant ❖ Primary graft dysfunction after heart or lung transplant Elective periprocedural support: ❖ During lung transplantation or tracheal surgery Cardiac arrest from any cause: ❖ Bridge to decision ❖ Underlying treatable disease Air leak syndrome Failure to wean from cardiopulmonary bypass	

154) Which of the following items is **not** one of the three most common allergies in children (often referred to as the "triad of allergies")?

A) Fish

B) Wheat

C) Peanuts

D) Sponges

D – Sponges (especially those that wear square pants and have been incredibly popular with children for over 20 years) are not a common allergen for children. A child can be allergic to any food, but there are eight allergens which account for 90% of all reactions in kids:

Top Three most common allergens (accounting for over 2/3 of the reported reactions in kids):
- Milk
- Peanuts
- Wheat

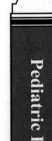

Certified Pediatric Emergency Nurse (CPEN) Review IV

The other top allergens which, in addition to the top three mentioned, account for the vast majority of allergic reactions (Allergens in **BOLD** can cause some of the most severe reactions):

- Eggs
- **Fish** (these can cause some of the most severe reactions)
- **Shellfish** (clams, lobster, shrimp)
- Soy
- **Tree nuts** (almonds, cashews, pecans, walnuts, etc)

Although many children "outgrow" some of their allergies, allergies to peanuts, tree nuts, fish, and shellfish may be lifelong. For adults in the ED, we commonly ask about "allergy to shellfish" prior to administering IV contrast dye for a CT scan. But when it comes to allergic reactions and peds, Peanuts are probably the Primary Perpetrator!

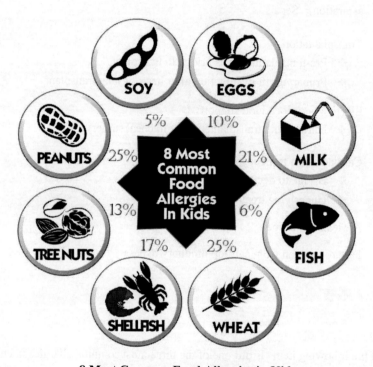

8 Most Common Food Allergies in Kids

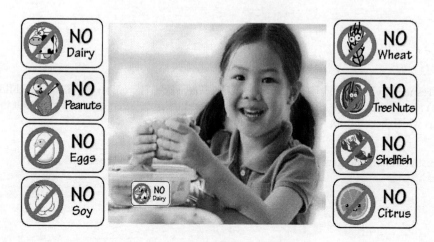

155) Parents bring a semi-conscious, 18-month old child to the emergency department. The parents report that they found the child on the floor next to a half empty bottle of hand sanitizer. Prior medical history is unremarkable and no allergies or medications were identified. The initial set of vitals showed HR 122, RR 12, BP 96/63, oxygen saturation on room air of 91%, and rectal temp 98.0 F (36.7C). Based on this presentation, the ED nurse should anticipate the need for customary lab work, respiratory support including possible intubation, and which of the following?

A) Serum alcohol level

B) Lumbar puncture for CSF glucose

C) CT scan of the head without contrast

D) Blood cultures followed by broad spectrum IV antibiotics

A - In addition to customary lab work, which should include a rapid point-of-care glucose test and respiratory support including preparation for possible intubation, obtaining a serum alcohol level should be anticipated. The key to this question is the fact that most liquid hand sanitizers have a very high <u>alcohol</u> content as the "kill 'em all" ingredient.

In addition to using soap and water, the portable nature of alcohol-based liquid hand sanitizers has made them an essential weapon in the antimicrobial arsenal. As hand sanitizers have become far more commonly utilized in homes and commercial buildings as well as traditional healthcare settings, the number and nature of incidents involving them has also increased.

There have been several case reports of adults (based on age rather than maturity) who intentionally ingested large quantities of sanitizer as a source of alcohol. But in an 18-month old, that's probably not the case. Why would an 18-month old drink hand sanitizer? Because they are 18-months old! Making these alcohol-based hand sanitizers even more attractive to kids is the fact that the options for colors and smells have grown exponentially. The Texas Poison Control Center estimates that a child this size would only need to ingest about 4–5 squirts of sanitizer to produce effects requiring medical attention. So over the teeth and past the gums, look out stomach (and bloodstream), here it comes!

156) Propofol (Diprivan®) is considered to be in which category of analgesics?

A) Non-opioid analgesics

B) Weak opioid analgesics

C) Strong opioid analgesics

D) No-analgesia analgesic

D – OK, this is either a trick question or an easy question. Propofol (Diprivan) is a sedative-hypnotic agent and does a great job of quickly putting the child to sleep, and it quickly wears off, but Propofol does NOTHING for pain (and therefore is NOT an analgesic).

But, since the question did ask specifically about analgesia, let's talk about ketamine, which seems to have taken the world of emergency medicine by a storm. It not only provides sedation, but also pain relief and amnesia. Wonderful! But ketamine does has side effects, most notably nausea and emergence reactions, aka., waking up seemingly possessed by demons. Not so wonderful. Wouldn't it be nice to have Miley Cyrus (during her Hannah Montana days) jump in and tell us about "The Best of Both Worlds." So, without further ado, here's Ketofol.

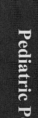

Ketofol is a mixture of ketamine and Propofol and is commonly given in one of two ways. Option one involves one syringe of ketamine and another syringe of propofol. That way, if the child needs more pain meds, give some more ketamine. If they need more sedation, give more propofol. The other less commonly utilized option is to mix ketamine and propofol in the same syringe. Slowly push, and when they drop, stop.

In theory, the potential benefits of combining these two medications include:

- Reduced vomiting
- Less hypotension
- Improved pain control
- Reduced dosage of both medicines versus one or the other
- Less emergence reactions (post-ketamine nuttiness)

Clinical research on this combination of medications continues, but the mixture appears to work as well, if not slightly better than ketamine alone. Experiences are including slightly faster recoveries, less vomiting, similar efficacy and airway complications, and slightly higher provider and patient satisfaction scores. Whether the differences between ketamine and ketofol are enough to choose one or the other is likely based on provider experiences and preferences.

157) When calculating a Glasgow Coma Scale (GCS), the child reaches **towards** the site of a trapezius squeeze. This is an example of:

A) Withdrawal

B) Localization

C) Decorticate (Abnormal Flexion)

D) Decerebrate (Abnormal Extension)

B – Purposeful movement **toward** the site of a stimulus is called "Localization." One of the three elements of the Glasgow Coma Scale is an evaluation of "Best Motor Response." If the patient is unable to follow movement commands (verbal or visual), the other possibilities (in decreasing point value) are: localization, withdrawal, flexion (decorticate posturing), extension (decerebrate posturing), or no response. When it comes to the Glasgow Coma Scale, several areas are simply confusing and difficult to remember unless you work in a neuro ICU. One of the big areas of confusion involves localizing vs. withdrawing. So, with that in mind, here are a few tips to help clarify the confusion.

Localizing (5 points on the GCS) occurs when a noxious or painful stimulus is sent to the brain, which then appropriately sends a message/impulse back to the body to try to stop or remove the source of the stimulus. While we most commonly associate this with a painful stimulus, we exhibit localizing movement in many different situations. Dr. Lou Romig reminds us that if we swat at an insect that lands on our arm or if we wave our hand in front of our nose when in the presence of a cloud of freshly expelled intestinal gas, we are making a purposeful, localized movement. In the clinical setting where we try to avoid insects (and freshly produced intestinal gas), we can test for localization by applying a trapezius squeeze or supraorbital pressure and evaluating the reaction. If the patient brings his or her arm up to the level of the chin or across the midline to the site of pain, or if the patient moves either arm above the neck to try to stop the mean nurse from pressing on the nerves right above the top of their eye socket, we are seeing localization. Pediatric Neurosurgery NP, Judie Holleman, teaches that if you can reach out and "locate" the area of stimuli, you are localizing.

Remember, the GCS is looking for the "best" score, the highest point response. It is not cumulative. Start at the highest point response and work down until you get an appropriate response. If the patient doesn't respond to instructions but does appear to be making deliberate attempts to pull out an endotracheal tube or IV, you have evidence of localization. You DO NOT need to use pain to further test for localization. You can see that they are localizing already.

Withdrawal (4 points on the GCS) occurs when a stimulus is sent to the brain, but the best that the patient can do is simply withdraw, or move away from the stimulus. The patient withdraws and/or recoils in response to a noxious or painful stimulus, but makes no direct attempt to remove the source of the painful stimuli. Using the example of the intestinal gas, turning one's head away from the source of the odor is withdrawal, waving the hand in front of the nose (the source of the stimulus) is localizing. Or again, in a clinical setting, if nail bed pressure is applied and the patient simply pulls away but doesn't do anything beyond that to stop the painful stimuli, that's withdrawal.

Purposely trying to LOCATE the area = Localizing

Moving away from the stimulus = Withdrawing

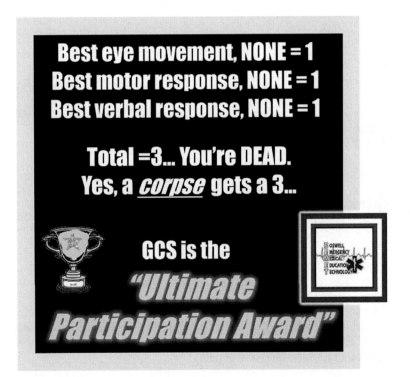

Courtesy of Mark Boswell MSN, FNP-BC, CEN, CFRN, CTRN, CPEN, TCRN

Boswell Emergency Medical Education

www.boswellemergencymedicaleducation.com

158) When assessing neurologically impaired patients for response to pain, which of the following techniques is **NOT** currently recommended?

A) Trapezius squeeze

B) Supraorbital pressure

C) Sternal rub

D) Nail bed pressure

C - Though it is still commonly utilized, neurosurgery professionals do **not** recommend performing sternal rubs for several reasons: 1) Technically, a sternal rub must be applied for 30-continuous seconds before you can say the patient is unresponsive to pain. 2) It hurts during application, and for quite a while after. 3) If it is done on a very regular basis, which, depending on the status of the patient may be as frequently as every 15 minutes, it leaves bruises which really look bad.

To take this concept a bit further, the different techniques mentioned above involve different neurological pathways when pain or pressure is elicited, specifically peripheral (extremity) pain/sensation versus central (brain) pain/sensation.

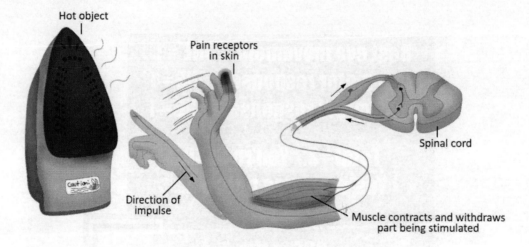

Reflex Arcs

Peripheral Pain: Remember, the intent is not to cause pain, but to evaluate neurological status. If there is a response to command/instruction, or if simple touch or pressure elicits an appropriate response, we don't need to go further. But if the motor response is less than normal, we may need to evaluate the response to more significant sensation (pressure or pain).

Nail bed pressure can be used to evaluate peripheral pain. This is elicited when a pen is rolled over the area just proximal to the fingernail bed for up to 15 seconds. The appropriate response? OUCH! Or if they can't say ouch, to hopefully localize (reach for the area) or at least withdraw away from the pain. The problem is... we need to determine if the response is real or reflex. (Is it real or Memorex? Remember that?) Think about a 2-year old who touches a hot stove. The impulse goes from the finger to the brain so that the child hopefully learns not to do that again. But it also goes from the finger via a reflex arc to the spinal cord and right back to the finger, telling it to pull away so the finger isn't cooked while the brain figures out what to do. That's important, as we need to differentiate in unconscious patients whether the impulse is getting interpreted by the brain or only to and from the spinal cord. So, while peripheral pain with pens is still used, neurosurgery teaches there's got to be a better way.

Certified Pediatric Emergency Nurse (CPEN) Review IV

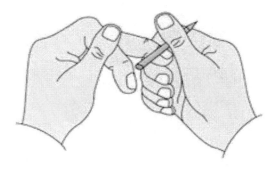

Nail Bed Pressure to Determine Response to Peripheral Pain

Central (Brain) Pain: There are some techniques for evaluating motor response that were used in the past, but are no longer recommended, such as the sternal rub and mandibular pressure. Mandibular pressure involved applying pressure to the back of the jaw (TMJ) area. One of the problems with this technique was that was very practitioner dependent. Simply put, the who was as much a factor as the what. In addition, adult case studies report that overzealous mandibular pressure produces subsequent bruising.

So, if sternal rub and mandibular pressure are no longer recommended, what other options are out there? One possibility is the trapezius squeeze, aka., the Vulcan neck pinch. This is performed by grabbing a nice chunk of the neck/shoulder muscle and gently squeezing. The appropriate response displaying "localization" would be if the patient identifies the local area with the opposite arm and reaches across the midline to the shoulder. A withdrawal response would be seen when the patient withdraws and/or recoils away from the point of stimulus. Another possible technique is applying "Supraorbital" pressure. "Supra" means above and "orbit" means eye socket. The supraorbital groove is found near the medial end of the eyebrows. Just under the skin, in that groove, several nerves are found. Pressure applied to that area reliably produces a painful stimulus.

For peripheral pain (remembering the influence of reflex arcs), think pens and pinkies. For central/brain pain, trap the trapezius or gently go for the groove.

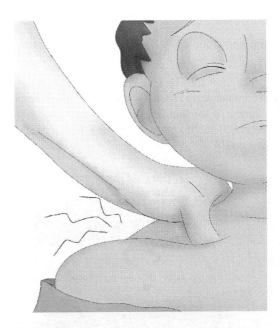

**Trapezius Squeeze Technique to
Determine Response to Central "Brain" Pain**

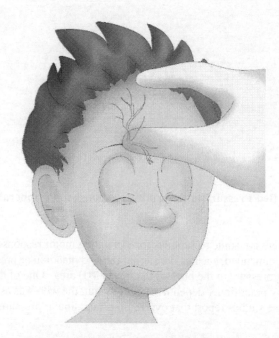

**Supraorbital Pressure Technique
to Determine Response to Central "Brain" Pain**

159) An adolescent patient presents to the triage nurse in your Emergency Department. Among the first things mentioned by the patient is the statement, "I am transgender." In order to establish effective communication and trust with the teen, which of the following would be the **most** appropriate question to ask?

A) "What was your sex at birth?"

B) "Which bathroom do you use?"

C) "When did you begin your sex change?"

D) "What is your preferred name and pronouns?"

D - Asking a patient (or family member/caregiver) who has identified as transgender what their preferred name and pronouns are is the recommendation of the Emergency Nurses Association (ENA) as well as the American Academy of Pediatrics. If for some reason you cannot ask a transgender person about their preferred pronouns, try to use a gender-neutral pronoun or identifier, or use the last name, as in "Patient Smith."

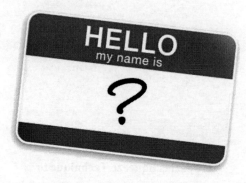

Certified Pediatric Emergency Nurse (CPEN) Review IV

The following chart is from a highly recommended resource published by the ENA, "Care of LGBTQ Patients in the Emergency Care Setting Toolkit." The publication is available free-of-charge to ENA members.

Do Not Use	Appropriate Terminology
Sex change	**Transition** Gender confirming (Affirming) **Surgery** Gender Reassignment Surgery
Hermaphrodite	Intersex
Transvestite	Cross-dresser
Transsexualism / Transgenderism	None – using those terms is always offensive
Sexual Preference	Sexual orientation
Gay Lifestyle Transgender Lifestyle	None – there is no such thing as a gay or transgender lifestyle. The word lifestyle implies that one's sexual orientation or gay identity is a choice.

Courtesy of the Emergency Nurses Association
www.ena.org

Another excellent resource comes from HealthyChildren.org and provides the following definitions:

- Gender diverse: An umbrella term to describe an ever-evolving array of labels people may apply when their gender identity, expression, or even perception does not conform to the norms and stereotypes others expect.

- Gender identity: One's internal sense of who one is, based on an interaction of biological traits, developmental influences, and environmental conditions. This may be male, female, somewhere in between, a combination of both or neither. Self-recognition of gender identity develops over time, much the same way a child's physical body does.

- Sexual orientation: One's sexual identity as it relates to who someone falls in love with or is attracted to. A person who is transgender still identifies as straight, gay, bisexual or something else. Like gender identity, an individual's physical and emotional attraction to a member of the same or the opposite sex cannot be changed and is very difficult to predict early in childhood.

- Transgender: Usually used when gender diverse traits remain persistent, consistent, and insistent over time.

HealthyChildren.org is sponsored by the American Academy of Pediatrics

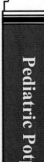

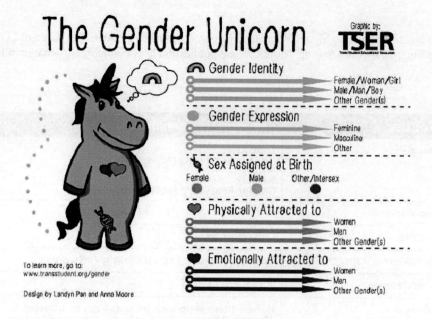

The Gender Unicorn
Courtesy of TransStudent.org

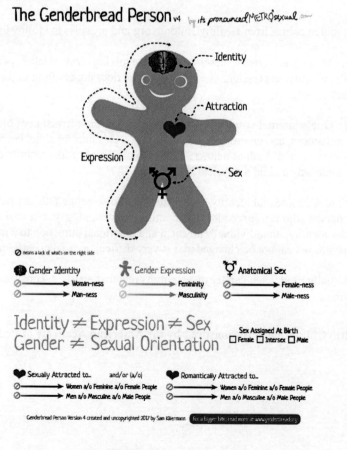

Genderbread Person v4
Courtesy of Sam Killermann and Genderbread.org

160) The ER nurse is asked to administer intranasal midazolam. It is important to remember that the dead space in the MAD Nasal™ Intranasal Mucosal Atomization Device is:

A) 0.15-0.16 mL

B) 0.5-0.6 mL

C) 1 mL

D) There is no dead space

A - Intranasal medication administration simply has changed the world of emergency pediatric care. Though initially used by EMS professionals for adults with opiate overdoses, atomized nasal medications have entered the world of pediatrics and the indications and medications continue to expand and evolve.

But there is a crucial, and often little-known technical detail about the atomizers. The devices have a "dead space" that must be accounted for when drawing up medication. For example, the MAD Nasal™ Intranasal Mucosal Atomization Device has 0.15 to 0.16 mL dead space depending on the model. *This seemingly insignificant amount of dead space is a very significant issue for little patients.* The medication getting atomized, aka., sprayed, into the nose, goes from the syringe, through the atomizer, and into the nose. That means the volume in the syringe will indeed be given, MINUS the dead space volume. So, if you are administering fentanyl 50 mcg (1 mL) to a teenager, if you don't account for the dead space, they really will only receive approximately 42.5 mcg of fentanyl. Perhaps that's not a huge deal. But, if you are giving fentanyl 5 mcg (0.1 mL) to a little one, if you do not account for the dead space, they won't receive any of the medication. That's a huge deal!

The *ideal* volume for intranasal administration is 0.2-0.3 mL per nostril, with a maximum recommended volume per nostril of 1 mL. Ideally, if the dose is greater than 0.5 mL, divide the dose and administer in each nare to allow for maximum absorption. Always accommodate for the dead space when calculating the final volume drawn up in the syringe, especially in dealing with little ones. This way, whether for seizures, sedation, or analgesia, kids actually get the medication!

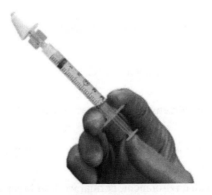

MAD Nasal™ Intranasal Mucosal Atomization Device
Image Courtesy of Teleflex
www.teleflex.com

161) According to the Pediatric Assessment Triangle (PAT), which patient should receive the **highest** priority?

A) Interacting with environment, increased work of breathing, skin is pink, brisk capillary refill

B) Not interacting with environment, normal breathing, skin is pale, brisk capillary refill

C) Not interacting with environment, increased work of breathing, skin is pale, delayed capillary refill

D) Interacting with environment, normal breathing, skin is pink, brisk capillary refill

C – According to the PAT, patient C should be the highest priority. Patient D is not showing any signs of immediate concern. Patient A has one side of the triangle abnormal, so is a higher priority than patient D. Patient B, with two sides of the triangle which is certainly worrisome, is a higher priority than both A and D. But, patient C has issues with not one, not two, but all three components of the PAT, and is therefore the highest priority of those presented.

Beyond recommending which of these patients should you see first, the Emergency Nursing Pediatric Course (ENPC) briefly discusses the idea of Sick, Sicker, or Sickest. However, these terms are not specifically defined in other common pediatric emergency/critical care courses such as Prehospital Education for Prehospital Professionals (PEPP), Pediatric Fundamental Critical Care Support (PFCCS) or Pediatric Advanced Life Support (PALS), but they are a component of ENPC. So, here's a really short and sweet summary of Sick, Sicker, Sickest *according to ENPC*:

- There is not a "not sick" category. A patient who does not have any abnormal findings is still considered to be "Sick" if the caregiver is concerned enough to seek care.

- If there is one component of the PAT that is abnormal, then the child is considered to be "Sicker."

- If there are two or more components of the PAT that are abnormal, then the child is considered to be "Sickest."

162) According to the Pediatric Assessment Triangle (PAT), which patient should receive the **highest** priority?

A) 3-year old, interactive with environment, increased work of breathing, skin is pink, brisk capillary refill

B) 2-year old, not interactive with environment, normal work of breathing, skin is pale, delayed capillary refill.

C) 4-year old, interactive with environment, increased work of breathing, skin is pale, delayed capillary refill.

D) 5-year old, interactive with environment, normal work of breathing, skin is pale, brisk capillary refill

B – Patient B is the highest priority. Remember: Appearance – Breathing – Circulation. Patients B and C both have alterations with two of the three components of the PAT, and that's bad. However, patient B is noted to be not interactive and unless its nap time, nothing good comes of a 2-year old being not interactive... Interacting with the environment is part of "A for appearance," and when "appearance" looks bad, it's bad! Then look at breathing and circulation.

Certified Pediatric Emergency Nurse (CPEN) Review IV

163) According to the Pediatric Assessment Triangle, (PAT) which patient should receive the **highest** priority?

A) 8-year old, not interactive with environment, increased work of breathing, skin is pink, brisk capillary refill

B) 5-year old, interactive with environment, increased work of breathing, skin is pink, brisk capillary refill

C) 4-year old, interactive with environment, normal breathing, skin is pale, delayed capillary refill

D) 5-year old, interactive with environment, normal breathing, skin is pink, brisk capillary refill

A – Patient A has two alterations with the PAT; Not being interactive with environment and working to breathe. Patients B and C each have one alteration with the PAT, while Patient D sounds cute. Again, *per ENPC*, if someone brings a child to the ED for evaluation, they are considered to be sick. One alteration with the PAT per ENPC is sicker, while two or more issues with the PAT are sickest. "Sick or Not Sick" is commonly taught in many pediatric courses and ENPC introduces "Sicker or Sickest." Beyond preparing for the CPEN exam, when it comes to what's important for our patients, being able to quickly recognize this child is truly "Sick" and should be seen quickly is the real answer!

164) A 6-week old infant presents to triage with the caregiver who reports a rash to the infant's face and torso for the past three days. The infant is awake, alert, and interacting with the environment. There is normal work of breathing, and the skin color is pink, but with a maculopapular rash to the face and torso. According to the ENPC textbook and course, which category of the Pediatric Assessment Triangle would this infant fall under?

A) Sickest

B) Sicker

C) Not sick

D) Sick

D – Even though none of the PAT parameters are abnormal, per ENPC, this patient would be considered sick since the caregiver was concerned enough to seek medical care. Rashes in and of themselves are not an indicator of perfusion status. Since the overall color of the skin is pink, circulation to the skin would be considered normal. It's common for some people to get confused and want to call circulation abnormal due to the rash when in fact, it doesn't count against circulation, **unless it's petechial** (little red or blue blotches) or purpuric (big blue blotches), in which case they are at risk of having abnormalities in all three categories!

Crucial Reminder: Just because all three PAT components are "normal," that doesn't necessarily mean that the patient isn't sick or at high-risk (i.e., febrile little ones under 30-days of age with rule-out sepsis).

Additional Insights from a Pediatric Emergency Medicine Attending Physician involved in the initial applications of the PAT in the Pediatric Education for Paramedics course, which later became PEPP:

Appearance: The original PAT designates only "sick" and "not sick" categories, based on how the child's body is compensating for compromised physiology. If the General Appearance is good (meaning adequate oxygenation, ventilation, circulation and fuel for complex brain function and no problem with the brain itself, such as meningitis, intoxication or brain injury), the patient is

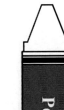

compensating and "not sick." If the General Appearance is not good, the brain isn't getting something (or multiple things) it badly needs; therefore, the body is not able to compensate physiologically, and the child is "sick." So, "not sick" means compensating well for any acute illness or injury, while "sick" means decompensating. Outside of the ENPC course, "Sick" is not commonly used by emergency healthcare providers to describe a kid that is in urgent care or the ED purely because someone perceives that the child needs some kind of medical evaluation and treatment. How many times have we seen kids brought for care who look better than we do and say "What's she doing here? She's not sick!"

Breathing: Don't forget that increased work of breathing is better than inadequate work of breathing. Don't be fooled by a child who's too tired to generate retractions and other signs of increased work of breathing. Decreased work of breathing/inadequate respiratory effort is a signal of impending respiratory failure and is usually accompanied by altered "General Appearance." I recommend using descriptions such as "normal" or "adequate" work of breathing, as writing "no increased work of breathing" could also mean decreased respiratory effort or inadequate work of breathing. The PAT, when taught correctly, recognizes both inadequate work of breathing and increased work of breathing as being bad.

Perfusion: Pallor is not the be all and end all of perfusion. The original PAT leaned on capillary refill and pulse quality, not just skin color. Pallor can just mean that someone is nauseated, tired, or cold. It doesn't necessarily mean there is systemically decreased perfusion pressure. There is a need in healthcare to address the "pale versus poorly perfused" issue in education.

Most importantly, remember that the PAT is NOT full triage; it's merely a quick snapshot of the child's current physiology to determine "sick or not sick," or when it comes to ENPC and the CPEN exam… "Sick, Sicker, Sickest."

165) A 16-year old with known congenital heart disease and a permanent pacemaker presents to the Emergency Department. He tells you that it feels like his heart is "not beating right." He is immediately placed on continuous cardiac monitoring, a 12-lead ECG is done, and a pediatric cardiology consult is called. The ECG shows what appear to be random pacemaker spikes. The ED nurse locates a cardiac magnet anticipating that it might be needed in order to do which of the following:

A) Magnetically disconnect the pacemaker battery from the leads that go into the chambers of the heart

B) Shut the pacemaker off

C) Change the device from the pacemaker setting to the ICD (Internal Cardiac Defibrillator) setting

D) Revert the pacemaker to an asynchronous mode

D - Placing a cardiac magnet, (aka., "the donut") over the center of the pacemaker will usually cause it to revert to an asynchronous pacing mode. This means the pacemaker is now pacing without regard to the patient's own atrial or ventricular activity.

It is important to know that the magnet <u>does not</u> shut the pacemaker off, nor should it be used to try to disconnect the leads from the battery (a surgical procedure). An ICD (Implantable Cardioverter Defibrillator) or as it sometimes referred to as an AICD (where the "A" stands for Automatic) functions differently from a pacemaker and is designed to recognize and correct arrhythmias.

Certified Pediatric Emergency Nurse (CPEN) Review IV

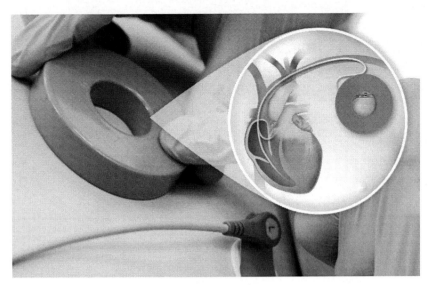

"Cardiac Magnet Donut" for Pacemakers and AICDs

166) Pacemaker spikes should be visible on the ECG:

A) Before the P wave for atrial pacing

B) After the P wave for atrial pacing

C) Before the P wave for ventricular pacing

D) After the P wave for ventricular pacing

A – Pacing isn't pushing, so it leads the way. A pace car at the race track is in front of the pack and literally set the pace or the speed of the rest of the cars. So, once you've established that pacing is "before" and not "after," it's just a matter of remembering basic cardiology. P waves are the atrial activity, not the ventricular activity.

Another way to think of it is that "Pacing" begins with "P" and the spikes should be "P"rior. Spikes prior to a P wave indicate atrial pacing. Spikes prior to a QRS wave indicate ventricular pacing. Spikes with no P or QRS waves indicate "P"rofound badness, i.e. asystole!

Special note about pacemaker spikes on a cardiac monitor: On many monitors, they will not show up unless the monitor is put in the appropriate mode. Check with your facility and the specific equipment manufacturer for more details.

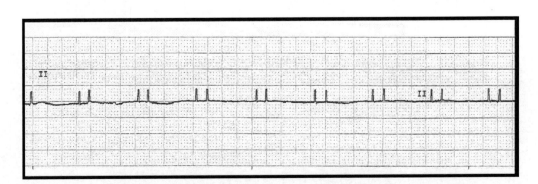

Asystole with Atrial and Ventricular Pacing Spikes

POSITION 1: CHAMBER(S) PACED	POSITION 2: CHAMBER(S) SENSED	POSITION 3: RESPONSE TO SENSING	POSITION 4: PROGRAMMABILITY	POSITION 5: MULTISITE PACING
0 = none	0 = none	0 = none	0 = none	0 = none
A = atrium	A = atrium	I = inhibited	R = rate modulation	A = atrium
V = ventricle	V = ventricle	T = triggered		V = ventricle
D = dual (A + V)	D = dual (A + V)	D = dual (I + T)		D = dual (A + V)

Pacemaker Codes

VOO: The ventricle is paced asynchronously

- Ventricle will be paced regardless of native cardiac activity

VVI: The ventricle is sensed and paced if necessary

- Ventricle is paced at a set rate
- Pacing is inhibited if pacer senses intrinsic ventricular activity

DDD: Both the atria and ventricle are sensed and paced

- The pacemaker will either trigger or be inhibited based on whether it senses native cardiac activity
- Atrial pacing is inhibited if a native atrial beat is sensed
- Ventricular pacing is inhibited if a native ventricular beat is sensed
- The pacer will trigger a ventricular beat if it senses an atrial beat (either paced or native) and there is no intrinsic ventricular beat within a programmed amount of time

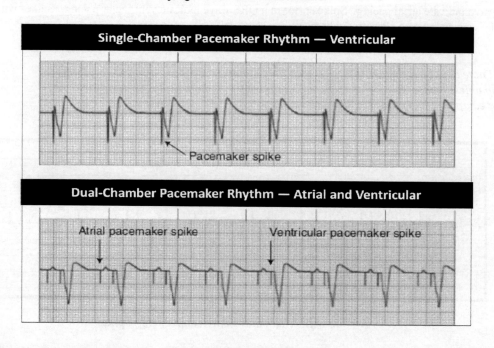

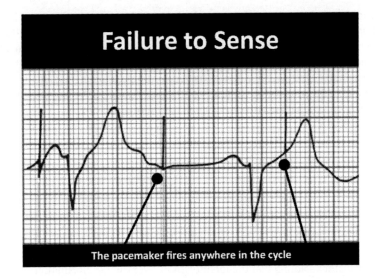

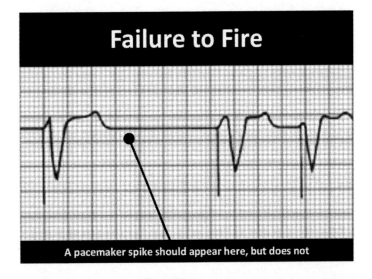

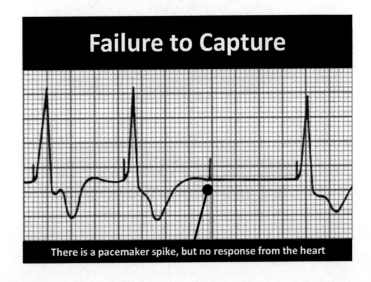

Additional Critical Care Transport Educator Insights: When it comes to paced ECGs, the old rule of thumb was that unipolar devices had big pacing spikes and bipolar devices had smaller (maybe even scarcely visible) pacing spikes. While this is still true of paced ECGs obtained from a programmer, many ECG monitors and other equipment today offer spike enhancement. This enlarges the pacemaker output spike so that even bipolar systems offer clinicians very prominent pacing spikes. If you do not put the monitor into this mode, the monitor could filter out the pacer spikes. With today's technology, many of the pacemakers produce spikes that are extremely small and normal filtering applied to a monitor could mask or "eliminate" the pacer spike. The selected lead on the patient's ECG monitor needs to be configured to the pacemaker detection or pacemaker tracking mode. Basically, you need to set up the bedside monitor to be in a lead that clearly shows the pacing spike.

167) A 14-year old with a history of Long QT syndrome is brought to the Emergency Department in full arrest. She has a medic alert bracelet which indicates that she has an AICD (automated implantable cardioverter defibrillator). Noting that the monitor shows ventricular fibrillation, the nurse should be prepared to immediately:

A) Defibrillate

B) Cardiovert

C) Externally pace

D) Wait for the patient's AICD to kick in

A - She's in full arrest and the monitor is showing V-fib. Therefore, treat her just like any other patient who is in V-fib and shock! Her own internal defibrillator didn't fix the V-fib, so you have to fix it!

Additional Pediatric Cardiac Surgery NP Insights: Most patients with pacemakers/AICDs carry a wallet-size card and/or have some sort of "Medic Alert" identification which would provide details about the type of device implanted as well as the contact information for the cardiologist and device representative.

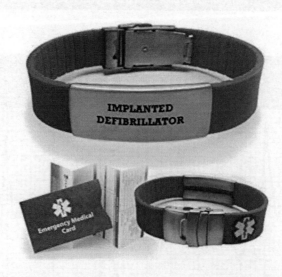

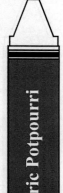

	Implantable Defibrillator		
	Patient Identification Card		
PATIENT:	ROMEO MONTAGUE		
	MODEL NUMBER	SERIAL NUMBER	IMPLANT DATE
ICD	CD3201-36	123456	29/JUL/1976
LCV	11581/86	ABC12345	29/JUL/1976
RVA	7122/65	XYZ54321	29/JUL/1976
PHYSICIAN: MARCUS WELBY VERONA, CA 94566		PHONE:	888-280-PEDS

168) A 16-year old presents to the Emergency Department with a complaint of flu-like symptoms for several days. His medical history is significant for a seizure disorder that required the implantation of a Vagal Nerve Stimulator (VNS). While awaiting lab results, he experiences a sustained tonic-clonic seizure. The ER nurse knows that the vagal nerve stimulator:

A) Is obviously malfunctioning as a seizure is occurring

B) Should immediately be deactivated

C) Magnet should immediately be swiped over the left upper chest

D) Should immediately be surgically removed

C – When a patient with a Vagal Nerve Stimulator (VNS) experiences a sustained seizure, a one-second swipe of the stimulator magnet over the implant area will provide an extra stimulation which may stop the seizure activity. Just because a seizure occurs does not mean that the device is malfunctioning, nor that it should be deactivated. And immediate surgical intervention to remove the device seems a bit drastic, don't you think?

When a child not only has repeated seizures, but seriously difficult to control seizures that are refractory to customary medications and/or surgical options, then placement of a Vagal Nerve Stimulator (VNS) (FDA approved in 1997) is an option. In many cases these devices are implanted on an outpatient surgery basis and happily <u>without</u> brain surgery. A small incision is made in the upper chest (generally on the left side) for the pulse generator (like a cardiac pacemaker) and another small incision is made on the left side of the neck where a lead is wrapped around the vagus nerve. *Fun fact*: Placement is generally on the left side to avoid interfering with the right vagus nerve which supplies the sinoatrial (SA) node.

The VNS sends an electrical impulse to stimulate the vagal nerve on a regular basis which can greatly reduce the frequency of seizures and seizure-related issues. The device is programmed to go on (give stimulation) for a certain period (for example, 7 to 30 seconds) and then to go off (stop stimulation) for another period (for example, 20 seconds to 5 minutes). The newer models can also be programmed to give stimulation automatically in response to a change in heart rate (called auto-stimulation).

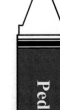

But here's what ER nurses need to know regarding patients with a VNS:

- Each person who has a VNS device is given a set of magnets, commonly worn as a bracelet/watch band. These can be used to give stimulation at a different time to stop a seizure or to temporarily turn off the VNS. The magnet is the key (similar to an AICD/automatic implantable cardioverter defibrillator).

- Patients who have focal seizures or auras may abort or shorten seizures themselves with the magnet.

- Family members (or other healthcare providers) may also help abort seizures via the magnet.

- X-rays and CT scans are fine, but if an MRI is being considered you need to check with the MRI tech and/or neurosurgeon. Some VNS devices are fine with MRIs... others not so much.

To stop a seizure:

- Swipe the magnet over the generator in the left chest area for <u>one second</u>

    - Usually, counting one-one thousand while it's swiped works well to make sure you are doing it correctly

    - Each time the magnet is swiped this way, an extra burst of stimulation is given and hopefully the seizure stops

- If the magnet is <u>held or taped</u> over the upper left chest pulse generator site, the VNS is temporarily DEACTIVATED. However, once the magnet is removed, then the VNS should quickly resume normal functioning. To paraphrase Mr. Miyagi's instructions from *The Karate Kid*... Swipe On, Seizure Off. But leave magnet on, then stimulator off!

Moral of the story: These toys have made a seriously positive impact on the lives of children and adults with repeated, really icky, seizures. If they are seizing, swiping the magnet over the generator for <u>one-second</u> will give a burst of stimulation, which often stops the seizure. If they are still seizing a short time later, then try the one-second swipe again. If no luck, then traditional anti-seizure medications are certainly an option, remembering that these patients may be on lots of seizure meds already. But in many cases, a simple <u>one-second swipe</u> will stop the seizure!

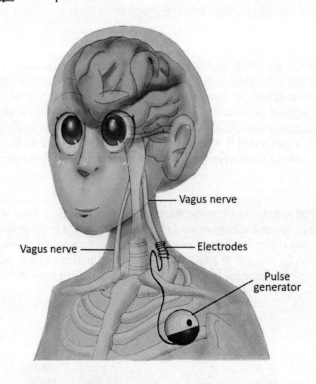

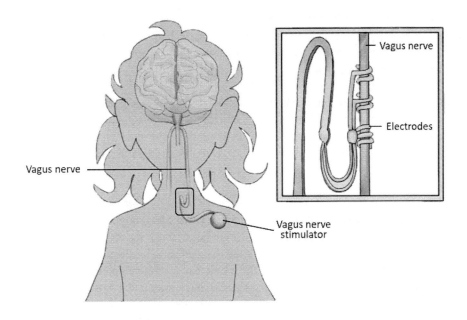

Vagal Nerve Stimulator As Seen From The Front Of The Patient

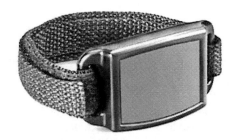

Vagal Nerve Stimulator Magnet (Bracelet/Watch Band Style)

169) The Zika virus is predominately spread by bites from:

A) Bats

B) Mosquitoes

C) Raccoons

D) Deer ticks

B – The Zika virus is spread by bites from mosquitoes; not all mosquitoes, just those that are infected by the virus. If you were hoping for a choice of "Vampires" or "Zombies," well, sorry to disappoint. While it may be the preferred bite in all of our favorite movies, those would have just been dead giveaways. (Did you see what we did there?)

Deer ticks carry the bacteria that cause Lyme Disease. Bites from bats and raccoons are particularly dangerous because those types of critters are the primary carriers of rabies. Yes, that's right, bats and raccoons, not dogs, are the favorite biter among the "I want to get rabies" group.

Although the Zika virus isn't front-page news anymore, the virus is still out there. More importantly though, the babies and young children infected with the virus before birth are very much still out there. Once a human is infected, only 1 in 5 experience common viral symptoms significant enough to prompt a visit to the Emergency Department.

Symptoms of Zika infection include rash, fever, conjunctivitis, muscle pain, and headache. These symptoms usually clear up in less than one week and rarely require admission to the hospital. Though the symptoms themselves do not point to Zika, this is another case in which the initial triage history about recent travel, especially to South America or Africa, can play an important role in helping diagnose a patient.

Why is Zika so dangerous? Humans get Zika after being bitten by an infected mosquito. It can then be passed on through sexual contact, blood transfusions, breastfeeding, possibly urine and saliva, and definitely during pregnancy! The issues with Zika are not so much for the adults or even little kids who have a run in with a Zika infected mosquito, but the real danger is for the unborn babies who can develop Congenital Zika Syndrome. Congenital Zika Syndrome has several components, and none are good. Most notably, newborns infected with Zika in utero can have profound microcephaly (small heads) and decreased brain tissue, and other complications leading to seizures and severe developmental delays. In the ED, the diagnosis is made by history, physical exam, and send-out-and-come-back-long-after-discharge blood or urine tests. In pregnant moms with a history of travel to specific areas, combined with viral symptoms, the ominous diagnosis and effects on the unborn baby can often be confirmed with fetal ultrasound or fetal MRI.

Pediatrics and prevention seem to go hand in hand, and for Zika this is very much the case, as no Zika virus vaccine currently exists. Recommendations for reducing the risk of contracting Zika include minimizing the chances of mosquito bites with appropriate clothing and insect repellants. Pregnant women are urged to avoid travel to endemic areas.

Most people across their lifespan will get mosquito bites countless times, and it's generally no big deal. But when the patient history includes travel to South America or Africa, exposure to mosquitoes, and pregnancy.... Zika is still out there and should be considered as a diagnosis.

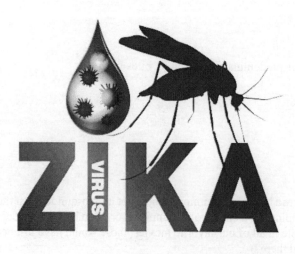

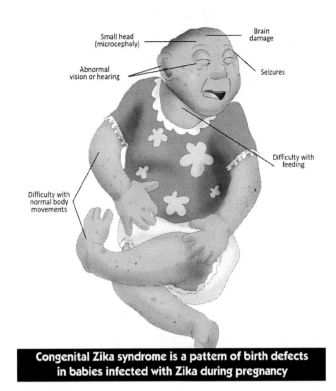

Congenital Zika syndrome is a pattern of birth defects in babies infected with Zika during pregnancy

170) EVD (Ebola Virus Disease) can be transmitted via each of these modes **except**:

A) Contact transmission via blood or body fluids

B) Airborne transmission

C) Infected bats

D) Contact transmission via inanimate objects

B - Ebola virus is transmitted among humans through direct or indirect physical contact with infected blood, bodily fluids, or skin. The <u>most</u> infectious vectors of transmission are blood, feces and vomit. Ebola virus has also been detected in breast milk, urine, semen, and, in lesser amounts, saliva and tears. Pretty much if it involves a bodily fluid, it can transmit Ebola. And just to really freak us out, yes, it is possible to be transmitted indirectly by contact with previously contaminated dry surfaces and objects, (i.e. bloody bed rails, laundry, etc.) for several hours.

Past clinical experiences have shown that spread of the virus via coughing or sneezing is rare (if at all.) Unlike measles, chickenpox, or TB, Ebola virus disease is <u>not</u> classified as an airborne infection. However, common sense and current protocols highly recommend wearing a surgical mask & lots of other PPE items. Previous Ebola outbreaks show that all cases were infected by direct close contact with symptomatic patients.

In regard to "kill all the bad bug wipes," the CDC recommends:

- The use of an EPA-registered hospital disinfectant with a label claim for use against a non-enveloped virus (e.g., norovirus, rotavirus, adenovirus, poliovirus)

- The product label use directions for the non-enveloped virus or viruses should be followed when disinfecting against the Ebola virus

- The product label will *not specifically mention* effectiveness against the Ebola virus. Instead, it will mention effectiveness against a different virus, such as norovirus, rotavirus, adenovirus, and/or poliovirus.

What this means in real life is actually pretty simple. Assume everything is dirty and clean everything. Chances are, hospital based "kill all the bad bug wipes" do what they are supposed to do, which is "kill all the bad bugs," including Ebola, but make sure to pay attention to the manufacturer recommended "kill times." If no wipes are available, bleach is your best buddy!

171) Waste generated by a person who has confirmed EVD (Ebola Virus Disease) is considered:

A) Category A waste

B) Category B waste

C) General biohazard waste

D) Regulated medical waste

A - Waste contaminated (or suspected to be contaminated) with Ebola virus is classified as a Category A infectious substance and is regulated as a hazardous material under the U.S. Department of Transportation (DOT) Hazardous Materials Regulations (HMR; 49 CFR, Parts 171-180). But don't worry if you didn't know that, it will probably never appear as a test question on the CPEN exam. That being said, there are a couple of key points worth remembering as a healthcare professional. Category A waste is defined as being capable of posing an unreasonable risk to health, safety, and property when transported in commerce. It has a very specific way of being disposed of (type/number of bags, closure technique, holding containers, autoclaving, permits, etc.).

Ebola-associated waste that has been appropriately incinerated, autoclaved, or otherwise inactivated is <u>not</u> infectious, does not pose a health risk, and is not considered to be regulated medical waste or a hazardous material under federal law. Therefore, such waste no longer is considered a Category A infectious substance and is not subject to the requirements of the Hazardous Materials Regulations.

172) If you suspect one of your patients might have EVD (Ebola Virus Disease), what information should you quickly obtain from them?

A) Current medications

B) Allergies

C) Last meal eaten

D) Travel history

D – Travel and exposure history is increasingly seen as an essential element in the initial assessment process. This should include the patient's travel as well as any contact with, or exposure to, an individual with EVD within the previous 21 days. Signs and symptoms of EVD are usually nonspecific with a patient presenting with complaints such as fever, diarrhea, or just generally not feeling well. Without having a travel/exposure history obtained and documented, these symptoms may not be suggestive of Ebola Virus Disease because of another infectious or noninfectious condition, such as flu, gastroenteritis, etc. Relevant travel and exposure history should be discussed early on at triage to determine if Ebola should even be considered. Most kids in the ER with flu or gastro symptoms probably have the flu or some gastrointestinal ailment. But, if they just came back from West Africa or another area with an Ebola outbreak, that's a whole different story!

173) While taking the initial triage assessment, you have concerns that a patient may have Ebola Virus Disease (EVD). Which of the following actions should be taken next?

A) Ask them to sit back down in the waiting room while you call for help

B) Place the patient in a private room or separate enclosed area while you call for help

C) Ask them to stay at the triage desk while you walk/run away to find help

D) Initiate a point of care test (or walk the patient to the Lab) for a Rapid Respiratory Virus Panel (RRVP)

B – Isolating a suspected Ebola Virus Disease patient in a private room or separate enclosed area with private bathroom or covered, bedside commode is an appropriate action. Your goal is to prevent transmission by direct or indirect contact (dedicated equipment, hand hygiene, and incredibly restricted patient movement). The patient should not be in contact with other patients to avoid potentially infecting others. You will also want to limit room entry to only staff who are essential to the patient's care and who have proper personal protective equipment (PPE). And when it comes to PPE, remember, "Ebola PPE" is very different than "chicken pox, meningitis, or measles" PPE. The CDC (www.CDC.gov) has great videos that review the necessary equipment and steps involved in PPE

So, that's the test answer. But, let's be honest. If you are at triage and someone mentions Ebola, your initial reaction might well be to try to find a reason to immediately be needed elsewhere... preferably miles away! But placing this patient immediately in a private room and calling for the cavalry are certainly appropriate.

Don't be distracted by something that sounds fancy like RRVP (which may or may not be a real thing). Safety for yourself, your colleagues, and other patients is the real priority.

174) Your patient is suspected to have Ebola Virus Disease (EVD) and is clinically stable. At a minimum, what personal protective equipment (PPE) should you, as the ED nurse, wear?

A) Powered air-purifying respirator (PAPR), coverall/full body suit, three pairs of gloves

B) Face shield, surgical mask, fluid-resistant gown, two pairs of gloves

C) Face shield, N95 mask, fluid-resistant gown, three pairs of gloves

D) Powered air-purifying respirator (PAPR), coverall/full body suit, two pairs of gloves

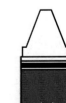

B - All healthcare workers who have contact with the patient should put on appropriate PPE based on the patient's clinical status. If the patient is clinically stable and is not actively bleeding, having diarrhea or vomiting, then the emergency healthcare workers should, <u>at a minimum</u>, wear: 1) face shield, 2) surgical face mask, 3) Single-use, fluid-resistant gown and 4) two pairs of examination gloves where the outer gloves have extended cuffs. Powered air-purifying respirators (PAPRs), coveralls, N95 masks, and three pairs of gloves are above the minimum recommendations of the CDC. Of note, if the patient is not clinically stable, actively bleeding ,etc. (often referred to as "wet" in Ebola-specialist speak), then that's a whole additional level of CDC recommended PPE.

Additional Insights from a Peds ICU Ebola Nurse Expert:

A full body suit or coverall is one that covers the arms, torso and legs. This may or may not have a hood as well as integrated socks. They must be made with fabric and seams/closures that passes ASTM F1671 (13.8kPa) or ISO 16604 ≥ 14 kPa. Testing by an ISO 17025 certified third-party laboratory is recommended by the CDC. It is <u>NOT</u> a patient gown, hospital isolation gown, or surgical gown.

175) What symptom is **most common** in a patient with suspected or confirmed Ebola Virus Disease (EVD)?

A) Diarrhea

B) Vomiting

C) Fever

D) Bleeding

C - Unexplained fever (greater than 101.5F (38.6C) is the most common symptom in suspected or confirmed cases of Ebola Virus Disease (EVD). Fever **may or may not** be accompanied by abdominal pain, diarrhea, muscle pain, severe headaches, vomiting, and of course, unexplained bleeding. This is a reminder as to why, at triage, screenings regarding exposure and travel history are essential. Even in pediatrics!

With EVD, the time interval between infection and symptom onset is from 2 to 21 days per the World Health Organization website. A person infected with Ebola is not contagious until symptoms appear.

Additional Insights from a Peds ICU Ebola Nurse Expert:

Most kids that come to your ED will not have Ebola, but some other disease. Ebola looks just like many influenza-like illnesses. It is important that you do your screening with due diligence to be able to catch a travel or contact history. It's not like the movies where someone with Ebola will come in bleeding out of everywhere. They will come in looking like every other kid in your ED, especially if its flu season or the stomach bug of the week is going around.

176) When a child with autism spectrum disorder (ASD) presents to the ER, the immediate and best source of information is:

A) The facility's electronic medical record system interoperability application

B) Mom or Dad

C) The local Health Information Exchange (HIE)

D) The patient portal application

B – Mom or Dad has spent more time with the child than anyone else. They understand and have developed unique communication skills with and for their child. Trust them!

Let's talk about why people with autism spectrum disorder (ASD) are commonly referred to as being "on a spectrum." At one end of the spectrum is a severely disabled, non-verbal child who is flapping and rocking in the corner. At the other end of the spectrum is a child with ASD who may appear uncomfortable or ill-at-ease in social situations. But the thing that all children with ASD have in common is that Mom or Dad tends to be the experts in their child's case. They, or the patient's caregivers, are with the child much more than we are and they know what works and what doesn't. More importantly, they also can tell us what the child's norm looks like. Especially with severe ASD, whereas rituals and routines are everything, simply... ASK MOM OR DAD!

Emergency departments, inpatient units, and more recently, prehospital EMS agencies, are now actively taking measures to better address the needs of these special needs children and their families. These initiatives range from portable sensory kits to completely redesigned sensory-friendly emergency department rooms.

Fortunately, new methods are being developed to help autistic patients and their families avert and avoid over-stimulation in the healthcare world. With insights from parents, patients, child-life specialists, and other experts, we now see specialized educational offerings, programs, and products designed to help these patients in stressful situations. You can help your facility by considering things like:

- Portable sensory kits (for EMS agencies and the ER) which commonly include noise-canceling earmuffs, sunglasses, weighted blankets, sensory toys and fidget devices

- Special rooms or areas which utilize soft colors such as gray, purple and light green for walls

- Padded walls to prevent injury in case an agitated child bumps into them

- Crash mats on the floors

- Exercise balls

- Changing the fluorescent light fixtures, which can buzz or hum, to LED (Light Emitting Diode) lighting and adding a dimmer function to lower the brightness to the child's comfort level

- Projectors for alternating soothing patterns of light onto the ceiling

- Adjusting the monitors so that alarms and alerts ring at the nurse's station instead of in the patient rooms

- Supplying softer gowns and softer arm identification bands

- Red, yellow, green, and blue emoji shaped pillows with different emotions (happy, sad, angry, and scared) throughout the room to help non-verbal children express their feelings

Additional Insights from a Parent of an Autistic Child (2020):

"We have been in three different hospital ER rooms with our son on more than ten occasions over the years. In general, our experiences waiting in the emergency room have not been positive. We have found that there really are no accommodations for a child on the spectrum. Please understand that our child with autism also had a serious and unstable mental illness happening at the same time, prompting us going to the ER as often as we did. Unfortunately, our reality was that our son had to be forced to receive treatment in the ER by the police on multiple occasions. One time, he even ran out of an ER, running all the way down the street in freezing snow until the police retrieved him. Having a self soothing sensory area would have been a great resource for us to placate him while we waited to be assessed. We have only come across one children's hospital that had an autism dual diagnosis treatment unit, however their waiting room had absolutely no accommodation for children on the spectrum. Once we were placed in an ER bed, the TV provided some distraction to prevent aggression and meltdowns. The children's hospital had more children's programming and games which temporarily helped until admission into the unit."

Certified Pediatric Emergency Nurse (CPEN) Review IV

Additional Insights from Autism Speaks (autismspeaks.org)

"It's exciting that more businesses are approaching kids with autism and realizing that, even though there's a neurodiversity, it doesn't mean they are defective. It means they just see the world differently. We need to be able to adapt and help them harness all of their talents and strengths; it would be a waste not to."

The Autism Program at Boston Medical Center

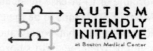
AUTISM FRIENDLY INITIATIVE at Boston Medical Center

Autism Support Checklist

Patient Name: _____
Patient Date of Birth: _____
Date Completed: _____

Communication

1. Does the patient communicate using spoken language?
   - ☐ Yes
   - ☐ No
   - Please explain: _____

2. What other ways does the patient communicate?
   - ☐ Pictures
   - ☐ Written Words
   - ☐ Electronic Communication
   - ☐ Gestures
   - ☐ Other: _____

3. What would help the patient understand information?
   - ☐ Spoken language
   - ☐ Pictures
   - ☐ Written Words
   - ☐ Electronic Communication
   - ☐ Other: _____

4. How does the patient communicate pain?
   - ☐ Spoken language
   - ☐ Crying/Screaming
   - ☐ Self Injury
   - ☐ Aggression
   - ☐ Other: _____

Sensory Needs

5. Does the patient have sensory triggers/needs?
   - ☐ Avoid bright lights
   - ☐ Avoid loud noises
   - ☐ Avoids touch
   - ☐ Seeks pressure
   - ☐ Other: _____

6. What items/actions would be helpful?
   - ☐ Sunglasses
   - ☐ Headphones
   - ☐ Stress Ball
   - ☐ Other: _____

Interacting with the Patient

7. What would help the patient understand the procedure/exam?
   - ☐ Talk the patient through the exam
   - ☐ Demonstrate on another person
   - ☐ Show a picture schedule
   - ☐ Other: _____

8. Are there particular actions or phrases that are likely to trigger the patient? (e.g. people speaking loudly)
   - ☐ Yes? Please explain:
   - ☐ No

9. Does the patient engage in behaviors that could be a safety concern?
   - ☐ Bolting
   - ☐ Self-injurious behaviors
   - ☐ Hitting, kicking etc.
   - ☐ Other: _____

10. What other information should we know to help make the patient more comfortable?

Please mail completed forms for BMC patients with autism to The Autism Program 72 E. Concord St. Vose, Boston MA 02118, or fax it to us at 617-414-3693. For questions, contact us at autismfriendlyinitiative@bmc.org.

Autism Support Checklist
Courtesy of Boston Medical Center
www.bmc.org

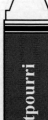
Pediatric Potpourri

Certified Pediatric Emergency Nurse (CPEN) Review IV

177) A 15-year old patient who identifies as a transgender male comes to the ED with a complaint of right foot pain for the past month, but denies any trauma or difficulty with ambulation. During the triage interview, the parent reports that he has missed several days of school, on and off, due to the pain in his right foot. What would be the **most** appropriate question for the primary nurse to ask?

A) "Do you feel safe at school?"

B) "How does your other foot feel?"

C) "What is the name of your best friend?"

D) "Can I get you an ice pack for your foot?"

A - Transgender youth are at a high risk for bullying, especially at school, so a question about the patient's safety should be very high on your priorities. These patients may often present with vague or chronic complaints and a history of frequent absenteeism from school. A variation on the safety concern might be to consider that the patient may not feel comfortable discussing the school situation in front of his parents, but that was not one of the options.

Though an appropriate question, asking about the patient's other foot does not really focus on the problem. Asking the name of the patient's best friend would not be appropriate and also does not focus on the problem. An ice pack would probably not be helpful since the pain has been going on for a month. Remember, the question specifically mentioned the teen identifying as transgender and missing several days of school for what sounds like a non-acute foot complaint. This should be a clue on the test that the answer is not going to involve the foot, but something more psychosocial in nature.

178) An adolescent has been receiving threats of violence on social media networks. This would be an example of which of the following?

A) Indirect bullying

B) Direct bullying

C) Traditional bullying

D) Cyberbullying

D - Cyberbullying involves using electronic communication or social media to threaten, harm, intimidate, or otherwise bother another individual. This type of bullying can be especially harmful and intense due to the anonymity of the perpetrator and an instant exposure to a wide audience. Direct bullying includes the use of physical force, while indirect bullying consists of gossiping, exclusion, and spreading rumors. Both direct and indirect bullying are examples of traditional bullying. Parents only need to spend a few minutes with their young and teen-aged children to see the unbelievable levels and depth of bullying that is widespread across social media sites.

179) An elementary school wants to initiate a bullying prevention program. Which strategy would likely be the **most** effective?

A) Providing high levels of playground supervision

B) Keeping the bullies separate from the other students

C) Providing martial arts training for the victims

D) Scheduling a one-day bullying awareness campaign

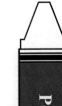

Pediatric Potpourri

A - Effective bullying prevention strategies for schools typically include focusing on the immediate problem and includes high levels of supervision at locations where bullying is likely to happen. Parent and teacher training activities and implementing school wide rules pertaining to bullying (that are enforced!) are also effective. Separating the bullies from the rest of the students is not effective and would not be appropriate. Providing karate, judo, or Mortal Kombat/ninja warrior training for the victims would single them out and encourage violence. Scheduling a one-day bullying awareness campaign may be informative, but would not solve the problem in such a brief period of time. As we have learned with drowning prevention, there is nothing that can replace eyes on supervision!

180) Parents bring a 4-year old child to the ED because "one of the tubes in his ear fell out." The child is alert and playful, with normal vital signs. History is significant for several past ear infections and the placement of "tubes in the ears" 9-months ago. The ED nurse should anticipate:

A) Immediate live ENT consultation and rapid surgical replacement

B) Immediate tele-health ENT consultation as well as sedation and pain management orders

C) NPO, STAT CT of the head, and placing the child in 23-hour observation status

D) Possibly an ENT phone consultation, but most likely reassurance and discharge home

D – There are several important things to know about myringotomy and tympanostomy (the surgical incision and placement of "tubes" in the ears). 1) While it may sound scary, it is a commonly performed procedure for children with frequent or chronic ear infections. 2) These tubes are expected to fall out in less than a year.

While the parents in this case may have been exhibiting a variety of symptoms, the patient seems pretty normal. No need for surgery, diagnostics, pain management... just reassurance and education.

The goals of the procedure are primarily three-fold: 1) To keep the air in the middle ear refreshed, 2) To allow for drainage, and 3) To equalize the pressure inside the ear with the air pressure outside the body. Pressure, especially in sensitive areas like the ear, means pain. And kids with lots of ear infections tend to be much happier once they have recovered from this brief outpatient procedure. *So what do parents want and need to know?*

> **Pain**: In most cases post-op pain is easily managed with just a few days of oral Tylenol® (acetaminophen) and/or Motrin® (ibuprofen.)
>
> **Ear infections**: Can the child get an ear infection even with tubes in the ears? Yes, but happily not nearly as easily or frequently as before the surgery.
>
> **Swimming**: Can the child go swimming after having tubes placed in their ears? As you can imagine, this is guided by ENT preference, but many peds ENT physicians now allow kids to go swimming, without ear plugs, after the very small ear drum surgical site has healed. As long as the kid swims in a chlorinated pool, it's all good. Swimming in a swamp, to no surprise, is probably not the best choice.
>
> **Falling out**: When it comes to myringotomy tubes, they are supposed to fall out. They commonly work and wiggle their way out between 6 and 9 months after placement. That's good, and to be expected. In fact, that's what they are supposed to do. If they fall out one week after initial placement, that's worth a call to the ENT. Nine months later, when the tubes fall out, that's a good thing. Just make sure that mom and dad don't try to put them back in!

Pediatric Potpourri

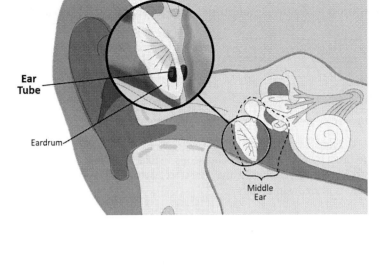

181) Which of the following formulas are recommended for selecting the size of a pediatric uncuffed endotracheal tube?

A) (16 + age) / 4

B) 1+2+3+4

C) E=MC^2

D) 8675+309=Jenny

A - 16 + age / 4 is one of the most commonly used pediatric ETT size formulas. Another way to come with the same answer is to use the formula [(age/4) + 4]. It's crucial to remember a few key things about using formulas. First, remember these formulas are for <u>uncuffed tubes</u>. Many pediatric ICU physicians are now recommending <u>cuffed</u> tubes be placed in sick children. So, if you are looking for a cuffed ETT, select a cuffed tube that is 0.5 - 1 mm <u>smaller</u> than what the formula suggests.

Second, using a formula involves doing mental math. Is mental math something that you want to do, especially in a high stress situation? Pocket cheat sheets and mobile phone apps are plentiful and most importantly, the calculations have already been done by people who are not stressed. So, when you are stressed because the kid is crashing, it's not cheating to use a cheat sheet!

182) A patient has arrived at the Emergency Department after their gastrostomy (G-tube) has been out for approximately 30-minutes. The largest temporary catheter able to be placed was an 8 French. What is the **most definitive** test to determine that the catheter is appropriately within the stomach?

A) An abdominal x-ray

B) A contrast/fluoroscopy study through the catheter

C) Aspiration of gastric contents from the catheter

D) Auscultation of the abdomen while air is being injected through the catheter

B - Contrast/fluoroscopy study through the catheter is the most definitive test to determine that the catheter is properly placed. An abdominal X-ray can visualize the G-tube, but cannot confirm if the tube is definitively within the stomach. Aspiration of gastric contents provides strong evidence for placement into the stomach, but is not as definitive as a contrast study. Though commonly done in clinical practice, auscultation of air into the G-tube <u>cannot</u> determine if the tube is within the stomach.

183) How quickly does a gastrocutaneous fistula or gastrostomy close when a tube is not present within the tract?

A) 30-minutes

B) 60-minutes

C) 4-hours

D) It is impossible to predict how fast a gastrocutaneous fistula will close

D - It is impossible to predict how fast a gastrocutaneous fistula will close. Just like with many body piercings, the longer tubes are out, the harder they are to reinsert. The most reliable way to keep the fistula open is to ensure a tube is placed within it.

184) A patient arrives to the ED after their G-tube has been out all night. The fistula appears closed, but there is a small dimple present and the mother thinks she saw a drop of milk come out of the stoma. You are going to attempt to place a tube to assess the fistula for patency. You have a variety of tube choices, including Foley urinary catheters (6-20 French), red rubber catheters (8-20 French) and low-profile balloon G-tubes in various French sizes and lengths. What is the **most appropriate** strategy?

A) Start with the smallest Foley catheter available to see if the fistula can be accessed successfully

B) Attempt to place the same tube the patient had before it came out

C) Call the operating room and book the patient for a surgical procedure

D) Have the patient drink some milk and see if anything comes out of the fistula

A – In this scenario, it is best to start with the smallest tube available to see if the fistula can successfully be accessed.

Attempting to place the same size tube that had come out could lead to site trauma and stomach detachment (that's bad!). Booking the patient for the operating room should be considered only if tube placement fails and the fistula has closed completely. Eating or drinking may or may not produce leaking through the fistula, even if it is open.

When it comes to G-tubes, or really any tube or catheter for the fistula… Foley catheters, red rubber catheters, regular G-tubes… Just keep the hole open.

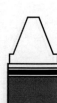

185) You are able to place a temporary Foley urinary catheter in a patient whose G-tube came out earlier in the day. The largest tube size you can place is a 10 French and the patient's bolus feedings pass through without resistance. However, the patient previously had a 12 French low-profile G-tube before this happened. What is the **most appropriate** plan for upsizing their G-tube back to a 12 French?

A) Secure the urinary catheter with a drain tube stabilizer device, discharge the patient home and make an appointment for them in 1-3 days for tube replacement by Pediatric Surgery or Gastroenterology

B) Admit the patient overnight for observation and attempt to replace the G-tube with a larger size in the morning

C) Send the patient home with a 12 French low profile G-tube and have the family replace it at home the next day

D) Tape the tube in place and ask the family to make an appointment in the next 10 to 14 days

Certified Pediatric Emergency Nurse (CPEN) Review IV

A - Secure the urinary catheter with a drain tube stabilizer device, discharge the patient home, and make an appointment for them in 1-3 days for tube replacement by Pediatric Surgery or Gastroenterology. This option allows the family to continue feeding through the current (but not long-term) catheter for a few days while you get an appointment for it to be replaced.

Additional Insights from a Pediatric Surgery Nurse Practitioner:

Despite the substantial amount of education that the pediatric surgery service gives to parents and patients with gastrostomy tubes, it is inevitable that when issues arise, families will turn to what's familiar to them... the Emergency Department.

It is not uncommon for G-tubes to come out unexpectedly. Over time, G-tube balloons may degrade and if severe enough, they may break. The one-way valve that allows for the induction of water into the balloon may also fail. If that happens, the water may leak out and cause the balloon to collapse. Collapsing of the G-tube balloon may create a favorable condition that could lead to the G-tube falling out.

Because of the common problem of G-tubes dislodgment, it is acceptable for the family to learn how to replace the G-tube at home, if possible. As ideal as that sounds, some families are either unwilling or afraid to replace the G-tube by themselves.

When the patient arrives in the ED for a G-tube concern, it is imperative that they be triaged immediately in order not to waste precious time. A delay in time may promote the fistula to close and make replacing the tube that much more difficult. Different size catheters ranging from small to the size that patient had before should be available at the bedside. The catheter preference is unimportant, as the goal is to prevent the fistula from completely closing. Red rubber catheters are a good choice because of their cost and flexibility. However, this flexibility may also make them difficult to place. Urinary catheters have several advantages over a red rubber catheter. First, they come in sizes as small as 6 French. A practitioner may be fooled in thinking that the fistula is completely closed, when in fact, a minute opening may still be present. The minute opening may be able to accept the small catheter. Second, the tip of a urinary catheter is tapered. A tapered catheter is easier to pass than a blunt-ended tube. Finally, a urinary catheter has a balloon. If a urinary catheter needs to remain in place, it can be secured and used as a feeding tube (G-tube) until the patient is seen again. But, a quick reminder regarding balloons and G-tubes; the amount of sterile water needed to inflate a Foley urinary catheter balloon is often far more than needed for a G-tube. You just need to make sure it's secure.

Once a tube is in place, the connection between the outside of the abdomen and the stomach is secured. Even though the original G-tube was unable to be placed, the patient may be able to go home, use the temporary tube for nutrition, and return the following day to "upsize" the tube. Sequential up-sizing is preferred over placing a larger tube immediately. Attempting to force a tube in place may lead to stoma trauma or even detachment of the stomach from the abdominal wall. And remember; always ensure that the tube you place is compatible with the equipment the patient has at home. Make sure that the attachments used to feed the child fit the replacement tube before sending them back home.

There are different types of G-tubes available, but the most popular tube amongst practitioners and patients are the button-type G-tubes. These are "low profile" G-tubes that sit close to the skin and do not hang out like other tubes. They require a feeding extension to be attached in order to infuse feedings. Patients like these tubes because: 1) They are less conspicuous, 2) They tend to leak less than other tubes, and 3) They are easier to manage.

If a G-tube needs to be replaced in an emergency situation, you'll need to have a same size replacement (or slightly smaller) G-tube (or, in a pinch, a urinary catheter), water soluble lubricant and a syringe with tap water. Inflate the G-tube balloon with water to check for leaks, then deflate it completely. Lubricate the G-tube stem and gently slip it into the stoma. Ensure that the tube spins freely 360 degrees and fill the balloon with the recommended amount of water. Before you use any G-tube that was replaced, you should **ASPIRATE GASTRIC CONTENTS** from the feeding tube. Once this is done, the tube is now able to be used. If there are <u>**ANY DOUBTS**</u> about the proper position of the tube, a contrast fluoroscopy study should be obtained.

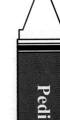

The majority of problems associated with G-tubes come from a lack of simple maintenance. Basically, if you want your car to run correctly, you need to fill the gas tank, change the oil, rotate the tires, etc. Just like with your car, G-tube site problems most often occur when regular maintenance is not addressed. These regular tasks include: 1) Not changing the tube on a regular (3-4-month) interval, 2) Ensuring there is a proper amount of water in the balloon, and 3) Detaching the feeding extension when the G-tube is not being used.

But when everything looks okay and you're still having doubts about whether it's in the correct position, simply go "**BLUE!**"

                                            (**B**)alloon

                                            (**L**)ength

                                            (**U**)pper GI

                                            (**E**)xtravasation

(**B**)alloon – Check the balloon to make sure that there is the recommended amount of water. The side of the G-tube should indicate the recommended volume. Simply grab an empty syringe, insert the syringe into the water port (facing laterally), and aspirate the water out of the balloon. Just reverse this step-in order to refill the balloon with the appropriate amount of water. And yes, tap water is just fine. <u>Do not</u> use saline in a G-tube balloon. Read the instructions, or in this case, read the G-tube fine print. It will indicate how much water is needed to properly inflate (and not burst) the balloon. Usually it's only a few mL (i.e. less than a Foley urinary catheter.) Read the instructions and look at the tube.

(**L**)ength – Take a look at the length of the tube to see if it looks appropriate. Appropriately fitting tubes are ones that are close to the skin with very little gap beneath the G-tube. A loose tube will have an obvious gap between the skin and bottom of the tube. An over tight tube will appear "sucked" into the abdomen. Obviously, loose tubes may leak, and over tight tubes may cause skin breakdown. Even if the tube looks appropriate and there is a proper amount of water in the balloon, things may be VERY wrong. There is one test that can quickly and easily confirm proper position of the G-tube.

(**U**)pper GI – X-rays (anterior/posterior and lateral) taken while the radiologist pushes contrast through the G-tube will light up the stomach. This test is essential if you want to verify that the G-tube is positioned within the stomach.

(**E**)xtravasation – This is the word that you **don't** want to hear from the radiologist right after that study. What you do want to hear is… "There is NO extravasation of contrast noted on the exam." Extravasation means that the contrast the radiologist pushed through the tube is in the wrong place. For G-tubes, this means the tube may be in the abdomen, but not in the stomach. The presence of feedings and contrast within the peritoneum will lead to serious illness and even septic shock. Infant formula is meant to go inside the intestines, so anything that should be in the stomach, but ends up flowing and floating outside the intestines, is a really bad thing!

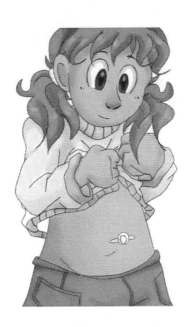
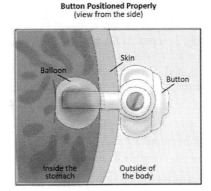

186) The attending physician will be ordering a number of lab tests for an infant in your Emergency Department. You know that blood samples for each of the following tests can be routinely obtained via heel stick **except**:

A) Complete blood count

B) Basic metabolic profile

C) Blood culture

D) Type and cross match

C – Of the common lab tests listed above, you would not expect to obtain a blood culture from a routine heel stick. On the other hand, for children who have not yet begun to walk, a properly performed heel stick can be a valuable time saver as well as a potential life saver.

That's great, but wait, there's more! If you continue to read on right now, we'll add even more information at no extra charge! There's more to a heel stick than just sticking the heel - actually, much more! Here's our special offer. Read now and you can receive this handy dandy proverb comparison, as well as the "Top Five Heel Stick Tips and Tricks" contributed by pediatric emergency nurse educator, Rosanne Conliffe.

A Rolling Stone Gathers No Moss
(English Proverb)

A Cold Heel Giveth No Blood
(Peds Proverb)

<u>Warm</u> the heel. If you remember nothing else prior to performing a heel stick, warm the heel. A commercially available warm pack held in place with a sock or a warm, wet washcloth (not too hot!) will do a great job of warming the heel in short order. In other words. Cool *your* heels for a few moments while you *warm* the patient's heel.

Warm the heel and … let **gravity** be your friend, not your worst enemy. In addition to warming the heel for several minutes, positioning really makes a difference. If the baby is flat on the bed and their heel is held up in the air, it should be no surprise that it's difficult for blood to get to the heel. But wait, it gets worse. If the child is really sick, where shunting away from the feet is expected, obtaining a good specimen will be even more difficult. Ideally, and of course, illness-dependent, having mom, dad, or caregiver hold the baby chest to chest not only provides comfort, but also allows gravity to do its work and be your friend.

Warm the heel and... Use the **right equipment**. In other words, use a heel stick device that is actually intended for infant heel sticks. Though a blood glucose lance that is used with adults and kids for finger sticks can certainly be used, there are heel stick lances specifically made for sticking heels of small children. Using the right equipment increases the chance of getting the amount of blood needed. Use the right equipment for the job and "letting it drip" (avoid milking) are the keys to minimizing hemolysis and rejected samples.

>Bonus Question: What lab result is most likely affected by "milking" the heel?

>Bonus Answer: Potassium! Squeezing and squashing the heel squeezes and squashes the red blood cells, and ruptured blood cells can leak potassium into the blood sample. This may easily lead to a falsely elevated potassium level.

>If this sounds familiar, it should. The rupture of red cells, and the subsequent release of the contents of the cells (especially potassium) into the serum, is called hemolysis.

Warm the heel and... **where** you stick, makes a difference. In real estate, the mantra is Location, Location, Location. When it comes to heel sticks, the mantra is Location, Location, Location. In little feet, the major arteries and nerves tend to be located towards the middle of the foot, so when you stick, stick to the sides.

Lastly, lest there be any confusion, before you stick... **Warm** the heel (are you noticing a trend here?) and if possible, a little ingested **sugar** in the form of breastfeeding or oral sucrose solution (Sweet-Ease®, SweetUms®, etc.) goes a long way to help the hurt heel.

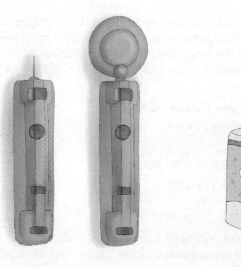 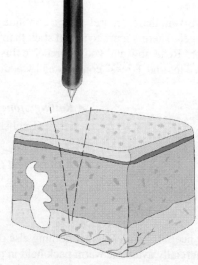

Traditional "Finger Stick" Lance   //   Skin and Finger Stick Lance = One Drop of Blood

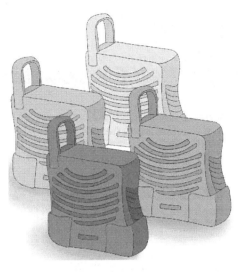
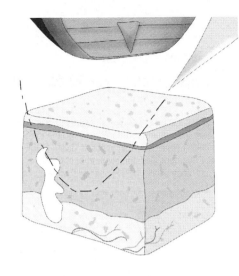

Heel Stick Device   //   Skin and Heel Stick Device = Several Drops of Blood

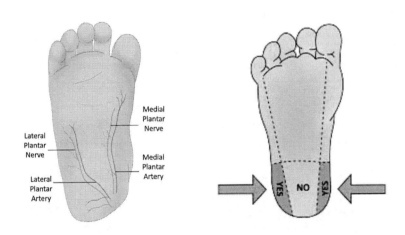

187) The proper way to chart administration of morphine sulfate is:

A) MS

B) MS04

C) Morph

D) Morphine sulfate

D - The Institute for Safe Medication Practices (*ISMP*) *List of Error-Prone Abbreviations, Symbols, and Dose Designations* contains abbreviations, symbols, and dose designations which have been reported through the ISMP National Medication Errors Reporting Program (ISMP MERP) as being frequently misinterpreted and involved in harmful medication errors. These abbreviations, symbols, and dose designations should **never** be used when documenting medical information. For example, the use of the abbreviation "MS" has resulted in the very serious error of magnesium sulfate being given instead of morphine. The ISMP has produced a variety of publications to help reduce the chance of preventable medical errors caused by such things as medications the "Look alike" and/or "Sound alike." ISMP advocates the use of "Tall Man" lettering such as with "predniSONE" and "predniSOLONE" to avoid confusion and errors. Other ISMP publications address the recommended use of standard concentrations especially in neonatal drug infusions and the identification of "High alert medications" in a variety of care settings. Best practice? Use the complete name of the medication and watch out for auto-correct!

Certified Pediatric Emergency Nurse (CPEN) Review IV

Institute for Safe Medication Practices

ISMP's List of *Error-Prone Abbreviations, Symbols*, and *Dose Designations*

The abbreviations, symbols, and dose designations found in this table have been reported to ISMP through the ISMP National Medication Errors Reporting Program (ISMP MERP) as being frequently misinterpreted and involved in harmful medication errors. They should **NEVER** be used when communicating medical information. This includes internal communications, telephone/verbal prescriptions, computer-generated labels, labels for drug storage bins, medication administration records, as well as pharmacy and prescriber computer order entry screens.

Abbreviations	Intended Meaning	Misinterpretation	Correction
μg	Microgram	Mistaken as "mg"	Use "mcg"
AD, AS, AU	Right ear, left ear, each ear	Mistaken as OD, OS, OU (right eye, left eye, each eye)	Use "right ear," "left ear," or "each ear"
OD, OS, OU	Right eye, left eye, each eye	Mistaken as AD, AS, AU (right ear, left ear, each ear)	Use "right eye," "left eye," or "each eye"
BT	Bedtime	Mistaken as "BID" (twice daily)	Use "bedtime"
cc	Cubic centimeters	Mistaken as "u" (units)	Use "mL"
D/C	Discharge or discontinue	Premature discontinuation of medications if D/C (intended to mean "discharge") has been misinterpreted as "discontinued" when followed by a list of discharge medications	Use "discharge" and "discontinue"
IJ	Injection	Mistaken as "IV" or "intrajugular"	Use "injection"
IN	Intranasal	Mistaken as "IM" or "IV"	Use "intranasal" or "NAS"
HS	Half-strength	Mistaken as bedtime	Use "half-strength" or "bedtime"
hs	At bedtime, hours of sleep	Mistaken as half-strength	
IU**	International unit	Mistaken as IV (intravenous) or 10 (ten)	Use "units"
o.d. or OD	Once daily	Mistaken as "right eye" (OD-oculus dexter), leading to oral liquid medications administered in the eye	Use "daily"
OJ	Orange juice	Mistaken as OD or OS (right or left eye); drugs meant to be diluted in orange juice may be given in the eye	Use "orange juice"
Per os	By mouth, orally	The "os" can be mistaken as "left eye" (OS-oculus sinister)	Use "PO," "by mouth," or "orally"
q.d. or QD**	Every day	Mistaken as q.i.d., especially if the period after the "q" or the tail of the "q" is misunderstood as an "i"	Use "daily"
qhs	Nightly at bedtime	Mistaken as "qhr" or every hour	Use "nightly"
qn	Nightly or at bedtime	Mistaken as "qh" (every hour)	Use "nightly" or "at bedtime"
q.o.d. or QOD**	Every other day	Mistaken as "q.d." (daily) or "q.i.d. (four times daily) if the "o" is poorly written	Use "every other day"
q1d	Daily	Mistaken as q.i.d. (four times daily)	Use "daily"
q6PM, etc.	Every evening at 6 PM	Mistaken as every 6 hours	Use "daily at 6 PM" or "6 PM daily"
SC, SQ, sub q	Subcutaneous	SC mistaken as SL (sublingual); SQ mistaken as "5 every;" the "q" in "sub q" has been mistaken as "every" (e.g., a heparin dose ordered "sub q 2 hours before surgery" misunderstood as every 2 hours before surgery)	Use "subcut" or "subcutaneously"
ss	Sliding scale (insulin) or ½ (apothecary)	Mistaken as "55"	Spell out "sliding scale;" use "one-half" or "½"
SSRI	Sliding scale regular insulin	Mistaken as selective-serotonin reuptake inhibitor	Spell out "sliding scale (insulin)"
SSI	Sliding scale insulin	Mistaken as Strong Solution of Iodine (Lugol's)	
i/d	One daily	Mistaken as "tid"	Use "1 daily"
TIW or tiw	3 times a week	Mistaken as "3 times a day" or "twice in a week"	Use "3 times weekly"
U or u**	Unit	Mistaken as the number 0 or 4, causing a 10-fold overdose or greater (e.g., 4U seen as "40" or 4u seen as "44"); mistaken as "cc" so dose given in volume instead of units (e.g., 4u seen as 4cc)	Use "unit"
UD	As directed ("ut dictum")	Mistaken as unit dose (e.g., diltiazem 125 mg IV infusion "UD" misinterpreted as meaning to give the entire infusion as a unit [bolus] dose)	Use "as directed"

Dose Designations and Other Information	Intended Meaning	Misinterpretation	Correction
Trailing zero after decimal point (e.g., 1.0 mg)**	1 mg	Mistaken as 10 mg if the decimal point is not seen	Do not use trailing zeros for doses expressed in whole numbers
"Naked" decimal point (e.g., .5 mg)**	0.5 mg	Mistaken as 5 mg if the decimal point is not seen	Use zero before a decimal point when the dose is less than a whole unit
Abbreviations such as mg. or mL. with a period following the abbreviation	mg mL	The period is unnecessary and could be mistaken as the number 1 if written poorly	Use mg, mL, etc. without a terminal period

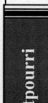

Pediatric Potpourri

Certified Pediatric Emergency Nurse (CPEN) Review IV

Institute for Safe Medication Practices
ISMP's List of *Error-Prone Abbreviations, Symbols*, and *Dose Designations* (continued)

Dose Designations and Other Information	Intended Meaning	Misinterpretation	Correction
Drug name and dose run together (especially problematic for drug names that end in "l" such as Inderal40 mg; Tegretol300 mg)	Inderal 40 mg Tegretol 300 mg	Mistaken as Inderal 140 mg Mistaken as Tegretol 1300 mg	Place adequate space between the drug name, dose, and unit of measure
Numerical dose and unit of measure run together (e.g., 10mg, 100mL)	10 mg 100 mL	The "m" is sometimes mistaken as a zero or two zeros, risking a 10- to 100-fold overdose	Place adequate space between the dose and unit of measure
Large doses without properly placed commas (e.g., 100000 units; 1000000 units)	100,000 units 1,000,000 units	100000 has been mistaken as 10,000 or 1,000,000; 1000000 has been mistaken as 100,000	Use commas for dosing units at or above 1,000, or use words such as 100 "thousand" or 1 "million" to improve readability

Drug Name Abbreviations	Intended Meaning	Misinterpretation	Correction
To avoid confusion, do not abbreviate drug names when communicating medical information. Examples of drug name abbreviations involved in medication errors include:			
APAP	acetaminophen	Not recognized as acetaminophen	Use complete drug name
ARA A	vidarabine	Mistaken as cytarabine (ARA C)	Use complete drug name
AZT	zidovudine (Retrovir)	Mistaken as azathioprine or aztreonam	Use complete drug name
CPZ	Compazine (prochlorperazine)	Mistaken as chlorpromazine	Use complete drug name
DPT	Demerol-Phenergan-Thorazine	Mistaken as diphtheria-pertussis-tetanus (vaccine)	Use complete drug name
DTO	Diluted tincture of opium, or deodorized tincture of opium (Paregoric)	Mistaken as tincture of opium	Use complete drug name
HCl	hydrochloric acid or hydrochloride	Mistaken as potassium chloride (The "H" is misinterpreted as "K")	Use complete drug name unless expressed as a salt of a drug
HCT	hydrocortisone	Mistaken as hydrochlorothiazide	Use complete drug name
HCTZ	hydrochlorothiazide	Mistaken as hydrocortisone (seen as HCT250 mg)	Use complete drug name
MgSO4**	magnesium sulfate	Mistaken as morphine sulfate	Use complete drug name
MS, MSO4**	morphine sulfate	Mistaken as magnesium sulfate	Use complete drug name
MTX	methotrexate	Mistaken as mitoxantrone	Use complete drug name
NoAC	novel/new oral anticoagulant	No anticoagulant	Use complete drug name
PCA	procainamide	Mistaken as patient controlled analgesia	Use complete drug name
PTU	propylthiouracil	Mistaken as mercaptopurine	Use complete drug name
T3	Tylenol with codeine No. 3	Mistaken as liothyronine	Use complete drug name
TAC	triamcinolone	Mistaken as tetracaine, Adrenalin, cocaine	Use complete drug name
TNK	TNKase	Mistaken as "TPA"	Use complete drug name
TPA or tPA	tissue plasminogen activator, Activase (alteplase)	Mistaken as TNKase (tenecteplase), or less often as another tissue plasminogen activator, Retavase (retaplase)	Use complete drug names
ZnSO4	zinc sulfate	Mistaken as morphine sulfate	Use complete drug name

Stemmed Drug Names	Intended Meaning	Misinterpretation	Correction
"Nitro" drip	nitroglycerin infusion	Mistaken as sodium nitroprusside infusion	Use complete drug name
"Norflox"	norfloxacin	Mistaken as Norflex	Use complete drug name
"IV Vanc"	intravenous vancomycin	Mistaken as Invanz	Use complete drug name

Symbols	Intended Meaning	Misinterpretation	Correction
ℨ	Dram	Symbol for dram mistaken as "3"	Use the metric system
♏	Minim	Symbol for minim mistaken as "mL"	
x3d	For three days	Mistaken as "3 doses"	Use "for three days"
> and <	More than and less than	Mistaken as opposite of intended; mistakenly use incorrect symbol; "< 10" mistaken as "40"	Use "more than" or "less than"
/ (slash mark)	Separates two doses or indicates "per"	Mistaken as the number 1 (e.g., "25 units/10 units" misread as "25 units and 110" units)	Use "per" rather than a slash mark to separate doses
@	At	Mistaken as "2"	Use "at"
&	And	Mistaken as "2"	Use "and"
+	Plus or and	Mistaken as "4"	Use "and"
°	Hour	Mistaken as a zero (e.g., q2° seen as q 20)	Use "hr," "h," or "hour"
Φ or ∅	zero, null sign	Mistaken as numerals 4, 6, 8, and 9	Use 0 or zero, or describe intent using whole words

**These abbreviations are included on The Joint Commission's "minimum list" of dangerous abbreviations, acronyms, and symbols that must be included on an organization's "Do Not Use" list, effective January 1, 2004. Visit www.jointcommission.org for more information about this Joint Commission requirement.

© ISMP 2015. Permission is granted to reproduce material with proper attribution for internal use within healthcare organizations. Other reproduction is prohibited without written permission from ISMP. Report actual and potential medication errors to the ISMP National Medication Errors Reporting Program (ISMP MERP) via the Web at www.ismp.org or by calling 1-800-FAIL-SAF(E).

www.ismp.org

Images courtesy of Institute for Safe Medication Practices (ISMP)
www.ISMP.org

188) A young child is brought into the emergency department by parents who seem uneasy as they speak to the nurse. They explain that they don't like going to the hospital and that despite many attempts to make the child better using other methods at home and with relatives, the child continues to complain of a fever and some problems with his breathing. Upon physical exam, you note that the child has several round bruises of the same shape, color, and size on his back, neck, and shoulders. The parents have difficulty explaining the bruising until a translator arrives. Based on the information presented, which of the following explanations by the translator would be **most** reassuring?

A) Cupping

B) Dodgeball

C) Non-accidental trauma

D) Allergic reaction

A - In the above question, there are a couple of key components that lend crucial clues as to the correct answer. The uneasiness dealing with what we would consider traditional "western" medicine, the mention of "other methods" (think alternative medicine), and difficulty with communication, all point to a cultural component to the situation. The fact that the bruises were all the same shape, color, and size is also very significant. Cupping, a traditional (alternative medicine) therapy originated in China and is believed to help increase blood flow and life force. Cupping will produce bruises as described above. These bruises are from a relatively common cultural practice.

Nothing in this scenario points to Dodge Ball, so hopefully you eliminated that option quickly. Allergic reactions seldom produce uniform bruising as described.

Of course, abuse/non-accidental trauma is a possibility with multiple bruises, and the reactions and explanations of the parents need to be taken into consideration. Inconsistent stories that don't "fit" the history or physical findings are troublesome, but that doesn't seem to be the case here. Emergency nurses should always be on the lookout for possible abuse, however, having a basic understanding of religious and/or cultural implications – also known as cultural competency – is crucial.

> *"Ignorance is one of the greatest barriers to understanding between two peoples. If we do not understand each other, if we do not know the culture, the language, or the history of each other, we are unable to see each other as human beings with value and dignity."*
>
> *William C. Wantland*

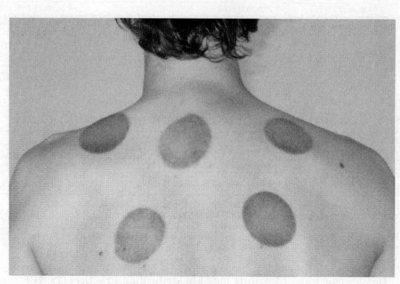

Cupping

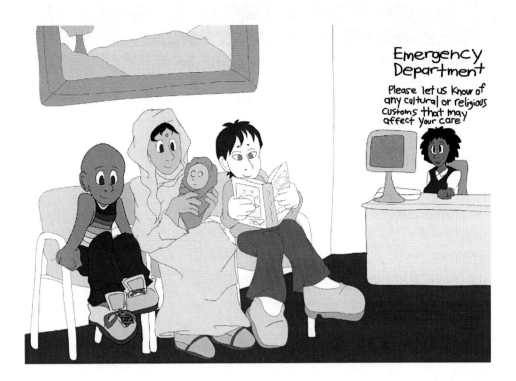

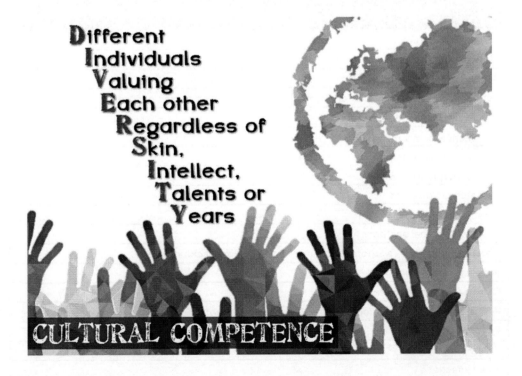

Risk Factors for Child Maltreatment

CAREGIVER OR FAMILY CHARACTERISTICS

- Domestic Violence
- Family history of abuse, neglect, and/or violence
- Inappropriate expectations of the child/development
- Low self-esteem
- Mental health problems (eg, anxiety, depression)
- Negative attitudes toward parenting
- Poor Impulse Control
- Poverty (especially for serious neglect and physical abuse)
- Social Isolation
- Substance abuse

CHILD CHARACTERISTICS

- Age younger than 4-5 years (especially for fatalities)
- Female gender (sexual abuse)
- Handicaps
- Irritable temperament, colicky infant
- Prematurity

Mimics of Child Abuse / Non-Accidental Trauma

Accidental fractures
Alopecia areata
Benign external hydrocephaly
Confusing cutaneous lesions (eg, hemangiomas, Mongolian spots, molluscum contagiosum)
Congenital coagulation disorder
Conjunctival hemorrhages*
Connective tissue disorders
Hair tourniquet syndrome*
Hematologic diseases
Intracranial bleeding*
Irregular hymenal anatomy
Metabolic disorders (eg, homocystinuria, methylmalonic aciduria)
Metastatic bone tumors
Osteogenesis imperfecta
Perinatally transmitted infection with *Chlamydia trachomatis*, bacterial vaginosis, etc
Periostitus
Thrombocytopenia
Tinea infections

* These conditions may be accidental or nonaccidental in etiology

Adapted from: Hicks, R. & Melvin, S. (2004, June 1).
Child abuse: An overview for the primary care physician. Primary Care Reports.

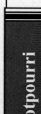

189) Which of the following mnemonics does the Emergency Nursing Pediatric Course (ENPC) use when obtaining an initial health history in the emergency department?

A) ABCDE

B) PQRST

C) SAMPLE

D) AVPU

C – In past versions of ENPC, the CIAMPEDS mnemonic was used. However, in the most recent course update, it has been replaced with the more commonly utilized initial history mnemonic, SAMPLE.

For pre-schoolers, ABCDE is a great way to literally learn their ABC's. PQRST is a mnemonic utilized when eliciting additional information regarding pain, while AVPU is the mnemonic for a short/sweet determination of level of consciousness. At the CPEN exam buffet, before you decide on a main course, SAMPLE the various options first!

	DESCRIPTION	QUESTIONS TO ASK
S	**Symptoms** Patient's chief complaints	"What's wrong?" "What brought you to the hospital?"
A	**Allergies** Seeking to know what type of allergic reaction they experience	"Are you allergic to anything?" "What happens to you when you use something that you're allergic to?"
M	**Medications** Prescribed, OTC drugs, herbal meds, etc.	"Are you taking any medications?" "What are you taking the meds for?" "When did you last take your meds?"
P	**Past Medical Hx** Seeking to know the previous state of health, and previous illnesses	"Have you had this problem before?" "Do you have other medical problems?"
L	**Last Oral Intake** Seeking what are the last oral intakes of the patient	"When did you last eat/drink anything?" "What is it that you last ate?"
E	**Events** Events leading up to the illness or injury	Injury: "How did you get hurt?" Illness: "What led to this problem?"

190) Rapid sequence intubation is being attempted in a child utilizing sedation with Versed® (midazolam), pain management with fentanyl, and neuromuscular blockade (chemical paralysis) with Zemuron® (rocuronium). However, shortly after the medications are administered, the situation quickly spirals into the worst-case scenario of "Can't Intubate, Can't Ventilate." Rocuronium may be reversed with which medication?

A) Anectine® (succinylcholine)

B) Bridion® (sugammadex)

C) Romazicon® (flumazenil)

D) Narcan® (naloxone)

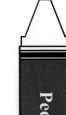

Certified Pediatric Emergency Nurse (CPEN) Review IV

B –The neuromuscular blockade (chemical paralysis) effect of Rocuronium (or vecuronium) can be reversed with Bridion (sugammadex). If a high dose of sugammadex is given IV (or IO), it can "block the blocker" and allow the patient to begin breathing again within just a few minutes.

Narcan (naloxone) is used to reverse the effect of fentanyl and other opiates, and Romazicon (flumazenil) reverses the effect of Versed (midazolam) and other benzodiazapines. (**Memory tip**: the "z" in the reversal agent works on the "z" in the benzos). And please remember that Anectine (succinylcholine) is a depolarizing paralytic, so more paralytics wouldn't help the situation at all.

Rapid sequence intubation is indicated when a sick child needs to be asleep and intubated right now (or at least pretty darn quick). To achieve optimal intubation conditions, many practitioners utilize a "consciousness cocktail" involving a sedative (Etomidate, Versed, Propofol, etc.) to put the child to sleep, an analgesic (fentanyl, etc.) to take away pain (being intubated hurts), and a neuromuscular blocking agent (paralytic), to relax the airway structures so tissues can be moved around to find the right hole, i.e. the trachea.

When it comes to the paralytic part of the cocktail, there are really only two kinds of neuromuscular blocking agents in common practice out there: Succinylcholine ("Sux") and everything else. Succinylcholine has been used for decades with emergency airway management as it "kicks in fast and goes away fast." This means that in most (*but, not all*) patients, the onset to chemical paralysis is less than a minute and it's worn off in less than 10 minutes. So, if the patient were unable to be intubated, they would be breathing on their own in less than 10 minutes. However great that sounds, succinylcholine has several serious side effects, most notably in patients with spinal cord injuries, burns, crush injuries, renal failure, and children with diagnosed *or yet undiagnosed* Duchene's Muscular Dystrophy (the most common form of muscular dystrophy). When succinylcholine is administered to these children, life threatening hyperkalemia can be the result, with serum potassium quickly going from normal (around 4) to lethal (around 14).

For the vast majority of children and adults requiring emergency intubation, "Sux" has been used for decades, producing optimal intubation conditions safely and quickly. Following administration of the initial medications and once proper tube placement has been confirmed by waveform capnography, longer term chemical paralysis is often needed. That's where Norcuron (vecuronium or "Vec') and more recently Zemuron (rocuronium or "Roc") come into play. They take a little longer to "kick in" (1-3 minutes), but they also last longer (20-30+ minutes) and don't have the hyperkalemia potential that is associated with "Sux." If the initial dose of rocuronium is on higher end, then the onset time gets really close to that of succinylcholine. In the critical care units, another longer term neuromuscular blocking agent Nimbex® (cisatracurium or "Cis"), is commonly used.

So, going back to our scenario, let's say the tube doesn't go in, and even worse, despite using a backup/alternate airway (Laryngeal Mask Airway, King Airway, i-gel airway), air can't go in or out, what do you do? Remember, if succinylcholine was given, in most (*but, not all*) patients, the paralytic will "wear off" in less than 10 minutes. That seems like a long time. What is the reversal agent for "Sux" if you don't want to wait that long? The bad news is that reversal agent for succinylcholine is called "Time." Time, along with patience and prayer are your only options until the "Sux" wears off. This is yet another reminder as to why bag-mask ventilation is an essential and lifesaving skill!

For rapid-sequence intubation in children, put them to sleep, take away their pain, and then BRIEFLY paralyze them until the tube is confirmed to be in the correct spot. Once the tube is in, give them more sedation, more pain medicine... Are you noticing a trend? If longer term chemical paralysis is required, either for producing optimal intubation conditions, or for maximizing ventilatory support (for ARDS, etc.)... remember, rocuronium rocks, but Bridion (sugammadex) breaks the blockade and helps take some of the terror out of tubing tiny tots.

Pediatric Potpourri

Certified Pediatric Emergency Nurse (CPEN) Review IV

191) A 15-year-old female is brought to the emergency department (ED) with several weeks of severe, repeated bouts of nausea and vomiting, and periumbilical abdominal pain. The patient states that the only thing that relieves her vomiting is to use marijuana daily and take long, hot showers several times a day. The nurse should expect treatment to be based on which of the following conditions:

A) Avoidant/Restrictive Food Intake Disorder (ARFID)

B) Cannabinoid Hyperemesis Syndrome (CHS)

C) Gastroesophageal Reflux Disease (GERD)

D) Intrauterine Growth Restriction (IUGR)

B - This patient is most likely experiencing Cannabinoid Hyperemesis Syndrome (CHS). CHS can occur when an individual uses marijuana approximately 20 or more times a month and develops acute nausea and vomiting unrelieved by standard antiemetic methods. Methods for reduction of the symptoms include long, hot showers, sometimes lasting several hours (difficult to perform in the ED), OTC capsaicin cream applied topically (yes, the same stuff that's in hot sauce and pepper spray), and the administration of Haldol® (haloperidol).

In situations where a digestive or eating disorder is suspected, it is important to evaluate the patient's dietary and nutritional status. In this case, the question doesn't ask about what to evaluate; rather, it asks what to *suspect* based only on the limited information provided. When treating any female patient under the age of 90, pregnancy is certainly a possibility, but as the question specifically mentions vomiting (emesis) and marijuana (aka., cannabis) use, an answer involving both those concepts is a good choice! **Be aware that CHS is relatively uncommon. Testing for other causes may be indicated, especially if the symptoms are of acute onset.**

192) After multiple trips to the emergency department (ED) where extensive workups have been negative, a previously healthy 16-year old male presents yet again with abdominal pain, significant nausea, and repeated vomiting. A working diagnosis of cannabinoid hyperemesis syndrome (CHS) was determined after the patient revealed that he recently moved to Colorado and has smoked marijuana several times every day for the last few months. While in the ED, an initial treatment plan with the least amount of unintended side effects for CHS would be:

A) Use marijuana the next time an attack occurs

B) Take a long, hot shower several times a day

C) Apply capsaicin cream to the abdomen area

D) Administer Haldol (haloperidol)

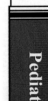

C - There are two important elements to this type of question: 1) the mention of "while in the ED" and 2) patient safety (minimal side effects). Given those parameters, and while all of the above treatments have shown varying degrees of success, the application of capsaicin cream is the best answer because it can be initiated in the ED and appears to have the least amount of side effects, beyond a not unexpected "burning sensation" on the skin (it contains the same active ingredient in many hot sauces, after all). Application of a 1-mm thick coating of 0.025% to 0.075% capsaicin cream to a clean, dry area of the abdomen is most commonly reported. The cream may be covered with a transparent plastic dressing, such as cling wrap. Additional application of capsaicin cream to the back and arms has also been described in some case reports. Onset is rapid, within 5- to 10-minutes, but duration and recommendations regarding repeat applications in the ED or home settings are unclear. Gloves should be worn while applying the cream, to prevent skin irritation to the provider. Patients should be cautioned to avoid touching their face, eyes, or mucous membranes (ouch!).

Capsaicin tips from an expert provider:

- The cream tends to "melt" into the skin; you or the patient can rub it in
- Use gloves to protect the person applying, and remember not to touch eyes or open sores!
- Try a light cling wrap covering over all four quadrants, covering at least 80% of the abdomen
- Leave on at least four hours, then remove with a warm cloth and reapply

The potential for dermatologic reactions to a topical cream exist, but systemic side effects of topical capsaicin are unlikely. Just like at your local restaurant when you dare to order "Are You Really Sure You Want Them That Hot" wings, if excessive skin irritation occurs to either the patient or provider, wash the area with cold milk (or another dairy product such as cream or yogurt) to quickly relieve symptoms.

Repeated use of marijuana has shown to work in the short-term for CHS, however, it then begins to have a paradoxical effect, intensifying the nausea and repeated vomiting effects (bummer!). Long, hot showers can initially help, and yes, cleanliness is next to Godliness, but the time and expense of this treatment (many, many hours per day and potentially multiple hundreds of dollars in gas/electric bills) pose serious (though non-medical) side effects. Haldol (haloperidol) as well as some benzodiazepines have been reported as producing positive results, but the potential troublesome side effects of these medications (especially dystonia, extrapyramidal reactions, and neuroleptic malignant syndrome with Haldol) is significant.

Studies have shown that typical antiemetic medications have <u>little or no</u> effect in stopping the repeated vomiting. Though normally "Zofran® (ondansetron) and saline" fixes just about everything for vomiting and dehydration, when it comes to CHS, capsaicin cream on the belly with some cling wrap is where it's at!

193) Johns Hopkins Medicine states that "among youth, e-cigarettes (vaping) are more popular than any traditional tobacco product." Vaping commonly involves the inhalation of nicotine and/or which of the following?

A) Marijuana

B) Ketamine

C) Fentanyl

D) Alcohol

A – Marijuana is a common addition to the vaping experience. Some of us are old enough to remember kids enjoying "candy cigarettes" or "bubble gum cigarettes" and an advertising campaign aimed at getting women to smoke a particular brand of cigarettes by telling those women that "We've come a long way baby." Well, we certainly have come a long way. Kids are no longer "smoking" candy and tobacco is no longer advertised on television. Initially introduced as an alternative to cigarette smoking and to assist with smoking cessation, vaping has become all the rage. This technique involves a small hand-held, battery powered heater which vaporizes (hence the term, "vaping") the liquid to be inhaled. Though there are vaping liquids available without nicotine, far more common and far more popular, are the legal options with nicotine, or depending on location, legal/illegal options with nicotine and marijuana.

From the kid's perspective, product marketing was the key. These devices allowed the ability to "smoke" without the cigarette odor and discolorations to teeth and fingers. It is cheaper overall than cigarettes. And as a bonus, vaping cartridges come in various flavors ranging from sour patch kids to cotton candy.

So, what's the problem? Several actually. First and foremost, one vape cartridge can be the nicotine equivalent of an entire pack of cigarettes! This amount of nicotine can easily result in anxiety, tachycardia, and hypertension. And in children, it can also lead to seizures from nicotine toxicity.

And if this wasn't enough, now there is the diagnosis of EVALI, (E-cigarette or Vaping Associated Lung Injury). First reported in 2018, EVALI has resulted in hundreds of deaths and thousands of hospitalizations from pulmonary failure in previously healthy teens. These issues appear to be primarily in patients who are vaping not only the nicotine liquid, but specifically those using the combination of nicotine and marijuana/THC. Vitamin E liquid is used in the "black market" preparation of some of these products and appears to be a "culprit" in EVALI. Think for just a moment about the appearance of a Vitamin E Softgel. It's soft and squishy and made for swallowing into the stomach, not being vaporized and inhaled into the lungs. Respiratory therapists remind us that just about everything can be given via a neb. Albuterol... Morphine... Lasix... Antibiotics... Absolutely. Nicotine, marijuana/THC, and Vitamin E ... not the best choice if you want to avoid EVALI!

Vaping 101 – Additional Insights from a <u>Non-Medical</u> "Former Vaper"

> Lord,
> Give Me Coffee
> To change the Things I Can,
> Wine,
> to Forget the Things I Can't
> and 30 mils of E-juice
> so I can Sit Back and Vape
> until I Can Figure Out The
> Difference
> ~ VL

What's the difference between vaping/e-cigarette devices and "Dab pens" (i.e., marijuana vaporizer devices)?

- Vapes, JUULs, Dab pens..." These can be confusing at times with the ever-evolving terms. It is hard to keep up with all the terms kids are using nowadays. But here's a quick breakdown of the common terms:
    - Vape: Smokeless tobacco that vaporizes liquid, <u>not</u> THC/marijuana. It most commonly contains nicotine.
    - JUUL™: A popular, commercially available, brand of e-cigarette.
    - "Dab pen": A vaporizer device that <u>does</u> contain THC/marijuana components.

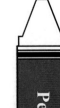

Certified Pediatric Emergency Nurse (CPEN) Review IV

Why are kids using e-cigarettes to begin with?

- According to the American Lung Association, and my personal experience knowing several young smokers, here are a few common reasons:
  - Peer pressure (Friends are doing it, so they want to fit in and be cool).
  - They think it's a safe alternative to tobacco so there's no long-term harm.
  - They use nicotine to help manage stress.

Why are kids using vaping or ENDS (Electronic Nicotine Delivery Systems) vs. regular tobacco, particularly if they have the same effect?

- The tobacco industry has lobbied to make it seem that vaping is a safe alternative to using tobacco. The FDA sent out warning letters to several companies, including JUUL, explaining that marketing vapes as a "safer alternative" to smoking is unacceptable.
- You can't get gummy bear, graham cracker, or cotton candy flavored cigarettes. There are a myriad of flavors available with e-juice, aka., what vapes are filled with, as opposed to traditional tobacco or menthol.
- Discreteness:
  - The odor dissipates quickly along with the smoke itself, leaving no trace that someone was vaping. This discreteness makes it popular among youth who don't want others, especially parents or teachers, to know that they're using vaping devices.

So, what's needed to vape anyways?

- For disposable e-cigarettes, such as Blu™ (An all-in-one e-cigarette you throw away after it's empty; commonly sold at gas stations/tobacco shops/superstores), all you need is the device itself.
- On the other hand, here is what's traditionally required for a vaping device:
  - E-juice: You choose the flavor of liquid (and there are countless flavors out there), fill up the vaporizer portion, activate the battery, and vapor is created. Another common option is JUUL pods.
  - Battery: This may be included as part of the kit.
  - Vaporizer: The part that vaporizes the liquid. Some companies offer plug and play devices that have the vaporizer component combined with the e-juice portion, example: JUUL pods. A JUUL pod contains the vaporizer and e-juice in one device. It's similar in concept to the Blu cigarettes, but you can replace the pod on the top instead of throwing away the entire unit/battery. For advanced users, those who are looking for a more customized experience, you can use "Tanks and Mods." Tanks, as the name alludes to, hold a lot of e-juice, while Mods are the part that vaporizes the juice.

Types of E-cigarettes

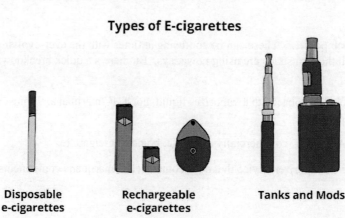

Disposable e-cigarettes   Rechargeable e-cigarettes   Tanks and Mods

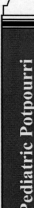

Pediatric Potpourri

If the legal smoking age in the United States is 21, then how are kids getting these vaping devices anyways?

- I interviewed a 14-year old user, and asked him where he and his friends got the products:
  - Vapor shops/head shops: These businesses specialize in e-cigarette products, but, as they are scrutinized heavily by regulators, tend to religiously check ID. The selection in flavors at these shops is spectacular, however, again, they won't let you in the door, not to mention purchase anything, if you are under 21.
  - Gas stations/convenience stores: These may be more lax due to higher volume of general business as well as perceived less intense scrutiny.
  - Online websites: Legally, websites that sell vaping devices/liquids are required to verify the age of the purchaser. However, some sites do not have age verification at all, which allows minors to buy the products. Kids talking with other kids can quickly figure out which sites are the best options for non-age verified purchases.
  - P-2-P: People selling to people. High schoolers/adults buy the vapes (with nicotine primarily) and sell to minors.

How long does an e-cigarette tend to last for?

- It all depends on the user. For some, it can last for a week or even two, and for others, only one day. This is just like the difference in a cigarette/day vs. a pack/day traditional cigarette smoker.

Up in Smoke: Let's talk marijuana:

- A marijuana cartridge is a system to vaporize marijuana concentrate for medical/recreational purposes. Like e-cigarettes, they come in multiple forms:
  - Disposable cartridge: The battery and cartridge are in an all-in-one form. You use it until it's empty and then throw it away.
  - Battery + disposable cartridge: The cartridges and battery component are separate, and when a cartridge is empty, you throw away the cartridge, but not the reusable battery.
  - Dry herb/concentrate vaporizer: These are higher-end devices that are meant to vaporize the actual plant/concentrates. "Wax, resin, batter, and butter" are all concentrates created using solvents to remove the plant matter from the marijuana plant itself and leave behind almost pure THC. They tend to produce more benefits, aka., a better high, versus their cartridge counterparts. But, to no surprise, these are significantly more expensive.

How do kids get these?

- Kids can't purchase marijuana products from a legal dispensary. It would be easier to walk into Fort Knox than for an underage minor to walk into a dispensary. THC products are not legally sold in gas stations or vape shops. However, in some states, if you are over 21 years of age, marijuana products can be bought at dispensaries, via online delivery services, and can even be shipped directly to your door!

So, why are kids getting sick from the use of these products?

- These "cartridges" and "concentrates" from legitimate dispensaries aren't the issue. I've personally used many dispensary cartridges and never been sick from one or heard of someone being sick from one.

- Enter the world of "CARTNIGHT," "Exotic cart," or "Mario Carts." Black market/illegally manufactured marijuana cartridges are filled with "Concentrate," not marijuana and sold for temptingly low prices. The last time I bought one at a legal dispensary, a traditional marijuana pen was $50 for a 0.3-gram pen. A 0.3-gram pen for an average user will last about a week or so. The last time I bought an illicit cartridge (before the vaping epidemic started), was $20 for a 1-gram cartridge. Three times the amount of concentrate for half the price. Spoiler alert: It wasn't really marijuana concentrate and gave me hallucinations that aren't associated with the use of marijuana. What was it? Who knows? But it certainly wasn't marijuana!

- These cartridges are manufactured in dealers' garages, basements, or wherever. They use packaging that looks remarkably like legitimate marijuana products and, in some cases, copy and print the real labels from legitimate products. You can't buy these from a dispensary. You buy them from drug dealers off the street. When you buy "dab pens" or "carts" from a dealer at a school or on the street, you really never know what you're going to get!

So why are teens using them?

- Simple. It's cheap and provides a decent high, albeit at the expense of the user's health.

- Teens aren't choosing high-quality marijuana or seeking the medical benefits with these products. They probably don't have glaucoma. They're just chasing a high.

- Just like with e-cigarettes, teens think that these are safer because there's no actual smoke.

- The odor dissipates quickly along with the smoke itself, leaving no trace that someone was vaping. This discreteness makes it popular among youth who don't want others, especially parents or teachers, to know that they're using vaping or even worse, marijuana devices.

Summary of the Smokes:

- E-cigarettes were initially marketed as a "safer alternative" to traditional cigarettes or as a smoking cessation aid, but when they also came in various "kid friendly" flavors, that changed the game completely. Now, JUULs are only available in "cigarette" flavors, but a whole lot of kids "got hooked" on the nicotine.

- Marijuana used to be only available from your local drug dealer, but with the introduction of medical marijuana, many states legalizing marijuana, and of course, the internet, the game changed yet again.

- So, when it comes to "vapes, dabs, and carts," unless you purchase the product from a reputable/licensed shop, you never know what you are going to get!

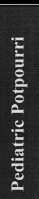

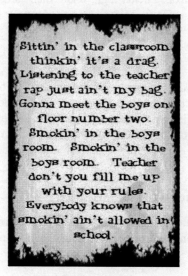

Motley Crue

Certified Pediatric Emergency Nurse (CPEN) Review IV

Up in Smoke? Dangers of E-cigarettes and Vaping
Laurie Romig MD, FACEP, BC-EMS

Most of us have heard about the on-going epidemic of fatalities related to the use of opioid drugs, but another public health emergency is gaining increased attention, at least partly because of the recognition of a pattern of severe lung damage among users of e-cigarettes and vaping devices. As of January 2020, the Centers for Disease Control and Prevention (CDC) had identified 2668 cases of and 60 deaths attributed to E-cigarette or Vaping Product Use-Associated Lung Injury, or EVALI. While there is a lot of formal research yet to be done to understand all the short and long-term effects of EVALI and other complications related to e-cigarettes and/or vaping, we do have some information to help you understand currently known issues and hazards.

Role in substance abuse disorders

The use of e-cigarettes and vaping devices are both highly addictive behaviors, even for people who smoke conventional cigarettes. Nicotine is the primary cause of addiction, but other substances such as tetrahydrocannabinol (THC) may be present; these additives may or may not be listed on the label and may be added by the user. Like alcohol, nicotine addiction is a common feature of multi-drug substance abuse and can complicate both medical care and substance abuse treatment.

History and basics of e-cigarettes and vaping

E-cigarettes and vaping devices are collectively known as Electronic Nicotine Delivery Systems (ENDS). There are many legally manufactured ENDS products with relatively minimal federal or state oversight, but there are also many, many illegal and illicit devices and liquid preparations available to the public. For example, as of 2014, there were more than 7,700 flavorings available for use with ENDS devices. This diversity of materials makes it difficult to thoroughly understand related health issues. Today's understanding of ENDS use and potential complications is probably at about the same level as knowledge about conventional tobacco/nicotine use was in the 1970s.

The e-cigarette was invented in 2003, primarily as part of the search for a safer delivery system for nicotine and a potential aid to smoking cessation. Conventional cigarette smoke is known to contain a large number of products of combustion (burning), many of which are known to cause various cancers or other types of damage to the body. E-cigarettes and vaping products attempt to address these dangers, at least partly, by avoiding the actual burning of tobacco leaves, using lower temperatures, and adding liquid extracts that can still release nicotine. Nicotine-containing vaping liquids contain varying amounts of nicotine; for example, a single JUUL brand vape cartridge contains the same amount of nicotine found in a full pack of conventional cigarettes. Other brands are following suit. Nicotine and other additives are found in the resulting vapor, so it's possible that second-hand smoke effects may still be an issue. Unfortunately, the short and long-term effects of specific components of the vapor are not yet well understood. Research does seem to show that use of ENDS decreases the incidence of lung cancer compared to conventional cigarette smoke inhalation, but many other effects are poorly understood and possibly very risky.

Another complicating factor is that, in some cases, the contents of the fluid (also known as e-juice) can be modified by users or distributors. This can be used to alter amounts of nicotine, flavorings, and THC, the psychoactive component of marijuana. Among other problems, THC can permanently affect brain development, not just in children and juveniles, but in young adults into their mid-20s.

Students by the numbers

Middle school and high school students are an especially concerning group of ENDS users who may be putting themselves in danger of both long and short-term health problems. Here are some interesting numbers:

- In 2017, the Food and Drug Administration (FDA) released survey statistics showing that more than two million middle and high school students were using ENDS.

Pediatric Potpourri

- Approximately 80% of these users believed that ENDS use was either totally or relatively risk-free.
- Between 2017 and 2018, high school student use nearly doubled and middle school student use increased by 700%.
- Of students who use ENDS but not conventional tobacco, 72.2% of high school students and 59.2% of middle school students use flavors.

Many people feel that advertisements for various ENDS products have been designed to appeal specifically to minors, even though a growing number of states specifically forbid sales to minors. Others feel that the development of flavored e-liquids specifically targeted young people. Interestingly, mint is the most popular flavor. The leading manufacturer of e-cig and vaping products, JUUL, has very recently agreed to stop manufacturing or distributing flavors other than tobacco and menthol. Media coverage includes a growing number of student ENDS users who have suffered various complications or who agree that student-focused marketing was a factor in their decisions to use ENDS.

E-cigarette or Vaping Product Use-Associated Lung Injury (EVALI)

While there had been some concern over the many "unknowns" associated with e-cig or vape use, the factor that has recently stood out is the recognition of a pattern of extremely serious and sometimes fatal lung problems found in some ENDS users. The condition has been named "E-cigarette or Vaping Product Use-Associated Lung Injury (EVALI)." In October 2019, 1,299 cases of EVALI were reported, with 26 deaths. About one month later, the case count was up to 2,290, with 47 deaths, including an increase of 118 cases and 5 deaths in just one week. Fortunately, as of January 14, 2020, these case reports peaked in the week of September 8, 2020 and have been decreasing since then.

EVALI patients mostly have breathing-related symptoms, but they may also have fever, chills, weight loss, and nausea/vomiting, abdominal pain, or diarrhea. Some patients require a ventilator and ICU care; others may be treated without admission to the hospital. ENDS users who are over age 50, who are pregnant, or who have heart or other lung disease are at higher risk. It appears that, at least in serious cases, lung tissue is destroyed and function can't be recovered. One patient required a double lung transplant!

What do these EVALI cases have in common?

- All have been in people who use e-cigarettes or vape pens
- 82% vaped THC (the component of marijuana that causes euphoria and other desired effects) either with or without nicotine
- 76% were aged 35 years or less, with a range of 13 to 85 years.
- Compared to ENDS users who have not had EVALI, these lung injury patients had higher odds of:
  - Using only THC products
  - Frequent use (5 or more times a day)
  - Obtaining vape fluid from informal sources (not legally obtained or regulated)
  - Use of "Dank Vapes," an illicit THC product that comes in 31 flavors

What causes EVALI?

The cause of EVALI continues to be uncertain, but several possibilities have been proposed. The current leading thought is that inhalation of vitamin E acetate causes the lung damage. The chemical is often used in the ENDS industry as a thickening and butter-flavoring agent. It is harmless when eaten but causes lung tissue damage when inhaled. Another chemical, diacetyl, is another suspect. There may be other causes or other factors that combine to cause EVALI. There may be other ingredients of e-liquids that cause medical problems or injuries related to the heating process used. Further experience and research are required.

Pediatric Potpourri

Other hazards of ENDS

- Becoming addicted to nicotine or worsening already established addiction
  - Although the e-cig/vape concept was created with the purpose of helping people to stop or decrease conventional smoking, the current vaping liquids often have higher levels of nicotine than regular cigarettes.
- Heart problems
  - ENDS effects on the heart may be mixed and are believed to be due to the nicotine content, just like conventional smoking. Some research suggests that these include the bad effects on cholesterol and blood sugar, and decreasing blood flow in the heart even more than regular cigarettes. Other studies have had conflicting results.
- Pediatric exposure
  - Between 2013 and 2017, over 4000 children under age five years were evaluated by Poison Control Centers or emergency departments for nicotine exposure related to ENDS. Over 90% of these were due to swallowing e-liquids. Hundreds of cases needed emergency department evaluation and treatment each year. Fortunately, that number is dropping slightly now because of special state and federal legislation that requires child-resistant packaging and special labeling of nicotine-containing products.

What now?

This crisis is so significant that the CDC Emergency Operations Center has been activated to the same level that has been employed for public health emergencies like the Zika virus and hurricanes. Congress and the FDA have collectively increased the minimum age for tobacco sales to 21 years of age and the FDA has prioritized enforcement of their previously authorized power to require authorization of e-cigarettes and vaping products prior to sale. To date, no products have been authorized; as of the end of January 2020, the FDA is expected to enforce a ban on the of sale of:

- Flavored, cartridge-based ENDS products other than tobacco or menthol flavors. This is the most commonly used type of product by minors.
- All ENDS products for which the manufacturer has failed to take adequate measures to prevent access to minors. These measures may include monitoring retailer compliance with age-verification requirements and sales restrictions and the use of enforcement measures for violations.
- Any ENDS product that is targeted to minors or likely to promote use of ENDS by minors

There are some exceptions to this enforcement, mostly related to the sale of refillable ENDS products that are mostly used by adults.

Various states have already enacted or are in the process of enacting legislation restricting e-cigarette and vaping products. Check with your state government.

Further study and public education programs are also in the process of production and implementation.

Advice for individuals and medical providers to follow comes from the CDC and is updated as further information becomes available. As of November 2019, the recommendations of the CDC for the general public include:

- Avoid vaping, especially if you aren't a smoker. Consider completely avoiding e-cigarettes or vaping products.
- Children, young adults, and pregnant women should not smoke or vape at all.

- Avoid smoking THC, even if the product is legal.
  - A very high percentage of EVALI patients vaped THC.
- Don't use modified or street-bought vaping products.
  - You just don't know what you're really getting.
  - A very high percentage of EVALI patients use modified or street-bought products.
  - Do not use products that contain vitamin E acetate.
- Don't use e-cig/vapes as part of an attempt to stop smoking.
  - You could be exposing yourself to even higher levels of nicotine and other harmful chemicals.
  - Stick to FDA-approved nicotine replacement products.

Conclusion

Our understanding of ENDS-related issues is progressing rapidly. Recommendations may change, even as frequently as on a monthly basis. Whether you are concerned for yourself or someone else, you can keep your information up to date via social media and news sources, but for the most accurate official information, go to the CDC.gov website.

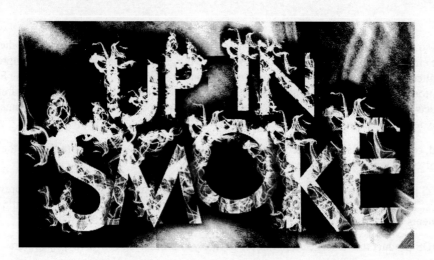

194) You have just received four patients from a multi-vehicle crash. According to the Pediatric Assessment Triangle, which patient should receive the highest priority?

A) 2-year old, quiet and non-interactive, increased work of breathing, pale skin/brisk capillary refill

B) 7-year old, crying, normal breathing, pink skin/brisk capillary refill

C) 9-year old, alert, normal breathing, pink skin/brisk capillary refill

D) 12-year old, moaning but alert, normal breathing, and pale skin/delayed capillary refill

A – According to the pediatric assessment triangle, a 2-year old who is calm after a car crash and in a strange environment is abnormal, as are tachypnea and pale skin. Remember, *a quiet pediatric patient is a scary pediatric patient*, and the quiet pediatric trauma patient is one that should absolutely make you pay attention!

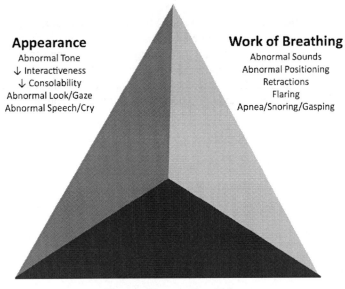

Appearance
Abnormal Tone
↓ Interactiveness
↓ Consolability
Abnormal Look/Gaze
Abnormal Speech/Cry

Work of Breathing
Abnormal Sounds
Abnormal Positioning
Retractions
Flaring
Apnea/Snoring/Gasping

Circulation to the Skin
Pallor
Mottling
Cyanosis

195) Which of the following is a warning sign of suicidal ideations in a teenage patient?

A) Reporting nicotine use

B) Expressing the need for acceptance from peers

C) Loss of interest in usual activities

D) Feelings of depression after failing a test

C – In addition to the loss of interest in usual activities, another warning sign of suicide might be signs of depression; however, periodic feelings of depression are not necessarily a warning sign of suicide. Reporting nicotine use is commonplace, and the desire for peer group acceptance is common among nearly all people in a social environment.

Other signs or observations associated with possible suicidal ideations can include:

- Changes in eating or sleeping habits
- Loss of interest in usual activities or school
- Alcohol and drug use
- Neglect in personal appearance
- Preoccupation with death and dying
- Withdrawal from friends and family
- Acting out in behavior or running away from home
- Difficulty concentrating, even during previously enjoyable activities
- Feelings of wanting to die
- Internet searches on suicide or ways to kill yourself

Recognition and early interventions are keys to preventing the tragedy of suicide. Parents can help by taking steps such as keeping medications and especially firearms away from children, getting help from a mental health professional, supporting your child by listening, avoiding undue criticism, and becoming informed through further research and local support groups. Importantly remember, if you don't ask... they probably won't tell! Asking about suicidal ideations does NOT put the thoughts into their head and does NOT make teens more likely to attempt suicide. If you think about it, ask about it!

Some wonderful sources of additional information:

- The American Foundation for Suicide Prevention (www.afsp.org)
- Suicide Awareness Voices of Education (SAVE) (www.save.org)

Additional Insights from a Pediatric Emergency Medicine Attending Physician:

Remember that the deaths/suicides of other teens or celebrities may trigger suicidal thoughts and even copycat suicide attempts.

196) A 22-month old boy arrives in the ED after ingesting an unknown amount of a laundry detergent pod. The child appears lethargic, tachypneic, with obvious retractions. Upon further assessment, the child is irritable, inconsolable, drooling, and has visible burn areas on the lips and oropharynx. Vital signs: HR 142, RR 46, oxygen saturation 92% on room air. Upon auscultation, coarse lungs sounds are noted bilaterally with rhonchi and rales. What is the **most** likely primary cause of the child's presentation?

A) Visible oral burns

B) Ingestion of the detergent

C) Aspiration of the detergent

D) Allergic reaction to the detergent

C – Aspiration of detergent is the primary cause of the presentation. Laundry detergent pods present unique dangers to small children who place the colorful packets into their mouths. Laundry detergent pods tend to burst when bitten into or punctured. This sends a large volume of highly concentrated detergent throughout the entire oropharynx, which in turn startles the child and they instinctively inhale sharply. As they inhale, the highly concentrated alkalotic detergent is aspirated, leading to the pulmonary toxic effects described above. Aspiration of the alkaline detergent can cause mild to severe burns anywhere in the upper and lower airways. This results in swelling and edema and leading to the rapid onset of varying degrees of airway obstruction that will probably get worse before it gets better. Ingestion is a concern as well, as the esophagus and stomach can also be burned. This scenario is way too complex to suspect an allergic reaction. When a caregiver brings a child to the ED with detergent ingestion concern, it's always best to consider the possibility of aspiration and evolving airway developments.

> "All things are poisons, for there is nothing without poisonous qualities.
> It is only the dose which makes a thing poison."
>
> **Paracelsus**

Certified Pediatric Emergency Nurse (CPEN) Review IV

Contrary to what we see in certain "cult sci-fi" movies, hazardous materials are not green and glow in the dark, nor are they found only at high-tech warehouses or super-secret labs. In fact, every substance, from oxygen to water to phosgene can be a hazardous material. Oxygen, in too high a concentration, is toxic, especially to premature neonates. Oxygen is the "ox" in oxidizer, which literally causes other substances to burn. In fact, liquid oxygen is used as rocket fuel. Water is also toxic in high quantities by disrupting electrolyte balances. And phosgene, well, that just sounds like a bad chemical, and indeed, it is. It is used in the manufacturing of many plastics and pesticides. Phosgene is very toxic at any dose.

Even though there are thousands of known toxins, the list of antidotes is disproportionately small. And while antidotes or treatment guidelines pertaining to a specific toxin do exist, for the most part, your treatment will vary little from standard care. Below is a table of known toxins and their antidotes or reversal agents.

Toxic Substance / Poisoning	Antidote
Acetaminophen	N-Acetylcysteine (PO/NG Mucomyst), Acetadote (IV)
Benzodiazepines	Flumazenil (Romazicon)
Beta-Blockers	Glucagon
Calcium Channel Blockers	Calcium chloride
Carbon Monoxide	Hyperbaric or high-flow oxygen
Cyanide	Hydroxocobalamin (Cyanokit)
Digoxin	Digibind
Heavy Metals	Dimercaprol (BAL), Edetate calcium disodium (EDTA), or D-penicillamine
Heparin	Protamine
Hydrofluoric acid or Fluoride exposure	Calcium Gluconate
Iron	Deferoxamine
Methemoglobinemic Agents, Nitrates	Methylene blue
Opiates, ACE Inhibitors	Narcan
Organophosphate / Nerve Agent	Atropine & pralidoxime (2-PAM)
SSRI	Cyproheptadine
Toxic Alcohols (ethylene glycol, methanol)	Fomepizole (antizol) or ethanol
Tricyclic antidepressants	Sodium Bicarbonate
Warfarin (Coumadin)	Vitamin K, FFP, or Kcentra

Certified Pediatric Emergency Nurse (CPEN) Review IV

197) You are treating a 12-year old female after exposure to chlorine gas. From the EMS report, you understand the patient was not exposed to any other toxic substances. The child had a first round of gross decontamination in the field. She is awake and alert, but complaining of inability to breathe while lying flat, skin irritation, and chest discomfort. Your assessment reveals slight erythema in the hands, bilateral rales, and tachypnea. In addition to detailed contamination and supplemental oxygen, what is the recommended course of treatment?

A) Inhaled albuterol and rapid intubation

B) Rapid CPAP and IV steroids

C) IV steroids and inhaled albuterol

D) Rapid intubation and IV steroids

B – In addition to the detailed decontamination and supplemental oxygen already mentioned, CPAP and IV steroids would be part of the recommended course of treatment for a patient after chlorine gas exposure. If the question mentions chlorine – think pulmonary edema! This patient is exhibiting signs and symptoms associated with non-cardiogenic pulmonary edema (think orthopnea, like big people CHFers). After ensuring proper detailed decontamination, (more than what was done before arrival in the ER) and supplemental oxygen, the rapid addition of CPAP is the next most appropriate intervention when treating non-cardiogenic pulmonary edema in the conscious and alert patient. Some studies have shown that IV steroids may be beneficial for patients exposed to chlorine, but these should be administered after addressing the pulmonary edema. CPAP works quickly, but steroids take much longer to kick in. Inhaled beta-agonists, i.e. albuterol, are certainly beneficial with wheezing, but in this scenario, symptoms OTHER THAN wheezing are identified. Lastly, while intubation is indicated for severe respiratory distress and ARDS, at the moment, this child doesn't require better living through an endotracheal tube.

Additional Insights from a Pediatric Emergency Medicine Attending Physician:

Detailed decontamination, aka., secondary decontamination, consists of the decontamination and cleaning of every inch of skin and even inside some orifices. Decontamination in the field is usually limited to disrobing and walking under/through a water spray to remove gross contamination. And to no surprise, different substances require different levels of decontamination.

198) The **first** sign of exposure to a nerve agent tends to be:

A) Bronchorrhea

B) Emesis

C) Fasciculations

D) Miosis

D – The first sign of exposure to a nerve agent is typically miosis. When dealing with nerve agents, the route and amount of exposure are important factors. What part of the body is almost NEVER fully covered or protected? The eyes! The term miosis, comes from the Ancient Greek μύειν, mūein, "to close the eyes," and is the very first sign of a nerve agent exposure. Small vapor molecules of a nerve agent pass unaltered through the cornea and interact directly with the pupillary muscles, causing miosis (constricted pupils). Think of this as your body's way of saying "please don't come into my eyes (and brain/body)." Patients with nerve agent exposure often complain of dim or blurred vision because of this. Emesis, fasciculations (muscle twitches) and bronchorrhea (lots and lots of airway secretions) are all common symptoms of exposure to nerve agents, but miosis occurs first. Remember, when performing a neuro assessment or with nerve agent exposure, the pupils are the windows to the brain. **AND ALWAYS REMEMBER THAT IF A NERVE GAS VICTIM ISN'T PROPERLY DECONTAMINATED, YOU TOO MAY GET BLURRED VISION AND MUCH, MUCH MORE!**

Certified Pediatric Emergency Nurse (CPEN) Review IV

199) A 16-year old female arrives in the ED after a suicide attempt. EMS reports that the patient ingested an unknown amount of malathion, an organophosphate insecticide. If proper PPE is not utilized, the healthcare team is most at risk of **secondary** contamination by:

A) Vomit from the patient

B) Residual malathion around the patient's mouth

C) Needle stick contamination

D) Coughing from the patient

A – Vomit from the patient poses a serious exposure risk to healthcare workers without PPE. Emesis from a patient who has ingested malathion is toxic and highly contaminated. While potentially contaminated, it is unlikely there was a large amount of residual malathion around the patient's mouth since in this case there was intentional ingestion. A needle stick poses no threat to the provider from secondary contamination (at least from the poison). Coughing could potentially cause secondary contamination, but is less likely as the route of administration was specifically ingestion, not inhalation.

200) When irrigating an eye following exposure to an alkali substance, what is the **best** device to use?

A) Tonometer

B) Ocular irrigation device

C) Sterile Basin

D) Normal saline

B – An "ocular irrigation device," such as a Morgan Lens® is the best device for ocular irrigation. Tonometers measure ocular pressure, but are not used for irrigation, and a sterile basin isn't necessary. Normal saline or lactated ringers are the solutions often used for ocular irrigation, but. remember the question specifically mentioned a *device*, not a fluid, to help with irrigating an eye.

201) When irrigating an eye after an exposure to an alkali substance, what is the **best** indication that an adequate amount of irrigation has been completed?

A) Saponification

B) Dua Classification: Grade II

C) An ocular pH of 7.0 – 7.3

D) Pain of 0 on a 0 – 10 pain scale

C – The best indication that an adequate amount of ocular irrigation has been provided is a return of normal pH in the eye, which is between 7.0 – 7.3. Remember that a pH of 7 is "neutral," so something close to that is probably a good goal to shoot for, especially as the question specifically mentions exposure to an alkaline, not neutral, substance. Saponification is the liquefaction of fatty cells due to alkali agents and just sounds (and is) bad. Dua Classification is a fancy scale used by ophthalmologists to estimate the percentage of conjunctival involvement and is not used to determine treatment status. While absence of pain can be a great indicator of success, an alkali substance can continue to cause damage even if no pain is present. The question mentioned alkaline (not normal pH) exposure... Pick the answer that involves pH.

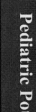

Pediatric Potpourri

202) A 14-year old female arrives in the ED approximately 40 hours after ingesting an unknown amount of Tylenol (acetaminophen). She is complaining of right upper quadrant pain and lab results reveal elevated AST, ALT, bilirubin, and an elevated PT. What organ is primarily affected with this type of overdose?

A) Kidney

B) Liver

C) Heart

D) Spleen

B – If the question mentions acetaminophen, think liver! We love taking acetaminophen for our aches because it is absorbed and acts quickly. The liver is tasked with breaking down the potentially harmful byproducts, and it does that quite effectively when the dose is appropriate and the liver is healthy. But in an overdose, the liver becomes overwhelmed! Liver enzymes (AST, ALT, bilirubin), and prothrombin time (PT) all begin to increase with hepatic injury from acetaminophen. Fatalities from acetaminophen poisoning generally occur as a result of fulminant hepatic necrosis. Ingestions > 150mg/kg are toxic. The antidote, *N-acetylcysteine*, aka., Mucomyst, provides little benefit if administered more than 24 hours post-ingestion, so time is tissue when it comes to strokes, heart attacks, torsions, and toxicology!

Unfortunately, by the time liver failure becomes evident (typically several days after the ingestion), it's far too late for any antidotes. Acetaminophen is so readily available that it's often taken with other medications in intentional overdoses. That's why it's so important to specifically ask about acetaminophen ingestion and try to estimate how much was taken and when. If the patient refuses to disclose what they took, always assume acetaminophen was potentially involved in toxic doses.

203) An infant arrives to the emergency department (ED) with a suspected ethanol overdose after his parent's added rum to the formula to "help the baby sleep." What complications should the ER nurse anticipate?

A) Hyperglycemia, hypothermia and seizures

B) Hypoglycemia, hyperthermia and CNS depression

C) Hyperglycemia, hyperthermia and seizures

D) Hypoglycemia, hypothermia and CNS depression

D – Ethanol, aka., alcohol (of any type), slows everything down. It's not a trick question. Alcohol inhibits gluconeogenesis, and therefore slows down energy production. A slower energy production depletes glycogen stores in the body. Alcohol also suppresses shivering, leading to hypothermia. It also inhibits the central nervous system. While an ethanol overdose may cause seizures, it does not cause hyperthermia or hyperglycemia. Think about your big people with ETOH abuse and everything slowing way down... babies with accidental (or intentional) ETOH exposure are the same way! (**Tip** – Have you also made sure the proper child protection contacts were made?)

204) You begin your assessment of a 13-year old female who is unconscious following multiple seizures of an unknown origin. During your assessment, you note the smell of wintergreen emanating from her breath. Which of the following do you suspect based on your assessment?

A) Methyl salicylate poisoning

B) Hypermethioninemia

C) Acetaminophen poisoning

D) Diabetic ketoacidosis

A – Methyl salicylate (oil of wintergreen) has a very distinctive odor which emanates from the breath of a patient poisoned by it. Methyl salicylate is contained in topical liniments to treat joint and muscular pain. However, in this case, it's more likely your patient ingested wintergreen oils, which is rapidly absorbed by the body and acts just like aspirin. Only one drop of the oil is roughly equivalent to a baby aspirin, so imagine the equivalent of a big swallow of wintergreen oils! Hypermethioninemia, wow that's a big word, is an excess of methionine, an amino acid, and may cause a patient's breath to smell of boiled cabbage (a unique aroma to say the least). Acetaminophen poisoning is not associated with the smell of wintergreen (or anything at all unless it was a flavored liquid) and diabetic ketoacidosis (DKA) often produces a fruity or sweet smell, but definitely not wintergreen.

205) A mother brings her 4-year old son to the ED after ingesting hand sanitizer. She states the child had ingested "2 or 3 pumps" before she could stop him. He is awake and alert and only complaining of burning in his mouth with no respiratory distress. You should suspect:

A) He has ingested a potentially dangerous amount of hand sanitizer

B) The hand sanitizer he has ingested is not dangerous

C) He will rapidly develop airway burns and needs immediate intubation

D) He has internal airway burns and needs immediate transfer to a burn center

A – Ingestion of just "2 or 3 pumps" of a hand sanitizer is a potentially dangerous situation because most hand sanitizers are comprised of between 40-95% ethyl alcohol (ethanol) or around 60% isopropyl alcohol. This is more than is present in most hard liquors. A small amount of hand sanitizer ingestion can cause alcohol poisoning in young children. Since the question specifically indicates that the child ingested the hand sanitizer, and had not inhaled or aspirated it, there is no immediate concern for any airway burns, compromise, or need for burn center evaluation.

Additional Insights from a Pediatric Emergency Medicine Attending Physician:

The alcohol in hand sanitizer should be absorbed quickly, so if the patient is brought in to get "checked out" several hours later and is fine, chances are that it was a nontoxic dose. If brought in very soon after the ingestion, the patient will need to be observed for at least a couple hours. Be sure to contact your Poison Control Center for guidance!

Pediatric Potpourri

Certified Pediatric Emergency Nurse (CPEN) Review IV

206) During a triage interview, an adolescent patient informs the nurse that he is transgender. What would be an appropriate question for the nurse to ask?

A) "What is your real name?"

B) "What are your preferred name and pronouns?"

C) "When did you decide to make this change?"

D) "Why are you telling me this?"

B – Asking a patient's preferred name and pronouns is not only the appropriate question, but also one which is important for all health care professionals to understand. It shows respect for all patients seeking care in the emergency department; patients in the LGBTQIA (lesbian, gay, bisexual, transgender, queer/questioning, intersex, and asexual/allies) population are no exception. Transgender patients may be wary and fearful of disclosing their gender identity. One of the best ways to establish rapport with these patients is to ask what their preferred name and pronouns are. Asking for the patient's "real" name will only make the patient (and caregiver) feel uncomfortable. Gender identification is not something that's decided, but is often realized at a very young age. Asking the patient why they are giving certain information is not appropriate and may make the patient feel even more uncomfortable.

207) A patient informs the nurse that they are a transgender female. The nurse understands that this patient:

A) Has transitioned from female to male

B) Is both female and male or neither

C) Has transitioned or is transitioning from male to female

D) Identifies as male, but dresses as female

C – The gender name in the title (female, male) refers to the identified gender that the individual has transitioned (or is transitioning) to – not their birth sex. In this case, the patient identifies as a transgender female, meaning that she has transitioned (or is transitioning) to female gender. An individual that identifies as both male and female or neither is referred to as gender fluid. The individual who identifies as one gender, but does not express that gender by conventional norms, is referred to as gender variant or gender non-conforming. An individual who identifies as one gender (typically male) but dresses as the "opposite" gender may consider themselves a cross dresser.

208) A young adult patient presents to the emergency department with a chief complaint of abdominal pain. During the triage interview, the patient informs the nurse that he is transgender. Based on this information, what part of the patient history would be the **most** important to obtain?

A) Surgical history

B) Current medications

C) Smoking history

D) Dietary habits

A – Although questions about medication, smoking, and dietary history are all intended to obtain appropriate information during a triage interview, the surgical history of any patient with abdominal pain is a high priority. This is especially true of a patient likely to have had surgical interventions as part of a gender transition (i.e., hysterectomy, salpingectomy, oophorectomy). If this transgender male patient still has their reproductive organs, those organs could be the cause of the abdominal pain.

209) A child presents to the emergency department with left lower leg pain and swelling for two days. Both the child and caregiver deny any recent trauma. Radiographic findings show a left tibia fracture with three other fractures of the same extremity in various stages of healing. What would be the priority action at this time?

A) Notifying Child Protective Services

B) Questioning the caregiver about the findings with security present

C) Talking to the child privately

D) Obtaining a thorough medical history

D - Although the findings of old and new fractures certainly may raise suspicion of child maltreatment, it is important to obtain a thorough medical history to rule out those conditions that may mimic abuse. Osteogenesis imperfecta (OI), aka., brittle bone disease, is a chronic condition that causes bones to fracture easily. Therefore, it is imperative to get as much information as possible from the caregivers, as well as ensure a thorough examination, review of previous injury visits and radiology reports before separating the patient and caregiver or going forward with any activities leading to a reporting process.

210) A child presents to the emergency department with symptoms of an upper respiratory infection (URI). During the assessment, the nurse notices uniformly patterned red streaks across the patient's back. What would be the next appropriate action?

A) Send the caregiver out of the room so you can speak to the child privately

B) Notify social services and Child Protective Services

C) Ask the family about cultural practices

D) Ask the physician to order a skeletal series to evaluate for signs of possible abuse

C – Certain cultural practices can easily be mistaken for child maltreatment, so asking about cultural practices might provide some critical information for moving forward. Coining, commonly practiced in some Asian cultures, involves rolling a coin that has been dipped in hot oil down the patient's back, causing reasonably symmetrical red streaks. The theory is that this will draw out the toxin causing the child's illness. It is important for the emergency nurse to obtain a thorough patient history, including cultural practices, to ensure a thorough assessment and appropriate examination.

211) Henoch-Schonlein purpura (HSP) may initially be mistaken for child maltreatment due to the presence of:

A) Petechiae on the face
B) Symmetrical bruises to both legs
C) Old and new fractures
D) Blistering lesions on the back

B - Henoch-Schonlein purpura (HSP) is an idiopathic condition typically occurring after an upper respiratory infection (URI). Symptoms of HSP include symmetrical bruises to the buttocks, arms, and legs – often similar to, and mistaken for signs of physical abuse. Petechiae often indicates a clotting problem i.e., idiopathic thrombocytopenic purpura (ITP). The presence of old and new fractures may be associated with osteogenesis imperfecta (OI). Epidermolysis bulosa (EB) presents with blistering lesions, mimicking partial and full thickness burns on an otherwise healthy child.

212) A toddler is to receive an intramuscular injection of Rocephin© (ceftriaxone). Which injection site would be the **most** appropriate?

A) Vastus lateralis
B) Dorsogluteal
C) Deltoid
D) Ventrogluteal

A – The vastus lateralis is a large muscle and is the preferred site for an IM injection in infants, toddlers, and small children. The deltoid muscle should be reserved for older children and should never be used to administer painful antibiotic injections. The ventrogluteal muscle can be used in older children for larger injected volumes, such as antibiotics. The dorsogluteal muscle is no longer recommended for any age group (adults included) due to the risk of sciatic nerve injury.

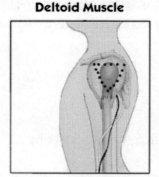
Deltoid Muscle

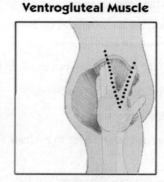
Ventrogluteal Muscle

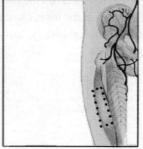
Vastus Lateralis Muscle

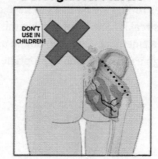
Dorsogluteal Muscle

213) An adolescent male comes to the emergency department with a complaint of increasing scrotal/testicular pain and a fever for the past four days. The patient also reports pain when voiding. The nurse suspects:

A) Testicular torsion

B) Pyelonephritis

C) Epididymitis

D) Paraphimosis

C – Epididymitis would be suspected when the patient presents with scrotal pain, fever, and pain on urination. Normally, when emergency department nurses see "teen" and "testicle" in one exam question, torsion is the answer. However, teens with torsions don't commonly have a fever or UTI symptoms, and with torsions, the acutely twisted testicles cause acute pain, as opposed to "increasing" pain. In this case, the gradual onset of scrotal pain, fever and dysuria in a male all point towards epididymitis; an acute bacterial infection that occurs in sexually active males. Pyelonephritis, a kidney infection, usually presents with UTI symptoms, flank pain and shaking/chills. Paraphimosis, occurs when the foreskin in uncircumcised males is retracted/gets stuck behind the coronal rim of the glans and can't be brought forward to the normal position. This would likely present with penile pain, not scrotal pain.

214) A 14-year old male presents to the ED with his parents. The patient complains of a sudden onset of left testicular pain and swelling "down there." Which additional finding would lead the nurse to suspect testicular torsion?

A) Positive cremasteric reflex

B) Normal urinalysis

C) Positive Prehn's sign

D) Yellow penile discharge

B – A normal urinalysis often accompanies testicular torsion, which typically presents with a sudden onset of acute unilateral scrotal pain and swelling, as well as nausea and vomiting. Since testicular torsion involves the testicle/spermatic cord, and not the urinary tract, a normal urinalysis would be expected. The cremasteric reflex, elevation of the ipsilateral testes when the inner thigh is stroked, is usually absent (negative) in this situation. Prehn's sign is pain relief when the testes are elevated. Twisted testicles are unhappy testicles and they will become even unhappier when they are elevated. The presence of fever, penile discharge, UTI symptoms, an intact (positive) cremasteric reflex and Prehn's sign are more typical with epididymitis. In this case, the age of the patient would also lead the nurse to suspect testicular torsion as 14 years is the peak age for that particularly painful condition.

215) A 3-week old neonate is brought to the emergency department by the caregiver who reports a 2-day history of poor feeding and irritability. On assessment, the baby is awake and crying with tachypnea and pale skin. The nurse knows that a **priority** initial intervention would be to:

A) Obtain vascular access

B) Prepare for a lumbar puncture

C) Offer a sucrose pacifier

D) Check a blood glucose level

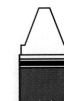

D – Checking a blood glucose level on a neonate who is anything but "sweet" is a priority. Neonates have high metabolic rates and extremely limited glycogen stores. Any stress, including illness or injury, can lead to hypoglycemia. Vague symptoms such as poor feeding and irritability in this age group should alert the nurse to possible hypoglycemia and the need to check a bedside blood glucose level. Obtaining vascular access may be indicated, but is not the priority. Preparing for a lumbar puncture might be indicated if sepsis is suspected, but checking a blood glucose level should be done first. Sucrose and pacifiers are useful for managing pain during any of these painful procedures, but checking a blood glucose level would be indicated before any form of sugar is given. You are probably noticing a pattern here.

216) A teenage mother has just given birth in the emergency department via vaginal delivery. After drying, stimulating, and warming the neonate, the newborn is noted to have slow, irregular respirations with circumoral (around the mouth) cyanosis. What would be the next appropriate intervention?

A) Suction the nose, then the mouth

B) Administer blow-by oxygen

C) Start positive pressure ventilations

D) Initiate chest compressions

C – If a neonate is apneic or has ineffective respirations after drying, warming, and stimulating, positive pressure ventilation with a bag-mask device should be started. If the heart rate is below 60, despite positive pressure ventilations, chest compressions should then be initiated. But remember, B before C means Bagging before Compressing. Blow-by oxygen would not be appropriate or effective in this situation as the baby is barely breathing. If suctioning is indicated, the mouth should be suctioned first, then the nose to avoid aspiration (M before N: Mouth before Nose, 1 opening before 2 openings). That being said, as the Bob Dylan song goes, "The Times They Are a Changin'," and with few exceptions, routine suctioning of the newborn's mouth or nose is no longer recommended.

217) A 2-week old neonate is brought to the emergency department by caregivers who report poor feeding and difficulty breathing for the past week. The oxygen saturation level is 83% on room air. After 100% supplemental oxygen is initiated, the oxygen saturation level is 81%. The nurse suspects:

A) Congenital heart disease

B) Pneumonia

C) Reactive airway disease

D) Pulmonary edema.

A – One method of differentiating between a possible congenital heart defect versus a respiratory condition is to look at the neonate's oxygen saturation response to supplemental oxygen. Respiratory conditions will often respond positively to supplemental oxygen. Increasing the oxygen delivery is expected to result in an increased oxygen saturation level. However, patients with cyanotic congenital heart defects will generally not respond to supplemental oxygen.

218) What blood test should be performed immediately for any child with acutely altered mental status?

A) Rapid bedside blood glucose

B) Rapid bedside complete blood count (CBC)

C) Rapid bedside type and screen

D) Rapid bedside complete cooties count (CCC)

A - Remember, your brain only wants three things to be "happy": Blood, oxygen, and glucose. And if the brain isn't "happy" nothing seems right. So, in the case of an acute mental status change, especially with children (and known diabetics), a rapid test for glucose is a must. A great way to remember this comes from a pediatric flight medic/RT, Stu McVicar. He reminds us that since before kindergarten, we are taught our ABCs. And in healthcare, especially with kids, we add DEFG... (**D**)on't (**E**)ver (**F**)orget (**G**)lucose). Brilliant!

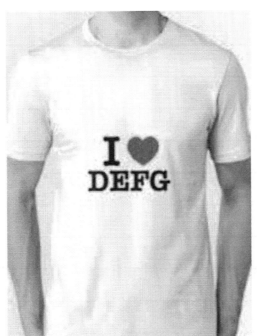

Pertinent Pediatric Ponderings (NOTES)

"If you want your children to be intelligent,
read them fairy tales.
If you want them to be more intelligent,
read them more fairy tales."
Albert Einstein

Certified Pediatric Emergency Nurse (CPEN) Review IV

Ten Commandments for Passing the CPEN

Preparing and passing the CPEN examination can be compared to my training and completion of the Chicago marathon. I trained sensibly (didn't try to run 20 miles the day before the marathon), and I completed the course because I did not let obstacles like uphill streets defeat me. You are NOT going to know EVERY single question with certainty, but you need to learn a strategy that will greatly increase your success.

Here's how:

You are motivated by the recognition and (possible) salary increases that comes from this certification. You are already part of an elite group because you are taking the test. In the marathon, there were six thousand runners, but there were tens of thousands of onlookers that I passed enroute. They recognized that what I was attempting was far beyond their capabilities. I had set aside time to train each day. Now those same people would see the results of my training, just as your fellow nurses will see your certification several weeks from now.

Let's talk about the "science" of the test:

1) Test questions have a specific anatomy, just as you do. The "stem" is the problem, stated in a question and the answer will be all of the following:
A) Reference validation of 5 years of less (i.e. no CPR done with victim on stomach and pulling on his arms, etc.)
B) Plausible, i.e. the answer makes "sense"
C) Usually two "distracters or "wrong answers" can be found. Eliminate these promptly, just as contestants can have two answers removed on TV's "Who Wants to be a Millionaire?"

2) No credible test preparer would have an obvious answer pattern for the test such as A, then B, then C, and then D. It may have worked for junior high teachers, but not for CPEN test item writers.

3) Is guessing allowed?
Yes, and so is prayer. Correct guess answers get the same credit as 100% certain answers.

4) Test makers include "qualifiers" like "usually", "commonly" "possibly" and "probably." How should I react to these?
They are "more likely" to be right than wrong.

5) What about "absolutes" like "all, always, none," or "never"?
These are more likely to be wrong. Just as grammar rules have exceptions. So do these "absolutes." Are you "absolutely sure" that the patient is a woman? Ever been fooled? You never really know until you place the Foley!

6) Can short answers also be correct? Do they have to be several sentences long to be the best answer? A shorter answer can certainly be the correct answer. Remember... everything in the answer must be correct. If one of the four facts stated are incorrect, it is the WRONG answer. You cannot be "sort of pregnant" any more than "sort of right." You are either 100% correct or 100% wrong. The correct answer is 100% correct in its statements.

7) What about "word fit?"
"Word fit" means "Do the words in the sentence sound correct?" A choice whose content or wording does not seem in the same class with the other choices is more than likely going to be wrong. Use this principle as an "eliminator." (See 1C)

Certified Pediatric Emergency Nurse (CPEN) Review IV

8) I want to prepare intelligently, not haphazardly; Suggestions?
A) Have a plan that uses these five keys:

> 1) The right study references such as this book, the ENPC and PALS textbooks, and the ENA peds core curriculum.
>
> 2) A time and place that minimizes distractions. Been to the library in a while? Librarians enforce the quiet atmosphere. There are no TV's or radios in the library.
>
> 3) Study for 20-30 minutes; then take a meaningful break away from study materials.
>
> 4) Everyone is not an expert at everything. Review your weak areas, i.e. what kind of patients you don't see every day.
>
> 5) Remember that the test is based upon evidence based practice, which means what your hospital does every day, may not actually be the correct answer.

B) Organize a study group of likeminded members. Each member will bring particular insights to the group.
C) Prepare flash cards on topics using 3 X 5 cards. Questions on one side; answer on the other. You can whiz through a section of anatomy or unfamiliar emergencies quickly with well thought out questions.
D) These steps may seem like Study Skills 101, but the principles are the same. Study smarter, not harder.

9) And the day of the test? What should be my focus?
A) You should have rested the night before, not indulged in a marathon "cram" session covering several anatomy and peds references. Preparation before the test involves weeks, not hours. You cannot chug-a-lug the materials in one night. You have a plan that has been followed. You could not read "War and Peace" the night before a World Literature final; don't try the equivalent for the CPEN.
B) Allow adequate travel time so that you do not arrive late. Test sites commonly schedule morning and afternoon sessions and if you are late, out of courtesy to the next person, they may not let you begin your examination. Yes, there can be accident sites on the way to your exam day; allow for the unexpected.
C) Arrive early. You can always engage in meaningless conversation with other test takers. Your calmness prior to the test will only add to their anxiety level as they think "Why isn't this person madly reviewing anything"?

10) And the test itself?
A) Make sure your answer is the "final answer." You have read through all the choices, you eliminated as many as possible; you looked for the most "correct" answer where nothing is incorrect.
B) Answer all the questions you are certain of first. All questions are of equal weight; do NOT throw away valuable time agonizing over one question.
C) Mark and come back to the unanswered questions; do the ones you are confident of first. This is making wise use of your time restrictions.
D) Unlike state board exams many years ago, in which you had to wait for weeks for your results, you will know that you passed immediately after completing the test.

Web based resources:
- www.bcencertifications.org

Thanks to Lynn Mohr PhD, APRN, PCNS-BC, CPN, FCNS and Larry DeBoer MA for their invaluable input with the creation of these test taking tips.

Requests from the Mother of a Catastrophically Injured Child

- My child had a full active life prior to this injury - Please ask them about it.

- Keep our family informed

- Answer questions to the best of your ability

- Whenever possible, provide information about possible outcomes

- Be ready for my child when he arrives on your unit / at your hospital

- I need some attention too - I am frightened and feel so alone

- Let me know how to get in touch with you if I need you

- Allow me to stay with my child whenever possible

- Help my child to not be in pain, please!

- Arrange it so he/she can get some sleep - Even in the ICU

- Try not to ask repeated questions for which there are answers in my child's chart

- Respect my child's need for privacy and modesty - Remember he's only a child

- Introduce yourself, write down your role - Better yet, give me your business card

- Document carefully so I don't have to clarify things

- Speak directly to my child

- Don't stand at the foot of his/her bed - Go the side, bend down he/she can see you

- My child is a bright child - Please don't talk down to him/her

- Notice non-clinical things (a new postcard, a photo of pet, etc)

- Help me to construct letters to my insurance company

- Allow my child to maintain a sense of self-esteem and some control over what is happening by giving my child some choices

- This may be the 100th child you have cared for with this type of injury - It's our first!

Good care is important - True caring is a gift!

The Miracle Toddler Diet

Over the years you may have noticed that most two year olds are trim. Now the formula to their success is available to all in this new diet... The Miracle Toddler Diet! You may want to consult your doctor before trying this diet. If not, you may be seeing him afterwards. Good luck!

Day One:

Breakfast: One scrambled egg, one piece of toast with grape jelly. Eat 2 bites of egg, using your fingers; dump the rest on the floor. Take 1 bite of toast, then smear the jelly over your face and clothes.

Lunch: Four crayons, any color, a handful of potato chips, and a glass of milk, 3 sips only, then spill the rest.

Dinner: A dry stick, two pennies and a nickel, 4 sips of flat Sprite

Bedtime snack: Throw a piece of toast on the kitchen floor.

Day Two:

Breakfast: Pick up stale toast from kitchen floor and eat it. Drink half bottle of vanilla extract or one vial of vegetable dye.

Lunch: Half tube of "pulsating pink" lipstick and a handful of Purina dog chow, any flavor. One ice cube, if desired.

Afternoon snack: Lick an all-day sucker until sticky, take outside, drop in dirt. Retrieve and continue slurping until it is clean again. Then bring inside and drop on rug.

Dinner: A rock or an uncooked bean, which should be thrust up your left nostril. Pour grape Kool-Aid over mashed potatoes; eat with spoon.

Day Three:

Breakfast: Two pancakes with plenty of syrup, eat one with fingers, rub in hair. Glass of milk; drink half, stuff other pancake in glass. After breakfast, pick up yesterdays sucker from rug, lick off fuzz, put it on the cushion of best chair.

Lunch: Three matches, peanut butter and jelly sandwich. Spit several bites onto the floor. Pour glass of milk on table and slurp up.

Dinner: Dish of ice cream, handful of potato chips, some red punch. Try to laugh some punch through your nose, if possible.

Final day:

Breakfast: A quarter tube of toothpaste, any flavor, bit of soap, an olive. Pour a glass of milk over bowl of cornflakes, add half a cup of sugar. Once cereal is soggy, drink milk and feed cereal to dog.

Lunch: Eat bread crumbs off kitchen floor and dining room carpet. Find that sucker and finish eating it.

Dinner: A glass of spaghetti and chocolate milk. Leave meatball on plate. Stick of mascara for desert.

How to Raise Mom and Dad (by Josh Lerman)
Instructions from an older sibling to a younger one

1) Always ask Daddy for candy, cookies, or lemonade. He'll give it to you; Mommy won't.

2) If Mommy says you can't have candy, cookies, or lemonade, do that thing where you change your voice so you're almost crying but not quite (Mommy calls it "whining.") Sometimes she'll give in.

3) If you ask Daddy to be a horse or to carry you or dance with you, and he says maybe later, that means he will really soon. If he says anything about his back hurting, that means he won't. Don't worry - His back doesn't really hurt, I looked once.

4) A lot of the time they're not listening, so always say things over and over.

5) The whole green-vegetable thing is pretty out of hand. So never admit you like them, keep changing the ones you'll agree to eat, and every once in a while claim that one of them makes you feel like throwing up.

6) If Daddy says, "Did Mommy say you could do that?" it means he doesn't want you to do it. Always answer "Yes."

7) If you wake up and you're lonely, call Mommy. She'll come in and might fall asleep next to you. Daddy will just kiss you and leave.

8) If there's a monster by the window, call Daddy - He can totally kill monsters. I don't think Mommy knows much about them because she doesn't even think there are any.

9) If you don't like your mittens, you can "lose" one and they'll buy you new ones.

10) When you get a toy with very, very small parts (like Barbie's shoes, Legos, Playmobil cuffs, collars, and hair thingies), put some in every room of the house. Mommy and Daddy will like finding this stuff because it reminds them of you.

11) Mommy and Daddy aren't so smart. If you just scribble all over a page, they'll tell you it's good. This has probably already happened to you.

12) This is what a minute is: It's the 200 or so hours between when Mommy says she'll do something (like come play dolls with you) and when she does it.

13) Mommy and Daddy are very rich - I think they earn like $40 or $100 a year - So if they don't buy you the toys you ask for, it's because they're mean.

14) Whenever Mommy and Daddy hug each other, always go and get in the middle because it's the best kind when it's everybody hugging.

God Created Children...

To those of us who have children in our lives, whether they are our own, grandchildren, nieces, nephews, or students... here is something to make you chuckle. Whenever your children are out of control, you can take comfort from the thought that even God's omnipotence did not extend to His own children. After creating Heaven and Earth, God created Adam and Eve... And the first thing he said was "DON'T!"

"Don't what?" Adam replied.

"Don't eat the forbidden fruit." God said.

"Forbidden fruit? We have forbidden fruit? Hey Eve... we have forbidden fruit!!!"

"No Way!"

"Yes way!"

"Do NOT eat the fruit!" said God.

"Why?"

"Because I am your Father and I said so!" God replied, wondering why He hadn't stopped creation after making the elephants. A few minutes later, God saw his children having an apple break and He was ticked! "Didn't I tell you not to eat the fruit?" God asked.

"Uh huh," Adam replied.

"Then why did you?" said the Father.

"I don't know," said Eve.

"She started it!" Adam said.

"Did not!"

"Did too!"

"DID NOT!"

Having had it with the two of them, God's punishment was that Adam and Eve should have children of their own. Thus the pattern was set and it has never changed!

But there is reassurance in the story! If you have persistently and lovingly tried to give children wisdom and they haven't taken it, don't be hard on yourself. If God had trouble raising children, what makes you think it would be a piece of cake for you?